1 MONTH OF
FREE
READING

at

www.ForgottenBooks.com

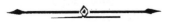

By purchasing this book you are eligible for one month membership to ForgottenBooks.com, giving you unlimited access to our entire collection of over 1,000,000 titles via our web site and mobile apps.

To claim your free month visit:

www.forgottenbooks.com/free804541

ISBN 978-0-483-12778-4
PIBN 10804541

THE

HALF-YEARLY ABSTRACT

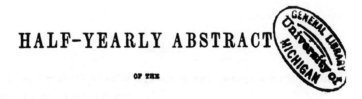

OF THE

MEDICAL SCIENCES:

BEING

A PRACTICAL AND ANALYTICAL DIGEST OF THE CONTENTS OF THE PRIN-
CIPAL BRITISH AND CONTINENTAL MEDICAL WORKS PUBLISHED
IN THE PRECEDING SIX MONTHS.

TOGETHER WITH

A SERIES OF CRITICAL REPORTS ON THE PROGRESS OF MEDICINE AND
THE COLLATERAL SCIENCES DURING THE SAME PERIOD.

EDITED BY

W. H. RANKING, M.D., Cantab.,

PHYSICIAN TO THE NORFOLK AND NORWICH HOSPITAL,

AND

C. B. RADCLIFFE, M.D., Lond., L.R.C.P.,

ASSISTANT PHYSICIAN TO, AND LECTURER ON MATERIA MEDICA AT, THE WESTMINSTER HOSPITAL.

Apparatu nobis opus est, et rebus exquisitis undique et collectis, arcessitis, comportatis.
Cicero.

NO. XXIII.

JANUARY—JUNE, 1856.

PHILADELPHIA:

LINDSAY AND BLAKISTON,

NO. 25 SOUTH SIXTH STREET.

1856.

TERMS.

Two Dollars per annum, free of postage, *if paid for in advance.*

LINDSAY & BLAKISTON,

Publishers.

NOTICE TO CORRESPONDENTS.

The Editors request that all communications be forwarded (free) to MR. CHURCHILL, *New Burlington Street, London.*

The Editors are compelled to remind their American correspondents, that no parcels are taken in, unless the entire charge be paid upon them.

No. XXIV. will appear on the 1st of January, 1857.

Books, &c., for notice, to be sent as soon as published (carriage free) to MR. CHURCHILL, *New Burlington Street; or to* DR. RADCLIFFE, 4 *Henrietta Street, Cavendish Square.*

C. SHERMAN & SON, PRINTERS,
19 St. James Street.

CONTENTS OF NO. XXIII.

PART I.—MEDICINE.

I.—*General Questions in Medicine.*

(a) *Hygiene.*

(b) *Acute Diseases.*

(c) *Chronic Diseases.*

II.—*Special Questions in Medicine.*

(a) *Concerning the Nervous System.*

PART II.—SURGERY.

I.—*General Questions in Surgery.*

(a) *Concerning Inflammation.*

PART III.

MIDWIFERY, AND DISEASES OF WOMEN AND CHILDREN.

(a) *Concerning Pregnancy and Parturition.*

REPORTS ON THE PROGRESS OF THE MEDICAL SCIENCES.

I.—*Report in Medicine.*

II.—*Report in Surgery.*

III.—*Report in Midwifery and Diseases of Women and Children.*

ABSTRACT OF THE MEDICAL SCIENCES,

&c. &c.

PART I.

PRACTICAL MEDICINE, PATHOLOGY, AND THERAPEUTICS.

SECT. I.—GENERAL QUESTIONS IN MEDICINE.

(A) HYGIENE.

ART. 1.—*The Atmosphere in relation to Disease.* By Mr. J. A. HINGESTON, of Brighton.

(*Journal of Public Health*, Dec. 1855.)

THE following remarks are taken from an elegant and admirable paper, the merits of which cannot be properly represented in any abstract. Mr. Hingeston agrees with many in thinking that the body sympathizes very closely with the electrical condition of the atmosphere, and he gives a hint which promises to be of much practical importance—that the clouds, which are, indeed, analogous, more or less, to Leyden jars, may serve as signs of the electrical condition of the atmosphere.

"We have some facts," Mr. Hingeston continues after many excellent remarks, "to show cause why we should connect disease with the greater or less amount of electricity, signified by the electrometer. It would seem that, in the non-electric states of the air, diseases of a low type prevail. Thus, in the Registrar-General's return for the week ending July 14th, 1855, we find it stated, at p. 232, 'weak positive electricity throughout the week;' and, on referring to the mortality of the same date, at p. 225, it is there recorded, that the chief deaths were from small-pox, hooping-cough, scarlatina, diarrhœa, and typhus. And thus, on the contrary, in the week ending Sept. 8th, at p. 296, the electricity is stated to be 'positive,' and the mortality, at p. 289, to be 'not high for the season.' During the prevalence of Asiatic cholera, the electricity is weak, or nothing: thus, in the week ending September 16th, 1854, on the 13th and 14th of September, when cholera was at its maximum, the electricity, p. 377, is stated, 'none was shown.' Thus, again, for the week ending September 22d, 1855, at p. 305, the mortality 'shows a decrease of about 100 in each of the three previous weeks, and indicates a satisfactory state of the public health;' while at p. 312, it is recorded that the electricity is 'positive,' 'strongly positive,' and 'active throughout the day.' Were we to connect health with positive electricity, as a settled thing, we might point out a curious connection between the deaths of the young and the continuance of a highly electric state of the atmosphere; but, as coincidence is not the same as cause and effect, we can only mention the isolated

fact, that, in the week ending October 13th, 1855, it is stated, p. 333, that out of
870 deaths (or 225 below the average), 449 (or about one-half) were in persons
under twenty years of age; the electricity (p. 340) being both positive and strong,
as it had been for several weeks past. It would be pushing the facts too far, and
laying ourselves open to the imputation of forcing a favorite theory to suit a particular purpose, were we to enlarge the number of our examples; but they are
endless, and we disclaim any theory whatever. Let the medical inquirer make
his own references, and judge for himself. Does positive electricity, long continued, predispose to inflammatory ailments? For, in the week ending October
27th, 1855, the electricity being, as it had been, both strong and positive, we
find, p. 319, three cases of peritonitis particularly reported.

   "If we consider that every living creature is as much an electrical machine
as each cloud; that the earth itself is the largest and most powerful electrical
machine of all; and that all things are always exchanging their electricities with
each other; and, furthermore, that a strong electro-galvanic current passed from
the nose to the tail of a living mouse, can kill it on the spot; that a simple electric stroke will abolish the life of a fly; and that lightning destroys myriads of
insects, as well as some animals and human beings, at a single flash, it is past
contradiction that electricity must be a grand actor in every form of life, whether
of health or disease. If we take an electrometer, and pass a powerful stream of
electricity into it from a large electrical machine in full play, the gold leaf within
the electrometer is whirled round with violence, shivered into atoms, and sent
flying in fragments to the inside surface of the glass, in desperate haste, to escape
and distribute the excess of electrical fluid to the nearest non-electrical bodies.
It is, in fact, a tornado within the bottle; like the tornadoes of the tropics, which
are, most likely, nothing else than convulsive equalizations of unequal electricities on a gigantic scale. The violence of the winds, if not their directions,
seems to be electro-magnetic. There are storms that disturb the magnet, or the
electrometer, or both at once. And the partial rarefaction of the air by heat, and
its condensation by cold, hitherto employed for explaining the force and current
of the winds, are, most likely, only striking parts of terrestrial electro-magnet-
ism. The tornado within the bottle is a practical exemplification of this supposition. Moreover, the sensorial effects of the electric fluid are proof paramount
of its pathological energy. The tingling produced by a shock from an electrical
machine in action, and the blindness, or loss of consciousness, or death, produced by lightning, exhibit the development of morbid phenomena too plainly
to be mistaken. We have, therefore, every possible reason for regarding the
kind of clouds as indications of the kind of atmosphere in relation to disease;
and the various forms assumed by the vapors condensing or dissolving in the air
may be considered, not only as picturesque beauties in the landscape we are
occupied in watching or sketching, but also as criteria for judging of some of the
most potent effects resulting from the operation of an experiment, silently and
delicately performed upon the functions and sensations of animated beings.
These signs only require reducing to some familiar characters, in order to render
them practically serviceable; and then, when once recognized, they might be
read off at a glance, and brought into daily use, as easily as the dial-plate of
the electric wire, the gauge that indicates the steam pressure of a locomotive, or
the minute hand of our watch in counting the pulse at a patient's wrist."

ART. 2.—*The season in relation to Disease.*
By Dr. B. W. RICHARDSON.

(*Journal of Public Health,* Dec. 1855.)

   "The distinguished Arbuthnot laid it down as an aphorism, that every season
has its special diseases. This is in some measure true; but as the seasons of
one year vary very much from the seasons of another year, and as the division
into seasons is, after all, arbitrary, the rule must be received with many exceptions.

   "The prevalence of diseases as a whole, and of the mortality arising from
them, is, however, well marked in various periods of the year. I made a careful analysis of the facts bearing on this subject two years ago, and obtained

very important results. The analysis refers only to the diseases of certain parts of England, and is made from mortality tables—viz., those published by the Registrar-General; but, from its wide basis, its results give a fair picture of the special season diseases of England.

"The analysis includes deductions made from not fewer than 139,318 deaths, occurring during years extending from 1838 to 1853, and arising from the following diseases—small-pox, measles, scarlet fever, hooping-cough, croup, diarrhœa, dysentery, cholera, influenza, ague, remittent fever, typhus, erysipelas, quinsy, bronchitis, jaundice, and carbuncle. The districts of deaths were London, Devon, and Cornwall.

"Out of the 139,318 cases thus chronicled as occurring from the above-named diseases, the percentage of mortality in the different quarters, and estimating the gross mortality according to the season, without reference to particular years, ran as follows:

In January, February, and March . . .	25 per cent.
In April, May, and June	21 "
In July, August, and September . . .	24 "
In October, November, and December . .	28 "

"Having learned thus much, I set about ascertaining, on the same large scale, whether the fatal diseases were in any way special to the seasons. The answer to this inquiry is to this effect:

"Whooping-cough, croup, small-pox, and bronchitis are most common to the first quarter. The percentage is:

	1st Quar.	2d Quar.	3d Quar.	4th Quar.
Small-pox .	27,352	24,551	22,824	25,272
Hooping-cough	32,704	27,825	17,116	22,354
Croup . .	27,523	25,100	19,919	27,456
Bronchitis .	36,793	20,301	10,327	32,570

"Pneumonia, I believe, might very properly have been added here.

"In the second quarter, quinsy only stands ahead—thus:

	1st Quar.	2d Quar.	3d Quar.	4th Quar.
Quinsy . .	21,762	30,596	21,231	26,410

"In the third quarter, diarrhœa, dysentery, and jaundice take the lead, in the following order:

	1st Quar.	2d Quar.	3d Quar.	4th Quar.
Diarrhœa .	10,196	10,717	58,519	20,567
Dysentery .	15,638	13,541	42,460	28,340
Jaundice .	24,877	24,030	26,967	24,109

"In this third quarter, Asiatic cholera, when epidemic, assumes a greater mortality and prevalence than at any other season. Sporadic cases of cholera are, however, possibly more prevalent in the fourth quarter, during which influenza, ague, remittent fever, typhus, scarlet fever, measles, erysipelas, and carbuncle take the lead:

	1st Quar.	2d Quar.	3d Quar.	4th Quar.
Influenza .	23,539	12,171	4,502	59,784
Ague . .	22,857	24,285	20,000	32,851
Remittent fever	23,077	26,315	23,481	27,125
Typhus . .	25,741	24,825	22,912	26,521
Scarlet fever .	20,809	18,978	26,234	33,976
Measles .	19,864	21,466	26,234	32,434
Erysipelas .	25,144	23,444	22,337	29,174
Carbuncle .	26,771	19,685	24,409	29,133

"In a pathological as well as in a statistical point of view, these results are most interesting; for they prove, in a great measure, that diseases analogous in their general characters group themselves singularly together at special periods. Thus we see that, in the autumn quarter, there are grouped together those diseases which have for one of their essential symptoms an exudation from the intestinal surface, or that large abdominal viscera the liver. In the first quarter, the diseases of the respiratory system—croup, hooping-cough, and bronchitis—stand forth prominently; while in the fourth quarter, a large family of diseases of the febrile or inflammatory order take the first position.

"It is not by mere accident that these divisions occur: they are the effects of fixed, though nearly unknown physical or chemical laws.

"It is worthy of special remark, that in the present quarter of the year—the fourth—the number of diseases which cause a prominent mortality is, as a general rule, greatest; and that next to it is the quarter commencing with the new year. During the third quarter of the present year, the mortality has been lower than is usual; a result due to the absence of any zymotic disease in a virulent form. As the cold of winter more decidedly sets in, we shall begin to see developed, almost of necessity, an increase of deaths from pulmonary diseases, and of low fever amongst the poor, if provisions become high in price and insufficient in quantity or quality.

"In public practice, it is almost always to be observed that diarrhœa is a common symptom amongst the poor during intensely cold weather. In this form it does not, however, prove very fatal; and hence it stands low at that time in the mortality returns."

ART. 3.—*The influence of Temperature upon Mortality.*
By Dr. BUCHNER.

(*Nederlandsch Lancet*, Feb. 1855: and *Medical Times and Gazette*, Nov. 10, 1855.)

The author's investigations, carried on during twelve years, from 1841 to 1852, on the influence of the temperature of the air on the mortality of the population of Amsterdam, have shown that the greatest mortality occurred in the month of March (on an average, 686 individuals), after which come January (685), December (651), April (591), February (589), October (573), November (567), May (564), September (554), July (553), June (509), August (489). The difference between the months, in which the greatest and least mortality took place, amounted for the twelve years to 2365 persons, or a yearly average of 197·08. Of the seasons, the greatest mortality belongs to winter (December, January, and February), the next to spring (March, April, and May), the next to autumn (September, October, and November), while summer (June, July, and August) affords the smallest number of deaths. The difference between the mortality in the winter and summer months amounts to 4500 persons, giving a yearly average of 375; that between spring and autumn is 1771, or 147·58 annually. On reviewing the several seasons, in connection with their average temperature, it appeared that, in the years in which the spring months were warm, the mortality was considerably less than in those in which the temperature was below the average. In the summer months, the mortality was highest during great warmth; this was also true of the warmer autumnal months, while, during the winter months, the mortality rose with severe cold, confirming for Amsterdam the position laid down by Moser, that elevation of the temperature above the ordinary range diminishes the mortality of winter, and increases that of summer. In very warm and very cold months, the mortality at Amsterdam appears not to be invariably great, while, on the contrary, in those which followed the hottest months, the mortality far exceeded the average. The coldest months of the several seasons are March, June, November, and January; the warmest are May, July, September, and December. As to the seasons, the mortality was greatest in the coldest winters and springs, and in the hottest summers, while the greatest mortality occurred neither in the warmest nor in the coldest month of the season. Great mortality appeared to coincide with high degrees of cold or warmth, in connection with relatively low ranges of the barometer and with drought. A comparison of the weekly mortality with the weekly range of the barometer, did not lead to the establishment of any rule as to the connection between the mortality and the pressure of the atmosphere.

ART. 4.—*The Comparative Mortality of a Manufacturing and an Agricultural district.* By Dr. J. BLACK.

(*Journal of Public Health*, Dec. 1855.)

"It is well known, from the Mortuary Registers, that there are considerable differences in the rates of mortality in the several districts of the kingdom; and that not only between communities widely situated from each other, but also between large districts in the same county. The principal causes recognized as producing this disparity of mortality, especially as it affects the comparative ages, are, the occupations of the people; their state in regard to habitations, numbers, residence in cities, towns, or rural villages; and the position of these towns, whether in the hilly interior of the country or upon the airy coasts of the neighboring sea.

"Among these several causes tending to produce the different rates of mortality, there are none more productive of the unfavorable balance, than the crowded and often ill-ventilated conditions of the factories and habitations of our manufacturing population, aggravated, as these evils are, by an ignorance and want of personal and domestic economy, occasioned greatly by the too early and continued employment of young and of married females in workshops and manufactories.

"Even where the rate of mortality is shown to be above the average of 23 in the 1000, it is seen, on examining the Register lists, that the excess is not generally found to exist at the ages above ten years, but in the years of infancy and childhood, *i.e*, up to the fifth or sixth year—those periods of life where, upon the mother's nursing and care, the life, the ill health, or death of the child depends. The too common ignorance and the want of these duties, among these classes of people have, in many communities, produced an awfully premature destruction of human life, even to one half of all born alive, before the little victims have attained the fifth year of their age.

"To illustrate the bearings of these different localities and modes of life in two districts, whose centres are within thirty miles of each other, I may cite the comparative rates of mortality, at two separate epochs of life, as they occur in the Registration districts of Bolton-le-Moors and that of North Meols, in which last is situated the rapidly growing town of Southport, on the west coast of South Lancashire.

"These returns were kindly furnished to me by the respective Superintendent-Registrars; and I herewith extract the following results from them, as bearing chiefly on our present subject.

"*Great and Little Bolton.*—The average number of deaths for each year of 1849 and 50 was 1770; and as the estimated population for the latter year was 59,050, this will give 1 in 33 62 of the population, or about 30 to 1000.

"The average mortality for the two years, at and under five years of age, was 52·22 per cent. of the whole deaths; and 17·5 per cent. of the same, at and above sixty years of age, one person being registered as having died at 99.

"*North Meols, including Southport.*—The population, calculated from the last census, was, in 1854, 8920, and in this year, 1855, at least 9000. The average number of deaths for each of the years 1853-54, is found to be 212; making 1 in 42·5 of the population, or at the ratio of 2·38 per cent., or 23·5 to 1000 living. The average mortality for each of the above years, at and under five years of age, was 38 per cent. of the whole deaths; and at and above 60 years of age, 23·1 per cent., the oldest person being registered as 95.

"From the above comparative enumerations, it is seen how much different localities and social conditions affect the relative ratios of mortality. Though the districts under notice are not very distant, one of them is the site of a large manufacturing town—a type of many others, which are held to be unfavorable to early and advanced life; while the other district is a perfectly flat rural country, once an extensive *tarburium*, but since covered over with deep beds of fine marine sand, and later still by loam, and is generally cultivated. On the sea verge of this plain, about six miles in diameter, are situated the three towns of Southport, Churchtown and Crossens, all of which are included in the District Registration, now embracing as noted above, fully 9000 inhabitants.

"Though the meteorological conditions of the two districts in question are nearly alike, modified only by neighboring hills in the one, and by the flat sea-coast in the other; producing inequalities of temperature between them, the average for both places is nearly the same, and the clothing, diet, and beverages of the people are alike.

"When we come, however, to observe the relative rates of mortality in the aggregate, and at the several ages of life, we see differences, not so marked as in some other districts compared with each other, but sufficiently obvious; for, while the rate of mortality in Bolton is 30 in 1000 of the population, it is in North Meols only 23·5 in 1000—neither of them showing the highest nor the lowest rate, according to Dr. Farr; for while in St. Savour's, Southwark, 33 die out of every 1000, in Lewisham 17 only die in the 1000; while the average of all England is 23 in 1000, the mortality of males in Manchester being 37 in 1000.

"The greatest disparity of ratio in the number of deaths, is seen at the several epochs of life; for while in the Bolton district, from a careful examination of the Registers for 1849 and 50, as many as 52·22 per cent. of the whole deaths occur at and under five years of age, only 38 per cent. obtain in North Meols at and under the same age. This excess of infant mortality in Bolton takes place to about the same extent in Manchester and Liverpool; and it is a matter for serious consideration to all social economists, how to diminish or ameliorate it, however well acquainted all practical observers are with the causes producing the evil.

"Again, while in Bolton 17·5 per cent. of the deaths occur at and above sixty years of age, in North Meols 23·1 per cent. happen at and above the same term of life.

"From the respective data of the above two districts, we may be led to infer that the lives of infants and children are, in the one case, taken prematurely away from the toils and evils to come, and, on the other hand, are spared to augment the ratio of deaths in old age. However much truth there may be in these views, it is proper to observe that there are many invalid people, who come from the interior to recruit their healths in the more equable and temperate climate of Southport and Churchtown, and where several of them end their days, and so add a little to the relative numbers of deaths in advanced life."

ART. 5.—*The influence of Vaccination on the rate of Mortality in France.*
By Dr. BERTILLON, of Montmorency.

(*L'Union Médicale*, Aug. 28th and Sept. 11th, 1855; and *Edin. Med. Journ.*, Dec 1855.)

The following is a *resumé* of a paper which has been submitted for examina-tion to M. Villerme, whose competence for such a task is well known, and upon which he has expressed his decided opinion of the correctness and legitimacy of the conclusions drawn by the author from the different documents and statis-tics made use of in its compilation.

The benefits of vaccination, tested with so much success for upwards of three quarters of a century, appear to be at the present day unknown to a great mass of the population, since, in 1850, nearly one half the number of children born were neglected in this respect, and that too at a time when every effort was being made by the Academy of Medicine and the practitioners of France, to extend and publish the advantages of the discovery. The opponents of vacci-nation rest their assertions upon statistics which are of a nature so deceptive that the doctrines founded on them will, upon-examination, be seen to be far from correct. It has been asked by M. Malgaigne, "Is it true that, previous to the discovery of vaccination, a greater proportion of individuals arrived at the age of maturity? The question is a simple one, and is a matter in which the data afforded, are well worthy of discussion. By the application of numbers to facts, observation becomes multiplied by itself. If the data be true, accept their signification; if false, at once assert and prove it." The new doctrine maintains that, since the last century, the mortality in France between the twentieth and thirtieth years is doubled, and attributes to the greater prevalence and fatality of *typhoid fevers*, this increase in the number of deaths. But there are no tables upon which this allegation can be justifiably based, as medical statistics, properly so called, are mostly confined to the present century, and there is scarcely a single document of this nature to be found relating to past centuries. To the labors of a few individuals, however, we are indebted for such statistics as will enable the question to be set at rest, so far as relates to the increased mortality between 20 and 30 years of age, during the present century, or in other words, since the introduction of vaccination. We have, as a mortality table for our own time, a work compiled during the period of 1840-49, by M. Heuschling, secretary of the statistical committee of Central Belgium. For the second half of the last century, we are less favorably situated, but we can confidently appeal to the labors of several esteemed authorities, such as Montyon, Messance and Duvillard.

Montyon, in 1774, published his 'Recherches et Considerations sur la Population de la France;' Messance wrote in 1766 and 1788 his 'Recherches sur la Population Française dans Diverses Généralites;' and Duvillard, so late as 1806, published his celebrated 'Analyse de l'Influence de la petite Vérole sur la Mortalite.' We have thus three tables exhibiting the mortality in France for the second half of the eighteenth, and one for the middle of the nineteenth century, and from these we subjoin the following extracts:

Tables of Mortality. (A.)

Ages.	Montyon. 1774.	Messance. 1788.	Duvillard. 1806.	Heuschling. 1840–49.	
0 to 5	470·15	400	416·85	340·30	
5 — 10	52·20	67·5	32	40·70	
10 — 20	44·70	59	48 90	47·85	
20 — 30	62·85	68	64	72	
30 — 40	72·95	64·4	68·80	59·40	
40 — 50	70·80	68·1	72·35	67	
50 — 60	71·80	74	83·50	77	
60 — 70	70·65	86·8	95·90	110·60	
70 — 80	61·69	73·5	83	118·90	
80 — 90	19·25	33·5	30·87	58·60	
90 — 100	2·96	4·8	3·62	6·90	
100 — 105	0·	0·4	0 21	0·15	
Total, . .	1000	1000	1000	1000	décès.
Vm. = P. N.	23·94	27·9	28 26	34·24	Vie Moy.

Tables of Population. (B.)

Ages.	Montyon.	Messance.	Duvillard.	Guillard after Heuschling.	Census of 1851.
0 to 10	254	241	214·40	197	185·25
10 — 20	193	180·50	186·30	175	176·20
20 — 30	148·75	158	165·60	157	163·15
30 — 40	135	134	141·40	137·60	147·50
40 — 50	123	110	116·75	119	124 70
50 — 60	76	84·75	89·40	98	101·50
60 — 70	49·45	55·75	57	70·70	64·70
70 — 80	18·15	27	24·40	36	30·20
80 — 90	2·04	79·0	4·50	8·93	6·34
90 — 100	0·61	1·03	0·44	0·76	0 45
100 — 105	0	0·07	0·01	0·01	0·01
Total, . .	1000	1000	1000	1000	1000

In calculating according to these tables, all that is necessary is to multiply any of the numbers indicating the *population* at any particular age·by the number marked v. m. (vie moyenne), and divide the product by the number in the other table indicating the *deaths* (décès) at the same age. This will give the *chance* of death at that age.

Upon this principle the following table is constructed:

Chance of Death at each Age. One Death in—

Ages.	Montyon.	Messance.	Duvillard.	Guillard. after Heuschling.	Census of 1851.
0 to 10	12	15	13·5	18	17
10 — 20	103	85	106	124	132
20 — 30	57	65	73	74	80
30 — 40	44	58	58	79	89
40 — 50	42	45	46	61	66
50 — 60	25	32	30	43·50	47
60 — 70	17	18	16	22	21
70 — 80	7	10	8·3	10·35	9
80 — 90	2·5	6·5	4·2	5·20	4
90 — 100	5	5·8	3·5	3·60	2·37
100 —	1	1	1	1	2

The result, as shown in this table, clearly demonstrates that the general mortality in France, between the twentieth and thirtieth years, far from having doubled, or even increased, has, not only at that period, but at all ages, diminished since the eighteenth century. Before such evidence the assertions of the opponents of vaccination fall to the ground, and it only remains for us to examine more specially the arguments upon which the statistics drawn up by them may be confuted.

In place of collecting their statistics in *all* the departments of France, the anti-vaccination party content themselves with those of *two*, namely of la Côte-d'Or, where most vaccination takes place, and of l'Aveyron, where it is least practised. And in order to exhibit the deplorable effects produced by its agency, they write to the Academy of Sciences (Comtes Rendus, 10th Sept., 1849) that in fifteen years the population of every age has increased twice as much in l'Aveyron as it has done in la Côte-d'Or, &c., &c. Other causes, however, can be adduced in explanation of the apparently great proportional increase of the population in l'Aveyron. First, the increase of a population occurs in the inverse ratio of its density; accordingly, l'Aveyron having a smaller population than la Côte-d'Or, with an equally great extent of surface, the number of its inhabitants should increase more rapidly: and, second, a population becomes more speedily increased with the advancement of trade and industry; and the extensive industrial establishments recently founded in l'Aveyron have led to the return in the census of 5920 workmen there, while only 3753 are returned for la Côte-d'Or.

In drawing these conclusions from only two departments, we are merely attacking our adversary on his own ground, but we cannot conclude without repudiating such a system for obtaining statistics to be employed in such general questions as the present. In all investigations of this nature, if anything like a scientific method is to be followed, *all* the departments should have been arranged, first according to the numbers vaccinated, and then according to the rate of mortality considered in connection with these.

ART. 6.—*The prevention of the spread of Cholera.*
By Dr. KÜCHENMEISTER.

(*Medical Times and Gazette*, March 15, 1855.)

Dr. Küchenmeister asks for co-operation in essaying how far the spread of cholera may be limited by the administration of small doses of preparations of iron in combination with salts of lime. Schmidt and others have shown that a large expenditure of chloride of sodium takes place through the stools and vomits in this disease, and that with this a retention of urea coexists. The latter is evidenced by the suppression of urine, and by the excretion of the urea, which should be discharged by the kidneys, in a crystalline form, by various parts of the body. Some observers have also succeeded in developing ammoniacal vapors from the blood in cholera. Thus, in cholera an expenditure of chloride of sodium goes hand in hand with the perversion of the excretion of urea. Unfortunately, the great difficulty attendant upon the examination of the excreta in general forbids the expectation of our easily ascertaining with exactitude the comparative conditions of the urea and sodium in the stools, urine, and sweat, in determinate individuals either in the prodromic stage or actual outbreak of cholera. In the absence of such exactitude, we must see whether we cannot utilize by analogy other practical facts. According to the author's experience the means best suited for bringing the excretion of sodium and urea into harmonious operation is the administration of iron with salts of lime. The iron acts as a direct local styptic and tonic upon the mucous membrane of the intestinal canal. Also those who have much to do with cholera patients, or in whose family the disease prevails, should assist the influence of the iron by the moderate use of red wine or bitter beer. No local tonic exerts such a powerful tonic influence upon the mucous membrane, without irritating it, as does iron. In this respect, as well as in its astringent power, it is superior to the nitrate of silver. From long personal experience, by testing his urine, &c., the author has ascertained that iron also much aids the favorable influence which the carbonate and phosphate of lime exert in regulating the excretion of urea. He proposes in any district where cholera prevails, and especially in families in which diarrhœa has manifested itself, the employment of the following formula :

R Ferri Lactici, ℨss—ℨj ;
Calc. Phosphat., ℨj ;
Calc. Carbon., ℨij ;
Sacch. Lact., ℨss—ℨj;
Pulv. Cinnam., Ɖj. M. Ft. pulv.

Of this a small teaspoonful should be taken at each meal time. A glass of good wine or beer, though not essential, may be allowed.

Dr. Küchenmeister begs for a trial of this simple means on a large scale in affected districts, especially as it does not prevent other means of a curative character being resorted to. Thus in persistent or relapsing diarrhœa, small doses of opium or ipecacuanha, may be given in the intervals of taking the powder. In cholera itself, he suggests also that advantage might be derived from the administration of real or artificial mineral waters, containing free carbonic acid, the carbonates and the salts of iron. Some practitioners have, during the after-treatment, administered chloride of sodium in order to directly replace the loss of this substance, but without the simultaneous employment of regulators of the chloride in the body, among which are iron and salts of lime ; but there is little utility in the practice.

(B) ACUTE DISEASES.

ART. 7.—*The pathology and treatment of Inflammation.* By Dr. J. HUGHES BENNETT, Professor of the Institute of Medicine in the University of Edinburgh.

(*Lancet*, March 8, 1856.)

The paper, of which we here offer an abstract, was read before the Edinburgh Royal Medical Society :—

Dr. Bennett, after some preliminary remarks, in which he alluded to the importance of the subject as a foundation for true pathology, defined inflammation as an exudation of the normal liquor sanguinis. Referring to other definitions, he calls their correctness in question. Mr. Paget had been unable to define inflammation. The view that inflammation might exist in non-vascular tissue he opposed by an examination of what occurs in so-called ulceration of cartilage, cornea, and epithelium ; the distinction being, that in inflamed parts there would be exudation of liquor sanguinis, in which new cells would form, but in non-

vascular tissues there would be simply increased growth, induced by endoge-
nous multiplication of pre-existing cells. Then, describing the various phenomena of inflammation, he divided them into preliminary, essential, and resulting
phenomena. The preliminary phenomena were contraction and enlargement of
the smaller vessels, increase and diminution in the flow of blood, and congestion.
The essential phenomenon was exudation of the liquor sanguinis, without which
no inflammation could exist. The distinction between it and effusion of serum
and extravasation he pointed out. The resulting phenomena were two: an
increase of growth by new cell formation, and absence or diminution of cell
growth. The theory of the preliminary phenomena consisted in spasm and
paralysis of the extreme vessels, operating sometimes through the nervous system, directly or by reflex action ; at other times the result of an injury, chemical
or mechanical, applied to the part ; in that of increased quantitative and diminished qualitative attraction exerted by the tissues on the blood ; the increased
spissitude of that fluid. The theory of the essential phenomenon consisted in
the attraction of the liquor sanguinis through the vascular walls into the surrounding parenchyma or neighboring cavities, where it coagulated to form a foreign
body. The theory of the resulting phenomena was, attributing to the exuded
matter, in one case, the properties of a living blastema, when it followed the
vital laws of cell growth ; in the other case, the properties of dead or dying matter, when rendered obedient to chemico-physical laws. Dr. Bennett then described the various ways in which the exuded matter, if it lived, was transformed ;
after which, he said, the disappearance of the exudation is brought about by the
breaking down and disintegration of the exudation, which is rapid according to
the amount of cell formation in it, by the passage of the disintegrated exudation
in a fluid state into the blood, and its elimination from the economy by the excretory, integumentary, intestinal, and renal glands. The exuded matter might
die suddenly or slowly ; if suddenly, its elements combined with those of the
atmosphere chemically, and caused inflammatory gangrene; if slowly, it gradually disintegrated, involved the surrounding tissue, and produced ulceration.
Then, remarking upon the symptoms of inflammation, Dr. Bennett noticed their
fallacious character. Heat, pain, redness, and swelling, might all be absent in
positive cases of inflammation ; hence the error in studying mere symptoms, and
how necessary to blend with it a knowledge of physical signs. These facts led
to the conclusion that all the healing phenomena of inflammation were reparative,
and depended on cell growth. From them was formed the induction "that the
treatment of inflammation to be successful, must be in harmony with those laws
which govern the formation, development, and disintegration of cells. The
treatment of inflammation bore reference to three orders of phenomena. The
symptoms of the preliminary phenomena when seen in medical practice could
not be separated from those of fever. In surgical practice they might be predicted to follow injuries and operations, but there were no means of arresting
them, and the treatment was expectant. The essential phenomenon was frequently observed taking place in surgical practice, but seldom recognized at the
moment of its occurrence in medical. In the latter case it is often most important to arrest exudation, but no remedies could ever be proved to have done
so ; this was illustrated by the effects of general and local bleeding. In surgical
practice, exudation was often necessary to cure, as granulation, adhesion, callus,
&c.; to check it then would injure. When thought advisable, the application of
cold was indicated. We could not cut short an inflammation once produced,
but merely conduct it to a favorable termination. Dr. Bennett then considered
the effects of various remedies—bleeding, mercury, antimony, diuretics, purgatives, sedatives, warmth, moisture, pressure, &c. He was altogether opposed to
bleeding, and mercury he maintained to be useless, in causing rapid absorption
of the exudation ; antimony and neutral salts favored secretion, and diuretics especially assisted the last stage of the process; the influence of sedatives was
exerted on the nervous system : but cold checked, whilst warmth was one of the
most powerful stimulants to cell growth, and favored suppuration. Moisture
favored the formation of independent cells, whilst dryness favored fibre cells ;
pressure was opposed to their expansion and growth, but when formed it favored
their disintegration and absorption. The action of counter-irritants was not under-

stood—it was probably excito-motory; but wine and nourishment were important when the febrile excitement had disappeared, in order to favor the transformation of the exudation. Dr. Bennett then described his mode of treating inflammation of the lungs on the principles he had brought forward, and its success. This consisted of antimonials and the acetate of potash during the febrile stage; then of wine and nourishment; and lastly of diuretics, to favor excretion of the absorbed fibrin, in the form of urates. Excluding complicated cases of pneumonia—i. e., cases connected with cerebral, cardiac, or renal disease, treated in the Infirmary,—there were forty-two in number during the last five years. Of these, two died; one, a boy, who had been wandering without food day and night; the other was a man, who had long been subject to a cough, ague, bloody expectoration, &c.; they died within three days. Of the others, 32 were single and double; the average duration of single pneumonias, counting from the primary rigor, was 15¼ days; the duration of the double, 17½ days; no case of double continued longer than 21 days, or shorter than 14 days. Of the single pneumonias—

1 case	.	.	.	.	lasted 29 days.
1 "	.	.	.	.	26 "
1 "	.	.	.	.	23 "
1 "	.	.	.	.	22 "
2 "	.	.	.	.	21 "
1 "	.	.	.	.	20 "
2 "	.	.	.	.	18 "
1 "	.	.	.	.	17 "
1 "	.	.	.	.	16 "
1 "	.	.	.	.	15 "
10 "	.	.	.	.	14 "
1 "	.	.	.	.	13 "
2 "	.	.	.	.	12 "
3 "	.	.	.	.	10 "
2 "	.	.	.	.	7 "

From all the facts referred to, Dr. Bennett deduced "that the most successful treatment of inflammation is that which is in harmony with those laws which govern the formation, development, and disintegration of cells." In reference to Dr. Alison's theory, in which he stated that acute inflammations have changed their type since the days of Cullen and Gregory, and that formerly they bore bleeding well, and were treated successfully, but that now bleeding was injurious, Dr. Bennett admitted that fevers had changed their type, owing to alterations external to the individual, either from locality, drainage, or malaria, a tropical climate, &c.; but with regard to inflammation as he described it, he said it was the same in all ages and places. According to Dr. Alison, the constitutions of men must have deteriorated, and have undergone a weakening process, by which they could not so well bear bleeding. Dr. Bennett could not agree with this theory. Dr. Alison had endeavored to point out the fallacy of statistics, but such fallacy told against him, as the fatal cases of pneumonia now were not those which possessed vigorous constitutions, and which formerly would have been bled, but they were those which were debilitated, and in which pneumonia occurred in a latent form. Hence he inferred that those cases which bore bleeding well in the days of Cullen and Gregory would do so now; and the expression "bearing bleeding well" was not a correct one, except in the sense that it does less injury to a strong man than a feeble one. Dr. Bennett said, in conclusion, that all important changes in practice must be gradual, and not influenced by the success of this or that empiric, but by the sober energies of those who investigate in the spirit of truth. Such seemed to him the only mode we possessed of improving our treatment of those mysterious processes hitherto involved in the word "inflammation."

ART. 8.—*Blackness of the Tongue without Fever.*
By M. BERTRAND, of St. Germain.

(*Gaz. Hebdom. de Med. et Chir.*, Dec. 7, 1855.)

M. Bertrand has met with four cases in which the human tongue presented the black discoloration which is met with naturally in the parrot and giraffe. The first case was that of a young girl, æt. 13, in whom extreme emaciation and increasing paraplegia gave evidence of serious mischief in the nervous centres. The second case was that of an asthmatic old lady, æt. 70, who was well in every other respect. The third case was that of an old man who appeared to have nothing the matter with him. The fourth case was that of a child, æt. 11, who was convalescing from typhoid fever. These persons complained of nothing but an extreme dryness of the mouth.

The black discoloration, which was perfectly like a pigmentary stain, began in the centre of the tongue, remained stationary for ten days, and then faded from the circumference to the centre—from forty to sixty days being occupied in this process. The color was not at all affected by any kind of washing.

Dr. Bertrand brought these cases before the Parisian Academy of Sciences, but they did not elicit any comment of value.

ART. 9.—*On the treatment of Fever.* By DR. WILKS.

(*Guy's Hospital Reports*, vol. i., 1855.)

We take the following remarks from an admirable report upon all the cases of fever which occurred in Guy's Hospital during the year 1854—a report to which we referred in our last volume for evidence respecting the typhus and typhoid distinctions of fever. Having related the cases, 187 in number, Dr. Wilks proceeds to comment upon the treatment.

"I know little of cutting short the disease by any powerful remedy, but in all probability it may sometimes be accomplished. The opinion, however, that its course when once commenced may be curtailed by ordinary judicious remedies, is one which the above cases will entirely refute. Their perusal will, I think, prove that the best plan of treatment is to guide the patient through the disease—not to endeavor to combat it, but to prevent the subject of it succumbing to its influence at urgent periods. These remarks, I would state, have especial reference to the treatment by stimulants, because it will be seen that in some of the cases which I have brought forward, the most extreme plans have been adopted with respect to them, both as to the time of their administration as well as to their amount. The plan of curing fever by stimulants has of late been strongly advocated, and this is not only by the administration of large quantities of wine, but by the early exhibition of brandy and other spirits; and, moreover, the method has been stated to be eminently successful. I have fortunately seen it adopted, and can judge somewhat of its merits. If the reader will refer, first of all, to the cases of typhus, he will see that Nos. 61 and 73 were two very bad cases with mulberry rashes, and yet each did well, like many others, with simple salines; on the other hand, No. 71, which took no wine, died. With reference to those who took stimulants, let him look at No. 64. This man came in at the very commencement of the fever; on the fourth day wine was at once had recourse to, but the patient continued to sink in the usual course of the disease. Brandy then was freely administered, so that a large quantity of wine and spirit was hourly poured into the system, but the patient died on the fourteenth day. As no morbid appearances were found after death, this must be regarded as a simple case of a patient succumbing to the fever poison in spite of stimulants. No. 65 will be seen to have recovered on the stimulant plan, wine being early given, and increased daily until twenty ounces were administered. In spite of this, however, the patient got lower and lower until the critical day, when the fever turned. No. 76 took all the stimulant that could be administered, but it produced no favorable result, as the case terminated fatally. We draw the same conclusion with regard to other remedies. No. 68 was ordered two grains of quinine three times a day, but the disease ran its usual course. In No. 69 it might appear that the same remedy did good, as convalescence occurred in four days; but then it will be seen that the patient was admitted on the tenth day of the fever, and recovery only occurred at the usual time. No. 90 was that of a man with no eruption, but desperately ill. He was ordered three grains of quinine every four hours, on the fourth day of the fever, and it was continued throughout. The remedy seemed to have the best effect in supporting the power of the patient, but had no influence in curtailing the course of the disease.

"If the reader will now refer to the typhoid case, he will see the same conclusions borne out. In No. 137, ten grains of quinine were given every four hours. This was taken for four days, and, producing no good effect, was discontinued. In reference to the administration of wine, in typhoid cases, it will be seen that deaths occurred in Nos. 108 and 114 where no stimulant was given; and, on the other hand, severe cases, as No. 117, were cured without any. Also some patients died where abundance of stimulants was given, as 131 and 161. The most important cases, in reference to this subject, are those which took a large quantity of stimulus early, but in whom the disease ran its usual course. No. 140 was that of a patient, ill five days with typhoid fever. The case was not more severe than many others that did well without any stimulant, but the plan was wished to be tried. Ten ounces of wine were given, and, in two days' time, increased to fourteen ounces daily. He still sank, and after four days twenty-two ounces of wine were administered. This amount he took ten days longer without any improvement in the symptoms, when at the expiration of this period he very slowly began to improve. The change then, though marked, was not so decided as in most instances. In case No. 142 the same plan was adopted. On the eighth day twelve ounces of wine were administered, and increased the next day to fourteen, and in two more days to twenty. The patient, however, rapidly sank; diarrhœa continuing until death. The inference then to be drawn from the above cases is clear, that fever, both typhus and typhoid, will run its course in spite of all remedies: that patients die with stimulants and without them, as well as recover on both plans. The fact is manifest that these remedies can in some cases be dispensed with, and that in others, although freely given, do not save the patient's life. With regard to their judicious use little can be said, for unless the reader had personally watched the particular cases under review he could not judge of their efficacy. From my own observation, however, I believe that the lives of a large number of cases have been saved by their timely administration. So far, therefore, am I from depreciating the use of stimulants in fever, that I believe the great success in its treatment of late years has been by their adoption; but at the same time I do strongly oppose the opinion that wine or brandy can be looked upon in the light of specific remedies or as antidotes to the disease. The cause which has given rise to this notion is no doubt to be found in the fact of the success which of late years has followed not only the abstinence from bleeding and other depletory means, but the administration of stimulants and support, and thus an opposite doctrine has been advanced, that we were not only to feed and nourish our fevers, but in all cases, even mild ones, to make use of stimulant remedies. Even supposing that this large amount of wine and spirits was not directly injurious, though I believe in many cases it is, a great evil dependent on the plan is, that the remedy is not given in proportion to the failing powers of the patient; and that when the time occurs that he wants all our attention, and requires every possible nourishment, the means for meeting them have been already exhausted; and another evil is, if the amount of stimulant be daily increased, it attains at last such a quantity that the patient is nauseated, and refuses altogether or very reluctantly takes it. At this critical time, when an energetic or powerful remedy is required, the increase of a remedy, already largely given, has but slight effect compared with one which is new; for then it is, when the powers of the patient are beginning to flag, that a judicious and timely use of a stimulant is seen to be followed by the best effect. To know when to give stimulus, and the amount, constitute the most important, and I believe the most difficult, feature in the treatment of fever. There are cases, no doubt, occasionally met with, and may be frequent in particular epidemics, where stimulants are early required, but in ordinary cases of typhus and typhoid fever I believe the most judicious plan has been to give simple salines at first, and towards the close, or the critical time, a moderate amount of wine, which may be increased if requisite. I believe a difference of opinion as to the administration of these remedies has been owing, in great measure, to a want of observation as to the age of the fever at the time of their use, and this strengthens the former remark upon the importance of studying the natural history of the disease. This opinion respecting the treatment of fever is fortified by my experience of dispensary practice; for having had many cases of typhus and typhoid under my care, and having met with but few fatal cases in the space of three years, I have been strongly impressed with the small amount of stimulants under which patients recover. Over and over again have I been surprised at the favorable termination of many bad cases of typhus, where little or no stimulant was made use of. Patients in whom I should have ordered a large quantity of wine had I had the opportunity, nevertheless recovered on the very small pittance they were able themselves to procure. In concluding this subject, let me again repeat that I am an advocate of the plan of nourishing cases of fever, and, if necessary, of stimulating them; but am opposed to the idea, as the reported cases negative it, that wine or spirit is antidotal to fever."

ART. 10.—*The treatment of Fever by "Cinchonism."*
By DR. PEACOCK, Assistant-Physician to St. Thomas's Hospital.

(*Medical Times and Gazette*, Jan. 5, and Jan. 19, 1856.)

In these papers, after relating the history of this mode of treatment, and criticising the views of Dr. Dundas, Dr. Peacock gives seven cases in which he treated fever by "cinchonism." The general result of the treatment is stated as follows:

"1. In one of the cases of typhus, the quinine was certainly not productive of any benefit, and probably added to the torpor and depression of strength. In the other case of typhus it produced the most marked depression, and the patient was only saved by its discontinuance and the liberal exhibition of stimulants. In both cases, though the patients recovered, the disease seemed to follow its natural course, and to be in no degree curtailed in duration by the exhibition of the remedy.

"2. In one case of typhoid, the depression of power and torpor increased under the use of the quinine, but the notes are too imperfect to allow me to speak confidently as to its effects. The patient recovered after an illness of average duration.

"3. In two other cases of typhoid, the remedy appeared to exert neither beneficial nor injurious effects; the disease followed its usual course, and the patients recovered.

"4. In another case of typhoid, it certainly added to the torpor and depression. The remedy was only exhibited in small doses, and for a short period, and was entirely discontinued after six doses had been given, in the course of a day and a half, and stimulants and other means were then freely had recourse to; the prostration and torpor, however, increased, and the patient died comatose.

"5. In the fifth case of typhoid, in which the affection was combined with bilious complication, the quinine was decidedly beneficial, the patient steadily improving under its use. The attack was certainly of shorter duration and less severity than might have been expected from the urgency of the symptoms when the treatment was commenced; but, in this case, the amendment was gradual, and no sudden improvement in the symptoms at any time occurred.

"In all the cases the patients had stimulus and support as required, and other accessory treatment, such as astringents, aperients, anodynes, &c. While also the quinine was exhibited in the various cases in different doses and at various intervals, the different results bore no relation to any of these circumstances.

"The facts and observations which I have now related must only be regarded as a contribution towards the solution of the question of the usefulness of large and repeated doses of quinine in the treatment of the continued fevers of this country. So far, however, as they go, they are opposed to the views of Dr. Dundas, that quinine possesses the power of cutting short the attack; on the other hand, they indicate that the remedy is, in some cases, beneficial; but only as an auxiliary to other measures. It remains to decide, by more extended observations, in what forms of fever, and under what peculiar circumstances, local and individual, the remedy may be advantageously employed; and whether the quinine is more useful in moderate doses at distant intervals, or in the large and frequently repeated doses which have been recommended.

"There is, doubtless, a mean between the results arrived at by different observers which correctly represents the usefulness of quinine in fever; and I am disposed to believe that the very discrepant statements as to its effects, before quoted, may be reconciled by reference to the various characters of fevers in different localities and seasons, and under different circumstances. From an observation before narrated, and from somewhat extensive experience of the use of quinine in smaller and less frequently repeated doses, I feel satisfied that the remedy is useful in the bilious type of typhoid, and also in cases which display a remittent character, or have a tendency to relapse. During the course of last summer, the fever which prevailed was very frequently followed by relapses, and in them quinine was eminently beneficial. There is also a form of typhoid which is of frequent occurrence, in which the fever, though never very intense, is extremely prolonged, day after day elapsing without any material change in the symptoms. In affections of this description, also, quinine is productive of marked advantage, and much accelerates convalescence. My experience, however, of the use of quinine in such cases, is only of its employment in doses of three to five grains three or four times daily. I am not able to say whether the remedy is more useful in such doses, or when exhibited so as to produce the markedly sedative operation on the vascular and nervous systems, indicating the full physiological action of the drug, and to which the term cinchonism has been applied. Possibly the different types of fever may affect the dose which it is desirable to employ—the larger doses being preferable, from their sedative effects, in the more sthenic forms; and the smaller, in the adynamic fevers which require a tonic treatment.

Art. 11.—*The prophylactic and curative treatment of continued Fever.*
By Dr. Semple.

(*Assoc. Med. Journ.*, March 8, 1856.)

The paper, of which the abstract is subjoined, was read before the Medical Society of London. The author commenced by remarking upon the great diversity observed in the nature of fevers, although the prominent and essential features—viz., cold, shivering, heat, and sweating—were the same in all cases. With regard to the proximate cause of fever, little was known with certainty; and perhaps the theory offered by Sydenham, which represented it as an inordinate commotion of the mass of the blood, on the change of that fluid into a new condition, was pretty nearly the same as that which is proposed in the present day; for modern physicians were now generally coming to the conclusion that fever is a blood disease, and that the "commotion" described by Sydenham is due to the introduction of some morbid matter, the exact nature of which, however, is not yet determined. In the present day there is a revival of the humoral "pathology" to a great extent; the belief that cancer and tuberculosis are blood diseases, is fast gaining ground; and that cholera, scurvy, purpura, and albuminuria, are of that nature can hardly be doubted; and in the whole series of inflammatory diseases, the blood is unquestionably affected in the first instance. This view is not merely theoretical, but is of the highest practical utility; for by admitting that numerous diseases are generated by the introduction of subtle poisons into the system, our legislators would be induced to examine the conditions of the atmosphere, of food, and of climate, likely to produce injurious effects upon the animal economy, and would thus materially prevent epidemic disease. With regard to the special treatment of fever, it could not be said that we possessed any one remedy which would positively cut short the disease; fever would run a certain course, and it is not possible to predict the exact length of time to which any given case would extend; but there was much reason to believe, although it could not be positively proved, that the duration of fevers was shortened by judicious treatment. The division of fevers by Cullen was shown to be inapplicable to the present forms of the disease; for the synocha of that

author was rarely, if ever, met with in modern practice, although it no doubt
existed even at the commencement of the present century. The division into
typhus and typhoid fevers was far more in accordance with modern experience,
and no one could study the subject of fever on a large scale without being impressed with the accuracy of the distinctions drawn between the two. The
opposition to this view of the division of fevers probably arose from limited
observation; and further experience would tend only to strengthen the diagnosis
which has been proposed. Admitting that in certain exceptional cases, the two
fevers presented characters in common, and might cause some difficulty in distinguishing them, the leading features were sufficiently striking; the typhus
being characterized by the abundant measly rash, the great tendency to delirium,
the rapid sinking, the absence of abdominal disease; the typhoid, on the other
hand, being marked by the scattered, evanescent, rose-colored spots on the
abdomen or chest, the less tendency to head symptoms, the insidious onset, the
presence of disease in Peyer's patches, the frequency of diarrhœa, a blown
condition of the abdomen, and gurgling in the iliac fossa. In reviewing the
remedies employed in the general treatment of fever, bloodletting, which was
formerly so strongly recommended, was now contra-indicated, in consequence
of the alteration which had taken place in the type of disease, although so lately
as 1830, bleeding was practised in fever with success. Putting the lancet out of
the question, even leeches and the cupping-glasses must be used with great
caution in modern practice; and it must be remembered that any mode of depletion was less easily borne by patients in an hospital than in private practice;
because in the former, the lowering influence of the poisoned atmosphere
affected the vital powers, and tended to produce collapse. Mercury, which was
once extolled as a remedy in fever, possessed very little power over that
disease, although in former years it may have been efficacious; and it was an
error in modern practice to adhere to the routine custom of giving mercury in
this and other diseases, when experience has shown that this mineral, indiscriminately employed, is more injurious than beneficial. Quinine, which is a very
valuable remedy in intermittents and remittents, could not yet be said to be
equally efficacious in continued fevers—at least, not in cutting short that disease;
and the treatment, by large and frequent doses of this alkaloid, had not been
found so successful in other hands as in those of Dr. Dundas, who strongly recommended its employment in this manner. Dr. Semple did not consider this
question as finally settled; but he placed great reliance upon the careful observations of Dr. Barclay and Dr. Peacock upon the subject. Purgatives were
also injurious when carried to any length in the treatment of fever; for they
always tended to produce depression, even if, as by irritating the inflamed bowel
in typhoid fever, they were not positively mischievous. The mildest aperients
should therefore be employed, and amongst the best of these were small doses
of castor oil. Typhus and typhoid fevers, as they were different in their nature,
required different methods of treatment. In the first, the tendency to depression
must be combated by wine, brandy, carbonate of ammonia, and other cordials
and stimulants; and to relieve the head symptoms the head should be shaved,
and a blister applied to the nape of the neck: in the second, or typhoid fever,
the necessity for stimulants at first is not so obvious; but the inflamed and irritated bowel should be an especial object of care, and constipation and diarrhœa,
which may alternately prevail, must be met by appropriate treatment; the former
by mild mercurials and alteratives; the latter by astringents, opium, and acetate
of lead. The prophylactic treatment of fever was even more important than
the curative, for when a fever was once established, its issue was doubtful, and
its treatment difficult. Typhus fever was certainly the most contagious, while
typhoid arose from local or endemic causes. The establishment of fever hosp
tals, he (Dr. Semple) regarded rather as a necessary evil than as a positive goo
they certainly diminished the danger of this disease in the localities from whic
the patients were drawn, but they spread it in the hospital itself; and probabl
the best hygienic treatment of fever was to isolate the patients, if that could b
accomplished, by placing them in situations which were airy, clean, well ven
lated, and remote from one another.

ART. 12.—*The treatment of Fever by Acetate of Zinc.*
By Dr. HEER.

(*Medicinische Zeitung*, No. 42, 1855.)

The cases treated in this manner (the numbers and particulars are not given) occurred in the second quarter of last year, and all presented either petechiæ, or the typhoid rash. Head symptoms predominated, but chest and abdominal symptoms were both frequent and urgent. Restless delirium, requiring the use of the strait-jacket, was very common, and often fatal, death being preceded by extremely rapid sinking of the physical and vital powers.

Dr. Heer did not trust exclusively to the acetate of zinc. On the contrary, he administered stimulants and antispasmodics wherever they were required, which was in almost every case. He speaks most undoubtingly, however, of the beneficial action of the sulphate of zinc, and says the great nervous agitation was frequently calmed by the very first dose. His mode of administering the remedy was to give, every two hours, a table-spoonful of a solution of one demigramme (nearly eight grains) in 250 grammes of water.

ART. 13—*Treatment of Typhoid Fever by Tar Water.*
By Dr. CHAPELLE, of Angoulême.

(*Charleston Med. Journal and Review*, March, 1856).

Having observed the favorable effect of tar in a certain case of typhoid fever, Dr. Chapelle was induced to pay particular attention to this remedy, in a series of cases occurring during the typhoid epidemic of 1854, 1855. His conclusion is, that liquid tar, if not an absolute specific, is yet incontestably the most efficacious agent yet discovered for the treatment of the above-mentioned disease. The tar should be administered internally as a drink, and in the form of an injection.

The drink is prepared in the following manner :—About two ounces of liquid tar are put into a vessel, containing nearly a quart of hot water; after it has stood a few hours, the patient commences to drink it, filling up with ordinary water after each draught, so that the same dose of tar will last during the whole treatment. The injection is prepared by rubbing up the yellow of one or two eggs with a tablespoonful of liquid tar, and diluting with a little more than a pint of warm water; this serves for two injections.

The patient should drink as much of the draught as he can ; as to the injection, that should be insisted on in proportion as the drink disgusts, for the intestines should be always kept supplied with a certain quantity. Sometimes six, eight, and even ten enemata, should be administered in twenty-four hours. Should the patient be taken with diarrhœa, these injections check it promptly.

This treatment, if continued for two or three days, generally triumphs over the typhoid state; typhoid fever of ordinary intensity, called usually mucous fever, needs double that time ; but typhoid fever, properly so called, of whatever form, is vanquished in its essential phenomena in eight to ten days. Each day the skin loses its dryness and heat, the tongue becomes clearer, abdomen presents less tension and susceptibility, the sleep is calmer, the fæcal matter acquires a more normal odor, and the digestive functions recover strength. When there exists only a simple typhoid state, the tar draught alone is commonly sufficient ; but when the general perturbation augments, the febrile reaction increases, and the functional disorder is excessive, a much stronger dose of the tar is required, and the injections are then indispensable. In all cases where the breast or the head has been affected with violent perturbation, the disappearance of the ordinary typhoid phenomena does not immediately produce a cessation of these complications. These functional disorders either disappear gradually of themselves, or need the application of treatment appropriate to the morbid state.

ART. 14.—*Case of Small-pox quickly recurring.*
By Mr. GASCOYEN, House Surgeon in St. Mary's Hospital.

(*Assoc. Med. Journal*, Feb. 23, 1856.)

This case occurred in St. Mary's Hospital, in a patient under the care of Dr. Alderson.

CASE.—J. W., æt. 23, laborer, was admitted into St. Mary's Hospital, December 28th, 1855, under the care of Dr. Alberson. Five months ago he was laid up with small-pox: from this he had recovered about a month, but for the last week he had suffered severely with pains in the shoulders and limbs, the joints having been much swollen. For this he was admitted. He now complained of pain in the shoulders and knees; the latter were slightly swollen, but he could walk tolerably; his skin was cool and perspiring, everywhere covered with cicatrices, exhibiting loss of substance, exactly similar to those left by variola. He had occasional chills and heats, with slight cough. Tongue clean. Pulse 96. Urine natural. He was placed upon full diet, with bark and colchicum, under which treatment he steadily improved till January 17, when his former symptoms returned, with violent headache, a furred tongue, and rapid, weak pulse. Salines were now given.

The next day he had nausea, rigors, and severe aching in his back and limbs.

January 9th.—The above symptoms continued unabated. His eyes were much congested, and his face thickly covered with an ill-defined eruption; over the limbs and body the skin around the old cicatrices was red and inflamed, forming bright red patches, with very distinct margins, giving a peculiar appearance; elsewhere it was of the natural color.

20th.—Over the forehead the eruption is more tuberculated, and feels like shot beneath the skin; the eyelids are much swollen; he has a sore throat, and is troubled with a short dry cough. He was very restless and delirious through the night, but now is quiet, and answers rationally.

22.—The eruption over the face is becoming pustular, and, in places, confluent; the eyelids are completely closed. He takes scarcely any nourishment.

23d and 24th.—He is not delirious now, but cannot sleep, and continues restless. Tongue brown, dry, and hard; throat very sore. He is ordered, as a gargle, and to drink, an ounce of port wine, with a drachm of yeast in half a pint of water, which is very grateful to him. The pustules over the face have all run together, incrusting it in one large scab. Over the rest of the body the skin is so thickly covered with pustules that it is impossible to place the tip of the finger on any part without touching some.

25th and 26th.—The pustules have become confluent over the scrotum, and down the inside of the thighs; and there are several large patches on various parts of the body. The eyelids are now inclosed, and there is a considerable discharge from the nose and mouth. The bowels not having acted for two days, he was ordered a small dose of castor oil.

27th.—The patient is very prostrated, and speaks with difficulty, in a husky low whisper, but takes more food, such as port wine, beef tea, or milk. He has considerable dyspnœa, and loud moist crepitations can be heard all over the front of the chest. Pulse so small it cannot be counted.

10 P.M.—He is quite conscious, but cannot articulate; he has mucous rattle in the throat. Pulse imperceptible. He swallows wine in small quantities.

28th, 3 A.M.—Died.

The autopsy presented nothing of the slightest interest.

ART. 15.—*Coma in Scarlatina.* By Dr. HENRY KENNEDY.

(*Dublin Quarterly Journal of Medicine*, Aug., 1855.)

On a recent occasion Dr. Henry Kennedy directed the attention of the Colleg of Physicians in Ireland to the coma which was known to be a frequent atte dant on scarlatina. The period of its occurrence was one of the points notices, and for this purpose he speaks of it as being observed under two different aspects, which it was well to keep in mind. In the first class of cases, the coma existed at the commencement of the disease; and here it might exist *per se*, and continue even without intermission till death. Of this he had known instances. In other cases, again, while the coma was a very early symptom, it was attended with convulsions, or, rather, the two occurred alternately. Of this, also, he had seen examples. But the most frequent occurrence was the presence of coma at the onset of the attack, and its gradual subsidence as the disease progressed. This, then, was the first way in which the coma was to be observed; that is, as ushering in the attack. In the second, however, matters were very different, for here the disease begins with the ordinary febrile symptoms, and it is only as it progresses that coma shows itself, and usually goes on increasing till the period of death. He thought it well to draw these distinctions as to the period at which coma comes on; for though ever a serious symptom, and occurring only in the worst forms of the disease, still there was this difference between the two classes of cases—that the first was a more favorable case to have to treat than the last. He stated that he had seen several instances where the disease had begun with coma, from which the child had recovered in a few hours. One such he had lately seen with his friend Dr. Denham, and they were not uncommon. But where the coma appeared at a later stage, and then only for the first time, matters went on very differently, and a case of recovery was a very exceptional one indeed. The remark applied not only to cases of scarlatina, but to all acute fevers, and more particularly to the ordinary fever of Dublin; in which latter it was well known that the approach of coma, and still more its actual occurrence and tendency to increase, were amongst the very worst signs which could appear. From profound coma, under the circumstances detailed, he had seen no recovery.

What could be done for the class of cases he had been speaking of? Unfortunately, but too little. Still, there was one remedy from which he had seen benefit when the coma was an early symptom. Though well known, it possibly might be used more generally than it is. He spoke of the cold effusion applied to the head, and under the inspection of the medical attendant. This, used with the ordinary care, and modified, as it could be, by taking the chill off the water, he had found very useful. Even when the coma appeared late, he had seen benefit from its use, but not at all equal to what occurred in the other cases. Many of the cases marked by early coma, on recovering from this state, exhibited symptoms of great depression, and which at once called for some modification of the antiphlogistic plan. Besides wine, he had seen marked benefit arise from the use of barm—a remedy which, though formerly much used, had latterly been nearly forgotten. In Cork Street Hospital it was, however, still employed by Dr. George Kennedy, and often with benefit.

ART. 16.—*On the relations between Scarlatina, Rheumatism, Carditis, and Albuminuria.* By Dr. WILLSHIRE, Assistant-Physician to the Charing Cross Hospital.

(*Lancet*, Dec. 1855.)

In a clinical lecture recently delivered, Dr. Willshire makes the following case the text for some remarks respecting the relation which exists between scarlatina, rheumatism, carditis, and albuminuria.

CASE.—Clara M——, æt. 10, admitted the 29th of October. On the 22d, the rash, sore-throat, and *malaise* of scarlet fever made their appearance. On the 23d, she was brought as an out-patient to the hospital. For six days nothing more was heard of her, but on the 29th her mother returned to say her daughter was very unwell, and that the day previously her limbs and joints had become very painful and seemed swollen. The child was admitted into the wards the same afternoon. On admission, the right knee and ankle-joint were swollen, slightly reddened by a blush, and painful; the tongue was coated, the bowels rather costive, and she looked a little puffy about the face; urine said to be passed in sufficient quantity. She was ordered the nitrate of potash mixture and compound powder of jalap. The urine to be preserved for examination.

On the 30th, she complained very much of pain; the limbs were too painful to be moved, and she lay on her right side, with the knees up towards the chin; the respiration was accelerated, the heart's action increased in frequency, and a slight bruit was heard, diffused, as it appeared, over the precordial region. The bowels had been slightly operated upon. No urine free from admixture could be obtained. Four leeches were ordered to be applied over the heart, and the bleeding to be somewhat encouraged, the compound jalap powder to be repeated, and the wine of colchicum to be added to the nitrate of potash mixture. Alkaline fomentations to the affected joints.

On the 31st, the patient seemed much better; the heart's action lessened, but the bruit was plainly to be heard. The countenance was more cheerful, and the position in bed could be changed. To continue the medicines as before.

November 1st.—Still improving; the pain of joints nearly disappeared; and cuticle freely desquamating. Could lie on right or left side indifferently. Complains of soreness of mouth. The tongue was red, with aphthæ upon it, and stomatitis was present; there was also a slight herpetic eruption about the lips. She was ordered the chlorate of potash mixture, and the application of the mucilage of biborate of soda to the mouth. Up to the 5th of November she went on improving, the skin freely desquamating, and the urine was found to be non-albuminous.

On the 5th, one of the wrist and ankle-joints again became painful and swollen, the heart's action increased, and the countenance somewhat anxious. At the base of the heart a sort of reduplication of the first sound was plainly to be heard, and over the apex a distinct systolic sawing souffle. Ordered to return to the nitrate of potash and colchicum mixture; to have a blister on the right side of the chest.

On the 8th she felt again better, the bruit over the apex continuing. Ordered to have two grains of mercury with chalk, and three of soda, every four hours. She went on generally improving; complained of no pain over the heart; no difficulty of breathing, or of pain of the limbs; the countenance was full of vivacity, but a loud sawing souffle beneath the nipple, and a slight roughness, with the first sound at the base continued.

9th.—Improves; apex sound as before, that at base less evident. Repeat the mixture.

10th.—Much better, but the pulse rather small; apex bruit as before, roughness at base less evident, but a reduplication as before heard of the first sound. To continue the mercury, but to take also cod-liver oil.

11th.—Improves; up and dressed; skin yet desquamating. To have a warm bath; and orders were given to the sister to have her skin well scrubbed.

12th.—Urine examined; not albuminous. To leave off the mercury, and to take cod-liver oil and quinine.

13th.—Was crying yesterday because not allowed to leave the hospital, being, she said, "quite well." Bruit at apex continues; skin still desquamates. To repeat the warm bath.

After relating this case, and after referring to the opinions of former observers, Dr. Willshire proceeds to make certain remarks, from which we take the following:—

" That there is some obscurity about the exact nature of a disease occasionally attacking not only children, but adults, and marked by arthritic pain and tension, often of a severe character, accompanied by a scarlet rash, is plain from the accounts given by some American and East and West Indian practitioners. For instance, in 1824, 1825, and 1847, outbreaks of a disease like the one I have just mentioned occurred in the East Indies. In the summer of 1828, the malady appeared epidemically in some of the southern cities of the American Union after having previously prevailed in some of the islands of the Gulf of Mexico. In Charleston it spread with great rapidity, ultimately attacking almost the entire population. In this latter city the last occurrence of it that I have found recorded was in 1850, and is alluded to by Dr. Dickson, of South Carolina. I Calcutta, again, during the hot and rainy season of 1853, a variety of the same affection prevailed, and has been well discussed by Dr. Goodeve in the first volume of the 'Indian Annals of Medical Science' for that year, and to which I must refer you. Now, this disease has been called *scarlatina rheumatica* b

Cocke and Copland, *exanthesis arthrosia* by Nicholson, and the strange cogno-
men of *dengue* has been popularly bestowed upon it. I have said that the first
account of this disease goes not further back than 1824; but it is proper that I
should mention that Dr. Dickson, of Charleston, writes as follows: 'I recognize
Rush's "breakbone fever" of 1780 in Philadelphia as the first notice of a malady
such as I have called dengue;' and Dr. Waring, of Savannah, alludes also to
dengue under the title of 'eruptive breakbone.'

"I cannot go into the details of this peculiar disorder; indeed, I have only
alluded to it to show you that there occurs a fever, accompanied by arthritic
pains and a red exanthem, whose true relations to scarlet fever yet require clearing up. However, I may just remark, that Dr. Dickson regards dengue as a
distinct contagious disease, giving immunity from second attacks, and that it is
not scarlatina; whilst Dr. Goodeve states that most of the symptoms characteristic of the latter affection found expression in some of the cases occurring in
Calcutta. He says, 'the fever eruption, reddened mucous membrane and tonsils, desquamation of cuticle, swelling of hands and feet, state of the tongue,
albuminous urine, are all such as go to make up scarlatina; but it would be
premature to assert that the cause is identical with that of scarlatina. I should
say that it would require a longer series of observations of several epidemics,
with careful examination of all the attendant circumstances, before we could
pronounce the diseases to be identical.' Again: Dr. Copland affirms, that the
disease called dengue 'was not a form of scarlatina is shown by the severity of
the rheumatic or neuralgic symptoms,' &c.; and 'that it was not a rheumatic
fever was shown by the undoubted propagation of it by infection,' &c. I see that
in some later observations by Dr. Mackinnon, in the third number of the 'Indian
Annals,' he doubts whether any of the epidemics of India described as attended
by red efflorescence of the skin can be identified with any of the varieties of
the scarlatina of Europe, denies the disease we have referred to to be contagious,
and for which, he says, the name of 'the red fever' is as good a name as any
other.

"On reviewing the different accounts given by Indian and American writers
of this puzzling affection, the disease appears, in certain places, and epidemics,
to have had more the characters of rheumatism; whilst in others it has had
more those of scarlatina. Our own case of M— may be said to illustrate, so
far as my own experience extends in respect to the relations between scarlatina
and rheumatism, one form of the arthritic complication—namely, that occurring
early in the course of the exanthematous disease. When it so occurs, the specific inflammation about the joints terminates, like primary or idiopathic rheumatism, in resolution or delitescence. But it may take place at a later period of
the disease, when all has been thought to be over. It occurs after desquamation has made some progress, and then may terminate in the suppurative crisis.
Now, this is peculiar about the rheumatic inflammation generally of young
children; unlike in adults or older children, it may lead to purulent effusion into
joints, and also about them. I have known this to occur in several instances,
and it is more liable, I believe, to ensue in the secondary rheumatism of scarlatina. This is a fact well known to others. If I recollect aright, Dr. Kennedy,
of Dublin, has published something upon it, and Trousseau, I know, states that
scarlatinal rheumatism is often more dangerous when localised to a single joint,
than when attacking several articulations at one time, as it is then more inclined
to terminate in suppuration, and even eventually to result in caries of the articulating surfaces. This circumstance, however, of the arthritic inflammations of
infants and young children, not unfrequently terminating in the formation of
matter, has led some pathologists to deny the true rheumatic nature of the disease in question. I must confess, too, it does seem to me not improbable that
the results of pyohœmia, or purulent infection, of phlebitis, umbilical or otherwise, may, along with other forms of abnormal action, have been occasionally
placed to the credit of ordinary rheumatic inflammation. But Mr. Henry
Lee, who has paid great attention to the subject of purulent infection, states
that he has seen, as the result of the absorption of sero-purulent fluid from an
ill-conditioned abscess, very severe rheumatism, affecting, in some instances,
the pericardium and dura mater. In these cases, there was occasionally more

fluid secreted than in ordinary rheumatism, but in milder examples there was no such distinctive mark; they are said to have been 'in every sign and symptom apparently identical.'

"I have undoubtedly seen cases in children, which I should not have known from rheumatism, terminate in the suppurative crisis. If it be said, then such cases therefore could not have been rheumatism, the argument is of course settled; but it appears to me only so by a *petitio principii*. In adults, again, rheumatism does occasionally, however rarely, terminate in the formation of matter. In M—'s case, some mischief has ensued certainly to the mitral, if not also to the aortic, valves. It may be but slight, still there it is, and may lay the foundation for changes in after years connected with the walls of the heart's chambers. The abnormal sound (which some of you have listened to) at the apex is very loud, but this you know is not proof of the amount of structural mischief at the mitral, for there may be much noise and slight change, and but little noise and great alterations. The former, I hope, is the case here; but from the pulse being so small at the wrists, my hope is not to be too much trusted to. A German pathologist affirms it to be a general thing in scarlatina for the first sound of the heart to be aspirated or blowing, and which is a result of the altered state of the blood, and not of the valves, and is a proof that scarlatina and all its complications arise from one common blood disorder. I presume he must mean to refer only to the sound at the base, and not at the apex (where our worst one is), of the cardiac region. Sounds at the base, you know, may be of hæmic origin, but at the apex they are, I believe, always of structural derivation.

"The liability of the heart to become affected during scarlatina has been known for some time. Roux in 1819, and Krukenbergius in 1820 are said by Rilliet and Barthez to have referred to the occurrence of pericarditis in connection with scarlatina and measles. Trousseau, says Bouillaud, pointed it out; but certain it is, Mr. O'Ferrall, in 1835, detailed it to Dr. Graves, of Dublin, how he was obliged to have recourse to leeching, calomel, and James' powder, to overcome acute pericarditis in connection with scarlatina. Several later writers, as Burrows, Willis, Joy, &c., have noticed this complication; and not long ago M. Trousseau stated it as his belief that 'many cases of organic disease of the heart, which only become evident at an after period, have had their origin in scarlet fever.' But, so far as I know, we are most indebted to Dr. Scott Allison for prominently bringing this matter before our notice, though it has been said that the frequency of the complication has been somewhat exaggerated. You will find Dr. Allison's original paper in the 'Medical Gazette' for 1845. The present case of M— makes the third one of heart complication during scarlatina that I have seen, and you perceive here it has occurred in connection with an arthritic affection. One might, à priori, suppose the sequence of the phenomena would always thus present themselves, but it seems that it is not so, as the involvement of the cardiac organ is alluded to by writers, as well as seen by myself, without the arthritic affection having preceded or accompanied it. I find it remarked that in the Stuttgard collection of papers on 'Children's Diseases' the occurrence of purulent collections in the pericardium during scarlet fever is mentioned by Von Ammon, whilst effusions of pus beneath the periosteum and in the substance of muscles has been recorded by others. It is, therefore, possible that the rheumatism in M—'s case had, in one sense, nothing in itself to do with the cardiac affection, but that both were but effects of one same and common cause, and that this cause was the same condition of the blood which gave rise to every other manifestation of the scarlet fever."

ART. 17.—*On some points in Epidemic Cholera.* By Dr. AYRES.

(*Medical Times and Gazette*, March 22, 1855.)

In a paper recently read before the Medical Society of London, Dr. Ayre after stating that he had no theory to support, went on to comment upon some of the symptoms of this disease, as observed by him during the epidemics of 1848–9 and 1853–4. In relation to premonitory diarrhœa, he observed that t' praiseworthy investigations of Dr. M'Laughlin, had led to his denial that colla ever occurred without premonitory diarrhœa of some hours' or days' durar

After adverting to certain recorded cases in which collapse occurred without premonitory diarrhœa, and the intestines were found after death gorged with the rice-water evacuations, Dr. Ayres observed that in a practical point of view, diarrhœa could not be correctly called premonitory, unless of sufficient duration to allow time for the action of remedies; and he detailed several cases in which collapse supervened so suddenly as not to give sufficient time for the exhibition of remedial agents. With reference to the evacuations, the author stated that neither chemical nor microscopical examination had thrown the smallest light on the cause of the disease. He explained the formation of the larger cholera bodies described by Drs. Swan and Budd, of Bristol, as one of the phases in the digestion of fats, and exhibited drawings of the cholera bodies of the rice-water evacuations, and the artificial cholera bodies, produced during the digestion of fat in a healthy animal. He also enumerated the microscopic objects discovered in specimens of rice-water evacuations from fifteen cases of cholera. Vogel and Heller had observed, that the addition of nitric acid to the distillate of rice-water evacuations produced a red tint in the liquids, and Simon had noticed the production of the same color by addition of nitric acid to the liquid motions in typhus. The author had, some years before, obtained the same roseate tint by the addition of this acid to the distillate of night soil. He repeated the experiment of Vogel and Heller, on cholera evacuations, with the same result, but being struck with the exact resemblance of the reaction of the distillates of cholera evacuations and night soil, he was led to ascertain whether fresh healthy fæces would yield the same results; and he found that such was the case in all minor degrees, thus proving that this peculiar reaction is not a pathological peculiarity of cholera, but a result of the putrefaction of fæcal matters. In reference to cramps, the author remarked, as a result of a somewhat extended experience, that this symptom was invariably absent in young children, and that the cramps were rarely severe before the age of puberty. He described certain peculiarities in the symptoms of collapse in children, as contrasted with those occurring in the same stage of the disease in adults. In relation to the cause and propagation of the disease, Dr. Ayres entered somewhat at large on the chief hypothesis on this part of the subject. He remarked somewhat severely on the conduct of the late Board of Health, for confounding the predisposing with the efficient cause of the disease, and for attributing to local causes, always present, the production of a disease which has only lately appeared among us, and at long intervals. He then proceeded to examine the hypothesis of Dr. Snow and Mr. Grove on the cause and propagation of the disease, raising serious objections to their opinions. Finally, in speaking of the treatment of the disease, the author stated that, among a very large number of cases of diarrhœa which came under his care during the epidemics of 1848-9 and 1853-4, he had only seen two or three cases in which the diarrhœa was uncontrollable by ordinary treatment, and then ran on into collapse. Considerable difference in relation to treatment was seen in the two epidemics; for while about two-thirds of the collapse cases recovered in 1848-9 under a treatment consisting of small doses of calomel frequently repeated, with chalk and catechu mixture rendered stimulating by the addition of tincture of capsicum; in 1854 nearly all the collapsed patients died under that, and other modes of treatment.

ART. 18.—*Meteorological Changes in relation to Cholera.*
By Mr. GLAISHER, F. R. S.

(*Report on the Meteorology of London, and its relation to Epidemic Cholera. Blue Book.*)

These are the conclusions of the report which was presented by Mr. Glaisher to the President of the Board of Health—a report which does full credit to the known ability of the writer.

"In the year 1854 the pressure of the atmosphere was great; the temperature generally high; sky overcast; direction of the wind northeast and southwest, and the velocity of the air was less by one half than its average for some time before; and at the time of the greatest mortality from cholera, the barometer reading was remarkably high, and the temperature above its average; a thick atmosphere, though at times clear, everywhere prevailed; weak positive electricity; no rain. In low places a dense mist and stagnant air, with a temperature in excess; temperature of the Thames water high; a high night London temperature; a small daily range; an absence of ozone, and no electricity.

"The three epidemics of 1832, 48, and 54 were attended with a particular state of atmosphere, characterized by a prevalent mist, thin in high places, dense in low. During the height of the epidemic, in all cases, the reading of the barometer was remarkably high, and the atmosphere thick. In 1849 and 1854, the temperature was above its average, and a total absence of rain, and a stillness of air amounting almost to calm, accompanied the progress of the disease on each occasion. In places near the rivers, the night temperatures were high, with small diurnal range, a dense torpid mist, and air charged with the many impurities arising from the exhalations of the river and adjoining marshes, a deficiency of electricity, and, as shown in 1854, a total absence of ozone, most probably destroyed by the decomposition of the organic matter with which the air in these situations is strongly charged.

"In 1849 and 1854, the first decline of the disease was marked by a decrease in the readings of the barometer, and in the temperature of air and water; the air, which previously for a long time had continued calm, was succeeded by a strong southwest wind, which soon dissipated the former stagnant and poisonous atmosphere. In both periods at the end of September the temperature of the Thames fell below 60°, but in 1854 the barometer again increased, the air became again stagnant, and the decline of the disease was considerably checked. It continued, however, gradually to subside, although the months of November and December were nearly as misty as that of September. By the close of the year diarrhœa and cholera had subsided, but a high rate of mortality still continued.

"The coexistence of cholera with coincident meteorological phenomena, is, to say the least of it, remarkable; so is the stagnant atmosphere prevalent during the time of cholera in each of the three periods, and which would seem to be a necessary condition to the activity of the disease.

"The inimical nature of the influence it exercises upon the public health, I regard as intimately connected with the state of the water and the marshes, which in the preceding pages are shown to be large evaporating surfaces for every description of poisonous exhalations. Impure water and impure air are inseparable, for the impurities of the former will be concentrated into the surrounding atmosphere, and there remain, unless rapidly dispersed under favorable atmospheric conditions.

"The agency of the river in fostering diseases is confirmed by the history of cholera just traced, and which we find to have been most fatal in low situations, and in London in those places on the south side of the Thames which afford an undisturbed lodgment for the reception of the air charged with the poisonous elements from evaporation and exhalation. The effect of a gentle wind is to float this atmosphere to enclosed spots, where its malignity becomes concentrated."

ART. 19.—*The chemical conditions of Cholera atmospheres.*
By Dr. R. D. THOMPSON, F.R.S.

(*Lancet, Jan.* 19, 1856.)

There is much food for reflection in the following facts:

"The chemical conditions of cholera atmospheres is a question of intense interest in the subject of public health; but with the exception of the unpublished experiments of Dr. Prout, during the epidemic of 1832, comparatively little attention appears to have been bestowed on it. One of the most striking circumstances connected with the occurrence of the disease is, that no change very palpable to the senses prevails; and it has even been remarked, that the weather has usually been exceedingly agreeable. In London, at St. Thomas's Hospital, the neighborhood of which afforded a large supply of cholera cases, the relative weight of the air, in August, 1854, a cholera month—and in August, 1855, when the metropolis was in an exceedingly healthy condition—is exhibited in the following table in grains per cubic foot:

1854. Week ending		Weight of cubic foot in grains.	1855. Week ending		Weight of cubic foot in grains.
Aug.	5th	522·9	Aug.	4th	516·9
	12th	526·7		11th	524·3
	19th	525·		18th	525·9
	26th	523·5		25th	519·2
Sept.	2d	525·2	Sept.	1st	523·0
	9th	530·3		8th	531·6
Mean		525·6	Mean		523·5

"The result, as deduced from this table, which has been calculated approximately from the barometric pressure, dry and wet bulb thermometers, is analogous to that obtained by Dr. Prout, in 1832, as I was informed by himself. Corresponding observations have been made by Mr. Glaisher, at Greenwich, and the same conclusions arrived at; from which it would appear that this superior weight of a given bulk of common air was not a local phenomenon, but was diffused to a considerable distance.

"Another character distinguishing September, 1854, from the corresponding period of 1855, was the absence of any atmospheric action on ozone test-paper in the former season; while during 1855, the oxidizing influence of the air has never been absent at St. Thomas's Hospital. During September, 1854, however, when no ozone could be detected in London, its action was sometimes faint, and often very strongly marked, at Lewisham, near Greenwich. Throughout the same periods the air was exceedingly stagnant; and it has since been observed by Mr. Glaisher, and also at Vienna, that rapid atmospheric movement is pretty generally accompanied by an oxidizing condition of the air.

"With reference to the chemical composition of the atmospheres of inhabited localities and malarious districts, experiments have usually been conducted on the constitution of the gases which enter into the composition of the air. But the results seem to have thrown little light on the possibility of the production from such causes of any disease characterized by a regular sequence of symptoms. So far as our knowledge warrants, gases can either act only as asphyxiating media by the exclusion of oxygen, or as slow or rapid poisons. The cause capable of inducing disease, formed on a peculiar type, analogy leads us to infer, must be in an organized condition, either in a solid form, or in a finely diffused, or vaporific state. The fact observed, that in malarious atmospheres sulphuric acid speedily becomes black, also points to the propriety of examining the air in such situations, with the view of filtering from it solid or condensible matter. In the epidemic of 1849–50, I examined the exterior air of an infected district with this object in view to the extent of many cubic feet; but the result was comparatively negative, and led to the inference that the examination of large masses of air could alone hold out any prospect of a successful issue.

"For this purpose, in 1854, air was passed through carefully prepared distilled water, contained in Wolfe's bottles, by means of a large aspirating apparatus, of the capacity of sixteen cubic feet, which was kept constantly in action during the day for several months. Occasionally freezing mixtures were applied to portions of the apparatus, and a tube filled with pumice moistened with sulphuric acid, placed near the aspirator, completed the series. A range of glass tubes conducted the air from a cholera ward into the aspirator. The ward was 32 feet long, 20 wide, and 9 high. The air was drawn from the centre of the ward, near the ceiling; and when the apartment was filled with cholera patients, the air, after traversing several layers of distilled water, speedily charred the sulphuric acid, and deposited a variety of solids in all the Wolfe's bottles, which could even be detected in some measure by the eye. The objects consisted of blue and red cotton fibres, from the dresses of the inmates, portions of hair, wool, fungi, sporules of fungi, abundance of vibriones, or lower forms of animal life, with particles of silica and dirt. In this and in all the experiments conducted on the air of closed apartments, the distilled water was rendered strongly acid, from the presence of sulphuric and sulphurous acids, derived from the products of gas and coal combustion. The distilled water used in these experiments was boiled for some time previous to being introduced into the apparatus, and was divided into two portions, one part being placed in a stoppered bottle, beside the Wolfe's bottles, through which the air was conducted, the sediment, if any, being afterwards examined and compared with that resulting from the experiment. When the ward was only partially filled, vegetable epiderm, vegetable cellular tissue, fragments of cotton, linen, vegetable hairs, sponge spiculæ, minute fungi, spiral vessels, sporules, spore cases, animal epithelium, oil-globules, and silicious particles were conspicuous, while vibriones were entirely absent, or at least mere traces could be discriminated. This is an interesting result, since, in the first case, only 98.6 cubic feet were examined, and of the partially empty ward 240 cubic feet passed through the apparatus. When the ward was empty, cotton fibres, wool, a trace of fungus, with carbonaceous and silicious particles, were alone observable, the amount of air examined being 304 cubic feet. The air external to the ward, and in the immediate neighborhood, afforded, from 560 cubic feet, one cotton fibre, one of wool, a crystalline body, probably a sponge spicula, sporules, beautiful mycelia of fungi in various stages of development, and some carboneous matter. The distilled water, in this instance, likewise yielded a strongly acid reaction, produced by sulphur acids. The possible influence of sewer atmospheres predicted interesting results from an examination of such air; and accordingly, it was found that the predominating feature of this experiment was animal life, in the form of swarms of vibriones, in various stages of advancement. The chemical reaction in this case, unlike that in the preceding experiments, was invariably alkaline, due to the evolution of ammonia from the nitrogenous matters contained in the sewage liquors. These experiments render it sufficiently obvious, that organic living bodies constantly surround us in close apartments, and particularly that animal matter, under certain circumstances, exists in the air. It is scarcely legitimate to infer, that the absence from the air of matter capable of communicating cholera has been proved by these experiments, since it is certain that nitrogenous materials, distinct from the germs of vibriones, must have been present, to supply food to these living beings. The researches show, that foreign animal matter, injurious to health, may speedily be concentrated in certain localities, which will undoubtedly assist, in conjunction with meteorological conditions, in the production and propagation of disease. Pathological investigation, carefully conducted by my colleague, Mr. Rainey, detected, in one case, an entozoon in the glottis, the only analogues of which have hitherto been found in the substance of the muscles of animals, a fact which would seem to indicate that the germ of this creature had been derived from the atmosphere, or at least directly from external sources. Careful pathological examination failed to detect in the mouth or air-passages sporules, germs, or living beings, in those patients who died of cholera.

ART. 20.—*On Yellow Fever.* By Dr. BLAIR, Surgeon-General of British Guiana.

(*Report of the Recent Yellow Fever Epidemic of British Guiana.* Churchill, 1856. Pamphlet, pp. 91.)

The following definition of yellow fever, and the account of the post-mortem appearances, are from a report upon which much care and labor has been expended—

"The efficient cause of yellow fever," writes Dr. Blair, "is an aërial poison, probably organic, which requires a certain temperature for its generation and existence, and affects special localities and persons. This poison attaches itself to the mucous surfaces of the human body. One of the primary effects of such contact, when the quantity is adequate, is to rouse the system into febrile reaction, and to excite through the stomach and intestines an effort to expel the noxious agent. There is reason to believe that this compulsory effort is sometimes successful unassisted, but is materially aided by the action of certain medicinal substances. In the event of the expulsory effort being unsuccessful, the effect of this poison is to act destructively on the epithelial structures of the body by inducing a specific irritation in the basement membrane, by which, and by allied consecutive lesions, the arterial and capillary tissues are impaired, the viscera become congested, the blood thereby contaminated by suppressed secretions, and fatal hemorrhages ensue."

With respect to the post-mortem appearances, Dr. Blair writes as follows—

"The first general anatomical fact in reference to the disease under consideration, is the almost universal *bloodiness* of the tissues of the body in a patient who has died from yellow fever, having been previously healthy, and not dying from actual hemorrhage. *Hyperæmia* does not express correctly the idea of this condition, for the dissection of the body shows not only too much blood, but also blood in the wrong place. It flows out from the subcutaneous areolar tissue; the mesentery is loaded with it; the areolar tissue forming the attachments of the windpipe and gullet is bloody; so is the mediastinum and the fat around the kidneys. The intestines appear, externally, slate-colored, or gangrenous-looking through the peritoneum, from congestions and extravasations in the mucous and submucous coat. The pleura costalis participates in the same sanguineous appearance as the connecting tissue of the throat, from the universal hyperæmia and extravasation beneath that membrane. If we look into the trachea and bronchi, and œsophagus, stomach and intestines, and coverings of the brain, and lining of the bladder, we find a similar condition in some, and it may be in all these surfaces. If we wash away the mucus or blood which obscures the view, we may find the part highly sanguineo-vascular, the capillaries in a state of distension, without breach of continuity; if in the stomach, leashes of them may be seen torn and disorganized; or the part may show structureless unvascular ecchymosis, and dots or wavy lines, or patches of greater or less extent, or splashes, as if red ink had been projected from a pen. The membrane of the stomach shows the most varied hyperæmia; sometimes it is arborescent, as if the arterial twigs were chiefly affected by engorgement. Sometimes it occupies the rugæ and villi in wavy lines; in other cases it is in rude hexagonals, as if the capillaries surrounding the mucous follicles were alone affected. At other times, the predominating appearance is a universal rosiness, or deep claret or purple, as if the submucous tissue had been infiltrated with pigment; but generally, most of these varieties of hyperæmia are blended together. If we examine the parenchyma of the great viscera, a similar condition of *bloodiness* obtains. The kidneys are sometimes ecchymosed below the capsule, and a section of them is *always bloody.* The liver is very frequently in the same condition, and is sometimes enlarged from general engorgement, and softened and friable in spots, as if from broken-down structure. The lungs are often apoplectic, with the interlobular spaces broken and infiltrated, so as to lose all physical appearance of pulmonary tissue, and resemble huge clots of blood. These conditions are generally found in the most dependent parts, but frequently the upper and front part of the lungs and liver, and pelvis of the kidneys, are so affected. The appearance is therefore clearly not hypostatic, although gravitation must exercise some localising power. Sometimes one viscus may be engorged, and a neighboring one anæmiated and dry. This relation sometimes exists between the kidneys and liver, as in the cases of Gibney and Morgan (Seaman's Hospital, 21st of September, 1852;) hemorrhage during the disease, and previous anæmia, have a similar modifying effect.

"The next general anatomical characteristic is the altered conditions of the mucous membranes. In the mouth, œsophagus, stomach, and intestines, it has suffered some serious alteration. The epithelium is peeled off, generally or partially, or the whole depth of the membrane is softened, as if acted on by an alkali, or is eroded through the sub-mucous coat.

"These are the two general facts common to all normal cases, and obvious to any careful observer. Inflammatory diseases seem congenial to the action of the yellow-fever poison; and during the progress of the disease we have frequently found them supervening as epiphenomena. We have also seen yellow fever apparently excited into action by their presence, and consequently the traces of these accidental complications will occasionally be found in the post-mortem examinations. But the lesions of yellow fever seem to have little or nothing in common with those of simple inflammation, and the only *quasi*-inflammatory condition which seemed a result of the disease was, in some instances, where the capsule of the liver—such as in the case of Ellwood (Seaman's Hospital, 21st of February, 1853)—was red and vascular, and, as if in incipient inflammation, excited apparently by the mechanical distension of the engorged parenchyma. It is likely that the suppurations of the liver, which

have occurred as sequelæ of yellow fever, were occasioned by the disorganiza
tion of tissue which follows the congestions and ecchymoses before referred to;
and that, had Macey lived, he would have suffered from an abscess in the softened part of the liver, as the only mode of reparation which nature could institute.

"In the post-mortem notes which follow in the reports of some of the fatal
cases, the terms 'blood congested' and 'bile congested' have been used, and
require some explanation. The first term is obvious enough, and means what
it says—engorgement with blood; but the latter does not always mean engorgement with bile: it has reference more to color than any other quality; and when
the liver was yellow, of whatever shade, the term 'bile congested' was applied
to it, in contradistinction to the dark purple or slate color which indicated
hyperæmia. Now, this yellow condition of the *enlarged* liver is not yet satisfactorily understood. It is no doubt true that the liver is found sometimes dry
and anæmic, from having been drained by hemorrhage, or vital or physical
determination to some neighboring viscus; and then the capsule of Glisson,
tinged by the bile, communicates the ochre, or straw or cream color, to the
whole mass. But where enlargement also is present, with or without anæmia,
the explanation is not sufficient. Of what does this yellow or ochre enlargement consist? This point has not yet received sufficient attention. But I have
found that, in these cases, a small portion of the parenchyma scraped off and
submitted to the microscope, showed an abundance of oil globules. In cases
which have terminated fatally after protracted illness or apparent convalescence,
the bloody condition of the kidneys has passed away, and the cortex is hypertrophied, and of a dull ochrey color. This condition seems clearly due to the
impaction of the tortuous tubuli uriniferi with the same epithelial and fibrinous(?)
matter which constitutes the sediment of the urine; and the presence of this
matter and fragments of tube-casts can be demonstrated by the microscope to
constitute a part of this yellow hypertrophy. But I have never been able to
detect oil globules in the kidney; and the instance narrated in the post-mortem
notes is undoubtedly a fallacy of observation, the oil most likely having been
derived from the blade of the knife. The congestion of the kidneys during life
seems to have been attended with no irritation: it is signalised only by albumi-
nosity of the urine. With one exception, nothing like diuresis was observed,
nor could have taken place without being noticed, till convalescence became
established. Neither was there pain in the congested organ but once or twice.
(Juan de Nolriga, 24th of December, 1852) The pain so often complained of
in the loins is lumbar, and in many of the best-marked cases careful pressure
failed in detecting tenderness of the kidneys. The lesion of the lungs was
seldom, if ever, attended by cough, or pain, or râle, or any sign to attract the
attention of the patient or physician until the blood extravasation demanded
expectoration. On the liver there seemed to have been induced an irritant
effect. The suppression of bile in the last stage had always been preceded by
an erethism of that organ, as indicated by the copious secretion of bile, independent (as in the case of the master of the *Undine*), although no doubt increased
by the action of the resolvent dose; and there was frequently tenderness of the
epigastrium towards the right side early in the disease, and before it could be
occasioned by, as it no doubt frequently is in the last stages, the distension of the
capsule: the kidneys and lungs, therefore, seemed to suffer passively, while the
liver suffered from active congestion. There was not always a perfect correspondence between the lesion of the kidneys and their functional disturbance
during life.

"Occasionally I have noticed the kidneys in an almost apoplectic state, and
yet their functions were scarcely interrupted; and, on the other hand, I have
been disappointed in the amount of congestion in instances of entire suppression.
In the former case, perhaps, the engorgement occupied less the secreting than
the ductal tissue; but this point requires much more investigation. In the post-
mortem notes, the weight of the several viscera is given. This precision would
have been enhanced had the total weight of the body in each case been also
given. Still the weights assist in forming an estimate of the condition; but
weight does not in all cases represent the proportional degree of congestion:
thus, in Maxwell's case (Seaman's Hospital, 12th of March, 1853), the kidneys

seem to have been naturally small; and although their weight was not extraordinary, yet the engorgement was so intense that their shape became altered to globularity. About one hundred dissections were made since the beginning of the epidemic; but the notes of the first series became confused, and are rejected; and several examinations were made of which no record was kept."

ART. 21.—On "Sudden and General Constitutional Decomposition." By Dr. R. D. LYONS.

(Dublin Hospital Gazette, Jan. 1, 1856.)

The following post-portem examination, and the comments which accompany it, are well calculated to illustrate the frightful manner in which the constitution was occasionally undermined by the trench and other duties of the campaign now happily terminated. Nothing is said of the antecedents of the case, except that it occurred in the Crimean practice of Dr. Howard, of the 20th regiment.

"The sectio cadaveris was made on the 7th of August, about twenty-two hours after death. The temperature of this and the preceding day I have noted at about 80° to 85°, the latter being the maximum in the shade. The gaseous distension of the body, and the frightfully distorted condition of the face, made it utterly impossible to recognize a feature, and would, I conceive, have put identification, if necessary for any medico-legal purpose, quite out of the question. The tension and distension of the abdomen were extreme, while numerous blobs or large vesicles existed on its anterior wall. There was immense tumefaction with extensive blue discoloration and large epidermic vesication of the whole of the upper part of the thorax and neck. The globes and lids of the eyes were greatly swollen, and discharged much sanies. Large arborescent veins were observable on the thorax, arms, groin, and upper parts of the thighs: the surface generally was emphysematous, and crackled on pressure.

"Gas escaped with great violence from the abdomen when first opened, and all the tissues were infiltrated with gas, while the intestines were distended to a great size.

"The lungs presented large vesicles on the surface, and broke down immediately on the least pressure or traction, the fingers passing through their substance on the least attempt to grasp them; the parenchyma breaking down at once, but leaving a sort of framework of the vessels and tubes.

"The pericardium was distended with gas, and the fatty tissue of the heart blown up; the heart itself was full-sized, round, and convex, but contained not a particle of blood; nor was there any in the great vessels.

"The liver was covered with blobs or vesicles under the peritoneal coat; its color was bluish black, while its tissue was soft, putrilaginous, and broke into a granular pulp on the least pressure. The spleen was soft and rotten; the kidneys on their surface, and to the depth of half an inch, were soft and pulpy, but the cones were a little more solid. The large intestines were of a dirty greenish black throughout, and were distended with a very fetid gas.

"The cava and iliac veins contained but little blood, but were full and round, being distended with gas: a couple of small transparent vessels crossed the lower part of the cava, distended in knot-like or beaded particles.

"A very small quantity of dark, quite fluid, semi-serous blood was found in the iliac veins, while a somewhat purulent-looking matter could be pressed with the edge of the knife from the swollen veins, both the tributaries of the iliacs and those of the surface of the thigh; there was some deposit of lymph in the lower three inches of the femoral vein; the femoral artery was pervious to the point of section.

"In the stump, very slight union had taken place at the external edge of the flaps, but within, the texture was converted into a blackish putrilage.

"The smell of all the tissues was very peculiar rather than intense. My researches on the curious subject of histolysis have made me familiar with all the phases of decomposition; and I can say, that I have never, under the highest .temperatures, seen changes, such as were effected in this and some similar cases within twenty-two hours after death, produced until after the lapse of very many days.

"On the day in which I inspected Dr. Howard's case, I also made other post-mortem examinations, and found the post-mortem changes at their normal standard, so to speak, notwithstanding the high temperature of both day and night. We have, therefore, to seek some explanation for the rapidity and intensity of the changes produced in the case under consideration. I am not satisfied, however, that I am enabled to do more at present than indicate the pathological category in which it is to be ranked.

"After very attentive consideration of a number of cases which have come under my observation, presenting many features in close parallel with those just detailed in Dr. Howard's case, I am led to believe that these very remarkable phenomena are the result of a process of sudden and general constitutional decomposition: the immediate origin of which decomposition is, I conceive, to be referred to a local, suddenly developed, but intense gangrene of the parts at the seat of injury or operation, which, by a sort of *pathological catalysis*, determines, in the first instance, the decomposition of the blood, and through this medium that of all the tissues with which it comes in contact. It is remarkable that the various tissues and organic parts not only seem dead and spontaneously undergoing decomposition as in ordinary cases, but appear to show evidence of a destroying agency, which I would seek the explanation of in the sudden and, it may be *explosive* decomposition of the circulating fluid, its chemical constituents assuming the gaseous form in a sudden and violent manner: the resulting gases in their expansion causing a mechanical separation and breaking up of the particles of the tissues.

"I have now unhappily witnessed many examples of this affection. It has generally occurred in cases which have undergone the graver surgical operations; as, more especially, amputations in the upper and middle thirds of the thigh: but, I have likewise seen it after less serious operations. After the affairs of the 7th and 18th of June, the final assault on the Grand Redan on the 8th of September, and the very lamentable catastrophe of the 15th of November, produced by the explosion in the French artillery park and English siege train of the Right Attack, several cases came under my notice, and from its effects, I, as well as others, had to deplore the loss of some of our very best surgical cases.

"It will be my duty in another place, and in full detail, to enter into the consideration of the clinical and pathological history of this very fatal affection, and I have reason to think that the profession will be favored with some valuable observations on it by my friend Dr. Mowatt, Staff Surgeon, 1st class, who has, with such distinction, presided over the General Hospital in camp, during the eventful period of the campaign which has just drawn to a close. I shall, therefore, not trespass much further on your columns than to state, that while the clinical features of these cases presented very great variety, the chief pathological characters bore in general a very close resemblance to those detailed in Dr. Howard's case, which may, indeed, be taken as a standard of the extreme result which may thus be produced.

"That it is a state beyond the remotest hope of the successful application of any curative means, when once it is established, is, I fear, but too clearly manifest. The suddenness with which, in many cases, it has been developed, and the all but total absence of premonitory symptoms, leave no room for therapeutic experiment of any kind.

"You have, perhaps, left your patient the night before, to all appearance doing well, and when, on the third day or after, you approach him at your hour of visit, you are quite struck by a peculiar fetor, which once perceived cannot be again mistaken: the pulse may be quiet, the countenance, perhaps, a little pale and anxious, and you are little prepared to find when you turn down the bed-clothes, that the entire stump is, for many inches, it may be through more of the limb even, entirely dead and its tissues irreparably destroyed. A few hours more, and your patient, who was perhaps himself the least conscious of any danger, is a decomposing and disfigured corpse. As already observed, however, the clinical features are very various. Those I have here attempted to describe are drawn from the phenomena presented in the cases of some of the most stalwart grenadiers that could adorn any army, many of them, too, our own countrymen, who succumbed after operations in the middle and upper third of the thigh on the third or fourth day, from the effects of this truly awful form of disease."

(c) CHRONIC DISEASES.

ART. 22.—*On Anæmia.* By M. BECQUEREL.
(Gazette des Hopitaux; and Dublin Hospital Gazette, March 15, 1856.)

The principal object in the following remarks (which were delivered in·a lecture at the Hôpital de la Pitié), is to show that anæmia and chlorosis are really distinct affections—distinct in their causes, character, and treatment required for their cure. M. Becquerel has only yet spoken upon anæmia.

"*Anæmia.*—This term is badly chosen, signifying as it does the absence of blood; it cannot however, now be changed, and must continue to be used with the acceptation so commonly attached to it by physicians. We may define anæmia to be: A morbid state, characterized by a notable diminution in the proportion of globules in the blood. Thus explained, we immediately see that anæmia is not, properly speaking, a disease in itself, but simply a morbid state consecutive to many others. And thus its history will include that of all those diseases with which it is found combined, and under whose influence it is produced. In order clearly to understand the state of the blood in anæmia, it will be well first to trace the relative composition of the healthy blood.

1000 parts of healthy blood contain:
 Water, from 830 to 770 parts.
 Globules, " 140 to 120 "
 Fibrine, " 2 to 3 "
In 1000 parts of serum there will be:
 Albumen, between 70 and 80 parts,
 Salts, extractive matter, 8, to 12 parts.

"The change which anæmia makes in the figures is the following: The quantity of water rises above 830, getting as high as 880, while the proportion of globules descends from 120 to 40. I consider there are three degrees of aœmia; 1st degree (slight anæmia), globules comprised between 100 and 120; 2d degree (decided anæmia), globules comprised between 80 and 100; 3d degree (aggravated anæmia), globules below 80. The proportion of fibrine seems to vary very little. The quantity of albumen also in the serum varies very little; when, however, the anæmia is considerable, the quantity of this principle is always diminished, descending to 65 in the 1000 parts. And when this is the case we find the salt, oily and extractive matter, augmented to their maximum physiological quantity. The albumen may, indeed, be notably diminished at the same time as the globules, but this is a morbid state, constituting a complication, examples of which we find in the dropsies.

"These modifications of the blood which we are considering are developed from several different causes. Amongst them are to be reckoned all the circumstances which tend to enfeeble the individual, to impair the vital powers, and to injure the organization. An insufficient quantity of food, particularly if continued for a considerable time, will produce anæmia. Strict regimen is, therefore, an exciting cause; it is in this way I account for the diminution of globules, which we found to exist after all acute diseases in our experiments with M. Rodier. We ought, then, to find a certain diminution of globules in convalescent patients. According to the researches of MM. Andral and Gavarret, there is, in certain cases of cancerous disease of the stomach, an inanition resulting from the incessant vomiting. This sort of forced abstinence brings on readily a diminution of the globules of the blood. Analogous results are produced by a course of diet composed exclusively, or nearly so, of vegetables.

"Privations and want act in the same way, and may be considered as the two great social conditions which most rapidly produce a state of anæmia. Want of proper oxygenation of the air, want of light, with minor degrees of privation, produce diminution in the globules. This I have observed in prisoners kept for a long time in obscure dungeons. Backe has admirably described an anæmia as it exists in the miners of Auzun, produced by causes of this kind. A prolonged residence in a damp situation will likewise produce the same result.

"I would also include amongst the causes of anæmia, acute and prolonged moral emotions; also long-continued grief, disappointed love, a sedentary life, excessive mental exertion : also too great muscular fatigue, venereal excesses, and, finally, excess of every sort."

Pathological causes.—Diminution of the globules of the blood, below their normal quantity, arises from a great number of morbid states, sometimes diseases, sometimes the means used to check disease. Both acute and chronic diseases may produce it; in the former a good deal will depend upon the strength of the patient, and upon the antiphlogistic means used for his cure. Thus it is much more rapidly produced in children than in adults. In a person of good constitution, previously in good health, it is with difficulty produced. In chronic diseases anæmia almost necessarily follows, but it will become much more aggravated when the fluids of the body have been sensibly diminished by hemorrhage, diarrhœa, or even an excessive secretion of urine. It is also developed with remarkable celerity when the disease is due to the development of some new organic formation, such as cancer or tubercle.

Certain therapeutical agents also produce anæmia, or at least diminish the globules of the blood. These are the following : *Bleeding*—Anæmia is more marked in proportion as the loss of blood has been copious, repeated, or accompanied by a strict abstemious regimen. *Purgatives*, when very active, giving rise to frequent and abundant evacuations, produce anæmia very rapidly. *Powerful diuretics*, and, lastly, mercury or iodine, when used for a long time, i. e., by their abuse, produce anæmia. Let us now examine the principal classes of the diseases ending in this constitutional affection.

" 1. *Inflammations.*—All that we have said of the acute and chronic diseases is applicable here, with the addition of these two facts, that inflammations of the intestines producing diarrhœa quickly cause anæmia, and that abundant suppuration, when prolonged for a certain time, continually produces anæmia.

" 2. *Hemorrhages* are the most frequent, the best marked, and the most powerful causes by which anæmia is produced, and the disease will be formidable in proportion as the hemorrhages have been frequent and copious.

" 3. *Dropsies* are frequently accompanied by a diminution in the proportion of globules in the blood. Thus, in Bright's disease this diminution is produced at the same time as that of the albumen in the serum.

" 4. *Organic diseases of the heart* are accompanied frequently by a diminution of the proportion of globules, chiefly when they have advanced to such a point as to produce peritoneal dropsy.

" 5. *Constitutional syphilis*, lasting for a long time and badly treated, often determines anæmia.

" 6. Certain nervous diseases, such as hysteria and hypochondriasis, when they are very obstinate, are accompanied by a diminution of the globules.

" 7. *Diseases of the spinal cord*, especially when chronic, produce anæmia.

" 8. Intermittent fevers lasting a long time, or even a residence in a marshy locality, produces a peculiar cardiatic state, of which a diminution of the globules is an essential element.

" 9. Certain poisons, especially lead, quickly produce anæmia.

" 10. *Involuntary seminal emissions, &c.—Symptoms.*—Anæmia frequently constitutes the only malady, and is then known by certain distinctive signs. But again it is often so mixed up with other affections, that it is by no means easy to decide what symptoms are to be attributed to the anæmia, and what to the coexistent disease. In order to facilitate its study we may divide anæmia into simple and complicated.

"*Simple anæmia.*—The morbid phenomena which simple anæmia gives rise to vary in intensity according to the degree to which the diminution of the globules have arrived, in proportion as the number of globules is represented by some number between 100 and 120, or between 80 and 100, or below 80. As the basis of our description we may take the medium anæmia, that represented by the figure between 80 and 100.

" The aspect of an anæmic patient is characteristic ; their countenance is expressive of suffering and weariness, the skin is pale, and their pallor is sometimes a dead white, sometimes of other shade of color. When the anæmia is very aggravated, we have a greenish white color, but this new particular belongs to chlorosis. In general in anæmia, especially in females, the eyes are surrounded by a bluish circle. With this want of color in the skin, there is almost always a general wasting, which at the first glance distinguishes it from the puffy swelling of the tissue, which is obscure in chlorosis. The loss of power, which is in direct proportion to the degree of diminution of the globules, produces in the patients a great susceptibility of fatigue, which is one of the characters distinctive of anæmia. Sleep is in general preserved : it seems as if the patients felt their need of sleep to restore their loss of power from the diminution of the globules.

"The appetite is in general preserved, sometimes augmented, accompanied by thirst, which becomes excessive in the aggravated cases. In the great majority of anæmic individuals, digestion in the stomach is carried on well ; there is no gastralgia, except in some rare cases.

" Constipation is an habitual phenomenon in the anæmic. We do not say the same of the development of gas, which we have observed but occasionally. We may sum up the symptoms observed in the digestive tube by saying, that in the greater number of cases of simple anæmia there is neither any disease very decided, nor any morbid phenomena very remarkable.

"In the respiratory apparatus we have nothing to remark but dyspnœa, which is one of the most constant symptoms of anæmia. When the globules are but little, or but in a medium degree diminished, this dyspnœa does not show itself, except when some exertion is made, such as going up stairs, &c. But in the worst forms of anæmia, where we find the figure expressing the proportion of globules come down to 50 or 60, the dyspnœa becomes considerable upon the slightest exertion, the patient not being able to turn in bed without suffering from dyspnœa."

SECT. II.—SPECIAL QUESTIONS IN MEDICINE.

(A) CONCERNING THE NERVOUS SYSTEM.

Art. 23.—*On some unrecognized forms of Mental Disorders.* By Dr. Forbes Winslow, D. C. L.

(Journ. of Psychol. Med., Jan. 1856, and April, 1856.)

The object of these very interesting papers is to show that there are conditions of the mind which are productive of serious, fatal, and irremediable mischief and misery, which do not come under the definition of insanity, and which persons, for the most part, are too slow to recognize as degrees of insanity, but which nevertheless, require very prompt treatment.

"The affections of which I speak," says Dr. Winslow, "are necessarily obscure, and, unlike the ordinary cases of mental abberation of every-day occurrence, they frequently manifest themselves in either an exalted, depressed, or vitiated state of the moral sense. The disorder frequently assumes the character of a mere exaggeration of some single predominant passion, appetite or emotion, and so often resembles, in its prominent features, the natural and healthy actions of thought, either in excess of development or irregular in its operations, that the practised eye of the experienced physician can alone safely pronounce the state to be one of disease." I do not refer to mere ordinary instances of eccentricity, to certain idiosyncrasies of thought and feeling, or to cases in which the mind appears to be absorbed by some one idea, which exercises an influence over the conduct and thoughts quite disproportionate to its intrinsic value. Neither do I advert to examples of natural irritability, violence or passion, coarseness and brutality, vicious inclinations, criminal propensities, excessive caprice, or extravagance of conduct, for these conditions of mind may, alas! be the natural

and healthy operations of the intellect. These strange phases of the understanding—these *bizarreries* of character—these vagaries of the intellect—these
singularities, irregularities, and oddities of conduct, common to so many who
mix in every day life, and who pass current in society, present to the philosophical psychologist many points for grave contemplation and even suspicion; but
such natural and normal, although eccentric states of the intellect, do not legitimately come within the province of the practical physician unless they can be
clearly demonstrated to be *morbid results*—to be positive and clearly established
deviations from cerebral and mental health. It has been well observed by Dr.
Coombe, that a brusque, rough manner, which if natural to one person, indicates
nothing but mental health in him, but if another individual, who having always
been remarkable for a deferential deportment and habitual politeness, lays these
qualities aside, and, without provocation or other adequate cause, assumes the
unpolished forwardness of the former, we may justly infer that his mind is either
already deranged or on the point of becoming so; or if a person who has been
noted all his life for prudence, steadiness, regularity, and sobriety, suddenly
becomes, without any adequate change in his external situation, rash, unsettled,
and dissipated in his habits, or *vice versâ*, every one recognizes at once in these
changes, accompanied as they are by certain bodily symptoms, evidences of the
presence of disease affecting the mind through the instrumentality of its organs.
It is not therefore the abstract feeling or act that constitutes positive proof of the
existence of mental derangement, but a departure from, or an exaggeration of
the natural and healthy character, temper, habits of the person so affected.

"These forms of unrecognized mental disorder are not always accompanied
by any well-marked disturbance of the bodily health demanding medical attention, or any obvious department from a normal state of thought and conduct
such as to justify legal interference; neither do these affections always incapacitate the party from engaging in the ordinary business of life. There may be no
appreciable morbid alienation of affection. The wit continues to dazzle, and
the repartee has lost none of its brilliancy. The fancy retains its playfulness,
the memory its power, and the conversation its perfect coherence and rationality. The afflicted person mixes as usual in society, sits at the head of his own
table, entertains his guests, goes to the stock-exchange, to his counting-
house or his bank, engages actively in his professional duties, without exhibiting
evidence, very conclusive to others, of his actual morbid condition. The mental
change may have progressed insidiously and stealthily, having slowly and
almost imperceptibly effected important molecular modifications in the delicate
vesicular nervous neurine of the brain, ultimately resulting in some aberration of
the ideas, or alteration of the affections, propensities, and habits.

"The party may be an unrecognized monomaniac, and acting under the terri-
bly crushing and despotic influence of one predominant morbid idea, be bringing destruction upon his once happy home and family. His feeling may be perverted and affections alienated; thus engendering much concealed misery
within the sacred circle of domestic life. His conduct may be brutal to those
who have the strongest claims upon his love, kindness, and forbearance, and
yet his mental malady be undetected. He may recklessly, and in opposition to
the best counsels and most pathetic appeals, squander a fortune, which has been
accumulated after many years of active industry and anxious toil. *He may
become vicious and brutal—a tyrant, a criminal, a drunkard, a suicide, and a spend-
thrift, as the result of an undoubtedly morbid state of the brain and mind, and yet pass
unobserved through life as a sane, rational, and healthy man.*

"We witness in actual practice all the delicate shades and gradations of such
unrecognized and neglected mental alienation. It often occurs that whilst those
so affected are able to perform with praiseworthy propriety and with scrupulous
probity and singular exactness, most of the important duties of life, they manifest extraordinary and unreasonable antipathies, dislikes, and suspicions against
their dearest relations and kindest friends. So cleverly and successfully is this
mask of sanity and mental health sometimes worn; so effectually is all suspicion disarmed, that mental disorder of a dangerous character has been known
for years to progress without exciting the slightest notion of its presence, until
some sad and terrible catastrophe has painfully awakened attention to its exist-

ence. Persons suffering from latent insanity often affect singularity of dress, gait, conversation, and phraseology. The most trifling circumstances rouse their excitability—they are martyrs to ungovernable paroxysms of passion, are roused to a state of demoniacal furor by insignificant causes, and occasionally lose all sense of delicacy of feeling and sentiment, refinement of manners and conversation. Such manifestations of undetected mental disorder are often seen associated with intellectual and moral qualities of the highest order. Neither rank nor station is free from these sad mental infirmities. Occasionally the malady shows itself in an overbearing disposition. Persons so unhappily disordered browbeat and bully those over whom they have the power of exercising a little short lived authority, and, forgetting what is due to station, intelligence, reputation, and character, they become within their circumscribed sphere, petty tyrants. aping the manners of an Eastern despot. They are impulsive in their thoughts, are often obstinately and pertinaciously riveted to the most absurd and outrageous opinions, are dogmatic in conversation, are litigious, exhibit a controversial spirit, and oppose every endeavor to bring them within the domain of common sense and correct principles of reasoning. Persons who were distinguished for their sweetness of disposition, unvarying urbanity, strict regard for truth, diffidence of character, evenness of temper, and all those self-denying qualities which adorn and beautify the human character, exhibit in this type of disordered intellect, states of morbid mind the very reverse of those natural to them when in health. The even-tempered man becomes querulous and irascible; the generous and open-hearted becomes cunning and selfish; the timid man assumes an unnatural boldness and forwardness. All delicacy and decency of thought is occasionally banished from the mind, so effectually does the spiritual principle in these attacks succumb to the animal instincts.

"The naturally gentle, truthful, retiring. and self denying, become quarrelsome, cunning, and selfish—the diffident bold, and the modest obscene. We frequently observe these pseudo-mental conditions involving only one particular faculty, or seizing hold of one passion or appetite. Occasionally it manifests itself in a want of veracity, or in a disposition to exaggerate, amounting to positive disease. It may show itself in a disordered volition, in morbid imitation, in an inordinate vaulting ambition, an absorbing lust of praise, an insane desire for notoriety, a sudden paralysis of the memory or impairment of the power of attention, with an obliteration from the mind of all the events of the past life. The disorder occasionally manifests itself in a depressed, exalted, or vitiated state of the reproductive function—in morbid views of Christianity, and is often connected with a profound *anæsthesia* of the moral sense. Many of these sad afflictions are symptomatic of unobserved, and. consequently, neglected cerebral conditions, either originating in the brain itself, or produced by sympathy with morbid affections existing in other tissues in close organic relationship with the great nervous centre.

"The majority of these cases will generally be found associated with a constitutional predisposition to insanity and cerebral disease."

The whole paper ought to be very carefully studied by all medical men, for all are deeply concerned in the subject of which it treats.

ART. 24.—*On the organic cause of Mental Alienation, accompanied by General Paralysis.* By M. BAYLE.

(*Journ. of Psychol. Med.*, Jan. 1856.)

The chief points in the paper are laid down as follows:

"1. There is a particular species of mental affection, of a symptomatic character, perfectly distinct from the essential forms of alienation, and forming a malady by itself, an individual malady, having its own causes, with symptoms and anatomical characters too distinct to permit of their being confounded with any other affection.

"2. Its causes have one common effect in producing slow or sudden congestion of the vessels of the pia mater and brain.

"3. The symptoms may be reduced to two, which commence and progress concurrently—viz., paralysis general and incomplete, and non-febrile delirium with great feebleness of the faculties. The paralysis makes constant progress in the course of disease, and terminates in almost entire privation of voluntary movements. The delirium has the peculiar feature of being characterized by ambition, and passing successively through the forms of monomania, mania, and dementia. Frequently, mania is wanting.

" 4. The anatomical characters are those of chronic inflammation of the membranes of the convexity of the cerebral hemispheres, often extending to the subjacent surface of the substance of the brain itself."

The proofs of these positions are deduced from the post-mortem examination of the brains of insane paralytics compared with the brains of sane individuals, and from the analogy of this disease with other inflammations of serous membranes.

" Among the lesions discovered in the examination of one hundred bodies, and which were characteristic of chronic inflammation of the membranes of the brain, some were met with in all cases, while others were absent in a certain number. The changes constantly met with were opacity, thickening, increased toughness of the arachnoid to such an extent that sometimes it was possible to suspend a slice of brain by its means without tearing it; extreme congestion of the pia mater; thickening of the arachnoid of the ventricles, which also was covered with granulations; considerable effusion of serum into the cavities of the ventricles and into the network of vessels of the pia mater.

" The morbid appearances less frequently met with were adhesions of the membrane, and the softening of the surface of the convolutions: false membranes, or extravasated blood. The substance of the brain, was softer in a few cases: in some it was firmer: in the majority it retained its natural consistence.

" These post-mortem appearances are not met with in other diseases than chronic meningitis; the slight opacities, &c., occurring towards the close of life in other forms of cerebral disease, do not offer even an analogy. They have always been found by M. Bayle after death from general paralysis, and never in the case of patients who have died from other maladies; hence it is inferred that chronic meningitis is the organic cause of insanity with general paralysis."

ART. 25.—*The Identity of Dreaming and Insanity.*
By M. Moreau, of Tours.

(*Annales Medico-Psychologiques*, July, 1855.)

The states of dream, delirium, and insanity, according to M. Moreau, are psychologically confounded. Madness is the dream of a man who is awake —" la folie est le rêve de l'homme éveillé." In madness, as in a dream, the thoughts wander in the same wild manner, and the power of controlling them is lost. In madness, as in a dream, there is often the same confusion as to personal identity. The intense mental pre-occupation of the madman is reflected in the lesser mental pre-occupation of the dreamer, and there is the same insensibility to external impression in both.

ART. 26—*The influence of Menstruation on Mania.*
By M. Clement Ollivier.

(*Jour. de Med. et de Chir. Pratiques*, Oct., 1855; and *Dublin Med. Press*, Nov. 7. 1855.)

" In reading the report of the discussion of the Academy on mania, I have been struck with a remarkable circumstance—namely, that not one member has alluded to the influence which chronic affections of various organs may exercise on the mind; each person attributing, on the contrary, all degrees of insanity to encephalic lesions.

" Every one is, however, aware of the influence of affections of the liver on mental diseases, and doubtless, none are ignorant of the essays of M. Brière de Boismont on the effect of menstruation on the same class of infirmities.

" In a small pamphlet entitled ' Supériorité des Emissiones Sanguines Directes dans les Affections Utérines,' published by me in 1847, I have quoted some remarkable facts tending to establish in an absolute manner the influence of affections of the womb on mental diseases. I have in particular brought forward two cases; one, that of a woman who was for twenty years chained in a dungeon in the hospital of Angiers, and was cured after having had a considerable loss of blood from the uterus.

" The second case was that of the daughter of one of our celebrities of the College of France, who was placed under my care by M. Récamier; this young woman was affected with an inflammatory congestion of the uterus; she had been eight years deranged, and at the menstrual period became so excited that she ran through the streets. The cure of the uterine affection removed the mental disease at the end of a two months' course of treatment.

" But the uterine affection which most commonly deranges the reason of women is ulceration, more or less severe, of the cervix uteri. So positive have been the results of my observations on this subject, that whenever a woman comes to consult me with any mental disturbance, or any disease of the imagination, I never fail to discover some irregularity in menstruation, or some ulceration of the cervix uteri, the removal of which is invariably followed by that of the mental affection.

" In a word, I doubt that an attentive observer can find a woman deranged in mind who is not or has not been under the influence of some uterine affection; I could bring forward an immense number of cases in support of this opinion, and I am surprised at the silence of the Academy on the subject.

" I shall not endeavor here to develop the theory of this influence of uterine disease on affections of the mind. Hippocrates long ago said, the womb is the whole woman."

Art. 27.—*On the Paralysis of the Insane.*
By M. Trellat, Physician to the Salpêtrière.

(*Annales Medico-Psychologiques*, April, 1855.)

The paralysis of the insane is an affection which invariably ends in death. It attacks man in his most vital centre, and simultaneously or successively, undermines and destroys the powers of thought and motion.

Wanderings of an ambitious character, and not symptoms of simple dementia, are among the earliest signs. Indeed, attentive observation will always detect hallucinations of this kind. Difficulty of speech, which is not caused by an acute malady, especially if this difficulty be accompanied with ideas of richness and grandeur, is a mortal sign.

The disease may progress with greater or less rapadity, and with occasional pauses or moments of amelioration, but it is never arrested. After difficulty of speech has manifested itself, the patient may die within the year, and he will not outlive three years.

This affection is very common in France, and apparently also in England, Belgium, and Germany. It is also found in Italy, and in warm countries, but less frequently than in countries further north, and where intemperance is a more common vice.

Art. 28.—*Statistics of Delirium Tremens.* By Dr. John Macpherson.

Indian Annals, Oct. 1855.)

In this paper, after some general remarks upon the nature of the disease, and after examining the statistics of other writers, Dr. Macpherson proceeds to analyze the statistics of two hospitals at Calcutta, especially the General Hospital. This evidence is of great value, for, as is well known, delirium tremens is a very common disease among the European residents in India, and among those who are especially under European influence. Thus, in Bengal (as Dr. Macpherson believes), more than 600 cases of ebrietas are annually sent to hospital out of an army of about 18,000 strong; and in Bombay and Madras it is not very different.

Dr. Macpherson's conclusions may be thus summed up:

1. The extreme discrepancy in returns as to the frequency and fatality of delirium tremens mainly results from cases of ebrietas and of delirium tremens not having been carefully distinguished and separated.

2. There is a good deal to show that the age of 40 to 45 or to 50 produces most

cases of delirium tremens, as it does of mania, and, though less certainly, that the greatest mortality occurs between 25 and 35, certainly above 25.

3. The disease is far less frequent in women than in men, but this results probably much more from difference of habits than from difference of sex.

4. The disease proves fatal oftenest within four days of the attack.

5. There is a presumption that heat favors the production of delirium tremens, and a still stronger one that it increases the mortality by it.

It would naturally follow as a corollary from this, that delirium tremens ought to be more fatal in tropical than in temperate climates. But the conflicting evidence afforded by the collection of facts under the head of general mortality, gives no support to this view. The experience of the future must be accurately recorded, before this point can be settled.

6. With reference to the morbid changes which have been enumerated, many are to be considered as the result of habitual indulgence in alcoholic potations. In cases, which are rare, in which the patient dies in the first or second attack, the appearances most likely to be met with are congestion of the cerebral vessels, some venous effusion, presence of more puncta than usual in the brain, carmine patches in the stomach. The brain and its coverings may appear quite healthy, but the latter appearance in the stomach is seldom absent.

ART. 29.—*On Apoplexy in relation to Renal Disease.* By Dr. KIRKES, Assistant-Physician to St. Bartholomew's Hospital.

(*Medical Times and Gazette*, Nov. 24, 1855.)

Dr. Kirkes's object in the present paper is to contribute a few additional facts in proof of the frequency with which the kidneys are found diseased in fatal cases of apoplexy, and to offer some suggestions towards explaining the connection between the renal and the cerebral affections. He says:

"An analysis of the fatal cases of apoplexy, which have fallen under my own observation, shows that in a large number the kidneys were extensively diseased. I have excluded from this analysis the cases of merely congestive apoplexy, for the same reason that induced me to omit those cases of apoplexy, with and without albuminuria, which have not died, or not been examined after death, namely, because without the visible evidence of extravasated blood within the cranium, it is just open to the objection that one or more of these cases might not be purely apoplectic. I have excluded, also, those cases in which the brain only has been examined after death, or in which but an imperfect inspection of other organs has been made, because with the object at present in view, it was advisable to make use of those cases only, in which a complete examination of all the important parts had been performed.

"With these exclusions, I find I have notes of 22 fatal cases of sanguineous apoplexy, in which the thoracic and abdominal viscera, as well as the contents of the cranium, were more or less minutely examined after death. Of these 22 cases, the kidneys in no less than 14, presented unmistakable evidence of disorganization; and with but few exceptions the disorganization amounted to the small, hard, shrunken, and granular condition so characteristic of advanced renal degeneration: the kidneys in the remainder of the 14 cases being generally large and soft, and greasy-looking. So large a proportionate number as 14 out of 22 seems clearly to indicate that the renal disease bears a very close relation to the apoplexy. In order to determine the nature of this assumed relation, however, the analysis of the cases must be pursued further.

"Of the 14 cases in which the kidneys were diseased, there was only one in which the heart was not enlarged. The enlargement in these, 13 cases, was principally, and often exclusively, confined to the left ventricle. In 5 there was no valvular disease whatever to explain the hypertrophy; in 4 there was slight, thickening, probably not amounting to inefficiency, of the mitral or aortic valves; and in 4 only was there sufficient valvular disease to account for the enlargement of the heart. So that certainly in 5, and probably in 9 cases, the cause of the enlargement was remote from the heart, and might, with probability, be referred to the coexistent disease of the kidneys. And, even in those cases in which the valves were extensively affected, the renal disease might be supposed to have contributed in some degree to the enlargement which the heart presented.

"This part of the analysis, while it confirms the opinion almost generally entertained, that hypertrophy of the left ventricle of the heart is among the most common of the sequences and results of prolonged disease of the kidneys, would also seem to furnish us with the true interpretation of the connection so obviously subsisting between advanced renal disease and apoplexy. For the researches of Dr. Burrows, and others, have placed it beyond a doubt that disease of the heart, especially hypertrophy of the left ventricle, has a most direct relation to apoplexy, constituting indeed, in many cases, the immediate cause of the attack.* And since hypertrophy of the left ventricle, independent of valvular disease is, as just shown, so apt to follow upon disease of the kidney, we seem to possess herein an intelligible explanation of the occurrence of apoplexy in connection with renal disease; the hypertrophied heart being in such cases the medium through which the affection of the kidney manifests itself injuriously upon the cerebral circulation. In no other way, I think, can we readily understand how the renal disease should give rise to apoplexy. The impure condition of the blood, resulting from the detention of the excretory principle of urine, is capable of explaining many of the complex and often serious nervous phenomena that are apt to occur in advanced diseases of the kidney, but it cannot be supposed to explain, at least directly, the rupture of the small bloodvessels of the brain, and the consequent occurrence of sanguineous apoplexy.

"A still further analysis of the 22 cases of sanguineous apoplexy, which form the basis of the present inquiry, will help to explain the mode in which hypertrophy of the heart, whether dependent on valvular or renal disease, or on the two conjoined, or on any other cause, may lead to the apoplectic attack. For of the 13 cases of associated cardiac and renal disease, there were 12 in which the coats of the cerebral arteries were more or less strikingly diseased, while they were diseased also in 5 other cases, in which the kidneys were healthy, and in 3 of these latter there was enlargement of the heart. So that of the 16 cases in which enlargement of the heart was associated with sanguineous apoplexy, no less than 15, that is all but one, presented disease of the cerebral arteries. Without bringing into this analysis any results of an examination into the frequency of disease of the cerebral vessels in conjunction with cardiac affection independent of apoplexy, the facts here given will suffice to show that disease of the vessels of the brain is even more closely associated with hypertrophy of the heart than the latter is with disorganization of the kidney.

"The intimate connection thus apparently subsisting between sanguineous apoplexy on the one hand, and diseased cerebral vessels, enlarged heart, and renal disorganization on the other, as deduced from the foregoing analysis, will, perhaps, be best apprehended by viewing the result of this analysis in a kind of tabular form. The 22 cases of sanguineous apoplexy may then stand thus:

Cerebral Vessels.	Heart.	Kidneys.	
Diseased	Diseased	Diseased	12 times.
"	"	Healthy	3 "
Healthy	"	Diseased	1 "
"	Healthy	"	1 "
"	"	Healthy	2 "
"	Diseased	"	1 "
Diseased	Healthy	"	2 "
			22

"From this it appears that—
The cerebral vessels were diseased 17 times.
The heart   "   17   "
The kidneys   "   14   "

"It cannot but be evident from this impartial analysis of 22 fatal cases of sanguineous apoplexy in which the different organs were carefully examined, that

* Burrows, "On Disorders of the Cerebral Circulation," 1846; see also for an interesting examination of the subject, Dr. R. Quain's "Observation on Cerebral Apoplexy," 1849.

disease of the kidneys, heart, and cerebral vessels stand in very close relation to the apoplexy; and this relation is the more evident when it is borne in mind that in more than half of the cases the kidneys, heart, and cerebral vessels, were found coincidently affected, while in only two cases was there absence of decided disease of any of these parts.

"Such being the principal information yielded by an analysis of these cases, two questions seem naturally to be suggested by it: first, what relation do the renal, cardiac, and arterial diseases bear to each other? secondly, what share do they severally take in the production of apoplexy? As regards the relation subsisting between the renal, cardiac, and arterial disease in sanguineous apoplexy, I believe that the affection of the kidneys is the primary disease, and that the other lesions are developed secondarily, and in the order just indicated, viz., hypertrophy of the heart, disease of the cerebral arteries, and extravasation of blood from rupture of these diseased vessels. That structural disease of the kidneys, of such nature as to interfere permanently, or for long, with their functions, has among its most frequent and prominent accompaniments an hypertrophied condition of the left ventricle is, as already said, a fact now almost generally admitted by pathologists. Of the various explanations of this pathological fact, the most probable perhaps is that which regards the blood as so far altered from its normal constitution by retained principles of urinary excretion, as to move with less facility through the systemic capillaries, and thus to require increased pressure, and consequently increased muscular growth of the left ventricle, to effect its transmission. To this, perhaps, may be added, among other additional causes, the direct influence on the circulation, resulting from the impeded transit of blood through two such large and vascular organs as the kidneys, in consequence of the structural change which has taken place in them. On whatever cause, or set of causes, it may depend, however, hypertrophy of the left ventricle of the heart, in consequence of prolonged renal disease, may, I think, be regarded as a well-established fact: and to the affection of the kidneys, therefore, may be referred the enlargement of the heart found in 9 of the 13 cases of associated cardiac and renal affections in the analysis above given, and part of the enlargement noticed in the 4 cases where the valves were considerably diseased."

And again:

"Sanguineous apoplexy, when associated with advanced renal disease, may, I believe, be generally found dependent on rupture of one or more of the cerebral vessels, which have been weakened by structural changes in their coats; and it may, I think, be held, that these changes in the coats are principally induced by continued over distension of the vessels, resulting from an hypertrophied state of the left ventricle, so commonly found in such cases; and lastly, that this enlargement of the left side of the heart when independent, as it often is, of valvular lesion, is the direct result of the renal disease. So that a primary structural lesion of the kidney may, in this manner, through the medium of the heart and cerebral vessels, which are secondarily affected, ultimately result in an attack of sanguineous apoplexy, which but for such renal disease might never have occurred. * * * *

"In all cases, therefore, of apoplexy or hemiplegia, it is advisable to test the urine for albumen, for beyond the direct information thus afforded of the probable state of the kidneys, an albuminous condition of this secretion may serve to explain, in the absence of any valvular disease, the hypertrophied heart which so frequently coexists with the apoplexy."

ART. 30.—*On the disease called Insolatio, or Heat Apoplexy.* By Mr. MARCUS G. HILL, Assistant-Garrison-Surgeon, Fort William.

(*Indian Annals,* Oct. 1855.)

The following extract will serve to explain the opinions which Mr. Hill is disposed to advocate in this long and elaborate paper:

"It seems to me," he says, "that there probably is a very close connection between these attacks of heat apoplexy and remittent fever, and there are indeed many good and substantive reasons for the assumption that it depends primarily upon a cause similar, if not identical, with that which excites remittent fever; nor do I think we wander far from the truth in supposing that it is due to precisely the same cause, and engendered by the same vagrant agency, though I am not forgetful that occasionally various and divergent forces seem to foster and give rise to it. But whilst willing to give due weight to these inexplicable circumstances, until we possess clearer views of, and know more definitely *all* of the sources of malaria—the possibility of its being wafted long distances, the actual period it may remain dormant in the system, its positive effect on the blood and other constituents of the body, and the peculiar constitutional state which alone creates the susceptibility to receive it in force—we cannot repudiate entirely this view, unless in the mean time we can alight on a more reasonable interpretation for the occurrence of the various concomitant phenomena. But, whilst adopting this view of its origin, I do not mean to allege that all attacks of what is called *coup de soleil*, heat apoplexy, insolation, &c., can without difficulty be brought under this category, for I rather incline to the belief of there being a distinct set of cases occasionally taking place in hot weather, and put under one or other of these names or a synonym, which are apparently the result of no poison, but are from simple vital exhaustion, and that these cases, though springing from a different cause, also at their commencement somewhat different from those properly coming under the head above mentioned, may nevertheless in their subsequent progress assume symptoms quite analogous to those of remittent fever.".

ART. 31 —*An analysis of* 100 *cases of Cephalalgia*. By Dr. SIEVEKING, Assistant-Physician to St. Mary's Hospital.

(*Assoc. Med. Journ.*, Nov. 9 and 16, 1855.)

One result of this analysis is that these 100 cases may be arranged under the following divisions:

Rheumatism. Cases 1, 2, 3, 13, 19, 24, 32, 44, 46, 54, 77, 81, 93,	Total,	13
Congestion. Cases 4, 10, 11, 12, 17, 20, 29, 33, 36, 37, 39, 40, 42, 51, 56, 58, 59, 62, 63, 65, 70, 72, 95,	''	23
Dyspepsia. Cases 5, 34, 55, 69, 74, 76, 79, 91,	''	8
Tænia. Case 6,	''	1
Anæmia. Cases 8, 9, 18, 21, 25, 28, 50, 52, 61, 68, 75, 78, 87, 97, 98,	''	15
Hyperæsthesia. Cases 7, 14, 22, 26, 30, 41, 45, 48, 49, 57, 60, 64, 66, 73, 80, 82, 83, 84, 85, 94, 99,	''	21
Asthenia. Cases 15, 16, 71,	''	3
Epileptiform. Cases 23, 27,	''	2
Catarrh. Cases 31, 88,	''	2
Syphilis. Cases 35, 43,	''	2
Intercranial Irritation (organic). Cases 38, 86,	''	2
Scrophulosis. Cases 47, 89,	''	2
Hæmorrhoids. Case 53,	''	1
Lithiasis. Cases 67, 100,	''	2
Morbus Cordis. Case 90,	''	1
Amenorrhœa. Case 92,	''	1
Dysmenorrhœa. Case 96,	''	1

ART. 32.—*The dependence of Facial Neuralgia upon Dental disease* By Mr. CLENDON, Surgeon-Dentist to the Westminster Hospital.

(*Assoc. Med. Journ.*, March 29, 1856.)

In the introductory lecture to his course of lectures on Dental Surgery at the Westminster Hospital, Mr. Clendon says (and we would call particular attention to his remarks)—

"Patients will complain to you of rheumatic pains in the face, of deep-seated pain in the jaw, extending to the orbit and temple, or to the ear; of pain, not in one tooth only, but 'in all the teeth;' of tic douloureux; of anything, in short, rather than admit the probable cause—a diseased tooth. In this, as in their history of cases generally, patients are not to be implicitly relied on; there is a natural tendency to magnify their sufferings, and they also deceive themselves, from an unwillingness to admit an unpalatable truth. Before you proceed to administer medicine in such cases, you must satisfy yourselves as to the condition of the teeth and gums. The patient will, of course, contend that the pain does not proceed from a tooth, and a cursory examination might possibly lead you to the same conclusion. But, you must remember, a tooth may not necessarily be decayed to occasion severe pain; some change may be taking place in the condition of its periosteum; there may be deposit of bone in the alveolus, displacing the tooth, or causing a corresponding absorption of its roots, or there may be ossific deposit on the root itself; either of these conditions is sufficient to give rise to the most painful and distressing symptoms, which may extend over a period of several years. Sometimes the pain is caused by the presence of a minute portion of root broken off from a tooth, deeply seated in the gum, and long since forgotten. Owing, perhaps, to the absorption of the alveolus, in which it hitherto quietly lay embedded, this being set free, may be slowly working its way to the surface, and giving rise to occasional paroxysms of the most acute character. In such cases. it is evident medicine is useless, and consequently injurious; relief can only be afforded by the removal of the tooth or root, which a careful and peculiar mode of examination—familiar to those who practise this branch of the profession—will alone enable you to detect. These occasional paroxysms in the face and jaws are not inaptly termed *tic douloureux*. Although a very fashionable complaint, it is by no means confined to the higher ranks; you will meet with it daily in every class of society. The pain arising from diseases of this character is sometimes so intense, and its cause so obscure, that patients naturally incline to give to their own sufferings the name which expresses at once the most acute and, as it seems to them, the most mysterious form of all such maladies. But when I tell you that in a tolerably wide field of observation, public and private, during a period of twenty years, I have only met with three or four cases of true idiopathic facial neuralgia—that is, neuralgia which would not yield to purely local treatment—you will at once perceive the necessity for a careful examination to satisfy yourselves most fully on this point, before you proceed to subject your patient to a course of medicine."

ART. 33.—*Paralysis of the Motor Nerves in Neuralgic Affections.*
By DR. C. HANDFIELD JONES, Assistant-Physician to St. Mary's Hospital.

(*Lancet*, Oct. 20, 1855.)

"Dr. Macculloch," says Dr. Jones, "is almost the only writer that I am acquainted with who distinctly states that paralysis is a mode of neuralgic disease. He considers that the action of malaria on the nervous system is essentially debilitating and prostrating, tending to produce numbness of sensory nerves, palsy of motor, and fatuity or mental debility when it affects the brain. Of the general correctness of his opinions I feel strongly convinced, although it must be admitted that the conclusion that the disorder is dependent upon malaria as an exciting cause is rather matter of inference than of demonstration in many cases. The recognition of the fact, that impairment of motor power may be owing to the cause just mentioned, seems to me so important that I offer the following histories in illustration."

CASE. 1.—R. B—, æt. 65, male, laborer, admitted June 18th. Had been ill three or four days. Is stout and healthy-looking; not subject to rheumatism; says he has lost the use of his right hand. can hardly grasp at all with it; the parts supplied by the median nerve are numb, but never in pain; has some stiffness extending up to the elbow; glands in the axilla not enlarged; the affection came on suddenly; no pain in the head; no giddiness; pulse large and full; skin warm; tongue large, moist, with long white papillæ; urine natural. His condition appeared so decidedly sthenic, that although I was much inclined to regard the disorder as of a neuralgic character, I thought it prudent to test as it were, the system I had to deal with by other agents, before administering the usual remedies for neuralgia. I gave him, therefore, bichloride of mercury, one eighth of a grain; nitrate of potass, ten grains; compound infusion of gentian, one ounce, three times a day.

June 25th.—Reports that he can close his hand better, but it feels stiff and numb; head rather giddy this morning; tongue large, quite clean, and moist. He feels the debility of the muscles of the forearm in the hand. I now thought I might venture upon tonics, and gave him citrate of iron and quinine, five grains; water, one ounce, three times a day. On this treatment—the iron and quinine being increased after a fortnight to eight grains—he improved steadily, and was discharged July 23d, having almost completely regained the power of his hand, as well as its sensibility. He said that at one time it had been so weak he could not use a knife or pen. Such a case as this illustrates very well M. Trousseau's remark, that "l'issue du traitément fait connaître la nature des maladies." Suppose cupping, blistering, and purging had been employed, would the result have been so favorable? His age, habit, and symptoms might well, however, inspire suspicions that the disease was of cerebral origin, and that an apoplectic attack was threatening.

CASE 2.—Is. E—, æt. 50, female, married, one child. Has been ill since Christmas; admitted March 22d; of short stature; complains of numbness and weakness of both arms, of the right especially; the arm, forearm, and hand are all affected; has pain mostly in the arms, and numbness in the hands; cannot scrub, or use her hand in anything that requires strength; is not worse at night; skin cool; pulse rather weak; digestion good; bowels regular; tongue clean; no catamenia for nine years; has much soreness in an old blistered spot on the right arm. Moderate doses of quinine and iron were given up to May 3d, conjoined at one time with tincture of Indian hemp, and at another with belladonna; but very little ground was gained. For the next two weeks she took ten grains of citrate of iron and quinine, with five grains of citric acid thrice, daily, but at the end of the week after (medicine having been omitted one week), she complained that her arm was weaker and all her limbs. I then began to give her larger doses of quinine (or cinchonine, which is supplied to out-patients), at first eight grains three times a day, and afterwards twelve grains. Under this she improved very much. By July 12th her arms were much stronger, and felt much less numb. I then gave her arsenite of iron, one-eighth of a grain, with Phosph. Amorph., one grain, to be made into a pill, and taken three times a day, which she did until August 23d, when she was discharged almost well, able to do needlework, or pick up a pin. There can be no question that this was a severe affection of the peripheral nerves, of a neuralgic character, and it is manifest that paralysis of the motor nerves was quite as prominent a feature of the disorder as pain, or numbness of the sensory. Large doses of cinchonine seemed to be most efficient in obtaining the cure; I have little doubt that still larger doses, and preferably of sulphate of quinine, would have produced more speedy benefit.

A circumstance which seems to me to invest with especial interest the occurrence of paralysis as a result of neuralgia is, that the heart itself is not very unfrequently the seat of a similar affection. I have been informed of the case of a man, who suffered from tertian ague, commencing with deadly faintings. I have seen a case in which attacks of syncope, apparently depending upon the action of malaria, were so severe as to cause much alarm. Patients convalescent from the Crimean fever are liable to attacks of a similar nature, sometimes so severe and so easily brought on, as to incapacitate the sufferers from performing their military duties. An officer, who labored under this form of neuralgia in a moderate degree, described it to me as "a sense of dead weight at the heart," attended with a feeling of exhaustion, and some failure of pulse, to relieve which, he was obliged to take ether or wine; it came on every second day or thereabouts, and was especially induced by any painful emotion or agitation, but not by cheerful exercise. Dr. Macculloch has noticed particularly *neuralgia of the heart* manifesting itself by palpitation, and also by paralysis more or less severe. In one case of this kind "the suffering was extreme, even frightful, as the sensation was always that of imminent or immediate death, and of death which nothing but a strong exertion both of the mind and body could have prevented."

ART. 34 —*On Atrophy of the Brain; with cases in which there were remarkable inequalities of the cerebral hemispheres, attended with hemiplegia, and contraction of
the limb on the side opposite the atrophied hemisphere.* By ROBERT BOYD, M. D., F.
R. C. P., Physician to the Somerset County Lunatic Asylum.

(*Lancet*, Jan. 19, 1856.)

The author commences this paper by alluding to the remarks of different writers, ancient and modern, on atrophy of the brain, more especially to Otto, Ca-
zawvieth, Andral, and Cruveilhier, as well as to papers previously published by
himself in the " Edinburgh Medical and Surgical Journal," and he then refers to
various cases of atrophy which have since fallen under his notice. Of the whole
of the cases referred to as having been observed by himself, he states that 33
were males, and 31 females ; one male only was below 30 years of age, and of
the other males, one-half were between 30 and 60 years of age, and the remainder above that age, the oldest being 84. The youngest female was 32 ; 12
were under 60, 18 above, and the oldest 98. The average weight of the brain
in the males was 43½ oz.; in the females, 39½ oz. The smallest brain in the
males was 30½ oz.; in the females, 27½ oz. The largest in the males was 52½
oz., and in the females, 50½ oz. Atrophy of the brain occurred in about 4½ per
cent. of the cases examined by Dr. Boyd at the St. Marylebone Infirmary. In
the insane he had found it at least twice as frequent, and males of this class are
very much more subject to it than females. Inequality in size between the cerebral hemispheres is common in epileptics. In 31 cases in the insane (21 males
and 10 females), there was a difference of one ounce between the cerebral
hemispheres in 7 males and 4 females; of 1½ oz. in one male; of 1½ oz. in 5
males and 4 females; of 1¾ oz. in 2 males and 1 female: of 2 oz. in one male.;
of 2½ oz. in 1 male; of 2½ oz. in 1 male and 1 female; and of 3 oz., 4 oz., and
6 oz., in 1 male each; and in these cases there was either general paralysis,
epilepsy, hemiplegia, with contraction of the limbs on the side of the body opposite to the atrophied hemisphere. The average weight of the brain in the 21
insane males was 45½ oz. ; in the 10 insane females, 41½ oz. In 10 males and
4 females, the atrophy was of the right cerebral hemisphere, and in 9 males
and 5 females, of the left. In 1 male and 1 female, the atrophy was general,
and in 1 male, local, being confined to the optic nerve. Dr. Boyd also states,
that amongst 32 male and 33 female epileptics, at present in the asylum, there
are 4 strongly marked cases of hemiplegia and contraction of the limbs, and in
1 there is a manifest depression of the cranium, on the side opposite the paralysed one. He concludes the paper by briefly describing the particulars of these
cases.

ART. 35.—*A case of " Paralysie musculaire progressive."*
By M. T. VALENTINE.

(*Prager Vierteljahrsch. für die Prakt. Heilk.*, 1855 ; p. 46)

In this case the anterior roots of the spinal nerves were atrophied in the manner which M. Cruveilhier has described, and, in addition to this (which is the
novel feature of the case), there was marked disease of the cord in the parts
adjacent. The symptoms and the muscular changes do not differ in any respect
from those which were observed by MM. Cruveilhier, Aran, Duchenne, Niepce,
&c.

CASE.—The patient, æt. 45, was a man living in respectable circumstances.
During two years the symptoms of the disorder had been making progress—fe-
bleness and emaciation, commencing in the hands and extending eventually to
the inferior limb,—tremulous movements, and then loss of all irritability, even
under the influence of galvanism: and last of all, difficulty of speech and swallowing. Symptoms of slight bronchitis showed themselves before death.

After death the muscles were found in every stage of fatty degeneration. The
anterior roots of the spinal nerves were all smaller than the posterior roots, in
the proportion of about one to six, and they were softer and redder as well as
smaller. These changes were most marked in the inferior part of the cervical
region, and in the superior part of the dorsal. Examined microscopically there

were evident signs of fatty degeneration, which were not present in the posterior roots.

In the region where the roots were most atrophied, the membranes of the cord were thickened, as by old inflammation; and the cord, where it corresponded to the last three cervical vertebræ, and to the first four dorsal, was manifestly softer in its centre, and contained more granular bodies than were met with elsewhere.

It is to be regretted that the microscopical symptoms are not given with any exactness.

ART. 36.—*Analysis of one hundred and thirty-one cases of Hydrophobia.* By Dr. J. LEWIS SMITH, Physician to the N. W. Dispensary at New York.

(*New York Journal of Medicine,* Sept. 1855, Jan. 1856.)

This analysis is appended to a case which recently fell under the notice of the author. Much care and labor has been expended upon it, and so far as we can see, the results are fully confirmatory of the generally received opinions upon the subject.

ART. 37.—*The etiology and treatment of Epilepsy.*
By Dr. HENRY HUNT.

(*Medical Times and Gazette,* Jan. 26, Feb. 9, March 1, and March 22, 1856.)

The theory which Dr. Hunt is disposed to uphold in these papers will appear in the following remarks, which are comments upon his first case:

"The primary cause of all the symptoms was a suspension, more or less complete, of the secretion of bile; and as bile contains, in its normal state, 'a considerable proportion of soda, in some very loose state of combination' (Prout), it follows that, when the functions of the liver were interrupted, an accumulation of an undue quantity of soda must have taken place in the blood. We may therefore infer, that the blood in the preceding case contained an excess of that ingredient of the bile.

"Now, according to Dr. Prout, whose accuracy of observation and skill in researches of animal chemistry are rarely questioned, it appears that an excess of soda or potash in the blood, which he calls 'the soluble incidental matters,' acts on the nervous system in a very deleterious manner, and he alludes to this subject in several places in the third edition of his work on 'Stomach and Renal Diseases,' but quite irrespective of the disease we are considering.

"He writes at page 280: 'The constitutional symptoms accompanying the various forms of urinary disorder now under consideration (those connected with the soluble incidental matters, soda and potash) partake of the characters of those accompanying the deposition of the phosphates, viz., nervous irritability displayed in various ways according to the idiosyncrasy of the patient. In some individuals it assumes the form of spasm of the respiratory muscles,' and other spasmodic affections. At page 223 he says: 'There are some individuals who cannot take alkalies in any form. The peculiar effects produced by them were great nervous disturbance, particularly of the *cerebral functions.* In one gentleman the excitement produced by alkalies was so great as to border on delirium or mania. They seemed to act like a poison, and there was reason to believe, from the effects produced, that if their use were persisted in they would even lead to a fatal termination.' Again, at page 224: 'The effect of alkalies at all times in large doses, and administered at improper times, is injurious to the system'—(they) 'produce serious disorder of the nervous system;' and it is worthy of remark, that the fits in the case I have related were much increased, both in severity and frequency, during the administration of the bicarbonate of soda and sulphate of magnesia.'

"If the correctness of Dr. Prout's observation be admitted, that an excess of soda or potash in the blood acts so injuriously on the nervous system, the next step is to inquire what is their *modus operandi.* To explain this point I shall again refer to the same authority, who states that, 'In certain habits and under certain circumstances, they (the alkalies) occasion a deposition of the phosphates in the urine;' at page 270, 'The long-continued use or abuse of alkaline remedies will, in irritable habits, likewise produce a tendency to an excess of the phosphates in general;' and at 312, 'The presence of magnesia (the phosphate of) in the urine is supposed to indicate destruction or malassimilation of a tissue intimately connected with the nervous tissues,' ' and the presence of phosphorus and its compounds to denote the destruction of the nervous tissues.'

"These disjointed remarks of Dr. Prout, when brought together, appear to have a very important bearing on the subject before us ; and if their correctness be admitted, and they are taken in conjunction with those before quoted, they seem to offer a plausible answer to the question, how a predisposition to epilepsy may be produced; for we may reasonably infer—indeed, it seems to follow, almost as a necessary sequence—that if an abnormal excess of alkali in the blood causes the deposition of the phosphates in the urine, and the phosphates are derived from the disintegration of the nervous tissues, or, as it has been recently suggested, of the phosphoric oil, of which the brain is partly composed, the alkalies produce this effect by acting on those tissues, as they are known to do on the other living solids, by promoting their softening and absorption ; and it is impossible that such a destructive process can take place, even to a limited extent, in the brain, spinal cord, or other nervous bodies, without exciting irritation, enfeebling their tone, and rendering them incapable of resisting the morbid influence of exciting causes of diseases. The post-mortem examination of the brains of epileptics somewhat tends to support the correctness of this hypothesis ; for in a large number of cases the brains of epileptic subjects are found so softened, that it is impossible to strip off the investing membranes, without tearing away portions of the gray substance with them ; while in other cases they are evidently shrunk and diminished in volume, and, although, in many instances, the epileptic brain is found to be firmer than natural, this may probably be the effect of the absorption of the softer, fluid, or oily portions of the nerve matter, which would necessarily cause the remainder to be relatively firmer than natural—a state equally abnormal and obnoxious to exciting causes of disease."

Again :

" It is also probable that a great excess of alkali may prevent certain normal changes among the various ingredients in the blood, which are necessary for the elimination of some of the noxious matters generated by, or derived from, the natural disintegration of the tissues of the body—the cyanide of ammonia, urea, for example. In confirmation of this hypothesis, I will quote a passage from the introduction to the work of Dr. Prout, so often referred to. In treating of urea, he says, 'Alkalies scarcely affect urea at low temperatures; but, when assisted by heat, they rapidly convert it (together with water) into carbonate of ammonia.' It is, therefore, a fair inference, that if alkalies decompose urea when formed, they will also prevent its elements combining so as to form it : an idea that is strengthened by the fact asserted by Dr. Prout, ' that the quantity of urea in the urine (of persons in whose blood there is an undue amount of alkali) is usually deficient, while the quantity of soda and ammonia is in excess.'

" These are points of great interest in investigating the causes of epilepsy, because in whatever form the elements of urea, especially the noxious ingredient cyanogen, may enter, they will, if retained in the system, probably account for many of the symptoms from which epileptics suffer so much, if not for the epileptic convulsion itself; for it is more than probable that when cyanogen or a cyanide has accumulated to a certain extent, it will act on the brain and spinal cord as it does in the form of hydrocyanic acid, which, according to Dr. Pereira, ' when given in large doses, but not sufficient to cause instant death, occasions convulsions;' and it would be likely, in smaller quantities, to produce those transient nervous symptoms, sudden faintness, momentary loss of consciousness, and those feelings of undefined terror and want of self-confidence so conspicuous in epileptics, especially as the period of recurrence of fits approaches, and which, together with feelings of general nervous irritability, progressively increase up to the moment of the convulsion, and usually subside after the fit : as if the cause, whether it be a materies morbi or not, having accumulated so as to produce an attack, is expended during the violent muscular and nervous action which constitutes a fit."

In this way Dr. Hunt is led to think that acids will be found to be important agents in the treatment of epilepsy, and he relates seven cases, of which we give two, in which this treatment seems to have been more or less successful.

CASE 5 —M. C., æt 11, was brought to me in September, 1853. He had been afflicted with epilepsy about two years. The first fit occurred at school, where he had been insufficiently nourished. It was attributed to a fright occasioned by a trick played on him by his schoolfellows. He was naturally quick and intelligent, but a sensitive child. Some time before the first fit he appeared dull, and unable to learn his lessons as well or as easily as he had been accustomed to do, and also to be unusually fearful. When I saw him he was pale and delicate, and his complexion presented the same transparency as in the preceding cases. He was very nervous and fearful, and showed evident terror at the idea of being left alone. His tongue was clean, his pulse quick and small, his eyes of a pearly whiteness. The bowels rather confined. The discharges were described as being pale, and the urine also pale, as well as clear. I prescribed the acid bath, and the internal use of the nitro-muriatic acid, and a sufficient quantity of an electuary, composed of equal quantities of sulphur, bitartrate of potash, and syrup of ginger, to regulate the bowels.

The child was brought to me again at the end of a month, when I learnt that he had a fit a few days after his first visit, but none afterwards. He appeared stronger, and much less nervous and timid; and he allowed himself to be left alone for a few minutes without hesitation. I recommended a steady use of the same treatment, and that he should spend as much time as possible in out-door exercise, and that lessons of every kind should be strictly avoided. I did not see this patient again, but I was informed that the treatment had been so successful, and had apparently effected so complete a cure, that his parents thought they might safely send him to school after the Christmas vacation. They did so, and he appeared to bear his work pretty well for a few weeks; he then began to feel confused, and soon afterwards he had a violent fit, in which he died.

This case, however, showed the power of these remedies to correct the state of the system on which the epilepsy depended; not only by the cessation of the fits, but by the removal of that morbid nervous terror from which epileptics so frequently suffer; and I think we may assume, judging from the other cases, that if the treatment had been continued longer, and more time had been allowed for the brain to recover strength before the intellectual faculties were again exerted, the epilepsy would have been permanently cured, and the child's life served.

CASE 6.—Miss D., æt. 56, had suffered for six years from dizziness, which generally came on walking out immediately after breakfast, sometimes so suddenly that there was neither time to return to the house, nor to sit down, before she would fall to the ground insensible, and on three occasions she remained unconscious for an hour and a quarter. I saw her in July, 1853. She was then slightly jaundiced; the tongue foul; the pulse feeble; the evacuations pale, sometimes nearly white; the urine pale and clear. I prescribed a course of saline aperients, with an occasional dose of Pil. Hydrarg. and Pil. Rhei Comp. Under this treatment she became much worse, especially as to the dizziness and faintings. She consequently again came to town in September, 1853, with a friend, from whose description I found that the faintness and other nervous symptoms, which I had supposed arose from bile, were epileptic. The urine was then examined, and was found to contain an inordinate quantity of the chloride of sodium (which, in the specimen analyzed, may have been partly derived from the soda given in her medicine), and less than a normal amount of urea, and there was a considerable quantity of the phosphates; specific gravity 1·020.

I prescribed the nitro-muriatic acid internally, and a dose of the compound rhubarb pill every other night. This plan was persisted in for six weeks; at the expiration of that time she appeared to have been restored to the same state as she was in before I first saw her. I then advised the acid sponging twice a day, and the drinking of strong lemonade, with a glass of sherry in it, both for luncheon and dinner, in addition to the internal use of the nitro-muriatic acid. The effect of this treatment was immediate and striking. She soon perceived a manifest improvement in her general feelings, as if more nervous vigour had been given her. The attacks of dizziness were evidently lessened. At the expiration of two months, she wrote me, that the dizziness had subsided altogether, and that she had not had a fit since she commenced the sponging. She further wrote, that she could not describe the improved state of her nerves better than by saying she had more the feelings of health than she had experienced for several years. She continued to use the acids for several months without interruption, and up to this time, February, 1856, she has remained perfectly well, although she has been exposed to severe afflictions since her recovery.

ART. 38—*Cases of Epilepsy.*
By Dr. RADCLIFFE, Assistant-Physician to the Westminster Hospital.
(*Medical Times and Gazette*, March 29, April 5, April 19, and May, 1856.)

These cases were related in some lectures which were delivered at the Westminster Hospital about three months ago. They exemplify, as it seems, the beneficial effects of a stimulant plan of treatment in this affection.

CASE 1.—Miss Henrietta W—, æt. 17.

The subject of distinct epilepsy for seven years. When a very young infant she had several attacks of convulsion, which were supposed to be dependent upon water on the brain. The first epileptic fit occurred at school, after having been frightened by a cow in the earlier part of the day. Before this time her health had been gradually failing,—failing, there is reason to believe, from the stingy dietetic arrangements of the school at which she was staying. After this time the fits recurred with considerable regularity at intervals of a month. The menses were established about two years ago without any sensible effect upon the fits. According to the aunt with whom Miss W—lives, there is much hysteria mixed up with the case, and the fits themselves are often of an hysterical, rather than epileptic character. The patient has never taken any stimulants.

November 17th, 1849.—Short and square built. Head somewhat large, forehead receding; eyes very prominent; pupils dilated, but not very sluggish. Expression of countenance sour, but not stupid. The memory not very defective, but very wanting in the power of application. Will often have fits of crying and sobbing for hours together, particularly after having had a long walk. Hands and feet constantly cold; pulse very small and weak, 72. The appetite fitful, but not defective on the whole. The tongue has been bitten several times. The aunt states that the fits occur now about the third day of the menstrual period, and generally in the night, and that the face is usually much discolored. Sometimes, but not always, there is foam at the mouth.

Ordered to be kept quiet and to be sent to bed early; to have an egg beat up in a glass of port wine at eleven o'clock every morning, and a glass of wine shortly before going to bed at night; to discontinue all studies for the present, and to take, three times a day, two table-spoonsful of the following mixture:

R   Ferri Ammonio-citratis, ℨj;   •
       Ætheris Chlorici, ℨij;
       Aquæ Distillatæ, ℨviij.   M.

29th—Much quieter, and in every respect better. No fit. No alteration in the treatment.

December 16th.—Three nights ago, about the usual time, a fit occurred in the night. This was very brief, and there was little depression and irritability the next day. The patient is stouter than she was, and she now eats with an appetite. Her countenance is more animated, and of a better color. No alteration in the treatment.

February 14th, 1850.—Until last night she went on very well, and then she had a fit of considerable severity after coming in from a long walk. This was two days after the completion of the menstrual process. This morning she is evidently depressed, and yawns very much. Her pupil, also, is considerably dilated. For the last three weeks, the medicine has not been given with any regularity, and she has been in the daily habit of taking long walks. She is growing very fast.

Ordered not to tire herself by walking, and not to neglect taking the mixture for the present. Ordered also to have a glass of wine or porter with her dinner.

March 16th.—Decidedly better. No fit since the last visit. During the last three or four weeks she has been a very persevering student at the piano, and this must be taken as a very considerable evidence of improvement, for when she was first put under treatment she had no power or no disposition to apply herself to this or any other pursuit. No alteration in the treatment.

June 12th.—No fit since the last visit, and a marked improvement in every other respect.

— This patient went abroad shortly after this time, and I saw her no more. Twelve months later, however, I learnt that her health continued to improve, and that she had had no fits; and a year after this time, when I lost all traces of her, I have reason to believe that she was still without the fits, and well.

CASE 2.—Mr William C—, æt. 19.

The subject of marked Epilepsy for six years. When sixteen he had formed an improper connexion with a young woman which ended in her pregnancy, and besides this, he had been guilty of other practices of an equally reprehensible character; and since this time there has been no material reformation in his habits in these respects. At first the fits occurred at wide intervals, but lately they have been of almost daily recurrence.

January 4th, 1850.—His appearance indicates great exhaustion. He is tall and thin, and very pale, perspiring profusely on the least exertion, and suffering from almost constant toothache and headache. He abstains, and always has abstained from alcoholic drinks, but he indemnifies himself by smoking excessively—even before getting out of bed in the morning. His memory, he says, is very bad, and he cannot bear the least contradiction. His fits occur generally at night. He dines in the middle of the day, and takes no meal of any moment afterwards. Often he lies awake half the night. The pulse is very feeble, 72. The hand is cold and clammy. The pupil is sluggish and dilated.

Ordered to be steady, to live more freely, to take more animal food, and make a good supper of one kind or another; to take a quart bottle of Guinnesse's stout in the course of the day, reserving the last glass for supper: to smoke less; to go to bed at half past nine, and to take the following draught three times a day:

R M. Ferri Comp., ʒj ;
Ætheris Chlorici, xx.

21st.—Much better. His appetite improved, and his sleep much sounder. The fits, however, have recurred every other day, and yesterday he had one of considerable violence. No alteration in the treatment.

February 8th.—Evidently improved. No fit for three successive days, and suffers now much less than he did formerly from toothache and headache. To continue as before.

21st.—Still improving. Has had three fits since the last visit. Appetite greatly improved. Pulse 70, a little stronger. Wakes frequently at night with cramp in his legs. He complains of feeling low and depressed in consequence of having given up (spontaneously) smoking. For three or four nights he has had a good deal of headache in bed. He proposes to go to Hastings for three or four months. Recommended him to sleep with his head upon a lower pillow, and to raise the head of the bed a little, so that the blood might gravitate into his legs, and prevent the cramp; but no alteration in other respects.

May 9th.—He has been at Hastings since the last visit, and is evidently much benefited by the change. He is both stouter and stronger, and he now suffers very rarely from headache. During the whole of his stay on the coast he only had three fits; and two of these, he thinks, were brought on by ascending the Castle Hill three times in the course of the same day. He has been taking no medicine during the last month, and he thinks himself not so well without it, though he has been taking wine in addition to the porter. He says that the wine and porter have the effect to make him less irritable and despondent than he used to be, and that he can now apply himself to reading without any great effort, which was not the case formerly. His mother's brother, it appears, was insane: and insanity, he thinks, may be his own fate, except he can get some thing to occupy his mind. At times he is much teased with flatulency. He was ordered to take ♏xxx of naphtha suspended in peppermint water, with a little mucilage, and to repeat the dose 3 times a day. No other alteration.

18th.—The medicine agrees very well. No fit since the last visit. The dose of naphtha increased from ♏xxx to ♏xl.

September 10th.—He has been in Scotland since May last, and during the whole of this time he had only one fit. Several times he had threatenings, but he succeeded in averting the fits by smelling at a bottle of salts which he carried in his pocket, or by taking a glass of wine if he had the opportunity. The fit which did happen appears to have been caused in the main by his having been kept waiting for food for some hours beyond the accustomed time, and then by being very sick in crossing a ferry. It was very violent, but he awoke almost immediately afterwards, and the next morning he felt comparatively well. His whole appearance is more satisfactory, but the expression of his countenance is jaded, and his pulse weak. He says, that when in Scotland, he generally took a glass of whiskey and water in the evening, and that he found no harm from the practice. He has again begun to smoke. He took the naphtha for two months.

October 14th.—No fit. Improved in general health. His memory, he says, now serves him very well, and it now requires more provocation to rouse his temper. He was desired to return to the naphtha for a short time.

December 1st.—This afternoon I was sent for to visit him at his home, and found him much worse. Three days ago, while amusing himself with joinering, he had plunged a sharp chisel into the palm of his hand, and lost a considerable quantity of blood before help could be obtained. The night following he had a fit during sleep, and again on the next night. He is now suffering from great mental depression and headache. I recommended him to take nourishment and wine, to be quiet, and to take an ounce of Griffith's mixture with half a drachm of chloric ether every four hours.

2d.—He is much relieved. No fit since the last visit.

4th.—He had a fit in the night, and now feels very much depressed. Ordered to take naphtha, ♏xxx, in a little peppermint water, every four hours.

12th.—He has been going about for the last three or four days, and he has now recovered his spirits and appetite. No fits since the 4th, and little or no headache. No alteration in the treatment.

January 8th, 1851.—Improving. Still no fit. No alteration in the treatment.

— August 15th, 1854.—To-day I have learnt, that very shortly after I saw Mr. Wm. C— last, he went out to act as a clerk in the office of a relative, a merchant in Calcutta; and that, upon the whole, he had had very good health. I could not learn any particulars, but my informant told me that my patient very rarely had a fit now, and that he was quite equal to all the duties which devolved upon him.

CASE 3.—Captain —, æt. 34.

For some years this gentleman was a "hard liver," and much addicted to very dissolute courses; but his health did not suffer, except in trivial matters, until about three years ago. The first sign of disorder was a fainting fit. This happened on parade on a hot summer day. About three months afterwards he fainted again. About this time he occasionally awoke with headache, and once his tongue was sore. Six months after the first fainting fit, he had a fit, in which he was convulsed and dark in the face. This was in a brothel. During the twelve months following he had three such fits, two of them under similar circumstances to those in which the last had happened, and one after a long and fatiguing walk on a very hot day. After this last fit he for the first time submitted to medical advice, which advice was to leave off his dissolute courses, to abstain from wine and spirits, to take less animal food, and to take regular walking exercise daily. He persevered in this treatment without any benefit. On the contrary, he became weaker and more dispirited, and he had several (he does not recollect the number) fits, fainting and others. After this he was urged by his comrades, the officers in one of Her Majesty's cavalry regiments, to return to the ordinary practices of the mess, and from this time, he says, he began to improve.

January 7th, 1850.—Slight made and rather tall. Complexion sallow and somewhat congested, particularly about the under eyelids. Pupil somewhat sluggish and dilated. Expression jaded. Pulse 58, weak. His memory, he says, was never good, but he does not think it is worse now than it was before he became subject to the fits. He further says, that the only change he can notice in himself is, that he is more easily " put out," and not quite so "plucky." When out with the hounds he "thinks" before putting his horse at a fence. His appetite is not amiss. He often makes large quantities of pale urine, and not unfrequently he is greatly teased with flatulence, particularly when he smokes.

I recommended him to take more animal and less vegetable food, with, at least, an average amount of wine and alcholic drinks—to leave off smoking, or else, to smoke very mild tobacco—to adhere to the strictest rules of celibacy—to go to bed early—and to take, three times a day, a pill, containing one grain of quinine and two grains of camphor.

February 12th.—He has had no fit since the last visit, and his countenance appears a little more cheerful than it did. There has also been much less flatulence. He has gone to bed early, and this is the only part of the treatment to which he objects. No alteration in the treatment.

March 25th.—Captain — went on well up to a fortnight ago, when he had a severe attack of diarrhœa, brought on, he thinks, by a stale lobster salad. This was eaten late at night at an evening party. This diarrhœa continued about twenty-four hours; and during this time he took little or no food, and nothing of a stimulating character. The day following he walked about three miles to see a friend, and then walked back again, and immediately upon his return he fell upon the dining-room floor in a fit. This dispirited him very much, and he had no dinner except a little soup. In the course of the evening he had another fit; and on the day after the next, he had another. At present he is far from having recovered, and he complains a good deal of flatulence and headache. He was recommended to continue his pills; and to take occasionally, in a little water, a small teaspoonful of a mixture, consisting of equal parts of chloric ether and sal volatile.

April 21st.—Since the last visit he has progressed favorably, and he is now in very good spirits. No fit as yet. No alteration in the treatment.

May 6th—No material alteration. No fit. The same treatment continued.

July 19th.—He progressed favorably, without any fits, until a week ago, when he had one. This was followed neither by headache nor sleep, and four or five. hours afterwards he went out to dine. He says that he cannot account for this fit, but that for a few days previously his appetite had not been quite so good as usual, and that he had been much teased with flatulence. The tongue is at present disposed to be dryish, and there is a little thirst. Ordered to have a grain of compound rhubarb pill added to the pills he is taking, and to go on as before.

September 14th.—He looks-to-day much better and stronger than he was when seen last, and there has been no return of the fits. He has just returned from a few days' partridge-shooting, and he says that he enjoyed his sport very much. Returning home one night he felt excessively tired and depressed, and he thought he should have a fit, but after dinner and a *few* glasses of wine he felt better. On this day he had forgotten to take any means of refreshment with him. He now thinks he is well enough to dispense with any more medicine.

December 5th.—The improvement noticed at the last visit still continues. The fits are still absent. Six weeks ago, he says he was troubled with headache and irritability, and these symptoms caused him to return for a few days to the pills and drops, and this was all. The pupil is certainly very much less sluggish and dilated than it was at first.

— This was the last time I saw or heard of this gentleman.

Case 4.—Mr. William H—, æt. 37.

The subject of epileptic fits for five years. Lately the fits have recurred as frequently as once a month, and generally with considerable regularity; but formerly they were separated by much wider intervals. The first fit occurred in the neighborhood of Calcutta, where he had been living for ten years. He never enjoyed good health in India, and more than once he nearly lost his life from dysentery. He had also suffered from three distinct attacks of remittent fever, and for six months preceding the first fit he had marked symptoms of tertian ague. The first fit occurred in the open air on a very hot morning; but he does not think he had been at all exposed to the direct action of the sun. For this he was bled twice. The week following he had another fit, when he was bled again. No purgatives were given him, for his bowels were then in a very loose state, but he was kept upon a very low diet for three or four weeks, and all stimulants were distinctly forbidden. During the next two months he had several fits, and at the end of this time, finding himself much weaker, he resolved to return to England. The voyage home, which was by the Cape, did him much good, and at its conclusion he felt much stronger. He had four fits while at sea, all in the night.

March 3d, 1850.—He has been in England about a fortnight, and feels the cold very much. He is short and well made, except that the head is perhaps a little larger than it ought to be. His countenance is somewhat wanting in expression, and his complexion is very sallow and much tanned by an Indian sun. There is no decidedly epileptic expression, and no epileptic petechiæ about the eyelids. The pupil is somewhat dilated and sluggish. The hand is cold, and he complains much of cold feet. In the night he had, for the first time for several months, a distinct attack of aguish rigor, followed with heat and thirst; but now his pulse is weak and slow (69). At the present moment he is suffering from what he says is a very common symptom—headache. The bowels are at present somewhat sluggish, and they have been in this state for four or five weeks; he complains, also, of a little dull pain in the right side and shoulder; but there are no other perceptible evidences of biliary derangement. The appetite is very defective, and there is no thirst. On the voyage home he was recommended by the captain to resume his former habits in the matter of stimulants; and after this time he always took wine or ale, or both, at dinner, and ended the day with a glass of warm whiskey and water. He had, he says, restless nights before he adopted this practice; but since he adopted it he has slept well, and finds himself refreshed in the morning. He says further, that stimulants do not now "get into his head as they once did." He still continues the practice.

I recommended him to keep quiet and warm, and to take three grains of quinine three times a day; and in other respects recommended him to live as he had lived on shipboard.

5th.—He had a bout of ague yesterday, but the rigor was not so prolonged as before. No alteration in the treatment.

11th.—He had another attack of ague in the night, and this morning upon getting out of bed, he felt faint, and fell upon the floor. He says he did not lose his consciousness; but there is some doubt upon this point. He is at present suffering from headache and depression of spirits. The tongue was not bitten, but it exhibits the scars of former bites. He was ordered to keep more quiet, and to continue as before.

29th.—He has been improving since the 11th, without any sign either of ague or epilepsy, and his appetite is now good, and his countenance much more cheerful. He talks about returning to India, and says he does not see why he should not be as well there as here, if he adheres to the same rules.

April 10th.—Much improved. For a whole month he has been free from headache, and this is a great evidence of improved health, for he has been an almost constant martyr to this affliction for years. The bowels act naturally. The quinine to be continued.

Feb. 6th, 1851.—Mr. — wrote to me from India to say that he had been quite well since he returned home, and that he still continues almost entirely free from headache. About three months ago he had some symptoms of ague, but these subsided in the course of a fortnight under the use of quinine. He still continues to take what he calls "a fair quantity of stimulants."

CASE 5.—Mr. Cæsar H—, æt. 27.

This gentleman has had occasional attacks of epilepsy for five years. These attacks have generally occurred during the night, but lately they have occurred several times during the day. He has also had repeated attacks of dizziness.

At one time he led a very debauched life, and he ascribes the fits to this cause; but now his habits are entirely changed. He has indeed for some time been a most rigid ascetic in every respect, not touching animal food on the days on which it is proscribed by the Romish Church, of which he is a very strict member, and never tasting any kind of stimulating drink. Every morning he gets up early to go to church before going to his ordinary duties, which are those of a clerk in a public office. For some time he has suffered from pertes séminales, and these occasion much physical depression and great moral distress.

March 7th, 1851.—Tall and thin. The face extremely pale, and the hands almost transparent. The pupils are both sluggish and dilated. His memory, he says, is not at all affected, and he has no difficulty in dealing with very complicated calculations. What he lays most stress upon is his moral depression, and this he considers as a proper punishment for his former misdoings. When at home he will lie brooding and desponding for hours together. He is unmarried, and studiously avoids all society. The pulse is exceedingly weak, 75. The tongue has not been bitten.

Ordered him to take animal food at least once a day; to take bottled stout; to go out occasionally to places of amusement; to go to bed early, and not to get up until nine o'clock; and to take an ounce of Griffith's mixture, with thirty drops of chloric ether three times a day. Ordered him also to have a biscuit and a glass of sherry at his office in the middle of the day.

30th.—His spirits are evidently improved. To continue as before.

April 10th.—He woke this morning laughing, and says that that laugh was the first he had been guilty of for at least three years. He now eats with an appetite, and begins to think the world not quite so dismal. Three days ago he had a slight fit on his return home, and thinks this was due to his having missed his biscuit and glass of sherry in the middle of the day, his stock being exhausted. This was followed by a good deal of sleepiness and headache, but the next day he felt pretty well, except a little uneasiness in his limbs.

May 5th.—He went yesterday to the Great Exhibition in Hyde Park, and became quite excited and delighted while there. After this he walked home with as much buoyancy as he had ever felt. He has ceased to fast on Fridays. He now takes upon an average three glasses of wine and two glasses of bottled porter in the course of the day. His countenance is still pale, but not so pale as formerly. No alteration in the treatment.

April 6th, 1852.—I met him to-day accidentally in the street, and was surprised to see the great change for the better which had taken place in his appearance. He said that he believed himself to have entirely got over his fits, and that he had not had one since he saw me a year ago, except once at the beginning of the past winter. This fit, if it did occur, occurred in the night. He thinks it did occur, because he felt in the morning as he used to feel after the fits; but he says that he had been smoking a good deal overnight, and that smoking always puts him out of order. Very shortly, after seeing me last, he removed into the country, and there he is at present. He says he now feels quite well and happy, and he hopes before long to be married.

Case 6.—Miss C—, æt. 38.

An epileptic of fifteen years' standing. The fits have always occurred frequently; but lately their frequency has considerably increased, and now rarely a week passes without one. Sometimes, but not invariably, two or three fits succeed each other before the consciousness returns. She suffers almost constantly from depression of spirits and great headache. She belongs to a very respectable family, but since the death of her father, which happened seven years ago, her circumstances have been much straitened.

October 29th, 1851.—Short and square-built. Head large; eyes large and prominent: pupils very much dilated and very sluggish; under eyelids large and bloodshot, with numerous minute spots of ecchymosis upon them. Expression of countenance dismal rather than melancholy. Pulse very small and weak, 56. Hand cold and clammy; tongue white; great flatulence; habitual diarrhœa; the catamenia profuse, and attended with much pain.

The directions given to her were, to take more animal, and less vegetable food, with a fair allowance of seasoning; to take beer, to avoid tea, and to take strong coffee instead; to avoid walking as much as possible; and to take, three times a day, a pill containing two grains of sulphate of iron and two of camphor, and occasionally a teaspoonful of a mixture containing equal parts of chloric ether and sal volatile. Her supper, for a short time, was to be a pint of milk, with half a wine-glassful of rum in it.

November 10th.—She looks a little more cheerful. The diarrhœa is stayed, but the bowels still act twice a day. The headache and mental depression are now a little relieved. She has had two fits. The pulse a little fuller, 62. No alteration in the treatment, except to take the drops a little more frequently, and to lie down for an hour after dinner, which is in the middle of the day.

December 1st.—A decidedly more cheerful expression in the countenance. She is now some hours without headache every day—a relief which she has scarcely known for four or five years, and her sleep is disturbed by fewer dismal dreams. The bowels now act only once a day. No alteration in the fits, one still occurring about once in seven days. No alteration in the treatment.

7th.—Not so well. Three days ago, having missed the omnibus, she had a walk of five miles. A fit followed in the night. The next morning the catamenia appeared with great profuseness and much pain, and during the day she had another fit. Her headache is almost constant; and the expression of her countenance is extremely desponding. Ordered her to keep in the recumbent position until the menstrual discharge ceased, to take bottled porter, and to continue the medicine.

26th.—Better again. She had a severe fit immediately upon reaching home after the last visit. Her headache is better, but her spirits are very desponding, and her dreams very distressing. Instead of the pills, to take, three times a day, the following draught:

R Naphthæ Purificatæ,
Spir. Ammon. Arom., āā ℈xx;
Mucil. Acaciæ, ʒss;
Aquæ Distillatæ, ʒxiss. M.

February 1st, 1852.—Since her last visit she has had two fits—one of considerable severity, and both during the period of menstruation. The menses were as profuse as ever. A fortnight later she had a good deal of headache, but she escaped the fit. During the last week she has been comparatively free from headache, and she says that her head is now comparatively comfortable, except after a disturbed and sleepless night. Hot coffee, she finds, will often relieve the headache now. The medicine, she thinks, has made her head feel lighter and clearer. Ordered to increase the dose of naphtha from ℈xx to ℈xl, and to go to bed not later than half-past nine o'clock.

March 16th.—No alteration of any moment. She had two fits during the last menstrual period, but these were less severe. The discharge, also, was less profuse, and there was less pain in the head and elsewhere. Her mother states that she wakes much sooner after a fit, and that there is less confusion and sleepiness afterwards. The dose of naphtha to be increased from ℈xl to ℈lx.

May 1st.—No material alteration. She believes, however, that she should have been much better if she had not had to bear some very distressing domestic losses. The medicine still relieves the headache, but it causes some nausea, and the patient has taken a strong dislike to it. Two fits occurred during the last menstrual period, and one a fortnight later—the latter being the termination of a fit of crying and sobbing, which continued for more than half the night. Ordered to take a glass of bottled porter or bitter ale before going to bed; to sleep with the head upon a lower pillow; and to take the following draught three times a day:

R Quinæ Disulphatis,
Ferri Sulphatis, āā gr. j⟨
Ætheris Chlorici, ℈xv;
Acidi Sulph., dil., ℈ij;
Aquæ Menthæ Pip. ʒj. M.

June 12th.—Looking better again. There has been only one fit since the last visit, and this occurred in the night about the end of the menstrual period. Much less headache than formerly. Ordered to persevere in all things, and to be particularly careful not to exhaust herself by walking or in any other way when she expected the next monthly period.

September 19th.—There has been no fit since the last visit, and the countenance has now become brisk and animated. Headache is now only an occasioual symptom. The mother also says that she is much less irritable, and enters more into the amusements and occupations of the family. This is a great change, for formerly she would sit for days in a moping, brooding condition, and never once lose the appearance of a person suffering from marked melancholy. She has fewer disagreeable dreams since she slept with her head upon a lower pillow. She has taken the medicine regularly up to this time, and now wishes to discontinue it.

December 8th.—Not so well. She went on well for two months after the time of the last visit, and during this time she had only one fit, which followed a long walk in the country. She says she could master her fits, she is sure, if she had less domestic anxiety to depress her. During the last fortnight she had three fits, occurring on successive days. These happened at the end of an unusually protracted menstrual period. Ordered to resume the last mixture, and to carry out all the old rules.

May 7th, 1853.—She has been staying for four months with a relation in the country, and the change has done her much good. During this visit she had every day three glasses of port wine, and this. she thinks, did her as much good as the medicine, which she was taking regularly. During this time she had two slight fits. These occurred at the first two menstrual periods.

— From this time I continued to see Miss C— at intervals. As the winter of 1853–54 came on, she began to flag, and she did not rally again until the summer. During this time the fits occurred about once in two months, and generally about the same time. Sometimes she got over two months. She is not now troubled very much with headache, and her spirits are much better. And this was her state about twelve months ago.

CASE 7.—J. W., æt. 30.

This patient, who was an out-patient at the Westminster Hospital, says he enjoyed good health until about two years ago, when he was turned out of his situation of groom in consequence of his sporting tendencies. Before this time he lived very well, and had abundance of malt liquors; but since this time he has been suffering from almost constant destitution. Soon after losing his situation he began to suffer from very frequent pertes séminales. The first fit occurred about eighteen months ago; and since this time the pertes and the fits have been very frequent. He rarely passes three days without a fit, and the fit generally occurs during a long walk. He walks a great deal, ostensibly with a view to finding work. His memory is very treacherous.

June 1st, 1853.—Tall, full, and flabby. His face is very stupid, and there are numerous epileptic ecchymoses upon the under eyelids and forehead. The tongue has been frightfully bitten, and it is now sore and raw from a recent bite. His pulse is remarkably small, 60. Ordered to live as well, and to keep as quiet as he could, and to take two grains of camphor in a pill every four hours.

7th.—No material alteration. The dose of camphor to be increased from two to four grains. One fit since the last visit.

14th.—Has had no fit since the last visit, and only one perte séminale. His pulse seems a little stronger.

21st.—He has now been ten days without either fit or perte, and his appearance is much more satisfactory. Ordered, in addition to the pills, an occasional dose of the ordinary carminative mixture of the hospital.

July 4th.—Still continues to improve, and still without a fit. He has now got employment in a livery stable, and he is already benefited by the better diet which he is able to command. He takes two glasses of bitter beer in the course of the day, and no more. No alteration in the medicines.

October 6th.—A week after my last seeing him, he considered himself well enough to be able to do without medicine, and the improvement continued until about a fortnight ago, when he had a fit in the night, and another on the night following. This was two or three days after marriage. These fits were followed by much headache, but his spirits were not so much depressed as formerly. He has again returned to the camphor pills and carminative mixture.

19th.—Considerably improved in appearance. No return of the fits.

— This was the last time this patient made his appearance at the hospital.

Art. 39.—*Cases of Chorea treated by leeches and cold.* By Dr. Malden, Physician to the Worcester Infirmary.

(*Amer. Med. Journal*, Nov. 2, 1855.)

The following cases are interesting, chiefly on account of the marked success of a plan of treatment not very frequently adopted, and opposed indeed to the views of many eminent authorities.

Case 1.—Emma B., æt. 12, a fresh-colored healthy-looking child, was admitted an in-patient, under the care of Dr. Malden, February 10th, 1855. Her mother states that, about three weeks ago, the girl had been frightened by some militia-men, and that in a few days she observed twitchings of the arm. The peculiar motions of chorea gradually extended, and increased in severity, till, on her admission, every limb was in constant motion, and the features were much distorted by the irregular and spasmodic action of the muscles. Her appetite is good, but she has some difficulty in swallowing food. Pulse and respiration norma.

Sumat. Pulv. Jalapæ co., gr. xv statim.
Mist. Ferri co., ʒj 4tis horis.

February 11th.—Bowels freely moved; spasmodic movements more severe.

Sumat Zinci Sulph., gr. ij; Ext. Hyos., gr. iij ter die.
Rep. Mist Ferri co.

12th.—She cannot now be kept in bed, unless constantly held or tied down: the movements are so violent. She had no sleep, last night. Bowels acting freely.

13th.—She appears now to be suffering from the constant irritation. Tongue dry and brown. She can take but little nourishment; spasmodic movements still more severe; gets no sleep. Ordered wine and beef-tea.

14th.—The nates and hips are excoriated from the incessant friction. She passes urine under her, and is rapidly emaciating. She is constantly held in bed, where she tosses about and moans, but says she is in no pain. Twenty minims of Battley's sedative failed to procure sleep last night; and, seeing the urgent necessity for procuring some cessation of the involuntary motions, I administered chloroform after repeating the opiate to-night. This was followed by about half an hour's repose.

15th.—She is now suffering greatly from four days' and nights' loss of sleep, and the consequent exhaustion. The sedative and tonic plan of treatment having had a fair trial without success, Dr. Malden carefully examined the spine, and in the lower dorsal region discovered a small spot, where percussion gave some pain, and immediately produced increase of the spasmodic action. Here six leeches were applied, followed by bladders of snow (which was lying on the ground at the time). There was at first great difficulty in the application, as it was necessary forcibly to restrain her movements; but in less than half an hour comparative quiet was produced, followed by more than four hours' tranquil sleep.

16th.—Convulsive motions less violent; tongue moister, but still brown. She expresses herself relieved; but as there was still some tenderness over the spine, the leeches and snow were repeated: and from this time she steadily improved, and in a few days was put upon the use of iron and the shower-bath, regained flesh and strength, and was discharged cured by the end of the month.

Case 2.—Hannah Holloway, æt. 12, admitted June 9th, 1855, also under Dr. Malden, with chorea of three weeks' standing. The disease arose without apparent cause, and, though gradually increasing in severity from the first, is not at present worse than the general run of cases. There is no spinal tenderness, nor abnormal cardiac action; and the bowels act regularly. She was at first put upon the usual plan of brisk purgatives, combined with ferruginous tonics, and the cold shower-bath; but by the end of the week the convulsive movements were much aggravated, articulation and deglutition were greatly impaired, and it was impossible to keep her in bed. She was placed on mattresses on the floor, where she lay tossing about for four days without sleep, rapidly emaciating, and the countenance marking the great exhaustion of the vital powers. Tongue parched and brown; pulse rapid and weak. Full opiates had failed to produce sleep; and, though the spine was repeatedly examined, no such evidence of tenderness could be found as was so well marked in the last case. On the 19th, however, a spot in the lumbar region of the spine appeared to be slightly more sensitive to percussion than others: and six leeches were applied, followed by ice in bladders. The relief was again most marked: four or five hours' tranquil sleep followed; and the improvement evidently dated from this point. The emaciation was very great, and the strength seemed to have been more diminished than in the former case. The excoriation of the elbows, ankles, and hips, was very severe. She was ordered wine, with beef-tea and eggs; and five-minim doses of Battley's sedative liquor every four hours. She became more tranquil, and the amendment was steady. On the 20th, she was able to use a cold douche to the spine, though she was obliged to be supported while using it, as she was unable to stand alone from debility. There are no remains of dorsal tenderness. Appetite good; tongue clean and moist; and bowels regular. The carbonate of iron completed the cure early in July.

Art. 40.—*Case of Cataleptic Hysteria.* By Dr. Ringland.

(*Dublin Quarterly Journal of Med. Science*, Aug. 1855.)

The following very curious case of cataleptic hysteria was communicated to the College of Physicians in Ireland, on April 4th, 1855.

Case.—Mrs. ——, an English lady, of literary taste and sedentary habits, about 30 years of age, and married eight years, had been very delicate from her earliest infancy. During the six years antecedent, and the year immediately subsequent to her marriage, she suffered from most intense headache. Two years prior to her marriage she was under treatment for spinal irritation, as she was informed by her then medical attendant. About this period, too, she voided several portions of tapeworm, and had frequently, both before and after her marriage, passed large quantities of ascarides. She was at all times subject to palpitation of the heart, and had on one or two occasions a slight hysterical fit. She suffers intense pain on touching the last dorsal vertebræ, which for some years has projected to about the size of a nut. A sound as loud as the snapping of the fingers is frequently heard proceeding from this locality whenever she is much fatigued, or has been standing for a considerable time; and this sound Dr. Ringland has more than once heard. She also experiences, since her first confinement, great pain on the least pressure being made against the coccyx, which has been slightly dislocated downwards and backwards, and has become anchylosed in that direction.

On the second night after she was married, whilst engaged at prayers, she was suddenly, and without the least premonitory indication, seized with the first of the series of fits about to be described; and this was shortly followed by a second, of a like character. An interval of six months then elapsed without their recurrence; when, however, being much about that length of time pregnant, she was again attacked, and, as on the former occasion, without any premonitory symptom, and whilst in a state of complete mental quiescence, having been previously engaged in calm, unexciting conversation with her husband. The headache from which she had previously suffered was greatly aggravated from this period until after her confinement, and she has described it as though a tight iron cap was violently pressed on the upper half of her head, to which the headache was strictly limited. The fits now returned with but very short intervals, and it was with considerable difficulty her medical attendant prevented a premature confinement.

Some little time after the fits became completely established, she observed that if she was engaged in conversation immediately antecedent to the access of one, she could not command the words she uttered, although fully aware of what she ought to say, and thus she frequently appeared to give expression to the most absurd ideas, and to opinions which were quite opposed to what she had intended to convey. Often, too, having spoken a portion of a sentence, she terminated it upon a subject quite different from that on which she had commenced her observations, or came to an abrupt close, finding herself totally deprived of further utterance.

Up to, and during her confinement, she had frequent attacks, sometimes so many as thirty in the twenty-four hours, and seldom less than fifteen or twenty. After her confinement, which was easy and natural, they were reduced to two or three in a day, and on very rare occasions one whole day has elapsed without their recurrence. Within the last eighteen months her health in this respect has considerably improved, as, repeatedly, days, frequently weeks, and sometimes even a month, has elapsed without a fit.

The origin of this affection she attributes to excessive fright, produced by witnessing very violent paroxysms of hysteria, almost amounting to insanity, in a female relative, with whom she was on a visit shortly before her marriage.

Fatigue, excitement—whether pleasurable or the reverse—or even music—if loud or prolonged—noise—the slightest start—the least pressure against the painful part of the spine, or against the coccyx, instantly induces a fit; they frequently, however, come on without any apparent exciting cause.

The duration of each fit is very variable; sometimes it lasts only three or four minutes, and sometimes it is prolonged to an hour and a half. Dr. Ringland has witnessed several which lasted from twenty minutes to half an hour each.

She has never had less than two fits when attacked, the second being of much shorter duration than the first, and invariably succeeding it after but a short interval.

She appears to have been obnoxious to the attacks at all times and seasons, in all postures, and under every circumstance. She has been liable to them in summer as well as in winter; has been attacked whilst in bed or at her meals; whilst engaged in reading, writing, or in conversation; whilst standing, walking or sitting; whilst alone or in the midst of strangers;—frequently with a word half uttered, or a piece of food partially masticated; and more than once has her life been placed in jeopardy by the fit occurring when she was near a fire, or whilst she was engaged in the act of deglutition. The presence or absence of menstruation has no apparent connection with the attacks, nor has that secretion ever been in the least affected by them, neither does the existence of pregnancy or lactation seem in any respect to influence this strange affection, excepting that the fits have been much more frequent from the moment of impregnation up to the period of quickening, than at any other time.

Instantly, on the access of a fit she falls backwards or forwards, according to the direction in which her head has been at the moment. Should she, however, have her baby in her arms at the time, she holds it firmly clutched in her hands, which cannot, without considerable violence, be opened; although, when the fit ensues at any other time, her hands, though closed, can be easily opened.

The particulars of this lady's case, Dr. Ringland learned from herself some months prior to her then approaching confinement—her fourth—and which took place early in December, 1854. Immediately after the birth of the child, which was mature and healthy, she had one of her customary fits, which was followed by a second, immediately after the expulsion of the placenta. The following is a brief description of the first fit witnessed by Dr. Ringland.

Without any previous indication whatever, she suddenly seemed to faint, and lay in a state of *apparently* total unconsciousness. She, however, was quite aware of every circumstance that occurred around her, and could afterwards detail the conversation which had taken place in the room. Her limbs remained in whatever position they were in at the time of the attack, or in any other to which they were subsequently changed. There was no alteration in the color of her lips, in her complexion, or in the appearance of her skin, which remained of the natural temperature. Her eyelids were closed, but when raised, continued open until closed again. The pupils contracted well on exposure to light. Her pulse was about 100, but very feeble. There were no apparent heavings of the chest nor movements of the nostrils. Repeatedly during the existence of the fit, but more violently towards its close, there were convulsive twitches of the muscles of the face, spasmodic clenching of the fingers, and forcible supination of the hands on the forearm. There were no convulsive movements of the lower extremities, although such occasionally occurred, as she informed Dr. Ringland, and were always present during the first few months of the existence of the fits.

No restoratives were applied during the fit, as she had previously intimated to Dr. Ringland that the employment of the most simple of these had always produced violent and prolonged hysteric paroxysms, which never presented themselves when interference was not had recourse to.

After the lapse of about five minutes she gave a deep sigh, then opened her eyes, looked about her, and feebly held out her hands. On this signal, which is well understood by her attendants, she was without delay raised into a sitting posture, and after a brief interval of quiet she was perfectly restored.

Had not her attendants, as she informed Dr. Ringland, at once placed her in the erect position, she would have relapsed again and again into the fit. She, too, is so conscious of this necessity, that instantly on the subsidence of the fit she holds out her hands, as described, thereby indicating her desire for the requisite assistance. Should she at this time be handled roughly, or should the tender part of the spine or the coccyx be touched, she at once relapses into the fit.

She is not able until after the lapse of considerable time, and not even then without the greatest effort, to utter a single syllable, the peculiar condition excited throughout the system appearing in her case to attach itself more firmly to the tongue than elsewhere.

After the subsidence of the attack she is greatly distressed with tremors of the whole body, which last sometimes for only a few minutes, but at times continue for several hours.

Before concluding, Dr. Ringland made a brief summary of this singular case, directing attention to its leading characteristics and points of interest; especially to the previous existence of spinal irritation; the occurrence of the attacks in summer as well as in winter; the existence of consciousness during the fits; the erect position being necessary at the close of the fit, and neglect in this respect causing relapse; the loss of speech being prolonged after the subsidence of the other symptoms; and, finally, to the fact that restoratives induced hysteria.

ART. 41.—*Mutism and Aphonia of twelve years' standing cured by electricity.* By M. FLAMANT, of Strasburg.

(*Dublin Hospital Gazette,* Feb. 15, 1856.)

On a recent occasion, M. Sedillot submitted to the Académie des Sciences, the case of a woman, 30 years of age, treated by M. Flamant, of Strasburg. The patient had, twelve years previously, been suddenly struck with dumbness and aphonia, in consequence of a sudden fright. Various plans of treatment had been adopted, without any benefit; hearing was unaffected, and the patient communicated with those about her by signs, but was unable to utter the slightest sound.

The tongue was found somewhat retracted upwards and backwards, the apex pointed to the roof of the mouth, and could, with difficulty, be depressed by the patient, who was wholly unable to press it against the back of the teeth. Deglutition was unaffected, but there were occasional hysteric attacks. The diagnosis which was formed was, that there was paralysis of the principal extrinsic muscles of the tongue, especially of the genio-glossi, with a similar condition of the muscles of the larynx which govern the action of the vocal cords. It was thought that electricity might be useful. [*Electricité par induction* was employed and the apparatus of Legendre and Morin was used.] From even the first application benefit was derived : after the third application, the power of speech was restored, but not the voice. For some time the attempts at pronouncing words caused a sensation of fatigue about the hyoid region. The voice gradually came back, and ultimately a complete cure was the result.

Similar cases are on record, but none in which the affection had lasted for so long a time. For example, in the "Mémoirs de l'Académie des Sciences" for 1753, there is a case very like this one. Three other cases are given in a German Journal of 1843 (" Canstatt's Jahresbericht"). One of these was a case of complete aphonia, the result of chronic syphilitic laryngitis, which got well after the third application of electricity.

(B) CONCERNING THE RESPIRATORY SYSTEM.

ART. 42.—*On the diagnosis of Fibrinous Concretions in the Heart in certain cases of Inflammatory Croup.* By BENJAMIN W. RICHARDSON, M.D., Physician to the Royal Infirmary for Diseases of the Chest.

(*Medical Times and Gazette*, March 8, 1856.)

" With regard to croup," says Dr. Richardson, " I take a decided and strong position, which has peculiar bearings ; first, on diagnosis, and, secondly, on treatment.

" My views are these : 1. That croup, like all other hyperinotic diseases, commences first as a general disorder. That, in the outset of the general symptoms, the respiration is quickened, the combustion of the body is increased, and the fibrinous constituent of the blood is made in proportions abnormally excessive.

" 2. In regard to the local mischief, I contend that this, in inflammatory croup, is a secondary effect, like all other local manifestations.

" 3. In croup of the inflammatory type death may and does occur, either from an obstruction in the heart (syncope), arising from the right cavities of that organ being the seat of a fibrinous deposit, or from obstruction in the windpipe (apnœa), arising from over-secretion ; or, lastly, from a combination of these causes, as happened in a case related to the Medical Society by Dr. Hawksley, where the local mischief produced death, while yet the fibrinous concretion was becoming developed, and before it had materially impeded the circulation.

" Holding, then, these views on the causes of death in croup, I am in no way prepared to deny the usefulness of tracheotomy in some forms of this disorder, nor have I ever denied it ; but I maintain that there are certain cases in which the death is clearly by syncope, the result of fibrinous deposition, and that in these cases the operation is simply absurd. I would further remark, that Mr. Smith has related cases where the symptoms, as he describes them, were those of syncope from this cause, and that the death in those cases was removed altogether from the operation—being death by syncope, not by apnœa.

" The symptoms which mark the cases of croup about to terminate in syncope the result of cardiac obstruction, are distinct from those arising from obstruction in the air-passages.

" The differences are these : In the cases of syncope from arrested circulation, the dyspnœa is not caused by obstruction in the larynx, but by the peculiar anxiety, and gasping desire to breathe incident to the want of blood in the pulmonic circuit. In this case, therefore, if the stethoscope be carried from the upper part of the windpipe downwards, and over the whole chest, the respiratory murmur is audible, and, it may be, clear throughout, so that the observer is prepared to say that there is here no such deficiency of respiration as will account for the severity of the symptoms. Again, the most common physical pulmonic sign in these cases, is that of emphysema, which is often accompanied, in very young children, by a peculiar prominence in the anterior part of the chest. This emphysema, when present, is strictly diagnostic of fibrinous obstruction, and is altogether subversive of the idea that the cause of the symptoms is an obstruction in the windpipe.

" In addition, there are, in these cases, the definite signs which mark the cardiac obstruction. The body is cold, and generally pale, almost marbly, but mostly so at the extreme parts. The lips are slightly blue ; the cheeks are occasionally the same. The jugular veins are distended. The pulse is irregular. The body is painfully restless. The heart-beats are feeble, quick, and irregular; the sounds muffled, with a bruit in some cases. No real convulsions of the limbs occur, but intense anxiety and constant movement.

"In those cases, on the other hand, where the death is really due to apnœa,—the effect of obstruction in the air-passages,—the symptoms are widely different. In these cases there is some point in the respiratory canal where an obstruction can be detected. The lungs show signs of congestion, but never of emphysema. The difficulty of respiration arises from an absolute inability to fill the chest. From the fact of the obstruction being in the respiratory circuit, such blood as passes through it is not arterialized, and the surface of the body, instead of being pale, as in cases of cardiac obstruction, is generally of a dark hue, with the veins more decidedly turgid. The muscles are not simply restless, but actually convulsed violently, the patient being unconscious of the fact; the heart-sounds are clear, and its motions, though feeble, are rarely tumultuous.

"Lastly, the breathing is the first to stop at death, while, in the former case, the heart takes the precedence in this respect.

"These broad and definite diagnostic signs, can never be mistaken, except in instances where there is a clot in the heart coincidently with obstruction in the windpipe. Here some difficulty may arise, but a careful inquiry into all the facts will indicate the existence of the complication.

"The points of practice which are to be gathered from a clear diagnosis in cases of this character are numerous, but in none so important as in settling the question whether tracheotomy should or should not be performed.

"If in any given case the practitioner shall find the symptoms referable purely to obstruction in the trachea or larynx, and the circulation unembarrassed, he will operate with good chance of success, granting that the point of obstruction is not too low, and that no further inflammation succeeds. If, on the contrary, he should diagnose the symptoms of cardiac obstruction, whether or not complicated with constriction in the windpipe, the operation is worse than useless; it will, of necessity, fail, because there are other fatal influences at work which the knife cannot affect."

ART. 43.—*On Tracheotomy in the last stage of Croup.*
By M. TROUSSEAU, Physician to the Hôtel-Dieu.

(*Medical Times and Gazette*, Jan. 5, 1856.)

After some preliminary remarks, M. Trousseau proceeds:

"I am firmly decided, for my part, not to be discouraged, but to advocate tracheotomy with so much the more conviction as the proportion of successful cases increase; and if that proportion remained even as it was ten years ago, I would still proclaim the necessity of tracheotomy, and I would not cease to uphold it as a duty, a duty as imperious for a surgeon as the ligature of the carotid artery after a wound of that vessel, even if death followed the operation as often as the cure.

"Here are the results of my operations for tracheotomy during the year 1854: I operated on nine children. Of these, two died, while seven were cured, and are now living in perfect health.

"Certainly the proportion of cured is not always so great; still, if I make the sum total of the operations I have performed in the last four years, I find twenty-four operations, and fourteen cures, equivalent to more than half.

"At the Hôpital des Enfans Malades, in the last five years, the proportion of cures has been nearly a quarter. Here are the official numbers, viz.:

1850	. 20 operations	. 6 cures,	about 1-3d.
1851	. 31 "	. 12 "	more than 1-3d.
1852	. 59 "	. 11 "	less than 1-5th.
1853	. 61 "	. 7 "	only 1-9th.
1854	. 44 "	. 11 "	only 1-4th.
Total 215 "		47 "	about 1-4th.

"This result is considerable, if we remember the social condition of the children who are brought to the hospital, the deplorable treatment they are subjected to by ' sage femmes,' quacks, etc. : in a word, those persons the poor generally consult in preference to doctors. We should bear in mind, too, the unfavorable condition of the hospital, where the children operated upon are placed in the midst of the most varied and fatal contagion ; so much so, that often when the operation for tracheotomy is succeeding as well as could be desired, the scarlet fever, measles, small-pox, or hooping cough, cause the most fearful complications.

" I do not doubt that half the operations performed out of hospital are successful, always provided tracheotomy takes place when the chances of cure are possible.

" This restriction is important ; for, if the diphtheritic infection is thoroughly rooted in the system, if the skin, and particularly the cavities of the nose, are invaded by this special phlegmasia ; if the quickness of the pulse, delirium, prostration, indicate a profound poison, and if the danger is rather in the general state than in the local lesion of the larynx or of the trachea, certainly the operation should not be tried, for it is invariably fatal ; when, however, the local lesion constitutes the principal danger of the disease, no matter at what degree asphyxia has arrived, even if the child has but a few moments to live, tracheotomy succeeds invariably, as well as though it had been tried three or four hours sooner."

Then M. Trousseau speaks of the mode of operating, and of the necessity of using a double canula ; and after this he proceeds to speak of the after-treatment. Upon this last subject his remarks are of extreme importance, and we copy them without abbreviation.

"The operation once performed, the first duty of the practitioner is to see to the nourishment ; that remedy above all essential in most acute maladies, and particularly in diseases of children. Certainly, abstinence, prescribed by Broussais, and ordered by those practitioners who still cling to the old school, and who keep up the prejudices of their early medical education, is one of the most pernicious helpers of disease ; it is the best means of prolonging the infection of the system, and the surest way of facilitating the absorption of exterior miasma and vicious excretions formed by the malady ; the surest opponent of that resistance which is the chief aid of convalescence and ultimate cure.

" Now, I do not mean that we must fall into the opposite extreme, that we must overfeed the little patients ; I only say, that we should satisfy the appetite, if they have any, and even force them to eat, if they show too much repugnance to food. Do not hesitate in employing intimidation ; in this case often have I assumed the air of severity, and obliged the child to eat, thus preparing the way to a cure I otherwise judged impossible. Milk, eggs, custards, chocolate, and soups are the aliments I most insist on. What I have here urged, sufficiently indicates that I most formally proscribe the continuation of those means judged more or less useful before the operation, viz.: calomel, alum, emetics, and purges, which are not compatible with the nourishment I advise.

" I need not add, that the application of blisters would be pernicious, inasmuch as they would establish a new surface when the specific inflammation would break out, and thus occasion a fatal absorption, which must be avoided at any risk.

" When this happens, as it often does, after blisters have been applied, we must as soon as possible dress the wound with extract of rhatany or Goulard's cerate, or else rub it with nitrate of silver, if diphtheritic concretions already cover the skin which has so uselessly been laid bare.

" I now come to the details of dressing, to which I seem to attach so much importance ; but the older I grow the more I am convinced that in medicine, the minutiæ hold a much more considerable place than is generally supposed. Great care must be taken in placing between the skin and canula a round piece of oiled silk, or india-rubber, in order to prevent the sides of the canula, and the strings which attach it, from irritating the wound.

" The patients must be taught to remove and replace the internal canula, which is to be cleaned every two or three hours.

" The child's neck must be enveloped in a knitted woollen scarf or large piece of muslin, so that he breathes in through the tissue which covers the neck, and inhales the warm air impregnated with the moisture furnished by the breath. This precept is excellent; we thus avoid the drying of the cavity of the canula and of the trachea; we prevent the irritation of the mucous membrane, and the formation of hard scabs, analogous to those which form in the cavities of the nose of persons attacked with coryza, scabs which, detaching themselves in complete tubes, or in fragments of tubes, cause terrible fits of suffocation, and sometimes even death, by the occlusion of the canula.

" Before Dr. Guersant and I had adopted this method, we lost numbers of patients by catarrhal pneumonia, and now this result is much less frequent. It is very probable that the introduction of hot and moist air into the bronchi is quite a favorable condition. There is still a practice, without which the cure is rare: I refer to the cauterization of the wound. The first four days the whole surface of the incision should be vigorously rubbed with nitrate of silver once a day; thus we avoid a serious result. I mean the diphtheritic infection of the wound which covers itself with thick and fetid false membranes. A specific inflamation seizes the surrounding cellular tissue, and developing often a bad species of phlegmonous erysipelas, which becomes the occasion of local gangrene, and at last of a violent symptomatic fever, and of a general infection almost always fatal. The fifth day the surface of the wound is so modified that the results above indicated are no longer to be feared. There now remains a last and very delicate part of the treatment, to which I wish to call attention for an instant—I refer to the removal of the canula and the definite occlusion of the wound. We must establish the fact that the sooner the canula is removed the better. This can rarely be done before the sixth day, as it is seldom necessary to scar it later than the tenth. However, there are cases when the larynx remains completely shut during fifteen, twenty, and even forty-four days, as I saw in the case of a young girl eventually cured.

" At the end of the first week we must remove the canula, taking care not to frighten the child or make it cry. The poor little sufferers are so accustomed to breathe with ease by artificial means, that when the canula is removed, in order to facilitate the passage of the air through the larynx, they are seized with excessive fear, expressed by agitation, cries, and in consequence there is an acceleration of the breathing. The larynx is still a little obstructed either by false membranes, by mucus, or by a slight tumefaction of the membrane; and then, perhaps, the laryngeal muscles have lost the habit of contracting in harmony with the wants of the respiration. There often results great difficulty from this circumstance. This difficulty disappears well enough in the great number of cases, if we succeed in tranquillizing the little patient: this is the province of the mother rather than the practitioner. The wound is closed with short strips of court plaster. If the sound of the cough or the respiration, or the nature of the voice, indicate that the opening of the larynx is sufficiently large, we leave the dressing there; but if the air only pass in insufficient quantity, the plaster must be put on; the wound should only be covered with linen and simple cerate, and we wait the next day before closing the wound; if the air do not pass at all, then we replace the canula, and, two or three days later, make the attempt again.

" So soon as the respiration proceeds well, notwithstanding the occlusion of the wound, we should renew the dressing two or three times a day; ordinarily, the opening of the trachea is shut in four or five days; then only remains the exterior wound which we dress with linen, and which in its turn soon heals.

" There is a serious difficulty which I have remarked to physicians for a long time, and to which Dr. Archambault has recently called attention, I mean that of swallowing. This difficulty consists in the passage of liquids through the glottis: each effort the patient makes to drink is followed by a violent and convulsive cough, and the liquids, which penetrate into the trachea and the bronchi, flow in abundance by the opening of the canula. Besides the serious inconvenience which may follow from the contact of food with the mucous membrane of the bronchi, there particularly results an insurmountable disgust, and children often die of hunger, in preference to taking their nourishment. So often this complication has been the cause of death after tracheotomy, that I have made great efforts to find a remedy. The best method is to forbid liquid food. I give to children very thick soup, vermicelli with milk, or with beef broth, so thick as to be eaten with a fork rather than a spoon, hard-boiled eggs, eggs with milk, occasionally meat in large pieces, and I forbid all drink. If thirst is too ardent, I recommend pure cold water, and I am careful to administer it either long after eating or immediately before, in order to prevent vomiting. I should remark, however, that the difficulty of which I speak scarcely manifests itself before three or four days after the operation, and that it lasts rarely longer than ten or twelve days. Nevertheless, I have seen it persist much longer with some children.

"It would seem that the larynx, which is so open to receive drinks and liquid aliments, should suffice also for the passage of the air necessary for the purposes of respiration ; this is not the case, however. If we remove the canula, we perceive that the opening is still insufficient, and even some days later, when we are able to close the wound with court-plaster, these difficulties continue with the same violence.

"It is almost impossible to discover the cause of this. Dr. Archambault holds that the child, who has breathed by the canula for some days, loses the habit of freely using those muscles which serve for the occlusion of the larynx, and those which push the food into the œsophagus, and he highly approves the following ingenious method, which consists in momentarily closing the canula with the finger, whilst the patient swallows ; thus the child is obliged to use its larynx, and the normal harmony of its organ is re-established.

"This little stratagem succeeds well in some cases, but in others it completely fails, and what I have said above proves it ; since even when the canula is removed, and the wound is completely closed, yet the difficulty of deglutition continues, although the breathing through the larynx may be perfectly free and regular."

ART. 44.—*The indication for Paracentesis Thoracis in Pleurisy.* By M. TROUSSEAU.
(*Medical Times and Gazette*, Jan. 26, 1856.)

These remarks are taken from a clinical lecture which was recently delivered at the Hôtel-Dieu.

"The indication for operating is to be drawn from the quantity of liquid, and not from the amount of functional disturbance, such as, for example, the oppression of breathing. Thus, the patient in No. 10 suffered four or five days ago from very considerable oppression, which then diminished so much as to cease to inconvenience him, although the operation furnished more than 7 lb. of fluid. So free had his respiration become prior to the operation, that he rose and went to the privy, fainting when he got there. You will meet with individuals with enormous effusion making no complaint of, and not perceiving, any oppression of breathing, although this is really in existence, as may be ascertained on examination of their inspiratory power. This defective impressionability, where so much cause for oppression existed, as in the case of the man in No. 10, is very remarkable, for respiration was carried on only by one lung, the play of which was also limited by the compression exerted by the heart and mediastinum. The same insensibility prevailed in cases seen by M. Trousseau at the Necker. M. Pidoux, too, in his monograph on latent pleurisy, relates the case of a patient who died suddenly under similar conditions. The same happened in a case in which MM. Trousseau and Chomel were about to determine to operate. We must, therefore, never take as the basis of our determination to operate anything but the quantity of fluid, the amount of which may always be judged of by inspection, percussion, and auscultation. The amount of febrile reaction will not serve us as a guide, any more than the oppression of breathing; for we find the effusion becoming excessive precisely in the subacute, the so to say hidden, form of pleurisy, in which the fever is slight, and the pain in the side almost insignificant. There appears in such cases something as much due to the fluxion as to the inflammation ; and, without professing to institute any exact comparison, they seem to differ as much from simple inflammatory pleurisy as a hydarthrosis differs from an arthritis, properly so called."

ART. 45.—*On Paracentesis Thoracis.* By DR DANIEL H. TUKE, Physician to the York Dispensary.

(*Assoc. Med. Journal*, Dec. 7 and 14, 1855.)

In this paper, Dr. Tuke relates three cases which illustrate the three principal terminations of cases after operation, viz, perfect recovery of health and lung, recovery of health with a contracted chest, and temporary relief but subsequent death.

Then follow statistics of the subject, with comments upon them.

"The three cases I have now detailed, added to those of which I have obtained the results (so far as the mortality is concerned), make a total of 246 on whom the operation was performed. In attempting to determine the success of the operation from the published cases, we are exposed, I am fully aware, to one source of fallacy, and that is, our ignorance, in a large number of instances, of the after-history of the patient. For instance, it is impossible to discover how many of these patients were living a year after the operation, yet this is surely a very important point in making any inquiry into its success, and our knowledge of it would, no doubt, add very much to our estimate of the mortality of the cases operated upon.

"The 246 cases alluded to have been collected from the practice of well-known medical men, as Dr. Hughes, physician to Guy's-Hospital; Dr. Hamilton Roe, senior physician to the Hospital for Consumption; Dr. Watson, Mr. Benjamin Phillips, and others.

"The following table will show the number of cases operated upon, and the proportion fatal under each; there being a total of 100 cases of genuine empyema, and 146 of serous effusion; the mortality of the former being 26, and the latter 33·7 per cent.; that is a mortality of 7·7 more than that which occurred in the cases of genuine empyema.

Table showing the results of Operative Interference in two hundred and forty-six cases. *

By whom observed or reported.	Fluid effused purulent.	Mortality.	Recovered.	Fluid effused serous.	Mortality.	Recovered.
Dr. H. Roe (collected by him), ...	20	6	14	19	5	14
Dr. H. Roe (observed by him), ...	10	2	8	14	4	10
Mr. Phillips, ...	31	5	26	91	29	62
Dr. Hughes, ...	10	2	8	19	10	9
Dr. T. Davies, ...	10	2	8	...	...	...
Dr. Watson, ...	6	3	3	...	...	...
"Med. Times and Gazette,"	9	4	5	1	1	...
Dr. Paley (Peterborough), .	1	1	...	2	...	2
Dr. Theoph. Thompson, 1 ⎫ The late Mr. Hey, of Leeds, ... 1 ⎬ Dr. Williams, of York, . 1 ⎭	3	1	2	...	...	...
Total, ...	100	26	74	146	49	97

* Vide "Med. Chir. Trans.," 1844; "Guy's Hosp. Reports," 1844; "Medical Gazette," 1847, &c.; "Med. Times and Gazette," 1854; "Association Medical Journal," Jan. 5th, 1856; Hey's Surgery;" Dr. Watson's "Principles and Practice of Physic," &c.

SUMMARY.—Total number of deaths,   -   -   -   -   - 75

Mortality per cent. in genuine empyema, -   -   26·0
      "   "   in serous effusion,   -   -   33·7
      "   "   in all cases,   -   -   30·4
Total recovered (more or less completely),   -   - 171

Grand total,   -   -   -   -   -   - 246

"I imagine the explanation of this is partly to be found in the fact, that the cases of serous effusion were more frequently associated with fatal diseases. This remark would apply especially to cases of mechanical hydrothorax. I believe, also, that a large proportion of cases of phthisis will be found among the examples of serous effusion operated upon.

"With regard to the real subsequent condition of the patient in those cases *in which death did not occur*, I find that, of 44 cases in which I have been able to determine this point, 33 appear to have recovered their health perfectly, and in 13 of these, the lung re-expanding, no contraction of the chest followed; 5 cases were progressing favorably when last seen, and 6 were not likely ultimately to recover: total, 44.

"Out of the 29 cases reported by Dr. Hughes, 14 recovered so far as regards the effusion ; 2 may be justly mentioned as having at least partially recovered ; one of these had, after seven years, a fistulous opening into the pleura, and the other had still some, though comparatively a very small quantity, of fluid in the right pleura (but so much better as to be in search of employment), when the cases were reported ; 1 remained under treatment. Twelve have ultimately died of other diseases, generally connected with that for which the operation was performed, but entirely independent of its performance. Of these 12 fatal cases, 6 have died of phthisis; 2 of malignant disease of the lung; 1 rather suddenly with hydrothorax of the other pleura ; 1 of gangrenous pulmonary abscess of the opposite side ; 1 died of chronic pneumonia ; and 1 (a case of pneumothorax, with effusion) of pneumonia and pericarditis."

Dr. Tuke's conclusions are these :

"1. It is impossible to determine the precise period when the lung becomes irremediably damaged by effused fluid—as this must depend to some extent upon the individual case ; but it can be proved to take place in a period certainly not more than one month and nineteen days. On the other hand, the longest time a lung was subjected to the pressure of a large amount of fluid, and yet recovered itself, was four months ; but, in the great majority of cases, the lung lost its power of re-expansion long before.

"2. That in regard to the danger of serum becoming converted into pus by delay, it can be shown that serum, the result of inflammation, may remain such for seven months ; but that, on the other hand, the conversion may take place in a very early stage of the effusion.

"3. That when the serous effusion has become purulent, we are not justified in expecting absorption, although such an event has occasionally occurred : but must expect the matter to make its escape either by ulceration of the walls of the chest, or of the pleura pulmonalis, producing pneumo-thorax and expectoration of pus.

"4. That the mortality per cent. in the cases operated upon (a large number of them apparently desperate cases) was 30 4, and only 26 per cent. in the cases of genuine empyema ; that with regard to the non-fatal cases, some would doubtless not survive long ; but that a fair proportion completely recovered, and that the most successful results were obtained when the operation was resorted to in an early stage. In some cases, immediate and permanent relief was obtained when death seemed imminent from suffocation. In none did the operation cause fatal results—facts which are much more encouraging than might have been expected from the experience of some other operators. Boyer performed the operation several times, but never saved a patient. Dupuytren saw only two successful cases in fifty. Sir A. Cooper saw only one successful case. Gendrin had not one successful case out of twenty in which he operated.*

* Dr. Bennett: vide "Lancet," Dec. 30th. 1843.

" 5. In regard to the main question of the essay—it appears to be incumbent to resort to paracentesis when the dyspnœa is so urgent as to threaten death, whether it be in an early or a late stage of the effusion, and whether that effusion be serous or purulent.

" Cases of mechanical hydrothorax, or cases in which the effusion is complicated with phthisis, malignant disease, &c , in which the symptoms of asphyxia are urgent, and in which an operation can afford only temporary relief, may perhaps be regarded as analogous to cases of phthisis, in which, from the larynx becoming involved, suffocation is imminent, and tracheotomy alone can prolong, though it cannot save life.

" It likewise appears to be reasonable to employ it when we feel satisfied that the effusion is purulent, and the patient is obviously losing ground. ' It is,' says Mr. Cock, surgeon to Guy's Hospital, ' from an early application of the trocar that a successful result must be anticipated, and it is the delay until the pressure of the fluid becomes indicated by external physical signs which has so often led to disappointment in the issue of the case.'

" How far, however, when a patient is in moderate health, and has a large collection of fluid in his pleura, uninfluenced by absorbent and other remedies pursued for many weeks; how far, I say, we are justified in endeavoring to anticipate the time when the lung will be irremediably compressed and bound down, by tapping the chest, is a much more difficult question; but, on the whole, I think that, unless we have strong grounds for believing the fluid has been converted into pus (judging of this more by the condition of the patient than the period of the effusion, important as this circumstance would be as an auxiliary), it would be rash to resort to paracentesis, especially when we know that occasionally large effusions are unexpectedly absorbed when remedial treatment has been regarded as hopeless. Dr. Hughes, however, says, ' My own experience and consideration induce me to believe that it is preferable to tap the chest as soon as all hope of the future beneficial operation of remedies has disappeared : and, if possible, before the effusion has been converted from serum into pus.' "

ART. 46.—*Prevention of reaccumulation of fluid after Paracentesis Thoracis.*
By M. ARAN.

(*Journ. de Med. et de Chir. Prat.*, Sept. 1855 ; and *Assoc. Med. Journ.*, April 19, 1856.)

" To prevent the reaccumulation of fluid after the operation of paracentesis thoracis, M. Aran administers a combination of nitrate of potash with digitalis. This produces a marked diuretic effect. The medicine is ordinarily given in powders or pills, containing from fifteen grains to a drachm of nitrate of potash, and from four and a half to thirty grains of powdered digitalis. Large doses at first are liable to produce a distressing feeling of *malaise*, and troublesome diuresis. Hence it is best to begin with fifteen grains of nitrate of potash and three grains of digitalis. If this is well borne, the dose may be rapidly increased. M. Aran usually begins with four and a half grains of digitalis, and doubles it the next day, if there is no vomiting. He also prescribes the medicine in a mixture with syrup; a form which he states to be a very good remedy in hæmoptysis."

ART. 47.—*Diagnostic value of a Microscopic Examination of the Sputum.*
By Dr. J. HUGHES BENNETT, Professor of the Institutes of Medicine in the University of Edinburgh.

(*Edinburgh Medical Journal*, Jan. 1856.)

" A proper appreciation of the structure of sputum requires a thorough knowledge of histology, as, mixed with the expectoration, may be found—1st. The natural secretion of the salivary and mucous glands, with the epithelial structures of the mouth, fauces, and pharynx. 2d. All the structures that enter into the composition of the bronchi and lungs, in various stages of disintegration. 3d. The results of various morbid processes, in different stages of development or disintegration, such as the inflammatory, tubercular, or cancerous exudations, extravasations of blood, earthy concretions, &c. And, 4th. All kinds of substances which enter into the composition of food, which adhere to the mouth and teeth, such as starch corpuscles, and the different elements which enter into the composition of the various vegetable and animal substances used as aliment. Great pains and considerable time are also required in the examination, so as to satisfy the inquirer that nothing of importance has been overlooked.

" Extensive examination of sputum with the microscope has, up to a recent period, served to persuade most scientific physicians that it was of little practical importance, inasmuch as percussion and auscultation yield us a more efficient and more exact means of determining the changes which go on in the lung. The recent careful examination of sputum, however, by Dr. Andrew Clark,* as well as a case which has come under my notice, may induce them to modify that o inion.

" Professor Van der Kolk of Utrecht,† was the first who directed attention to the fragments of the elastic fibres of the lung in sputum, as occasionally being of diagnostic importance. That such fibres were common in the sputum of consumptives, after ulceration of the lung has commenced, is easily proved, and has been familiar to myself for the last fifteen years. The important part of Van der Kolk's memoir, however, is contained in the following passage: ' But we ought to determine if these fibres are only observed when phthisis is already well advanced, and produced great ravages, or if they exist in expectorated matter at the first formation of vomicæ, so that they enable us to determine their existence when commencing. My conviction, with regard to this important problem, is, that it is exactly at the commencement of phthisis, and at the first formation of a vomica, that the elastic fibres were present in the greatest abundance, and that they may then be considered as among the most positive signs we possess of the presence of a cavern. Later, when the cavity has acquired a certain extent, these fibres become more rare in the expectoration, and are with difficulty distinguished.' This statement is supported by a case, in which very insignificant signs could be determined by auscultation, although the general symptoms indicated phthisis—yet, where the fibres existed in considerable numbers in the sputum, and led to a diagnosis, which was confirmed by the subsequent progress of the case.

" Such an instance as that described by Van der Kolk I believe to be very rare, and the question always arises whether the lungs were examined with sufficient care, so as to render it certain that, whilst fibres of elastic tissue, derived from those organs, existed in the sputum, no auscultatory sign could be detected. But that this does occasionally occur, I have now no doubt—1st, from the facts previously given, which show that advanced phthisis may exist without any positive signs; and, 2d, from the following case, which fully confirms the statement made by the distinguished professor of Utrecht:

" CASE.—In August, 1854, I was consulted when in London by a lady. Mrs. B., æt. 23, who had for some time suffered from cough, accompanied by muco-purulent expectoration. There was little emaciation, the general powers of the system did not appear to be much impaired, although she complained somewhat of weakness and diminution of appetite. Frequent cough, with expectoration, were the principal symptoms. Careful percussion and auscultation of the chest, (which was well formed) elicited positively nothing: the percussion note was normal and equal on both sides: the respiratory murmurs distinctly audible, soft with their usual rhythm, free from all abnormal murmur—no increase of the vocal resonance. Repeated examination, especially in both subclavicular and suprascapular regions, convinced me of this fact. The practitioner (W. T. Iliff, jun., Esq., of Kensington), who had previously attended her, and who was again subsequently called in, informed me. however, that she herself had an impression, that some time previously (in March). she was in the habit of spitting up fragments of her lungs. Mr. Iliff had taken portions of the indurated matter expectorated to Mr. Quekett, who, in fact, positively affirmed them to be pulmonary substance. At my request, Mr. Iliff was so good as to forward to Edinburgh a portion of the expectorated matter discharged the March previous to my seeing the patient—an oblong substance, about one-third of an inch long and one-sixt of an inch in thickness, presented all the characters of a piece of lung infiltrate

* "Trans. of Patholog. Soc. of London," vol. vi. p. 74.
† "Nederlandsch Lancet," 2 Sir. D. 1.

with tubercle. On examining sections of it under a magnifying power of 250 diam. linear, I, with some difficulty (the structure having been preserved in alcohol), determined the existence of circular bundles of areolar and elastic tissue, obscured by a mass of molecular matter in which tubercle-corpuscles were imbedded. That this tissue was really expectorated by Mrs. B , Mr. Iliff entertains no doubt, as he himself removed it from a tenacious mass of expectorated matter. Subsequent to our correspondence on the subject, he also submitted it to Dr. Beale, and Messrs. Quekett and Rainey, of London, all of whom agreed as to the fact of i's being a portion of human lung.

"During the winter of 1854–5, Mrs. B. continued tolerably well, and without medical attendance. Mr. Iliff, however, was again called in on the 7th of April, and found that the disease had been slowly progressing. The expectoration was now increased and more purulent, and she had sensibly lost flesh and strength. On the 25th of May, Dr. Latham was consulted. There was then flattening at the left apex, and in his opinion a cavity there. She had also hectic fever, copious night sweats, diarrhœa, haggard countenance, emaciation—in short the usual symptoms of the advanced stage. From this time notwithstanding the most judicious treatment on the part of her medical attendant, the disease progressed rapidly, and she expired, July 26th. An examination after death, revealed extensive tubercular disease in both lungs, with cavities in their apices; the left side being the one most affected.

"The facts of this case serve, in my opinion, to establish, that there are instances in which the occurrence of disintegrated lung tissue may be detected by the microscope in the sputum, *before* any auscultatory signs are audible. On this latter point, I may observe that Mr. Iliff could not detect such signs any more than myself, although he was in possession of the expectorated lung substance. There were also particular circumstances connected with my knowledge of the patient's friends, that made me unusually careful and anxious when making the stethoscopical examination, and certainly, in August, 1854, five months after pulmonary tissue was evacuated, there were no audible signs of phthisis pulmonalis. In reply to a question by me, as to how and when these signs first made their appearance, Mr. Iliff stated that he could not tell, as, for many months, he was not in attendance. But I need scarcely remark that, between August, 1854, and May, 1855, there was ample time for the disease to have progressed to the formation of cavities.

"All the circumstances of this case, therefore, have impressed upon me the importance of a microscopic examination of sputum. whenever the symptoms, and a suspicion of phthisis pulmonalis exist, without any clear evidence being present derivable from auscultation."

ART. 48 —*The diagnostic importance of Bronchitic signs as preceding and masking Phthisical disease.* By Dr. J. HUGHES BENNETT, Professor of the Institutes of Medicine in the University of Edinburgh.

(*Edinburgh Monthly Journal*, Jan. 1856.)

In this paper Dr. Bennett relates three cases which support the following conclusions:

"1st. That phthisis pulmonalis may exist and prove fatal. and yet, *during the whole of its progress*, only give rise to the physical signs usually considered as indicative of bronchitis with emphysema.

"2d. That such signs when persistent with all the symptoms of phthisis, should render the physician very suspicious of the existence of pulmonary tubercle.

"3d. That the analeptic treatment of such cases, and the avoidance of cough mixtures, or other means directed to the alleviation of mere symptoms, offers the surest means for procuring arrestment of the disease, and bringing about an ultimate recovery."

In explanation, Dr. Bennett suggests the probability that conditions of the lungs may exist in which the augmented sonoreity of emphysema will so counterbalance the increased dulness of tubercular deposition that the resulting note on percussion may assume a medium character and thereby approach that of health.

One of the three cases will serve in illustration:

"CASE 1.—I was consulted in the case of a young lady, æt. 11, in the year 1845. She had a short time previously recovered from a violent and prolonged attack of hooping-cough, and when I first saw her, complained of dry cough, and occasional difficulty of respiration. On percussion, the chest on both sides, presented its normal resonance. On auscultation, there was slight harshness of the inspiratory, and trifling prolongation of the expiratory murmur, very general over both sides anteriorly, but especially on the right side, with occasional sibilation. No increase of the vocal resonance anywhere. The patient was a well-grown girl, and had no other complaint or functional disorder, and the conclusion, of course, was bronchitis, with slight emphysema, following hooping-cough. This bronchitis, however, continued, the cough and occasional dyspnœa being sometimes very urgent. When eighteen or nineteen years of age, the latter symptoms sometimes attacked her when dancing, an exercise of which she was very fond, and obliged her to desist. In the autumn of 1853, expectoration of purulent mucus commenced, and the appetite began to fail, circumstances which excited my apprehensions, although nothing was to be heard but sibilation and prolonged expiration; percussion being everywhere clear. The most anxious care was now taken, by means of good diet and exercise, to support the general strength, and with such success that there was no emaciation, and little falling off in her bodily powers. In the spring of 1854, however, hæmoptysis commenced, at first slight, but subsequently more abundant, especially at the periods of menstruation. Now commenced, also, languor, weakness, dyspeptic symptoms, pallor of countenance, night perspirations, and other signs of debility, which gradually increased, notwithstanding the use of cod-liver oil and every conceivable means of support. All this time, although it was evident to me that she was consumptive, the most careful examination could elicit nothing but the physical signs formerly noticed, with the addition of occasional sonorous râle posteriorly and inferiorly, mingled with occasional mucous râle. Misty, foggy weather invariably added to her sufferings, while clear, dry weather, notwithstanding the cold, served to revive her. On the approach of winter in 1854, Dr. Christison saw her with me, and confirmed the results previously arrived at from physical examination of the chest, and it was then resolved that she should spend some months at Clifton. During the journey she had a severe attack of hæmoptysis, and this symptom prevented her going out for some time. Notwithstanding the assiduous professional care of Dr. Symonds, the disease progressed, and she died the very day of her return to Edinburgh.

"On examining the lungs, there was found great emphysema anteriorly on both sides, and considerable engorgement posteriorly and inferiorly. The middle and inferior lobes on the right side were hepatized from chronic pneumonia, and the upper lobes on both sides, but more especially on the right, contained circular patches of miliary tubercle, about three-fourths of an inch in diameter, irregularly scattered through the pulmonary tissue, communicating to it, when pressed on externally, a nodular character. Between these isolated patches the lung was, with the exceptions just noticed, quite healthy.

"In this case, which I occasionally saw during a period of ten years, I am satisfied that the ordinary physical signs of phthisis never were present. There was never dulness on percussion, or any indication of softening or of a cavity, and the post-mortem examination betrayed a condition of the lungs which proved that the signs of bronchitis and emphysema, which had been present throughout her illness, were true indications of what really existed. The pneumonia, the more immediate effects of which caused death, was of comparatively recent occurrence, and the time of tubercular deposition cannot be fixed with certitude, although, judging from the symptoms, I am inclined to consider that it dated from the spring of 1854. Here then we have chronic bronchitis and emphysema, terminating in phthisis, without any physical sign being manifested indicative of the latter lesion throughout the whole course of the disease."

Art. 49.—*On the Arthralgia of Phthisical patients.*
By M. J. H. G. Beau.

(*Presse Méd. Belge*, Jan. 3, 1856; and *Dublin Medical Press*, Jan. 30, 1856.)

"Under this term I comprehend settled pains in the limbs of phthisical patients. M. Tanquerel was the first to make use of this expression to designate the acute pains which affect the limbs in cases of saturnine intoxication, correctly remarking that the word αρθρον was employed by the Greeks to signify indifferently limb or articulation.

"The same name, arthralgia, might be given also to those pains in the limbs which mark the third degree of scurvy, and which have been pointed out by the different writers on that disease.

"In phthisis, then, as well as in saturnine poisoning and scurvy, we meet with pains of greater or less intensity affecting the limbs. It is those pains, which are nowhere described or even mentioned, that I am about to bring before my readers, by giving a succinct history of them under the name of the arthralgia of phthisical patients.

"I would first state that these pains show a decided preference for the lower limbs. During about two years that my attention has been directed to the observation of this symptom, I have only once seen the arthralgia settled at the same time in both the lower and upper extremities. I may add that it is very rarely confined to one lower extremity. Almost always it affects both limbs at once, although it is often less intense on one side than on the other. In like manner the arthralgia is seldom limited to the thigh, the leg, or the foot; it almost 'invariably occupies both lower limbs in their entire extent.

"The character of the pain varies a little in individual cases. Thus it is sometimes described as an intolerable sensation of rending or bending; at others it is lancinating, and appears to follow the course of the nervous branches.

"Its intensity is also very variable; some phthisical patients scarcely suffer from it, while in others it is insupportable. I have frequently known this arthralgia elicit groans from the sufferers, and completely deprive them of sleep. Sometimes the pain, especially when it is of recent occurrence, is excited only by pressure; but it soon becomes spontaneous, and in this case, when it is very intense, the slightest touch is sufficient to make the patient cry out.

"This pain is continuous, but it is subject to exacerbations, supervening chiefly during the night; it is never accompanied with convulsive movements of the muscles. I have remarked that when it is very acute, the limbs are flexed and the muscles relaxed; the patient can neither extend nor make use of his limbs.

"It is very difficult to localise these pains. They affect the lower limbs in a mass, without our being able to fix their seat in the nerves, the muscles, or the osseous tissue, either during life, or even after death.

"This arthralgia is met as a prominent symptom in scarcely more than a fourth of the number of those who die of pulmonary tuberculization. It generally shows itself along with the symptoms which constitute the third or colliquative period of pulmonary phthisis.

"It is observed particularly in the cases in which the emaciation is very great, where the fever is high, especially in young subjects of the female sex.

"Sometimes it is complicated with simple œdema of the lower limbs, and one would be tempted to diagnose a case of this kind as one of phlegmasia alba dolens, which is often enough observed in phthisical patients. This error may be avoided by observing that in phlegmasia the skin is tense and does not retain the impression of the finger, while in ordinary œdema it has not these characters; and, moreover, in phlegmasia it will often be possible to feel with the fingers the inflamed venous cord, while in the simple œdema, complicated with arthralgia, nothing of the kind can be observed.

"The prognosis of this affection is very unfavorable. I have never seen tuberculous patients who suffered from it, I will not say get well, but even experience an alleviation of their disease. It indicates that the subject of it labors under a fatally and rapidly progressive consumption.

"The treatment can, consequently, be only palliative. It consists in the external and internal use of the preparations of opium, which occasionally procure relief. Pains of this nature are often relieved by enveloping the limbs in hot cloths."

ART. 50 —*Hourly Pulsation and Respiration in Phthisis, with its relation to Sleep, Food, and Sunlight.* By Dr. EDWARD SMITH, Assistant-Physician to the Hospital for Consumption at Brompton.

(*Lancet*, March 22, 1856.)

The author commences this paper (which was read before the Royal Medical and Chirurgical Society on the 11th of March, 1856), by stating that this investigation was made in June, 1855, and embraced the rate of pulsation and respiration at each of 144 consecutive hours, or six days and nights, in three women and three men, aged twenty, twenty-two, forty, forty-one, and forty-five years, all of whom had cavities in the lungs, but were able to take sufficient food and exercise. The rate was ascertained in the recumbent position, and for this purpose the patients were required to lie down five minutes before each hour. The author first discussed the rate of pulsation, and then that of respiration; and under each head considered the rate both absolutely and as influenced by disturbing causes. The paper was accompanied by numerous tables and diagrams. He ascertained that pulsation is lowest from one to five A M., and highest from ten A M to ten P.M. The effect of sleep is to lower pulsation, and of food commonly to raise it; but the rate of the pulse was increased if the patient rose earlier than usual, without taking breakfast at an earlier hour. The variations in the temperature of the hospital at different hours were very slight, and did not appear materially to influence the pulse. Moderate and gentle exercise also produces little effect, while sunlight powerfully excites pulsation. Respiration in phthisis is constantly much more rapid during the night than in the day; food also produces a well-marked effect in increasing the frequency of respiration. There is a closer correspondence between the temperature and respiration than between temperature and pulsation, but the hours of maximum and minimum respiration did not accord with those of temperature. The effect of sunlight upon the respiration in phthisis appeared to be null. The ratio of the rate of respiration to that of pulsation in phthisis varies with every hour of the day and night, but it is highest in the night, when the pulsation is the lowest, and the respiration highest. The lowest ratio observed was 1 to 5 8, and the highest 1 to 1·4. The author inferred from his investigations that, as profuse perspirations occur in phthisis during sleep, and as in both day and night sleep the pulse is lowered, and to a very great extent in the night, he considers that the former may much depend upon the latter; and acting upon this impression, he has exhibited food during the night with great advantage in preventing perspirations. As day sleep does not depress the pulse so much as night sleep, the perspirations may be somewhat prevented by curtailing the former and encouraging the latter He also recommends early rising, care being taken to exhibit food accordingly. Too much sunlight should be guarded against in summer; while its deficiency in winter, and in close, dark streets and alleys is likely to maintain the state of low vitality which is so essential a part of the disease. The low state of pulsation maintained by many hours of darkness, with the increased ratio of respiration during sleep, indicate the necessity for the administration of nutritious food during the night, and this will also allow the meals taken during the day to be moderate in quantity, and so lessen the unnatural day elevation of the pulse. This might also be accomplished by exhibiting oleaginous substances, as the cod-liver oil, the last thing at night. The author thought that the aim should be, to increase respiration disproportionately to pulsation. This may probably be effected by remedies which give tone to the system, but it is shown to be accomplished by food, and especially by sleep. Hence the due cultivation of the horizontal posture, with frequent food and day sleep, are indicated: early retiring to rest had also the same effect. The author referred to the low ratio of respiration to pulsation, which had been found to exist in persons of unusual stature, and in the early stage of the disease.

ART. 51.—*On the correlation of Phthisis and Diabetes.*
By M. LEGRAND.
(*Gaz. Méd. de Paris*, Dec. 1, 1855.)

On a recent occasion M. Legrand brought before the French Academy of Sciences the notice of a case which was calculated to illustrate this correlation —a correlation which was first pointed out by Dr. Copland.

The particulars of the case are not given in the account to which we have access, but it appears that the patient had suffered from diabetes for some time, with considerable disturbance of the digestive functions, but without any obvious signs of pulmonary disorder. Under proper treatment the dyspeptic symptoms gave way, but there was no diminution of the sugar in the urine. On careful examination, afterwards, symptoms of latent phthisis were detected.

The inference drawn by M. Legrand is that the diabetes was caused in this case by the pulmonary disease—the sugar of the liver not being properly burnt up in the lungs, and so finding its way into the water; and he thinks that this is often the case in diabetes. He concludes, indeed, that, to be treated successfully, diabetes must be treated as a symptom of phthisical disease, rather than as a special affection.

ART. 52.—*Treatment of Hæmoptysis.* By M. ARAN.
(*Gaz. des Hôpitaux*, 1855, No. 94 ; and *American Journal of Medical Science*, April, 1856.)

M. Aran condemns the employment of bloodletting in the treatment of hæmoptysis, believing that it only temporarily arrests the bleeding, while it is dangerous from the debility and increased susceptibility to the intercurrent affections it gives rise to. He has for some time past been engaged in testing the efficacy of various hæmostatic agents employed in hæmoptysis; and in this paper he gives the results of his observations. He considers the essence of turpentine a most valuable remedy, given in doses of from 10 to 30 drops every hour, either in a spoonful of water, or mixed up with magnesia as a bolus. Marked amendment usually occurs in a few hours, and in from twenty-four to thirty-six hours the bleeding ceases. It is less suitable for young or plethoric subjects with febrile action, than in weak cachectic individuals, exhibiting atonic characteristics. Ergot of rye and ergotine are far less efficacious; but chloride of sodium, given in doses of 1 to $2\frac{1}{2}$ drachms proves very efficacious in some cases, and has the advantage of being always at hand. Among the astringents, tannin, and especially gallic acid, are to be recommended : the latter, while quite as efficacious, does not exert the same desiccating effect upon the tissues, or induce the obstinate constipation produced by tannin. As a mean dose, M. Aran gives 15 centigrammes (a centigramme is $\frac{1}{6}$ grain) every hour or alternate hour. He has had little experience in the use of emetic and nauseating remedies; but in three cases in which veratrine was employed, the bleeding ceased as if by enchantment. This class of remedies, indeed, would deserve to stand in the first class of hæmostatic agents, were there not others possessing like efficacy, and yet not giving rise to the painful nausea these produce. M. Aran has derived great advantage from the combined use of digitalis and nitre. In ordinary cases, he gives in the twenty-four hours, 30 centigrammes of digitalis, and $1\frac{1}{2}$ gramme (a gramme is 15 grains) of nitre, divided into four doses; but in very severe cases, these doses may be very much increased, so that the digitalis has been given to the extent of $1\frac{1}{2}$ gramme, and the nitre to 4 grammes, without injuriously affecting the action of the heart, while the effect produced on the hemorrhage has been remarkable. Its arrest never, however, takes place so suddenly under the use of these medicines, as when turpentine or gallic acid is employed.

In abundant, but not immediately dangerous hemorrhage, we can choose among any of the above-mentioned means. In extremely abundant hemorrhage, we must arrest the flow as speedily as possible, by agents which do not depress the powers of the economy too much, and which are not too slow in their operation. Neither ergot, acetate of lead, nor alum is sufficient to meet the danger. Turpentine, gallic acid, chloride of sodium, or nitre with digitalis can alone be trusted ; but the necessity of increasing the dose with the intensity of the hemorrhage may, perhaps, render the chloride of sodium, and especially the nitre and digitalis, dangerous, through the possibility of the production of a too great depression of the heart's action. It is, therefore to gallic acid or turpentine that we must chiefly trust in these severe cases; and we must not limit ourselves to their employment, but also endeavor to procure a temporary arrest of the hemorrhage by ligatures to the limbs and the application of ice to the chest, allowing the means employed internally to consolidate this temporary cure.

ART. 53.—*On the efficacy of small doses of Morphia in certain Chest diseases.*
By Dr. EDWARD SMITH.

(*Assoc. Med. Journal,* Jan. 19, 1856.)

The dose referred to by the author is from the $\frac{1}{24}$th to the $\frac{1}{16}$th of a grain for an infant or young child, and from $\frac{1}{10}$th to $\frac{1}{2}$th of a grain for an adult, repeated from three to six times in the twenty-four hours. The principle involved is the removal of excessive cough in those cases in which the cough resulted from nervous irritability of the structures of the air-passages, and the consequent prevention of the various ill effects which would follow from the continuance of the cough.

The author shows that the effect of minute and often-repeated doses of morphia was far more efficacious than occasional and larger doses; and that the sensorium remained quite unaffected, and the bowels nearly so, under its influence, and therefore that no disturbance to the general system was produced by its administration.

The author selects three diseases in illustration of the merits of the remedy—viz., hooping-cough, the ordinary and spasmodic form of chronic bronchitis, and phthisis.

Hooping-cough he regards as essentially a disease of the nervous system, quite apart from inflammation, and considers the principle of treatment to be the removal of the spasm, so that the cough might be reduced to the harmless state of a common cough. He believes the secretion to be chiefly due to the violence of the cough, and consequently that the aim should not be to increase the secretion by expectorants, but to stop the cough and allow the secretion to cease. He is also of opinion that the congestion of the lungs in more advanced cases, which often leads to other complications, is chiefly due to the spasmodic cough. The treatment recommended is, first, to remove all sources of irritation; to give nutritive food in small quantities, and very frequently; to expose the patient to cool pure air, and in general to place it in the best sanitary conditions, and then to administer morphia. The system adopted in giving the morphia is, to begin with a very small dose ($\frac{1}{24}$th of a grain to an infant four months old), and, if need be, to rapidly increase it until the slightest drowsiness was perceptible, and then to regard that effect as the measure of the dose, and to continue the dose and effect until the spasm subsided. Any dose less than sufficient to effect the sensorium in the slightest degree was insufficient for the immediate cure of the disease; and therefore the art in the administration was to produce and maintain that effect in the quickest way, and with the smallest dose. After giving the $\frac{1}{24}$th of a grain for three or four doses, without any drowsiness, he would then increase it to the $\frac{1}{16}$th of a grain for three or four more doses, and again, if need be, to the $\frac{1}{8}$th and the $\frac{1}{12}$d of a grain, until the slightest drowsiness appeared. Thus the proper dose would soon be ascertained, and within one or two days the spasm would be materially lessened.

He states that within four, and commonly within ten days, he has cured severe cases so far as to reduce the spasmodic to a common cough, and to prevent the occurrence of any complication. The points he especially urges are, the rapid increase of the dose to produce the desired effect, and the careful maintainance of the effect by regulating the dose. He insists upon the necessity of using a graduated measure in the administration of the remedy.

Chronic Bronchitis.—The attacks of this disease commonly seen, in the *habitués* of hospitals, Dr. Smith believes not to be inflammatory, but nervous or spasmodic, both in the cough and the dyspnœa, and also even in the sense of constriction of the chest; and that the aim should not be to increase the secretion, but simply and purely to remove the nervous condition on which the cough, secretion, dyspnœa, and tightness depend. The cough he believes to be much more than needful to remove detached phlegm, and, by its continuance, to excite the secretion; and he infers that, when relief was obtained with the increase of secretion, the former was not due to the latter, but both resulted from exhaustion of the nervous irritability by lapse of time. He therefore commonly banished expectorants, and administered small doses of morphia. The dose was usually $\frac{1}{12}$th of a grain, repeated three or four times a day. Very speedily the cough was relieved, and then the dyspnœa, and at the same time, or subsequently, the sense of tightness. He maintains that the same remedy which first relieved the cough only would, by continuance or increase, relieve the dyspnœa also. As a preliminary step, all sources of irritation are attended to, especially the liver, stomach, and bowels. The croton-oil liniment was efficacious only on the principle laid down by the author, and not upon the relief of any supposed inflammatory action.

Phthisis.—The exhibition of small doses of morphia in phthisis is not with a view to cure that disease, but to lessen or prevent the occurrence of certain important complications which the author believed to be in great part due to the cough; such were hæmoptysis, congestion on inflammatory action, vomiting after food, increase of night perspiration, disturbance of sleep, and the increase of the general irritability of the system. He is decidedly of opinion that, in all stages of the disease, the cough is commonly greater than is required upon the principle of relieving the system; and therefore, and because it leads to further evils, it ought to be arrested. He especially refers to two periods: first, in the early stage, when there is scarcely any secretion, and when the patient voluntarily adds to the cough to remove a little phlegm which he believes to be the cause of the cough. He considers it essential to disabuse the patient's mind of this error, and by that means, and by the aid of morphia, to arrest the cough. Second: he has ascertained that the vomiting of the food after meals was not usually due to disorder of the digestive organs, but to cough accompanying an irritable state of the general system, and a state of repletion of the stomach; and he had commonly prevented it by reducing the quantity of food at each meal (giving the food more frequently), and by administering $\frac{1}{16}$th of a grain of morphia immediately before or after a meal, as well as at the usual intervals during the day. A more tranquil sleep and less severe night sweats resulted from the small dose of morphia, repeated once or twice in the night, than when one large dose was given.

In some of the above conditions, he considered the cough to have the importance not merely of a symptom, but of a substantive disease, and, as such, to require especial attention in the treatment; but, as it was oftentimes associated with constitutional ailments, he frequently combined the morphia with vegetable bitters, and with the sesquichloride of iron. He preferred morphia to other narcotics, because its strength is more uniform than that of vegetable extracts, and more permanent than that of hydrocyanic acid; and, upon the whole, it was as easily capable of minute subdivision and increase in its dose, and was less dangerous in its administration.

ART. 54.—*On a self-adjusting double Stethoscope.* By Dr. POLLOCK, Assistant-Physician to the Hospital for Consumption at Brompton.

(*Lancet*, April 12, 1856.)

"Since the first discovery of auscultation, and its general use, many attempts have been made to obtain an instrument which shall combine simplicity of construction with a high conducting power, and various modifications of the ordinary stethoscope are familiar to all of us. To those most accustomed to the investigation of chest disease, the instrument is of but slight importance, and an accurate estimate of the chest sounds can no doubt be easily made with a simple cylinder, such as Laennec used, or by any of the ebony, cedar, deal, or mahogany tubes which abound in the shops. It is truly to the tact of the observer, and not to the medium applied to the chest, that we owe precision in auscultation; and provided that the instrument be simple, the bore true, the ear-piece easily adjusted to the ear, and the bell so expanded and flattened as to oppose a convenient surface of contact to the chest, we may leave the material of the single instrument to individual taste or fancy. Some will use a solid instrument with precision, whilst, strangely enough, others maintain that the air in the tube is the conducting medium: but on this point I will only stop to remark, that metal, deal, box, ivory, cedar &c., solid and perforated, may be used with nearly equal facility, and that, having acquired by practice the 'hearing ear,' the observer of chest disease may be content to leave refinements of construction to the instrument-maker.

"The increase of sound to be gained by using both ears at once, while all loud external noise is excluded, is, however, a means of obtaining new information on the exploration of the chest, which has excited the attention of several careful ausculiators. Many years ago, Dr. Williams used a double metal tube with two flat ear-pieces,* and adapted to the bell of an ordinary stethoscope, which, except for its inconvenience, would fully answer the above indications, and give great increase in conducting power. M. Landouzy, of Paris, in 1850, constructed an instrument having a number of gum-elastic tubes, by means of which several persons could listen at the same time. In 1851. Dr. N. B. Marsh, of Cincinnati, patented a stethoscope with two gum-elastic tubes, and a membrane over its objective end, which required both hands to keep it in position. More lately, in this country. Dr. Leard has made a double-instrument with gutta percha tubes.

"In January, 1855, Dr. Camman, of New York, had constructed with great care a double self-adjusting instrument, of which the engraving is taken from the 'New York Medical Times' for that month. Dr. Coulson, of Castle Doning-

Fig. 1.

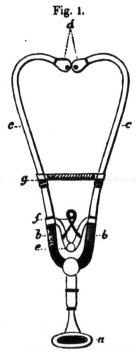

a. Objective end. b. Two gum-elastic tubes. c. Two metallic tubes. d. Two ivory knobs at aural extremities. e. Hinge joint. f. Spiral spring. g. Elastic movable spring.

ton. Leicestershire, having been favored by Dr. Camman with one of his instruments, the former gentleman most kindly placed it at my disposal for experimental purposes. The instrument is fourteen inches long; the tubes are of German silver, with a double curve towards the aural extremities terminating in ivory knobs, which, when applied, should rest closely against the external openings of the ears. The bore is two lines and a half in diameter, and smooth throughout. Dr. Camman dwells much on the accuracy of the curves, and conceives that the sounds conveyed are thereby increased; but it is doubtful if this be the case. Without these curves the instrument would not be capable of self-adjustment. The elastic band or spring retains the aural ends in contact with the ears, and leaves the hands free.

"It will be observed, then, that we have here a very perfect instrument, which conducts the chest sounds to both ears at once, and excludes all ordinary external sounds. The results of many experiments with it prove that it is a great intensifier of sound, acting to the ear the part which a powerful lens performs to the eye. All sounds are magnified many times, and some which were inaudible by the ordinary instrument are revealed to the ear. The healthy respiratory murmur heard through it is a loud blowing, almost like the entrance of air into a smooth cavity, as heard through the single stethoscope. In intensifying, it of course alters the *character* of chest sounds, which, generally speaking, are lowered in *tone* by it. Again, as many magnifying glasses of great power are bad definers, so the ear is apt to be confused by the loudness of the sounds heard, and some practice is therefore necessary to insure accuracy in estimating the modifications of healthy or morbid respiration.

* This and various ingenious modifications of the ordinary stethoscope, constructed for experimental purposes, were kindly shown me by Dr. Williams, on the occasion of his trying the powers of the American instrument now described.

"The dry sounds are more accurately conducted than the moist; and a pure friction, as in the early stage of pleuritis or pericarditis, is rendered very intense; and the dry crepitus occasionally heard in the eary stages of phthisis is greatly developed. The same remark is applicable to the wavy or interrupted inspiration. The healthy expiratory murmur, which (as heard in the single stethoscope) is in duration, when compared with the inspiration, as 1 to 5, becomes prolonged when conducted by this instrument; and, without a knowledge of this fact, the observer would therefore argue some solidification of the lung as the cause of its increased audibility. This observation will at once illustrate the power of the instrument as a conductor, and the special study of it which is necessary before drawing any inference from its use. The voice sounds are greatly intensified, an ordinary pectoriloquy becoming almost startling from its loudness. The heart's sounds are magnified, but more precision in their conduction is to be gained by the use of the ordinary stethoscope. Morbid cardiac sounds are never difficult to *hear*, though their origin may be occasionally obscure: it is therefore plain that a magnifier of sounds would not assist the diagnosis. Certain low and indistinct murmurs, in aneurisms within the chest, might possibly be revealed by its use, which would be otherwise unheard.

"Slight differences in the percussion note are rendered very manifest by applying this instrument to the ears, and holding the bell near the part of the chest percussed, which may be done either by the observer or another person, the self-adjusting power of the stethoscope leaving the hands free. It is obvious that the fœtal heart sounds, and the (so-called) 'bruit placentaire,' in pregnanc , may be heard at a very early period, and that in doubtful cases of fractures, crepitus, undistinguishable by the single stethoscope, would most likely be detected. In applying it to the chest, it is absolutely necessary to remove the dress, as the slightest friction masks all other sounds; its perfect adjustment, so that no air may enter under the edge of the bell, is also requisite.

"It is plain, from the above remarks, that some practice is necessary to enable us to profit by the increased p wers of this stethoscope, as all the sounds are exaggerated, altered in tone, and therefore unlike those which we at present recognize by the aid of the old instrument. It is also evident that it is not likely to displace the latter in daily use, the sounds in which, duly recognized, are sufficiently accurate, and, above all, so universally known, as, in the judgment of skilful observers, to lead to a satisfactory diagnosis. Nay, further, it is little likely that advances in our knowledge of affections are to come through improvements in mechanical devices for measuring or rendering manifest physical alterations in the respiratory organs; but there are various physiological and experimental uses to which such an instrument as this may be applied, and it may also prove a valuable assistance in the investigation of disease. I may add that Mr. Coxeter, of Grafton Street, has, under my directions, constructed with great care some of these instruments."

(C) CONCERNING THE CIRCULATORY SYSTEM.

ART. 55.—*A case of very extensive Suppurative Carditis.*
By M. OPPOLZER, Professor of Clinical Medicine at Vienna.

(*Wochenbl. d. k. k. Gesell. d. Aertze s. Wien*, No. 21, 1855.)

This case is sketched with very great brevity.

CASE.—A strong man, after violently exerting himself by dancing in the open air, experienced extreme precordial anxiety, and expectorated several clots of mucus streaked with blood. He remained almost pulseless until his death, which happened seventy-two hours after the occurrence of these symptoms. During life, the heart beat with extreme feebleness, and the beats were accompanied with to-and-fro rubbing sounds, which were supposed to be indicative of pericarditis; and after death, the entire substance of the left ventricle, and a part of the right ventricle, were infiltrated with pus. This is all that is said about the case.

ART. 56.—*Case in which the Pericardium was tapped, and Iodine injected successfully.* By M. ARAN.

(*Medical Times and Gazette*, April 12, 1856.)

M. Aran, physician of the Hôpital St. Antoine, at Paris, lately brought before the Academy of Medicine the case of a young man, 23 years of age, who was admitted under his care in July, 1855, with all the symptoms of severe pericarditis. The patient had been treated for pleurisy in the same hospital a few months before, and there was reason to believe that tubercles had formed in the lungs. As the young man was, on his second admission, very weak, and affected with diarrhœa, the antiphlogistic treatment could not be used with sufficient energy; and the inflammation of the pericardium, far from becoming subdued, was speedily followed by effusion. The liquid was so abundant, that very severe fits of dyspnœa came on, and M. Aran therefore resolved to tap the pericardium.

Though *physician* to an hospital, he performed the operation himself, with a small-sized trocar and canula, the direction being from below upwards, in the fifth intercostal space, a little below the spot where the dulness on percussion was well marked. The actual extent of the distended pericardium was figured by concentric lines drawn on the chest, and the actual situation of the heart carefully ascertained by auscultation. About twenty-eight ounces of a reddish transparent serosity escaped, with great relief to the urgent symptoms which had called for the operation. An injection was then thrown into the cavity of the pericardium, composed of an ounce and a half of water, half an ounce of tincture of iodine, and fifteen grains of iodide of potassium. The injection was well borne, and a few drachms of the liquid having been allowed to flow out, the wound was closed by compresses.

The symptoms, however, returned, and twelve days after the operation tapping was again had recourse to, when forty-nine ounces of a greenish albuminous liquid escaped. A stronger iodine injection was now used. The operation gave the patient neither pain nor uneasiness, and in the space of ten days the dulness had considerably diminished. But as the heart and pericardium improved, the lungs grew worse; symptoms of tubercles became more plain, and dropsical effusions in various parts of the body appeared. The latter symptoms were removed by blisters and vapor baths, and the patient finally recovered so far as the affection of the pulmonary organs would allow; but the bold treatment used for the pericarditis with effusion was completely successful.

ART. 57.—*On the effects of Lead on the Heart.* By Dr. CORSON, Physician to the New York Dispensary.

(*New York Journal of Medicine*, March, 1856.)

The evidence in this paper, in Dr. Corson's opinion, tends to establish the following conclusions:

1. That allowing a due excess of force to carry on the embarrassed circulation in organic affections of the heart, it appears that certain symptoms in slow poisoning from lead, as well as in cardiac disease proper, typhus fever, and apparent death from catalepsy or other causes, all tend to prove that as a rule the *impulse* may be termed the *pulse of the heart;* and that, its more careful study than heretofore may aid us in the general diagnosis and treatment of disease.

2. That the symptoms of weakening of the heart in lead poisoning, are confined to cases of *partial paralysis, or general muscular debility,* accompanied usually by the purple streak of the gums, indigestion, constipation, pains in the head, muscles, or joints, and sometimes by lead jaundice: and that commencing and emphasising with the most frequent, these heart symptoms from lead are: *weakened or soft tapping impulse; faintness on unusual exertion;* feeble and generally slow pulse; palpitation; cardiac uneasiness: and to these are occasionally added, great despondency or morbid fear of death; suspicions of organic disease of the heart, fainting fits, night-mare, or troubled dreams.

3. That these depressing heart symptoms are absent in the earlier and more acute stage of lead poisoning, known as "*lead-colic,*" when, on the contrary, the

stimulus of pain generally renders the impulse of the heart and the pulse at the wrist more firm than natural.

4. That skill in the detection of minute variations in the impulse of the heart, naturally requires a little careful attention and practice.

5. That these debilitating effects of lead most commonly occur in hearts previously sound, but they sometimes complicate existing organic cardiac disease from rheumatism or other causes.

6. That the agencies or causes of lead poisoning are very numerous, and often obscure ; and that slighter cases supposed to be ordinary dyspepsia, constipation, debility, or bilious colic, are frequently undetected.

7. That the above tests of the immediate influence of lead on the heart disease, are further corroborated by experiments upon animals; showing that, more mildly and slowly, *lead*, like digitalis, oil of tobacco, upas antiar, the woorara, and some other poisons, tends specially to paralyze the central organ of the circulation, and like these, ultimately to produce what Bichat termed " *Death by the heart.*"

8. That the remedies for the paralyzing influence of lead may be divided into two classes : *Disinfectants*, such as the iodide of potassium, and preparations of sulphur; and *Antiparalytics*, such as strychnia and electricity ; that the best treatment combines those two elements, and that, on the whole, the most convenient and efficacious are free doses of the iodide of potassium, and minute proportions of strychnia or nux vomica.

9. That the above conclusions are founded mainly on the evidence of ten cases, principally among the badly nourished and improvident poor finally resorting to public institutions; and they may possibly be somewhat modified in future by more extended observation in private and more favorable practice.

Art. 58.—*Obliteration of the Thoracic Aorta.* By M. Skoda.

(*Wochenbl. der Zeitschr. der k. k. Gesellsch. der Aertze zu Wien*, Nov. 5, 1855; and *Medico-Chir. Review*, April, 1856.)

" At a meeting of the Medical Society of Vienna, held on the 19th of October, 1855, Professor Skoda introduced a man affected with obliteration of the thoracic aorta. In illustration of the lesson, the Professor exhibited preparations of a five-months' fœtus and of a new-born child, in which he indicated the point at which alone this anomaly can take place or has hitherto been observed. It is the point at which the ductus botalli communicates with the aorta and the short space intervening between this point and the origin of the left subclavian artery. During fœtal life, this portion is commonly narrower than the remainder of the aorta, and only acquires the same calibre after birth.

" The individual in question was a man aged forty-seven ; a jeweller; of normal complexion, and throughout well nourished. On the whole, he enjoys good health, and has only come under clinical observation owing to his having, for three years past, suffered from some dyspnœa in making violent exertion. This is due to an insufficiency of the tricuspid valve, which has only been established for three years.

" The following are the grounds upon which Professor Skoda has diagnosed a coexisting obliteration of the aorta : In addition to the blowing murmur coincident with the impulse, and which indicates the above mentioned insufficiency, a 'peculiar vibration or whirring (schwirren) is to be perceived over the greater part of the thorax, partly by palpation, partly, as in the course of the intercostal arteries, by auscultation ; it follows the impulse, and for that reason has its seat in the arteries. The vibration of the arteries of the thorax is due to their dilatation, as may be shown by touching the superficial epigastric arteries, which are much dilated and very tortuous. The beat of the crural arteries at the groin is very feeble, and no pulsation can be felt in the abdominal aorta.'

" These are the indications characteristic of obliteration of the thoracic aorta ; the collateral circulation is carried on by the branches of the subclavian arteries which must therefore be dilated. A large volume of blood passes from the anterior intercostals to the posterior intercostal, and by centripetal movement reaches the descending aorta, which is thus filled with blood sufficient to supply the arteries of the intestines, but not sufficient to produce distinct pulsations. The inferior extremities probably also receive a supply by the anastomosis of the superior and inferior epigastric arteries. No cyanosis is observed, because nowhere venous blood is introduced into the arterial system.

"In connection with this case, Professor Skoda made the following remarks: 1. That in examining the heart, we occasionally perceive murmurs which give rise to the assumption of valvular disease, while the heart is afterwards found healthy; and that the murmur was produced in the coronary arteries or in other arteries, in the vicinity of the heart. Such errors can only be avoided by carefully attending, as in the case detailed, to the coincidence or non-coincidence of the murmur, with the movements of the heart. 2. The circumstances that the nutrition of the individual was unimpaired, although the circulation in most of the organs must be, doubtless, slackened, proves that the deranged nutrition, so frequently coinciding with impediments in the circulation, does not depend solely upon the latter.

"Professor Skoda was of opinion that the obliteration of the aorta was due either to a complete obliteration or absence of the corresponding portion of aorta in the fœtus, or to the contraction of the latter coincidently with the ductus botalli, owing to the exceptional extension of the tissue of this channel into the coats of the aorta. Professor Skoda maintained that the obliteration could not be set down to inflammation, as arteritis led, not to obliteration, but to aneurism. He referred to an analogous case which had occurred in his wards some years previously, where no disturbance of function was manifested until, accidentally, endocarditis supervened. Death occurred later from pneumonia; and the obliterated aorta has been preserved in the anatomical museum of Vienna."

ART. 59.—*Case of Rupture of the Aorta.*
By Dr. G. W. SMITH, Penang.

(*Edinburgh Monthly Journal*, Nov. 1855.)

This case is thus related:

CASE.—"31st July, 1855, I was called at half-past five P. M. to attend Mr. G. B—, æt. 47, married and having a family, who was said to be in a fit. He was upon a couch. looking deadly pale, very anxious, bathed in a cold, profuse perspiration, and with a weak, quick pulse. He complained of great weakness, of *severe* pain across the middle of the chest, and in the neck; but there were neither cough nor difficulty of breathing. He said that he had suddenly felt sick, giddy, and would have fallen, but for the support of a friend. During the previous part of the day, he had experienced no indisposition. and only a short time before had eaten dinner with usual appetite, but was a little fatigued from having been up all the previous night, watching a person in an apoplectic fit, and was taken ill when about to accompany the funeral of the body of that individual. On inquiry, he added that for some months back, he had felt short of wind on going up hill, but did not experience the same on ascending a stair, and had been subject to rheumatic pains (as he termed them) about the chest and neck, but was not liable to palpitation, and considered himself in the enjoyment of good health. He was a man of short stature, rather robust than square, and of quick, dogmatic temperament; a missionary by profession, and performed the duties of a preacher and teacher, and for some years had also been a little engaged in agricultural pursuits: his habits were strictly temperate.

" He was conveyed to his house, about half a mile distant; a mustard poultice was applied to the chest, a little spirit of lavender administered, and his damp clothes removed. He felt somewhat relieved, after the mustard acted, of the pain of the chest, but still complained much of that of the neck. At seven P. M., when I left him, the skin had regained a natural warmth, the pulse was improved, but the countenance was still very pale.

" I learned from Mrs. B—, that Mr. B—, although usually, to all appearance, in good health, had yet, during the last year and a half, repeatedly complained of being sick and faint, requiring him to lie down for a moment, to recover; and that this was especially the case after food; but in these attacks there was nothing that excited her alarm.

"I warned her that there probably was serious organic disease of the heart or arterial system, and advised that the usual medical attendant, who was then absent, should be consulted.

"1st August. at half after three A. M., was sent for in a great hurry, and on my arrival a few minutes after, found Mr. B— dead. It seemed that, about nine last night. the pain of the chest returned, that of the neck continuing persistent; but as they were deemed rheumatic, no particular alarm was taken. He continued to suffer in that way. more or less severely, up to three A. M , when, sitting up in bed, he suddenly called out, 'Another fit, a fit,' and dropped down. He was thought by Mrs. B— to have fainted, and she used such remedies as occurred to her for that, for some time before she discovered that he was dead.

"*Diagnosis.*—Internal hemorrhage, which had by some means been arrested for a while, and then returned with fatal effect.

"*Autopsy.*—Five hours after death, in presence of Mr. Williamson, of the Madras Medical Service, and of Mr. Rose, of the Bengal Medical Service, the medical attendant of the family. who could not be present at the beginning, but arrived during the course of the examination.

"The external appearance of the body bloodless. The thoracic and abdominal cavities being laid open, and the innominate vein being wounded in reflecting the parts, blood flowed from it, and oozed also freely from the sections of the swollen veins. There was a considerable deposition of fat between the layers of the abdominal parietes, and fat was also abundantly found deposited in the omentum. A cursory inspection only was made of the abdominal viscera, and all appeared healthy. There were some old adhesions of the pleura costalis and pulmonalis, at the apex of right lung. The left pleural cavity contained several ounces of serum. The pericardium being slit open, exposed to view a large amount of coagulated blood, which being removed, extravasation was observed beneath the cellular covering of the aorta. The lungs. heart, and pericardium, as well as the aorta and a portion of the innominate and left carotid and subclavian arteries, were all carefully removed from the body. The lungs being found healthy, were detached from the rest. The different cavities of the heart were then laid open, in succession, and were found empty; and all, as well as their respective valves, were, so far as we could see, free from disease. The pulmonary artery was then slit open, from its origin to its division, and exhibited nothing abnormal, nor did the valves between it and the ventricle. The cellular substance and pericardial covering having been dissected off the aorta, extensive extravasation was seen to exist between the external and middle coats of that vessel from its origin to the giving off of the large vessels of the neck, and to a small extent along their course. The aorta was then slit open from its origin to nearly where it perforates the diaphragm, to which extent it had been removed. Throughout the upper part. as far as the giving off the large vessels of the neck, there were numerous deposits of atheromatous degeneration in and beneath the serous coat, varying in size; some being mere points, two or three about as large as a sixpence, but none very prominent, so as to project much into the vessel; and the interior of the vessel was studded with small holes, some of which were sufficiently large to admit the round end of a surgeon's probe, which perforated the inner and middle coats, and admitted the probe to the extravasated blood, observed between the external and middle coats. A rupture of the inner and middle coats of the vessel, of several lines in extent, was discovered at the origin of the innominate artery, and another of smaller extent at the origin of the left carotid. Through these ruptures the blood had escaped, and separated the external from the middle coats, throughout the whole circumference of the aorta from the ruptures to its origin, and a thin congestion lay between them, but no deposit of fibrin. The external coat had given way near the heart, and allowed the blood vent into the pericardial sac. The aorta was not dilated throughout any part of the extent of it examined, and the valves at its mouth were perfectly healthy. The head was not opened.

"The immediate cause of death was, no doubt, loss of blood through the rupture in the aorta. One or both of these, in all probability, took place to some extent, the moment complaint was first made of sickness and faintness; but the external coat resisting for a time the escape of the blood, permitted the patient to rally; the strain, however, continuing upon that coat, and probably becoming greater from the extent of the ruptures increasing, it at length gave way, and permitted the blood to flow into the pericardium, at which moment the second and fatal fit happened—nine and a half hours after the first. The swelling, occasioned in the first place by the escape and lodgment of blood between the coats of the vessel, may perhaps explain the severe pain experienced across the chest and in the neck, by the pressure that would exert upon the recurrent branch of the vagus nerve of left side, which winds round the aorta in that situation The absence of dyspnœa is perhaps, too, accounted for by the absence of disease of the heart or lungs, or of any other disease that could seriously retard the circulation. It is probable that the disease of the coats of the aorta was of some years' standing; but with no obvious symptomatic indications, and with insufficient causes to produce marked physical evidence, I think it not likely that the disease could have been discovered during life. Could the fits of sickness and faintness, occasionally experienced, have arisen from a slight escape of blood through the holes noticed, which had afterwards been resolved?"

Art. 60.—*Case of Thoracic Aneurism ascending into the Neck, with permanent Contraction of the Pupil of the Left Eye.* By JOHN T. BANKS, M.D., King's Professor of Physic, Physician to the Whitworth and Hardwicke Hospitals.

(*Dublin Hospital Gazette,* Jan. 15, 1856.)

The case which Dr. Banks details is one which presents a feature of great clinical interest, and which, from its extreme rarity, is worthy of being placed on record, and added to the two previously reported examples of aneurism, in which the phenomenon of contracted pupil has been noticed in connection with the disease. That the state of the pupil existing in this case must be of very unusual occurrence, may be inferred from the absence of any mention of it in the works of many writers who have so largely contributed to our knowledge on the subject of cardiac and arterial disease. Dr. Banks proceeds: " I was not myself aware that contracted pupil had ever been remarked under similar circumstances to those in the case about to be narrated, until my attention was attracted to a communication from my friend Dr. Gairdner, in the August number of the 'Edinburgh Journal,' a periodical the pages of which are frequently enriched by highly valuable communications from the pen of this distinguished physician.

" The case, in which this condition of the pupil was observed by Dr. Gairdner, was one of aneurism of the aorta projecting into the neck: he observes that it is ' an interesting example of a pathological condition explicable by physiological laws.'

" Dr. Gairdner refers to the researches of Dr. John Reid on the vagus nerve, and also to the experiments of Valentin, and comes to the conclusion that these investigations are clearly applicable to the explanation of the case he communicates. According to Valentin, the iris is furnished with nerves from two sources. The section of the sympathetic trunk in the neck paralyses the nerves which act on the radiating fibres of the iris, from the spinal system *through the sympathetic,* and resigns the pupil to the exclusive influence of the circular fibres, or those which contract the pupil, and which are supplied from the inferior branch of the motor oculi nerve, and thus the pupil is kept permanently contracted. Budge and Waller's experiments are confirmatory of Valentin's views.

" Stimulating the sympathetic in the neck dilates the pupil, and cutting it causes contraction of the pupil more or less permanent.

" It appears that the records of medicine present only one case of aneurism, in which contracted pupil had been noted, previous to the case described by Dr. Gairdner. In the year 1838, Mr. Hare, the house-surgeon of the Stafford Infirmary, published, in the ' Medical Gazette,' a report of a case in which a scirrhous tumor, occupying the inferior triangular space on the left side of the neck, was accompanied by a *contracted state* of the pupil. On dissection, after death, it was found that the pneumogastric, phrenic, and *sympathetic* had passed into its substance, and were transformed into diseased structure.

" Dr. Gairdner refers to a case of aneurism at the root of the neck, noted by Dr. Walshe, in which the pupil was observed to be ' very notably smaller than the other.' "

CASE.—"A. F., a woman, æt. 24, was admitted into the Whitworth Hospital on the 27th of November, 1855. She stated she was a married woman and had four children, and it was afterwards ascertained that she was a person of dissolute and highly intemperate habits. She was rather delicate in appearance, and of slender form; but she said her health was perfectly good until twelve months before her admission into hospital. At this period she received severe injuries from blows inflicted by her husband. Her lower jaw was broken, and she fell heavily on her left shoulder. For some time after she experienced pain in the side of the neck and point of the shoulder, light at first, but gradually becoming more severe, and causing her to lean to the left side.

" The complaint for which she sought admission was bronchitis. Her breathing, she informed us, had been for a considerable time short. more especially on making any unusual exertion, but it had recently become more oppressed, and the cough had been accompanied by stridor. Aphonia did not exist. On proceeding to examine her chest the following condition of parts was observed: There was an obvious prominence, involving the left clavicular region, extending beyond the median line, and also above the clavicle, the sternal end of which was displaced forwards, and a little upwards. The superficial veins were enlarged over the infra-clavicular region. The jugular vein at the left side was also larger than the right. An impulse is visible at the upper sternal and subclavicular regions. The sternal half of the clavicle is dull on percussion, as is also the infra-clavicular region, to an extent of two inches beneath the bone at its sternal end. The upper third of the sternum is also dull, and over the tumor percussion gives a sensation of abnormal resistance. With regard to the acoustic phenomena, two sounds are audible in the same situation, resembling the cardiac sounds, but being less clear. Neither sound approaches in the least to the character of a murmur. No pulsation can be discovered in the left carotid, and the radial pulse is absent. The respiratory murmur is decidedly more feeble over the left lung than the right.

" Pain was experienced in the seat of the aneurismal tumor, and it extended along the inside of the arm to the ring and little finger. The arm was also numb and colder than the right arm; there had never been œdema. The first time this patient was seen by me, I remarked that the left eye was smaller than the right, and upon examination of the eye, I noticed also that the left pupil was smaller than the right. This condition of the pupil was constant, I mean its being always relatively smaller; it was susceptible of change, however; but in strong light. or in shade, the relation between the two pupils continued the same. The sight of the left eye was as good as that of the right. I repeatedly and most minutely made the eye the subject of investigation, and I called the attention of my clinical class to this singular phenomenon. I had intended to have made some observations on the effect of atropine on the eye, but I failed in my endeavor to induce the patient to remain in hospital, after she experienced relief from the symptoms for which she sought admission originally. At some future time I may be enabled to communicate the sequel of this highly interesting case; meantime I considered the case, incomplete as it is, worthy of publication, for taken in connection with Dr. Gairdner's case and the other, it may aid ' in fixing the attention of physicians on the state of the pupil in similar cases of disease.' To Dr. Gairdner is due the merit of bringing the contracted state of the pupil, as a result of pressure produced by aneurismal tumors on the nerves, in a prominent manner before the profession, and thus in his own words he has 'indicated a new source of functional disturbance in thoracic aneurism, as connected with the interference of such tumors with the nervous system.'

" In conclusion, I may refer to the fact not observed in the former cases, namely, that in the case under consideration, not only was there contraction of the pupil, but the eye itself was considerably smaller than the other."

ART. 61.—*On Factitious Heart Sounds, &c.* By (1) Dr. JENNER, Physician to University College Hospital; and (2) Dr. ELLIOTSON, F.R.S.

(*Medical Times and Gazette*, March 1 and April 5, 1856.)

(1) In a clinical lecture, recently delivered, Dr. Jenner makes some remarks of much practical value, upon the effects of pressure in producing, intensifying,

and modifying certain morbid sounds in the heart and great vessels, in the larynx and in the lungs.

"There are," he commences, "three patients still in the hospital, and others have recently left it, in whom I pointed out to you some facts illustrating the influence of pressure in the production, intensification, and modification of certain morbid sounds generated in the region of the heart.

"To the case of the lad Exley, suffering from pericarditis, I lately directed your attention at length; I will recall some of the points of the case to your memory; when the stethoscope was placed over any part of the præcordial region between the fourth and seventh costal cartilages, two abnormal sounds were heard with each beat of the heart—one systolic, the other diastolic—I say systolic and diastolic, though they were not completely synchronous in point of time with the heart's systole and diastole. Loud as were the murmurs, especially the systolic, over the heart, they were not audible when the stethoscope was placed at a very little distance from the præcordial region. In character the murmurs were rubbing. I pointed out to you at the bedside, that the case offered us a perfect example of the to-and-fro sound of Dr. Watson. Moreover, the sounds impressed on all who heard them the idea that they were generated very near to the stethoscope. As the parietes of the lad's thorax were tolerably flexible, a moderate force sufficed to bring the two layers of the pericardium more closely into contact, and so the friction resulting from the passage over each other of the roughened visceral and parietal layers of the pericardium, was increased, and consequently the murmur generated by the friction was intensified. At one time it was supposed (and is so still by some), that murmurs generated in the pericardium could always be intensified by pressure in the young; and, also that when a murmur, audible over the heart, could be intensified by pressure, that absolute proof was obtained that the murmur was generated in the pericardium.

"However, we now know that neither of these statements is true; for, Dr. Walshe has observed one or more cases in which a pericardial murmur was diminished in loudness by pressure, the free play of the surfaces being impeded by the pressure. And the girl Stone, and the boys Perrin and Whiting, afford us indisputable evidence that a murmur may not merely be intensified, but may even be generated at the base of the heart, by pressure. These children are aged respectively 7, 9, and 10; the girl was the subject of chorea, one boy is suffering from enlargement of the spleen, the other from a skin affection; all have well-formed chests, but in all the thoracic walls are very flexible. Moderate force causes recession of the sternum, and of the cartilages of the ribs, and consequently of the parts subjacent.

"In reference to these children, and several other cases of a like kind, which I have noted, I wish to impress on you the following facts:

"1. That no murmur was audible when the stethoscope was applied without force to the sternum, or to the cartilages of the ribs.

"2. That when a moderate amount of pressure was exerted, through the medium of the stethoscope, on the sternum, over the base of the heart, a systolic murmur was audible.

"3. That the loudness of the murmur varied with the degree of the pressure.

"4. That pressure on the base of the sternum did not elicit a murmur.

"5. That pressure on the sternum, opposite and above the fourth cartilage, and below the first costal cartilage, elicited a murmur.

"6. That the healthy sounds of the heart only were to be heard at the second right costal cartilage, whatever the amount of force to which it was subjected.

"7. That a moderate degree of pressure on the second left costal cartilages, or on the second left intercostal space, near the sternum, rendered a murmur audible.

"Judging, then, from the situations in which the murmur was producible, viz., over the base of the heart and upwards to the first left interspace: the period in the heart's beats which it occupied, viz., the systole; and the manipulation required to elicit it, viz., pressure, I think there can be no doubt—1. That in these cases the murmur was generated in the pulmonary artery. 2. That the murmur was produced by the passage of the blood through a narrow part of the vessel into a wider part. 3. That the direct force exercised on the thoracic parietes by the stethoscope, was the immediate cause of the local diminution of the calibre of the vessel.

"The only observer who has, so far as I know, recorded a case identical with those to which I have just referred, is Dr. Latham. You will find the case in his third Clinical Lecture; it is so admirably told that I must read it to you: 'A little boy, aged 8½ years, high-spirited and vivacious, but thin and out of health, was brought to me under a suspicion of disease of the heart. Its impulse was not felt beyond the apex, but there it was in excess; yet there was no larger space of dulness than natural in the præcordial region Upon auscultation, however, this remarkable peculiarity was made out: when the ear or the stethoscope rested gently upon the præcordial region, no unnatural sound whatever was heard; but when either the ear or the stethoscope was applied with such force as to cause the ribs to sink a little below their natural level, then a loud bellows murmur sprang up. The space at which it was heard, and not beyond it, was just so far as the mouth of the stethoscope covered, when it was placed upon the cartilage of the third rib as a centre. This case, which occurred to me,' continues Dr. Latham, 'five years ago, has made me watchful ever since, lest haply I might create the murmur I was in search of; and it is no needless caution where the patient is young, and the framework of the chest is yielding. Never, indeed, the chest being not deformed, never but in this single instance have I produced a murmur simulating that of valvular disease. But very often, when over-earnest in what I was about, I have ressed too heavily on the præcordial region, a sort of jarring sound has reached my ear, and brought with it the suspicion of disease; until setting the heart free from the weight and the restraint which I had inadvertently imposed on it, I have at once lost the sound and the apprehension too, which had arisen from my own awkward manœuvring.'

"Since, however, my attention was directed to the subject by hearing the produced murmer in the girl Stone, I have found that I have been able to produce a basic systolic murmur in a large number of healthy children, and I am satisfied that Dr. Latham's caution is highly necessary, viz.—that when examining a child you must be careful not to exercise much pressure at the base of the heart, lest you produce a murmur which may cause considerable anxiety in regard to the ultimate fate of your patient. For you will remember that the murmur produced by the weight of your own head on the stethoscope placed over the base of the heart, in the girl Stone, was infinitely louder than you or I ever heard in the same situation from mere anæmia, or spanœmia, as what we lately knew as anæmia is now often called. Had I not detected the cause of the murmur, I should have supposed the child to be the subject of congenital disease of the heart.

"In the girl May, lately admitted into Ward 3, because the subject of tape-worm, we found that pretty firm pressure on the thoracic walls over the pulmonary artery modified materially the first sound, and although we could not say that a murmur was produced by the pressure, we could not but admit that so long as the pressure was maintained the first sound was not healthy.

"This again confirms the accuracy of Dr. Latham's observations, recorded in the quotations I have read to you from his lectures.

"I have told you that the murmur produced by the pressure over the base of the heart, in the cases in the hospital, originated in the pulmonary artery; I must add, that I doubt much whether pressure can be exercised over the base of the heart, powerful enough to diminish the calibre of the aorta, and for these reasons: 1. Because of the relative situation of the aorta and pulmonary artery. 2. Because of the comparative thickness of its walls. I am inclined, then, to think, that systolic basic endocardial murmurs produced or intensified by pressure have their origin in the pulmonary artery. So when in doubt as to whether a systolic basic endocardial murmur is generated in the pulmonary artery or aorta, I have derived some assistance in arriving at a correct conclusion from a consideration of the effect produced on it by pressure.

"The little boy Perrin, now in Ward 4, and whom you can see after the conclusion of the lecture, affords us an example of a very common condition, viz.: one in which the patient can exercise pressure on his own pulmonary artery, sufficiently powerful to generate a murmur. So long as this child is inspiring there is no cardiac murmur, but at the termination of expiration there is a loud blowing, systolic murmur; this murmur has its point of greatest intensity at midsternum, opposite the third interspace; it is louder at the first left than at the first right intercostal spaces next to the sternum; it is not audible at the apex. These facts show the pulmonary artery to be the seat of the murmur. During forced expiration the anterior surface of the thorax is flattened, the antero-posterior diameter of the thorax is considerably shortened, and so the pulmonary artery is pressed on. This child, as you know, is remarkably anæmic, there is a very loud venous hum in his neck, and it is difficult to place the stethoscope over his carotid artery without compressing it enough to generate a systolic murmur.

"Compression of the pulmonary artery by the patient in expiration, or by the physician with his stethoscope, is a common determining cause of the basic systolic murmur so often heard in anæmia. In anæmia, too, the arterial walls appear to resist pressure less strongly than in health, and this is one of the reasons why it is sometimes almost impossible to place the stethoscope on the carotid artery of an anæmic young woman, without diminishing its calibre at the spot, and so generating a loud murmur."

Dr. Jenner then proceeds to show that the pulmonary artery may be compressed by the sternum, during expiration, sufficiently to produce a murmur when the patient is not anæmic, if the chest is very flat from before backwards, and if the walls are very flexible. Moreover, factitious sounds may be produced in the aorta and pulmonary artery, when the position of the heart is altered in relation to these vessels, by the pressure of fluid, as in ascites, &c. Prolonged cough may have a similar effect. Dr. Jenner also points out that the thrill which is felt by the hand in some morbid conditions of the heart and great vessels, may be diminished or extinguished by pressure, and that the natural fremitus which is felt over the larynx and chest generally may be changed in the same manner.

(2) Dr. Elliotson's remarks, apparently, were called forth by the preceding lecture of Dr. Jenner. Dr. Elliotson says:

"It is more than five and twenty years since I published cases of morbid sounds of the heart without disease at any of its openings. In the 'Lumleian Lectures,' published by me in 1830, I stated, at page 18, that—'I once witnessed a remarkable instance of the temporary occurrence of this (the bellows) sound. In this case there was ascites; and the bellows sound, which was in the region of the left ventricle, instantly ceased on the removal of the fluid from the abdomen, and was not heard for several weeks, when the fluid again accumulated, and it again became audible.' In my lectures on the practice of Medicine at University College, London, I invariably mentioned this case from 1831 to 1838 inclusively, and I find, in the editions of them published by Dr. Rogers and Mr. Lee, that I added the remark that, 'after death, the opening was found healthy, but the left ventricle dilated. It appeared to me that the diaphragm, being pushed up by the water, tilted the heart a little, so that the passage of the blood into the aorta was a little impeded.'

"I have never met with such an instance again, nor had I ever heard of one, and I was, therefore, pleased on reading one recorded by Dr. Jenner in the 'Medical Times and Gazette' of the 1st of last month. 'When the abdomen is enormously distended,' says this gentleman, 'the relation between the ventricles and the orifice of the pulmonary artery and aorta is altered, and a murmur may be the consequence. A well-marked case of this kind fell under my observation some time since; the patient was the subject of ovarian dropsy; at the base of her heart a loud blowing murmur was heard; whether generated in the heart or pulmonary arteries could not be determined; perhaps a murmur originated in both. She was tapped, and all murmur disappeared. In such cases the apex of the heart is tilted' (p. 204).

"As, notwithstanding my examination of the sounds of the heart in the numerous cases of peritoneal and ovarian dropsy, some of them of course enormous, that I have attended subsequently, I have not met with the same occurrence, I presume that the sound depended upon the tilted ventricle being morbidly dilated. In my patient the accumulation was not enormous, either in the first or the second accumulation of fluid. Dr. Jenner does not mention that he was able to learn whether the sound in his case returned with a return of the accumulation of fluid, or that the heart labored under dilatation—two important facts in my case; but he must be pleased equally with myself in recording his case in confirmation of mine, which he heard me detail in each course of my lectures attended by him in University College.

"Among the many cases which I have seen of effusion into the left pleura, and of removal of the apex of the heart to the right side, I have never heard a morbid sound of the heart. Nor was one to be expected, because, the apex of the heart being pushed to the right, there can be no impediment to the exit of the blood into the aorta; whereas, when the heart is pushed upwards by the diaphragm, the apex will incline to the left, and the course of the blood into the aorta be, in some circumstances, more or less impeded.

"In the same lectures, it will be found that I stated the observation made by me upon the similar effect of posture upon a morbid sound of the heart in some cases. 'A patient was, some months ago, in St. Thomas's Hospital, in whom the recumbent posture produced it. She was a young woman, with chronic bronchitis, dyspnœa, livid lips, and œdematous legs, and afforded no bellows sound while erect; but it became audible the moment she lay down.' 'I have since noticed the same fact in other cases of dyspnœa; and it shows the necessity of examining patients in both postures. By continuing the investigation of this point, I have ascertained that the preternatural sound heard with the pulse is generally louder, and often very much louder, in the recumbent posture; while the preternatural sound when articular is louder, if anything, in the erect. The cause of the ventricular bellows sound being less in the erect posture is, perhaps, that the ventricle is then drawn down more into a straight line with the aorta by the gravitation of the heart, and an easier exit given to the blood.' ('Lumleian Lectures.')

"At the period of my lectures, a difference of opinion existed as to narrowness of passage producing a morbid sound; and I therefore mentioned ' our being able to produce the bellows sound in the abdomen by compressing the abdominal aorta with a stethoscope; and to regulate its intensity by varying the degree of pressure.'

"In anæmia, the morbid sound in the neck may be increased, or even brought on altogether, by pressure with the stethoscope, or by turning the head very much round to the opposite shoulder; as is well known, and as I have done and do continually. I have, for several years since I ceased to lecture, been in the habit of increasing the morbid sounds of the openings of the heart, by making the patient, whatever his age, expire as forcibly as possible, and refrain from inspiring again as long as possible. This measure is useful in cases of doubtful morbid sounds of the heart; and I adopted it with the view of bringing the heart and the walls of the chest in as great proximity as possible, that its sounds might more perfectly reach my ear. But Dr. Peter Latham produced a morbid sound by pressing the walls of the chest upon the heart of a child, and Dr. Jenner has done it in many children, the parietes of whose chests are of course yielding, by moderate pressure with the stethoscope on the second left costal cartilage, or on the second left intercostal space, where the pressure would influence, he suggests, the pulmonary artery."

(D) CONCERNING THE ALIMENTARY SYSTEM.

Art. 62.—*Quinsy treated internally by Belladonna.*
By M. POPPER.

(*Prager Vierteljahr. f. d. prak. Heilk.*, 1855; and *Gaz. Hebdom. de Med. et Chir.*, Jan. 11, 1856.)

Resting, as he says, upon an experience of more than 500 cases, M. Popper asserts that small doses of the tincture of belladonna, frequently administered, will cure quinsy in twenty-four hours, if the inflammation be not of a syphilitic character, or associated with a diphtheritic condition of the mucous membrane. No particulars are given.

ART. 63.—*A case of Scirrhus of the Pancreas.* By Dr. WM. THORN.

(*Lancet,* Nov. 10, 1855.)

This case is related as follows:

CASE.—Mrs. C—, a lady 44 years of age, mother of three children, a native of, and long resident in, British India, who had suffered from fever and ague, from which she had recovered under the use of *mercury* and quinine, came under my care three weeks before her death. She said that she had been suffering from constant vomiting and purging for four months past, for which every kind of homœopathic remedy had been tried *without effect;* she was now complaining of excessive dryness of the mouth, there being an *entire suppression of the salivary secretion,* and a constant discharge of mucus and blood from the nostrils and back portion of the throat; she was in an excessively *anæmic state,* no doubt produced by the vomiting, which was of *an exceedingly acid character,* and purging of *a bilious and most offensive odor;* the bodily appearance gave the idea of a malignant disease, and the constant diarrhœa was considered to diagnose ulceration of the bowels; *still there was no pain,* either constant or occasional, not even when the stomach was sharply pressed; for after examining the uterus without effect, the scirrhus was looked for in that viscus. Having ordered injections of beef tea, and laudanum to cause them to be retained, several times daily, and the exhibition of the citrate of iron internally, and, by the advice of Dr. Elliotson, the sulphate of that salt, by enema, as an addition to the beef tea, and having run the patient through the gamut of copper, tannin. gallic acid, and strychnine, for the relief of the diarrhœa, without effect, she finally sunk into a deep sleep, apparently the result of the attention of a female mesmerist (for the injections had been omitted), for which the poor patient so urgently craved that her friends deemed it right to indulge her wish in that respect. This comatose state lasted about four days, during all which time the pulse was only 80, having dropped down from 96; the breathing 24, and perfectly regular, and the vomiting ceased entirely, the diarrhœa also ceasing in a material degree. Finally, at the end of the fourth day, life departed without a struggle, it really being a simple cessation of breathing without the least apparent pain.

The post-mortem revealed that the heart, lungs, *liver,* and spleen were perfectly *healthy:* perhaps under a magnifying glass, it might be said that there existed in the liver the slightest trace of fatty degeneration; the pancreas, however, was coverted into a dense white fibrous mass: and although the duct was pervious, it is quite evident (and I have the preparation before me while I write) that no fluid could have been secreted for a long time past; the colon was extensively ulcerated throughout, which, doubtless, accounted for the continuous and unsubduable diarrhœa.

ART. 64.—*On the nature of the change known as Fatty Liver.*
By M. LEREBOULLET.

(*Mém. de l' Acad. Impériale de Med.;* and *Medico-Chir. Rev.,* July, 1855.)

The following are the conclusions of the author:

" 1. The fatty degeneration of the liver is due to the accumulation of fat in the biliary cells themselves. 2. Special fatty cells are not formed, as biliary cells would then be found amidst the fatty ones, which is not the case. 3. Nothing authorizes us to admit that the fat becomes developed in the interstices external to the cells. 4. The biliary cells may, by the accumulation of fat, acquire double or triple their normal volume, this development of the cells explaining the increased size of the fatty liver. 5. These cells entirely lose their secretory character, and no longer contain biliary granules: the biliary secretion is obstructed. and the contracted gall-bladder contains but little bile. 6. The fatty degeneration induces a decolorized state of the liver which progresses from the periphery towards the centre of a lobule, giving the organ a spotted and reticulated appearance. 7. The decoloration arises from the development of the fatty cells compressing the portal vesicles, and impeding the circulation in them. 8. In the artificial fattening of geese, the liver only becomes loaded with fat after the other organs of the body, and especially the abdominal viscera, have become saturated with it. 9. The cells of the liver of fattened geese differ from pathological fat-cells, inasmuch as the fat that fills the former always retains the form of distinct droplets, accumulated in the cell, to which they give an irregular appearance on distension: while in the pathological cells the fat becomes united into larger and larger drops, until the cell is at last distended by a single one like a balloon. 10. The fatty cells in the goose resemble, as regards the deposition of the fat in the interior, the physiological fatty cells of the fœtus and those of the lower animals. 11. The nuclei of the normal cells, as well as the biliary granules, disappear when the fatty degeneration commences. 12. The degeneration takes place simultaneously throughout the organ, but all the fatty cells do not present the same degree of development. 13. This change of biliary into fatty cells is observed in tuberculosis, cancer, cirrhosis of the liver, &c. 14. The deposition of fat in the cells appears to be closely connected with a diminution of the nutritive process, and consequently of organic combustion, which is the primary condition of that process. When the quantity of oxygen absorbed is less than in the normal state (as in tuberculosis, cancer, and probably all diseases of nutrition); or, when the respiratory elements (fecula, &c.) are taken in too large proportions, the combustion of these substances is incomplete, and the chemical elements which enter into their composition combine so as to form fat, which is deposited in the biliary cells.

ART. 65.—*A case bearing upon the origin of Tape-worm.*
By Dr. GAIRDNER, Physician to the Royal Institutes at Edinburgh.

(*Edinburgh Monthly Journal*, March, 1856.)

At a recent meeting of the Medical and Chirurgical Society of Edinburgh, Dr. Gairdner narrated the case of a girl, at present under his care in the Infirmary, which seemed to support the views of Siebold and Kuchenmeister, as to the transformation of the cysticercus cellulosæ, found in the hog and other domestic animals, into the *tænia solium.* Nine yards of the tape-worm had been expelled under the action of the shield-fern oil. On inquiry, the girl admitted that she had been in the habit of eating quantities of raw pork and butcher-meat generally. This was from a peculiar liking or inclination of her own, and was not a habit contracted in consequence of the example of others. In other respects her diet had been similar to that generally in use in her station in life in Scotland. It was well ascertained, that in Scotland the occurrence of tape-worm was rare as compared with some parts of England, and very rare when compared with some other European countries. It was not less unusual in Scotland to indulge in the eating of raw flesh, which practice was believed to be a frequent source of the production of tænia. The occurrence of tænia was very common in Germany, where the practice of eating raw ham was also prevalent. On the other hand, Dr. Gairdner had reason to believe that tænia was rare in Holland, where the eating of raw animal food is very unusual. Dr. Gairdner alluded to a case lately published by Dr. Crighton ('Monthly Journal,' June, 1855), in which he had been able to trace the occurrence of tænia solium to the practice of eating raw meat, a practice which was common among the Lancashire operatives. Dr. Gairdner was inclined to attribute the rarity of the occurrence of hydatids in Scotland, to the small proportion of animal food, and especially of ill-cooked animal food, used by the laboring classes. During Dr. Gairdner's connection, as pathologist, with the Infirmary, he had opened not fewer than 1500 bodies, and he had never met with a single case of hydatids of the liver. Two cases had otherwise come under his notice; but in his dissections at the Infirmary, he had never seen one instance of the occurrence of the acephalocyst. In the London hospitals a considerable number were known to occur every year.

(E) CONCERNING THE GENITO-URINARY SYSTEM.

ART. 66.—*Case of Tubercle of the Kidney.*
By Dr. BASHAM, Physician to the Westminster Hospital.

(*Lancet*, Dec. 8, 1855.)

"Notwithstanding that diseases of the kidneys have been studied with results as advantageous to correct diagnosis as they have been beneficial to the general principles of treatment, there are, nevertheless, morbid conditions of these organs, which still, and perhaps ever must, except under very peculiar circumstances, present difficulties and obstacles to a correct diagnosis. Tubercle of the kidney is a disease of this character; it is of comparative unfrequency, and if the record of such a case does not assist in clearing away the obstacles to a correct estimate of the presence of this deposit in the kidney, it will, however, exhibit the group of symptoms, as well as the complications which may arise and become associated with tubercle in these organs. The following case will demonstrate that while the existence of pyelitis, probably from calculus in the pelvis of the kidney, as well as the sacculated and enlarged condition of the right kidney, was clearly made out during life, yet, on the other hand there was nothing in the urinary secretion or other symptoms that could suffice for the suspicion of the presence of tubercle. The amorphous organic granular matter, insoluble in hydrochloric or acetic acids, and associated with pus in the urine, which has been supposed characteristic of softening tubercle of the kidney, was in this case so masked by the presence of amorphous granular earthy (phosphatic) matter, but readily soluble in these acids, that tubercle was neither suspected nor recognized. And even after death, when the nature of the purulent contents of the kidney was known, and submitted to the microscope, the presence of this organic granular matter was very doubtful."

CASE.—"J. W—, æt. 29, a carpenter, was transferred from the care of Mr. Charles Guthrie, and admitted into Burdett ward on the 18th of May, 1855. He came under the care of that gentleman, suffering from irritable bladder, and doubtful symptoms of calculus. He was examined by Mr. C. Guthrie, Mr. Holt, and Mr. Brooke, and they were unanimously of opinion that there was no stone in the bladder, nor stricture, nor disease of the prostate. While under surgical treatment, samples of his urine were twice sent to me for examination. On the first occasion, the urine was faintly acid, slightly albuminous, natural in color, and depositing, when set at rest, a faint flocculent cloud; there were also small membranous shreds, one or two of which contained a minute coagula of blood. Under the microscope, there were seen the large pavement epithelial cells in abundance; many blood-corpuscles; some fibrinous coagula, quite amorphous, but stained of a reddish yellow; and a few of the smaller, spherical, glandular epithelium. The bottom of the glass vessel in which the urine had remained contained a few membranous shreds, which felt gritty, and which readily dissolved in dilute hydrochloric acid. The patient described his symptoms as of about some seven weeks' duration; he could not account for their origin, but described them as commencing with severe lumbar pain, of a sharp, pungent character, followed by frequent desire to pass urine, and inability to retain but a small quantity. This was followed by severe paroxysms of pain, referred to the perinæum and canal of the urethra. The irritability of the bladder increased; he passed urine every hour, day and night; he had never passed blood, but he had seen very minute threads of coagulated blood. The house-surgeon stated that he had once noticed the urine of a dark chocolate color; and a few days before he was transferred it became opaque and milky. As the pain became more urgent and distressing, his bodily strength failed, and he rapidly lost flesh. While under Mr. C. Guthrie's care, he had been cupped *in perineo;* he had taken, also, diuretics, with liquor potassæ: opium and ether had also been given; but from none of these remedies did he experience any relief. On being received into Burdett ward, the following were the chief symptoms recorded in the ward-book: there was great physical exhaustion and debility, much emaciation, and a careworn, anxious expression of countenance. The pulse was small and weak, the respirations natural, the tongue slightly coated, torpid bowels, deficient appetite, craving thirst, and profuse and exhausting perspirations. The patient complained of urgent pain, referred to the hypogastric region of the abdomen, and accompanied by darting, stabbing paroxysms in the perinæum. This pain, the patient states, is temporarily relieved by micturition, that for a few minutes afterwards he is comparatively easy, but that the uneasy sensation then commences, and continues augmenting in intensity till the distress becomes most urgent, and is again temporarily suspended by voiding the small amount of fluid collected in the bladder, which seldom exceeds one or two ounces. The pain is not increased by walking or exercise, and he has never known the urine to stop suddenly, and he is quite clear that the only interval of ease that he experiences is immediately after micturition. He has for many weeks suffered from a constant fixed pain in the small of the back, to the right of the spine, and referred to the posterior crest of the ilium. There is a greater degree of fulness in the right lumbar region than in the left; and pressure made on the former, by grasping this region with the right hand, the thumb resting on the lumbar muscles, and making pressure on the abdominal wall with the fingers, excites an increased amount of pain. An obscure sense of limited fluctuation is also elicited out of the same region. These conditions are absent on the left side.

"The urine passed last night is milky and opaque, which characters the patient now states he has noticed during the last week. On being set aside it separates into two portions; an upper, slightly clouded, but otherwise naturally looking urinary fluid; and a lower, distinctly separated precipitate of yellow pus-corpuscles. The upper portion is not ropy, but pours off naturally, is faintly acid, and a copious precipitate of albumen is obtained by heat and nitric acid. Examined by the microscope, the lower part is composed entirely of pus-corpuscles, with granular walls, and with addition of acetic acid these nuclei become distinctly visible. Some granular matter observed in another sample was readily dissolved by dilute hydrochloric acid. The supernatant portion before the glass exhibited large spheroidal epithelial cells, with many scattered pus-corpuscles.

"The opinion expressed after these facts had been elicited was that the patient was suffering from pyelitis of the right kidney, due in all probability to the impaction of the calculus in the ureter, or its lodgment in the head of that outlet from the pelvis; that the right kidney was enlarged and sacculated from this cause; and that the irritation of this concretion had set up inflammation of the mucous membrane lining the pelvis and extending probably to the calyces; and that the products of this inflammation (only partially retained by the body lodged in the head of the ureter, for the irregular shape of these concretions does not completely close the canal), on the one hand, passed as it were, *stillatim*, into the bladder; while, on the other, it was continually exercising a dilating or expanding pressure from within outwards, causing the kidney to become distended, and ultimately sacculated, with the entire loss of its tubular structure.

"The uvæ ursi was first administered, with a grain of morphia, night and morning; but, in a few days, the morphia appearing to fail in its anodyne effects, Battley's solution was substituted, and for a short time with apparent relief; for on the 29th of May the ward book states that the pain was neither so urgent or distressing, nor the desire to pass urine so frequent. The quantity passed each time, however, did not exceed two ounces; and the whole quantity during the twenty four hours at this time amounted to not more than sixteen ounces. The character of the urine continued the same; a dense well-defined purulent deposit, and a supernatant, now perfectly clear portion, faintly acid and albuminous. Emaciation continues; there were profuse perspirations; much thirst, and the tongue becoming brown and dry; pulse very small and weak.

"On the 2d of June he took quinine and sulphuric acid, the anodyne being continued; the former of these remedies seemed to check the perspiration.

"On the 12th of June, there was some apparent improvement in the general condition of the patient. The thirst was less, the perspiration less, and the tongue, although red, was moist, and the patient had slept better. The urine passed in the latter part of the day emitted a very offensive odor, and was for the first time alkaline, and contained a much larger proportion of purulent deposit; the upper portion was, however, clear and not ropy, and abundantly albuminous. There followed so much exhaustion on the next day that he was placed on ten ounces of port wine. Micturition became more difficult than at any previous period of the disease. The opium continued to procure slight mitigation of the symptoms.

"On the 14th there was much exhaustion, pallor of the countenance, and the urine passed involuntarily from him; the quantity could not be estimated, nor the character ascertained. On the evening of this day the nurse reported that he was suffering from loose watery diarrhœa.

"On the 16th the ward-book stated that although much more exhausted, yet the patient stated that he felt easier, and that the pain referred always to the neck of the bladder and perinœum had subsided. An opinion was expressed that in all probability a communication had become somewhere established between the enlarged and sacculated kidney and the intestines. by which the contents of the renal organ had been discharged, and relief for a time obtained. The condition of the patient was such that no examination of the loins and abdomen could be efficiently made. He lingered for two more days. The watery discharge from the bowels continued, and a turbid fluid escaped now and then in small quantities from the urinary passage. He died on the 18th of June.

"*Post-mortem examination, eighteen hours after death.*—The body was much emaciated. On opening the chest, the lungs only partially collapsed; a few scattered bands of old organized lymph united the pleuræ in both cavities. Both lungs were the seat of tubercular deposit in the form of small gray granules, not exceeding a pin's head in size, nowhere in a stage of softening, nor were they in any spot aggregated together, but were diffuse, distinct, and surrounded by elastic permeable lung substance; the bronchial mucous membrane was natural in appearance throughout. The heart was soft and flaccid, with two white opalescent patches on its surface; the interior cavities and valves were free from any morbid appearance. The cavity of the abdomen: the peritoneal surface of the intestines presented no inflammatory appearance, except at one spot, where a fold of small intestine, lying in contact with the fundus of the bladder, was covered with some recently effused lymph, and surrounded with a margin of injected vessels. The colon was traced from the cæcum, and on raising it the right kidney was observed much enlarged, of a somewhat quad-rangular shape, apparently sacculated, and fluctuating distinctly to the touch, from contained fluid. The large intestine was traced to the rectum, but no morbid condition was noticed; but the rectum, at a spot corresponding to the posterior and inferior third of the bladder, and a little to the left of the median line, was firmly united, and a fistulous communication at this point had become established between the bladder and the intestine, and by this channel the contents of the bladder had, since the commencement of the fluid dejections, been voided by the rectum. The mucous membrane of the bladder was of a dark slate color, the upper half presenting the usual corrugations, but below the fistulous opening, and surrounding it, were numerous granular deposits, presenting the character of tubercle; the prostate was also the seat of a granular deposit. The effused lymph thrown out on one fold of the small intestines lying in proximity to the bladder was not more than a finger's breadth in extent, and had been developed by contiguity to the fistulous opening between the bladder and rectum. Within the bladder, the edges of the fistulous passage had a ragged and gangrenous appearance, and immediately beneath, and filling the portion of the bladder inferior to the fistula, was a mass of fibrinous matter, gelatinous in character, and adherent, though not firmly, to the mucous membrane; there was much amorphous and gritty mater diffused through it, and in the most inferior part fragments of earthy, gritty matter, composed of triple phosphate and urate of ammonia. The two kidneys differed very materially from each other. The right was much enlarged; it distinctly fluctuated; and was lobulated. The left, though somewhat larger than natural, preserved its form, and presented no evidence of disease. The capsule of the right kidney was firm and dense, and was with some difficulty dissected from the cortical surface. When this was accomplished, the surface was found studded with white tubercular spots each surrounded by a faint-red areola. On a section being made, a considerable quantity, about ten ounces, of a purulent fluid, of a yellow color and creamy consistence, escaped, and displayed the interior of the kidney as a large sac, each of the calyces repsesenting a small cup-shaped cavity, constituting the walls of the dilated kidney. These smaller cavities, as well as the pelvis of the kidney, were covered with a rough, ragged fibrinous deposit. The ureter was much thickened, and throughout its extent was cord-like, its canal much narrowed, and its lining membrane of a slaty color. There was not complete occlusion of its passage, for a small probe could be passed into the pelvis of the kidney, and, before the sac was laid open, the purulent fluid from the interior could be expressed from it. All trace of the tubular portion of the kidney had disappeared. The cortical part, when examined under the microscope, exhibited only a fibrous material, with diffused granular and fatty matter. The urethra presented no evidence of disease. The mesenteric glands were enlarged, and were the seat of tubercle. The liver was natural in size and weight, but somewhat soft and greasy, and the hepatic cells were more loaded with fat than in health. A few scattered tubercles were present in the spleen."

ART. 67.—*On the use of Diuretics in Renal Dropsy.*
By Dr. BURROWS, Physician to St. Bartholomew's Hospital.

(*Medical Times and Gazette,* Nov. 8, 1855.)

The following remarks were made by Dr. Burrows at the bedside of a patient who was recovering from a very severe attack of the dropsy:

"'I wish, gentlemen, that you should notice the treatment which has been here pursued. I well recollect that long ago it used to be Dr. Latham's observation that this form of dropsy was often very efficiently treated by the tartrate of potash. That salt was, indeed, his favorite remedy. Then came the addition to our pathological knowledge, and the announcement of the fact that the disease was essentially one of renal disorganization. From this it was thought to follow clearly, that whatever stimulated or irritated the kidney must do harm. Diuretics, consequently, fell into almost universal disuse. Latterly, however, some of us are again coming back to the old practice; we find that no other remedies effect so much for the relief of the patients as diuretics, and we, therefore prescribe the latter. The matter is one of experience, and my own is to the effect that the kidneys, though in a state of chronic disease, obey diuretics well, and that no inconveniences are produced.' The prescription which the patient, in this case, has been taking was as follows:

R Potassæ Tartrat., ʒss;
Spirit. Æther. Nitr., ʒss;
Aquæ Piment., ʒj. Ft. haust. ter die.

The case was, of course, one of chronic dropsy, and the diagnosis as to its renal cause, had depended upon the absence of cardiac disease, and the presence of a large quantity of albumen in the urine."

ART. 68.—*Restoration of the Secretion of Urine after seven days' suppression, &c.*
By Dr. G. P. MAY, of Maldon.

(*Lancet,* Dec. 22, 1855.)

" It is a remarkable feature in this case, that complete restoration of the functions of the kidney should take place after a suspension existing for so long a period. That the suppression arose from mechanical impediments, rather than from defect in the secreting apparatus itself, appears probable from the following circumstances:

" 1st. The sudden and copious discharge of urine immediately succeeding the sensation experienced by the patient of 'something having given way in his side.' 2d. The presence of calculous matter in the calyces of the kidney and in the bladder. 3d. The absence of that complete uræmic condition of the system, to which the entire suspension of the function of the kidney for so long a period would give rise. 4th. The condition of the kidney, in a pathological point of view, would not prevent its discharging its peculiar office; such condition might perhaps be considered to be one of hypertrophy rather than of actual disease."

CASE —T. M—, æt. 39, a man of spare habit, and delicate and unhealthy appearance, had, for some months previous to his death, suffered occasionally from pain in his left side, with shortness of breath. This ailment was not deemed by him of sufficient importance to require medical aid, and he was able to pursue his ordinary avocation (that of a hawker), and was accustomed to walk a good deal in the country. In the month of April of the present year he was seized rather suddenly by acute pain, originating in the left lumbar region, and extending across the abdomen. He was confined to his bed a few days, but shortly recovered so far as to be able to resume his usual employment. At this time there was nothing remarkable either in the quality or quantity of the urinary secretion. On the 15th of August he was again attacked in a similar manner; the pain, as before, extended from the left loin across the left hypochondrium nearly to the umbilicus, and was much aggravated by an attempt to draw a deep inspiration. These regions were very tender and intolerant of pressure. On the 18th, the fourth day of his illness, it was observed that he had passed no urine; he felt no disposition to do so. There was no pubic distension, although there was considerable abdominal uneasiness and tension of the belly. From this date to the 25th, a period of seven days, he passed no urine. A catheter was introduced twice during this time, at an interval of two days; on the first occasion about an ounce of urine was abstracted, on the second, a teaspoonful, containing a few granules of uric acid. There was never any pubic tumor, or any indication of retention. For the first three or four days after the suppression he was cheerful and intelligent when spoken to, after which he became drowsy, and complained of heaviness in the head. When left to himself, he generally fell asleep, in which condition he frequently muttered and talked incoherently, but up to the last day of the suppression he was perfectly rational when roused. A large amount of fluid passed off by perspiration, with which he was almost continually bedewed. During the whole time he suffered more or less from uneasiness in the left side and abdomen.

On the 25th, after dysuria had existed seven days, he felt (to use his own expression) "something give way in his side." Very shortly after this, he passed spontaneously eight ounces of pale-colored urine. During the day the act of micturition was frequently repeated, and upwards of three pints of urine discharged. The latter portions exhibited a reddish brown tinge, and the sediment contained a proportion of blood-discs, many of them broken down and imperfect, and epithelial scales. On the following day, the urine, though discharged in sufficient quantity, was deeply tinged with blood. This condition obtained, in a greater or less degree, for a day or two, and then almost entirely subsided. His general condition was not at all improved after the restoration of the secretion. He was usually lethargic when left to himself. He became considerably emaciated, and his countenance assumed a worn and haggard aspect. On the 30th he died. He had not been the subject of ague. The treatment adopted in this case consisted principally in cupping on the loins, blisters, successive warm baths, diaphoretics, and anodynes.

Post-mortem examination.—The liver was much enlarged, being about twice its natural bulk. The spleen, enormously increased in size, encroached largely upon the left cavity of the thorax, and was strongly adherent to the costæ: it weighed four pounds and a half, and it had entirely lost its characteristics in shape, color, and consistence: it somewhat resembled in shape the larger lobe of the liver, when in its normal condition, was of a light mahogany color, and indurated throughout its substance. The left kidney measured in length nine inches, and in breadth three inches and three quarters; there was no appearance of mottling or granulation, but the cortical portion was much developed and encroached somewhat upon the tubular substance. Some white gritty matter was apparent in the calyces and infundibula, which was put aside for investigation, but was unfortunately lost. No lesion could be detected in any portion of the vesico-renal mucous membrane, nor any evidence of pyelitis. No trace whatever of kidney or capsule could be discovered in the right side. The bladder was quite healthy, and contained a little matter similar to that noticed in the kidney.

ART. 69.—*On Cystic Entozoa in the Human Kidney.*
. By Dr. T. HERBERT BARKER.

(London: Hamilton, Adams & Co., 1856, pp. 18.)

This essay was originally read before the Medical Society of London. It is founded upon a case which fell under the notice of the author, and it contains an analogous case by a friend of the author. The origin, the consequences, and the treatment of the disease are all carefully considered, and the whole essay will well repay perusal.

Dr. Barker's case is as follows:

CASE.—"A. F—, æt. 28, plumber, glazier, and painter, came under my care on 17th December, 1853, with dull heavy pain in the loins, particularly on the left side, frequent desire to pass urine, and slight difficulty in voiding it. The urine was not particularly high colored, and contained no deposit on cooling. The specific gravity was 1020. Treating the case as one of common lumbago, which at first sight it closely resembled, I prescribed simply ten minim doses of potash water, with thirty minims of sweet spirits of nitre in camphor mixture, together with an aperient of calomel and jalap, and an embrocation for the loins of ammonia, laudanum, and soap liniment. On the 22d December he observed to me, that during the early part of the past night he had experienced greater difficulty than ever in passing urine, and that for some hours he had been unable to pass a single drop. Early in the morning he passed some little jelly-like masses, four in number, which he called 'bladders,' and the emission of which gave him instantaneous relief. They were hydatid cysts. Subsequently he sufficiently recovered to follow his occupation through the summer of 1854, suffering nothing more than an occasional frequent desire to void urine.

" On September 10th, he passed six of these cysts, but with less pain and difficulty than on the former occasion—a result which he attributed to ten drops of the oil of turpentine, which had been recommended to him, and which greatly increased diuresis. The urine, after the passage of the cysts, being somewhat tinged with blood, I recommended merely a continuance of the medicine I had previously prescribed, adding only to each dose half a scruple of the sesquicarbonate of soda.

" On November 16th, he passed four of the cysts, the urine not being bloody afterwards. The passage of these cysts was, however, preceded by severe pain in the region of the left kidney, by the passage of several pieces of clotted blood, and by considerable difficulty in voiding urine. Indeed, for two entire days he passed no urine. On this occasion he took nineteen drops of turpentine within two hours, but in divided doses. Shortly after taking the turpentine, the pain in the left kidneys suddenly ceased, with a sensation which, to use the patient's own words, seemed to indicate that 'something had suddenly broken in the kidney.' He then complained of pain along the left iliac region, which continued for several hours, and ceased as suddenly as the previous pain had done. After this, all attempts to void urine were accompanied with pain along the urethra, premonitory to the expulsion of the cysts from that passage. The cysts passed on this occasion were larger than before, and after their emission, all pain ceased ; and he continued in good health, with the exception of an occasional dull aching pain in the lumbar region, especially on the left side, from the date I have named (November 16th), until the 9th December of the same year.

" On December 9th, he passed five cysts, but all of smaller size than those referred to in the preceding paragraph, and the passage of no others was observed until December 31st, when he awoke in the morning with acute pain in the loins, and all the other symptoms described previously as occurring on November 16th. During the day he passed not fewer than twenty cysts—one at 8

A. M., eleven at 1 P. M., five at 7 P. M., and three at 11 P. M. He had never previously passed so many as eleven with one effort: nor has he since. The cysts passed in rapid succession, and some were of a size as large as a small walnut. He felt tenderness in the urethra for a few days after this date, but considerably less pain in the loins.

"On January 1st, 1855, a single cyst was passed in the morning; on the 2d, two others, also in the morning; on the 3d, one in the afternoon; and on the 10th, two in the morning. From that date (January 10th) until July 23d, the peculiar class of symptoms to which he had been liable never left him entirely. He had frequent attacks of pain and difficulty in passing urine, followed often by the expulsion of cysts, between seventy and eighty of which he has brought to me on various occasions. He passed one large cyst on the 23d July. On the 9th November, he passed what appeared to be a portion of a very large cyst, and on the 11th November, he passed an entire cyst of moderate size. Since the last date to the present time (December 8th), he has passed no other cysts. He continues to take the diuretic medicines and occasionally, when the pain is more severe than usual, a dose of the turpentine. Before the 23d July, he frequently experienced an immediate cessation of the pain in the iliac region, upon what he called the 'dropping' of something which he distinctly felt, and which, as I take it, must have arisen from the escape of a cyst, from the ureter into the bladder. These sensations were always confined to the left side. The relief has not been so frequent or decided since that date, and he is daily expecting to pass more cysts. Latterly, he has also complained of pain in the region of the right kidney. Careful examination has failed to detect any abdominal enlargement.

"While these remarkable and well-marked symptoms were thus progressing, my attention was often directed very naturally to the urine, which was examined on various occasions. I have already remarked on the passage of blood in small quantities after the expulsion of the cysts; but as this was only a mechanical result, arising from slight lacerations in the canal, from the distension caused by a cyst, and the violent efforts made to expel it, the mere presence of a few blood-globules, which were often found in the urine, is easily accounted for. In addition, the urine was often loaded with the lithates and phosphates, and occasionally I detected microscopically the crystals of lithic acid. The same crystals were not unfrequently found attached to the outer surface of the cysts themselves.

"The man's general health having suffered but little interruption while the events now described were taking place, I have really already written a complete history of the symptoms presented, as well as the treatment pursued.

"For special reasons, to which I shall refer in the sequel, it is right to record the diet of the patient. For some years past he has rarely eaten either beef or mutton, having a natural aversion to these meats, and for one year, six years ago, he was a vegetarian. As an ordinary rule, however, he has lived on pork, and thinks that, on an average, he has taken 'pig's-fry,' consisting principally of the liver, at least twice weekly. He has on more than one occasion eaten 'measly' pork, and pig's chitterlings (the intestines of the animal) has been a frequent dish. He is also very fond of sheep's head, and especially of the brains, but does not know whether the brains he has thus taken were those of 'sturdy' sheep. He has likewise been accustomed to take in the morning herbal bitters, such as decoctions of horehound, wormwood, and agrimony. He is fond of coarse brown sugar. He does not remember ever having eaten meats badly cooked, and has not suffered from other forms of entozoa, except ascarides, which troubled him greatly in early life. His wife (since their marriage) has lived on the same diet, but has not shown symptoms of the same disease."

(F) CONCERNING THE CUTANEOUS SYSTEM.

ART. 70 —*Treatment of Lupus by the application of Iodide of Mercury, &c.* By Mr. M'WHINNIE, Surgeon to the Hospital for Diseases of the Skin, &c.

(*Medical Times and Gazette*, Oct. 20, 1855.)

A few years ago M. Cazenave published, in the 'Annales des Maladies de la Peau et de la Syphilide,' his experience of the effects of the red iodide of mercury in lupus. In obstinate cases of this disease, particularly of the non-ulcerated form, with or without hypertrophy, the most favorable results have been obtained at this hospital from the local application of that remedy.

The following case, treated by Mr. M'Whinnie, is selected :—R. H—, æt. 25, dressmaker, of nervous temperament, but in otherwise good general health, and of healthy parents, was admitted in January last.

The back of the right hand and fingers were beset with lupus of the tubercular form, amid much swelling of these parts from hypertrophy of the surrounding skin and subjacent cellular tissue. The unsightly appearance was further increased by the desquamation of the surface of the tubercles and the livid color of the integuments. The disease made its appearance about ten years ago upon the knuckles; it afterwards invaded the back of the hand; and she noticed that it happened to spread over points which were formerly occupied by warts. She experienced no relief from any of the remedies suggested by several surgeons both in England and France, when in 1852 she became for a short period a patient of M. Cazenave himself, who commenced the plan of treatment which, with some modification, has since been attended with so much advantage.

The topical remedies have consisted chiefly in the application of red iodide of mercury ointment (according to the formula introduced into the Pharmacopœia of the hospital by Mr. Startin),* at intervals of three or four weeks to the diseased surfaces; these were always blistered with the vesicating fluid on the day preceding the employment of the caustic. The consequent swelling and acute pain which followed (the latter continuing sometimes for thirty-six hours) being relieved by emollient hand-baths and poultices. After a few days, either the red precipitate ointment was applied, or the parts wrapped in bags wetted with dilute nitric-acid lotion, according to the convenience of the patient.

The reduction of the chronic hypertrophy is mainly attributable to the employment of well-sustained compression for a week preceding each application of the caustic ointment. The general health has been attended to, and cod-liver oil and mild mercurials administered. By steady adherence to this plan the improvement has been uninterrupted, and almost the only trace now left of this disease is the discoloration of the skin.

Equable and firm compression, patiently and perseveringly continued by means of strips of plaster and bandages, is a most valuable adjunct in the treatment of this form of lupus conjoined with hypertrophy, and is further assisted by the use of mucilaginous and vapor baths.

In this way the swelling and deformity of the limbs resembling elephantiasis, and the most hideous distortion of the features resulting from lupus, may be relieved. Such a case, Mr. M'Whinnie observed, he had witnessed in the wards of M. Brett at the Hôpital St. Louis. The whole head and face were swathed with bands and rollers as accurately as an Egyptian mummy; the occlusion of the nostrils, which may arise both from the hypertrophy and subsequent cicatrization, being guarded against by the introduction of tubes or of cylinders of prepared sponge.

ART. 71.—*On the treatment of Eczema.* By C. HANDFIELD JONES, M.B., F.R.S., Assistant-Physician to St. Mary's Hospital.

(*Assoc. Med. Journ.*, Oct. 19, 1855.)

" It never seems to be worthless in a science which is necessarily subject to so may causes of variety and uncertainty in its phenomena as that of medicine, to record definite results. For if they be true and good facts, they either give corroboration to the conclusions arrived at by others, or else they show that those conclusions are incomplete, and do not embrace the whole truth relating to the matter in question. These considerations lead me to state briefly what experience I have had of the treatment of eczema, which Dr. Burgess describes as ' perhaps the most frequent, as well as the most troublesome, cutaneous affection that the practitioner will meet with in practice.' The treatment advised by those who have written upon the subject varies a good deal. Mr. Hunt, premising antiphlogistic remedies if there be any inflammatory action, relies in the

* ℞ Hydrargyri Biniodi, ʒj; Adipis, ʒij; Emplastri Opii, ʒvj. Misce.

main upon arsenic, neglecting or altogether disapproving of local applications.
Mr. Startin uses arsenic alone, and in various combinations, as well as iodide of
potassium, colchicum, digitalis, bichloride of mercury, &c., internally, together
with various local applications, both ointments and lotions. Dr. Burgess holds
‘ greasy applications under any circumstances as barbarous and often injurious
remedies in the treatment of cutaneous disease ;’ he employs mineral acids,
liquor potassæ, and bicarbonate of potash, cantharides, iodide of mercury, arsenical preparations, especially Donovan’s solution; tonics, as citrate of iron and
quinine; as well as various washes locally. Professor Bennett, of Edinburgh,
believes that keeping the affected parts moist is all that is necessary, and only
employs an alkaline lotion on account of the hardness of the Edinburgh water.
Dr. Neligan employs also an alkaline lotion, or citrine ointment (the latter in
chronic and languid cases), administers alterative doses of Hydrargyrum cum
Cretâ, with iodide of mercury, and enjoins milk diet.

"I have notes of about forty cases, for the most part out-patients, at St. Mary’s
Hospital. Some of them might perhaps have been more properly classed as im-
petigo; but I do not love straining after subdivisions, and I group them together,
because they all had the same general easily recognized features; viz., the pouring out of an exudation, which was serous or sero-purulent, from a more or less
inflamed and excoriated or superficially ulcerated surface. Out of forty cases,
fifteen were below the age of five years, and twenty-three below that of ten. The
cases occurring in children have generally appeared to me by far the easiest to
manage; as indeed is the case with most of the diseases of the young frame,
yet sound and ‘ integan vitæ.’   The treatment which I now adopt invariably in
such instances (it being understood that active inflammation is not present), is
to give a minim of Liquor Potassæ Arsenitis three times a day to a child one
year old, desiring all scabs to be removed carefully, and dilute citrine ointment
(ʒiss to ʒvss) to be rubbed into the affected parts once a day. I have often given
a few drops of liquor potassæ, conjoined or not with a grain of iodide of potassium, with the above dose of Fowler’s solution; but it has not appeared to me
to be of any particular advantage; and I now mostly use the arsenic alone. Instead of the citrine ointment, I have used in several cases zinc ointment with
nitric-oxide of mercury (Ðj to ʒj), or Unguentum Hydrargyri Ammonio Chloridi
diluted, or bichloride of mercury lotion (gr. v-x to ʒij). I am not very sure, however, that one has any particular advantage over the other, except that the zinc
and nitric-oxide combination, especially if about a drachm of subcarbonate of lead
be added to it, seems to be best suited to irritable excoriated surfaces pouring
out much discharge. With this treatment, I have every reason to be quite satisfied; the only thing that I feel some hesitation about is, whether some amount
of relapse may not take place when the remedies are discontinued. However,
as I do not find that any discharged cases return again upon my hands, except
in rare instances, I think relapse cannot be very frequent. In one case, I tried
the effect of dilute citrine ointment alone, and it unquestionably did good; but
the eruption was not satisfactorily cured without the administration of arsenic.
In this class of cases, I have not attempted any particular restriction as to diet,
and have not found it necessary.   *   *   *   *

"In the class of cases of which I have been speaking above, the eczema is
supposed always to be in a chronic state, or at least that there is no sthenic inflammation. This condition is of absolute necessity, for if there be active inflammation arsenic will prove most injurious, increasing the vascular congestion, and
aggravating the disorder. Why? Probably for this reason, that arsenic exerts an
irritant action upon the tissues, as well as a toning one upon the vessels, and
may thus, if the former action predominate on account of the already morbid
condition of a part, increase existing inflammation. No one has appreciated this
better than Mr. Hunt. Arsenic (as he states) is by no means always necessary
to the cure of inflammatory eczema; saline aperients, with colchicum and magnesia, or alkalies, will alone subdue the disease. This is analogous to the case
of gastric catarrh in persons of high tonicity and sthenic system. All that is
necessary is to subdue the inflammatory action; as soon as this is effected, the
parts spontaneously return to their natural state; and far from needing, will not
even endure tonics.

"Between the chronic and the inflammatory cases there is an intermediate class, mostly made up of adults, in which the beneficial action of arsenic appears to be decidedly promoted by combining it with alkalies, iodide of potassium, neutral salts and colchicum, the whole dissolved in some bitter infusion. These, no doubt, promote excretion and elimination, previously defective, and bring the general system into a healthier state. One may compare their action with that of calomel in preparing the way for quinine in the treatment of ague complicated with hepatic and intestinal disorders. With regard to the dose of arsenic, I have generally found four or five minims, three times daily, quite sufficient even for adults. In the case, however, of a girl, aged nine years, I found it necessary to increase the dose of Fowler's solution up to fifteen minims three times daily. Under these large doses she was nearly well when I last saw her—no steady improvement having been produced by smaller. If prescribed alone, I follow Mr. Hunt's recommendations of giving the arsenic at meal-times; if conjoined with alkalies, I prefer to give it three hours after the meal. Out of all the cases in which I have given arsenic (no inconsiderable number, including the neural-giæ), I can remember but very few in which it has disagreed, and even in these it is very likely that a smaller dose would have produced no inconvenience. Almost invariably it is borne well by children, and improves their health decidedly. My experience of it, whether in neuralgic affections, or in skin-diseases, is, that it is a most valuable tonic, and I have yet to learn why we should be at all shy of giving it. So far from any disorder ensuing when the cutaneous discharge is checked, I have found the health materially improved. As to Mr. Hunt's pre-cept of producing some degree of conjunctivitis in order to obtain the full cura-tive power of arsenic, I cannot say that I have generally found it necessary to do so, though I am convinced that the healing process goes on very favorably when this has been the case; and I am sure that so long as the conjunctivitis is moderate, there is not the least reason for interrupting the use of the remedy. Scrofulous ophthalmia, with its attendant photophobia, I have not found to cause any impediment to the use of arsenic for a coexisting eczema. The state of the eye and of the face improved together in the case I allude to. The arsenic was combined with iodide of potassium and alkali; and cod-liver oil was given at the same time."

Then follow ten cases, of which we give the first two:

CASE 1.—A. Ph—, æt. 4, a female, was admitted on February 6th, with severe suppurating eczema of the ears, chin, and lips: she was cachectic in appearance, but was said to be strong generally. In my absence, a friend prescribed a weak alkaline lotion and oiled silk; but this was of no avail.

February 12th.—I directed the following ointment to be applied to the affected part:

> R. Unguenti Zinci, ʒj;
> Hydrargyri Nitrico-oxydi, ʒj. M.

A drachm of the following mixture was ordered to be taken three times a day:

> R. Liquoris Potassæ Arsenitis, ℈l;
> Aquæ, ʒiij. M.

19th.—The patient was much improved. The mixture and ointment were continued; and a drachm of cod-liver oil was ordered to be taken three times a day.

26th.—There was improvement: but a good deal of eczema was still present in the fold of the ear. The mixture and ointment were continued; and a drachm of the subjoined mixture ordered to be taken three times a day:

> R. Liquoris Potassæ Arsenitis, ℈lxxx;
> Aquæ, ʒiij. M.

March 1st.—Improvement continued; but there was some catarrhal affection of the chest. Three grains of citrate of iron and quinine were ordered to be taken in two drachms of water three times a day. An ointment was prescribed, consisting of—

   R. Unguenti Hydrargyri Nitratis, ʒiss ;
       Adipis, ʒivss. M.

26th.—The patient was quite well, having improved steadily under the use of the tonic and ointment. The local applications certainly did not do harm, and I am confident that they did amend the skin disorder.

Case 2.—Ch. W—, æt. 4, a male, was admitted May 25th. He had been ill seven months previously with an attack of typhus fever. He was very subject to diarrhœa. He had a patch of eczematous eruption in the fold behind the right ear, where the skin was very deeply fissured at one part. Other patches existed on the scalp. The urine was rather high colored, and offensive. He had had pertussis, measles, and variola. I ordered him—

   R. Liquoris Potassæ Arsenitis, ℳxxv ;
       Liquoris Potassæ, ʒiss ;
       Infusi Gentianæ co., ʒiij. M.
  Sumat ʒij ter die.

   R. Hydrargyri Bichloridi, gr. v ;
       Aquæ, ʒij.
  Solve ut fiat lotio.

June 1st.—The urine was absolutely colorless ; it deposited pale lithates in small quantity, with oxalates ; it was feebly acid, and not albuminous. Hydrochloric acid threw down no uric acid. This examination showed that the assimilative processes were very languid.

By the 22d he was quite well ; the only trace of the eruption was a little congestion of the integument. Debility was a marked feature of this case ; and the tonic influence of the arsenic told well.

Art. 72.—*Rapid treatment of Itch.* By MM. Dusard and Pellon.

(*L'Union Médicale*, No. cix. 1855 ; and *Medical Times and Gazette*, April 12, 1856.)

" The remedy here mentioned is the chloride of sulphur dissolved in sulphuret of carbon. The chloride, easily obtained by the action of chlorine of sulphur, was at first employed in its pure state in minute quantities, but this not acting promptly enough, the sulphuret of carbon was, after various trials, chosen as the best vehicle. Twelve grammes of chloride are dissolved in one hundred of the sulphuret, this being the utmost quantity required for an adult. The application should be made in a well-ventilated room, removing all copper articles liable to tarnish. The patient is placed quite naked on a stool, and his head is covered with an immense cone made of strong paper, opened only at the top, so as to protect the face from the effect of the sulphureous vapors which exhale. The whole surface is rapidly smeared over with the mixture, by means of a large badger's-hair brush or charpie, applying it especially to the parts where the acari most resort. Any hospital attendant can do this. A general sense of heat, without painful smarting, immediately follows, and the patient is thus cured in five minutes. The itching ceases as if by magic. After thirty-six hours a bath is taken, the patient being recommended to abstain from washing his hands and neck until then ; and baths on alternate days for a week, to complete the treatment. Complications that may have arisen may, however, require treatment ; but they soon subside. When eczema predominates, some gelatinous or starchy baths are employed, and porrigo is usually relieved by alkaline baths. When the complications are very aggravated, they should be somewhat modified before the treatment is commenced, or this may cause pain. After disappearing, the itching may return in five or six days, but it is of a different kind, dependent on persistent porrigo, and relievable by alkaline baths."

Art. 73.—*On a new Parasite in Man.* By M. Zenker, of Dresden.

(*Zeitsch. für Rat. Med.*; and *Dublin Medical Press*, Nov. 28, 1855.)

It was Professor Siebold who first demonstrated from the observations of Drs. Pruner and Bilharz, physicians in Cairo, the existence of a species of the genus

Pentastomum living in the intestines of man; Siebold gave it the name of *P. constrictum.* The author states that Egypt is not the only country which has the *good fortune* to possess a pentastome; another species, the *Pentastomum denticulatum,* Rud., which had hitherto been met with only in animals, is found in man, and is even very common in Germany. The author has observed this worm seven times, and always in the superior surface of the liver, under the peritoneum. It is contained in a dense fibrous capsule which adheres to the parenchyma of the liver and to the peritoneum, but which admits of being easily detached; it appears under the form of a little tubercle of from 2·25 to 3·37 millimetres (·0935 to ·1326 of an English inch), usually filled with a calcareous deposit with which the animalcule is itself encrusted. The capsule is proportionally very thick, and it is difficult to extract the worm from it uninjured; sometimes, however, the capsule separates easily from the earthy concretion, and the worm can then be withdrawn.

The author gives a detailed description of the animal, and the description is accompanied with figures to exhibit more clearly the form of the worm, and especially that of the tentacula with which the head is furnished.

PART II.—SURGERY.

SECT. I.—GENERAL QUESTIONS IN SURGERY.

(A) CONCERNING INFLAMMATION.

ART. 74.—*On Carbuncle and Boil.* By Mr. SYME, Professor of Clinical Surgery in the University of Edinburgh.

(*Lancet*, March 8th, 1856.)

"CARBUNCLE," says Mr. Syme, in a Clinical lecture, "is a circumscribed, inflammatory condition of the true skin. It begins with a small red point, which gradually and rapidly extends with a peculiar tingling and pungently painful sensation, much greater than might be expected from the degree of morbid change apparent to sight. The skin becomes loosened in its texture, and swollen, so as to be an inch or an inch and a half in thickness. Small yellow points appear on the surface, and are presented by a section of the dermoid texture, interspersed in the interstices of its substance. These local changes are attended with a more than corresponding amount of constitutional disturbance, the patient being unable to sleep or eat, having an anxious expression of countenance, and presenting all the characters of excessive irritation. If the evil be permitted to pursue its course, it terminates in sloughing of the affected skin, and either death of the patient from exhaustion, or a very tedious recovery from the loss of substance which has been sustained. All sorts of internal remedies and local applications have little or no control over the progress of a carbuncle, and the only effectual method of cutting short its advance is to make a free crucial incision completely through the whole extent of inflamed skin. Immediately upon this being done, the redness disappears, and the pain ceases, the constitutional disturbance soon subsides, and the affected skin, unless already deprived of its vitality, quickly resumes its natural thickness and healthy action, so as to remove all obstacle from the healing process.

"Reason and experience being so decidedly in favor of the practice here employed, I should consider it unnecessary to say a word now upon the subject were I not aware that the most erroneous ideas in regard to the pathology, as well as treatment of the disease, are extensively diffused; and as my duty is not merely to inculcate what seem to me sound principles of practice, but to counteract and extirpate the misleading notions which you may have elsewhere acquired, I deem it necessary to warn you against the four following errors, which are very generally entertained, and which may, perhaps, in some measure, account for the large numbers of deaths connected with carbuncle in some bills of mortality.

"In the first place I beg to remind you that the disease is not subcutaneous, but seated in the skin itself. Secondly, that the object of incisions is not to allow room for the escape of matters confined under the skin, but to extinguish the inflammatory action, through discharge of blood and the relief of tension, by dividing the texture in which it is seated. Thirdly, that the application of caustic is the extreme of absurdity, since it directly insures what the great object of treatment should be to prevent, and by destroying the skin affected, instead of restoring it to a healthy condition, necessarily protracts recovery, and renders it less perfect. Fourthly and lastly, I beg to warn you against giving the patient wine and nourishing food, or employing local applications of a stimulating kind, so long as the inflammatory tendency continues in operation.

"It may here not be out of place to say a few words in regard to boils, which are very nearly connected with carbuncle. Like it they are seated in the skin, begin by points so small as to be hardly perceptible, and extend from the centre in a circumscribed form, with local and constitutional symptoms of disturbance greatly disproportioned to their extent. They are distinguished by being restricted to a smaller size, by presenting a more convex surface, and by tending to suppuration rather than to sloughing. It is true that they contain a white substance, named their core, which looks like, and is often mistaken for, merely dead cellular substance, but is chiefly the result of a morbid deposition. Fomentation and poultices may soothe the uneasy symptoms proceeding from boils, but the only effectual mode of checking their progress is to make a free crucial incision through the whole extent of inflamed skin which constitutes their base. It is often said that 'opening' boils does no good, and this may be true, since the incision, like that for the remedy of carbuncle, must be directed, not with a view to evacuation, but to free division of the affected skin. The opinion generally entertained at present, is, that boils should be allowed to pursue their course, under palliatives, with a liberal diet, and patients are frequently met with who have suffered for months, or even years, from their successive formation. Now it seems to me that nothing can be more injudicious than such a procedure, since each boil, instead of being extinguished by a timely incision in its infancy, is allowed to go through the whole of its irritating course, with attendant constitutional disturbance, which instead of benefiting the patient's system must increase its derangement and liability to similar formations. Between two and three weeks ago a medical man of great respectability in this city called upon me, complaining of a boil upon his arm, which he had been poulticing, and did not wish to remedy by incision. Two days afterwards I was asked to visit this gentleman, found him in bed, and was told that he had been deprived of sleep throughout the preceding night by a large boil on his haunch, which, if allowed to pursue its course, threatened to produce a great amount of distress, and seriously to disturb his health. Having been requested to do what seemed best, I made a free crucial incision, and restricted the diet to milk and farinaceous food. Next day I found the patient down stairs, sitting in his library perfectly comfortable, as he had been ever since submitting to the incision. I have no doubt that if the system at present in fashion had been pursued in this case, my friend, instead of enjoying perfect health, would now have been fairly entered upon a course of annoyance no less distressing than unlimited in its duration."

(B) CONCERNING TUMORS.

ART. 75.—*The effect of Creosote on Warty Growths.*
By Mr. RAINEY, Lecturer on Anatomy at St. Thomas's Hospital.

(*Lancet*, Dec. 8, 1855.)

"In order to secure the full effect of the creosote on the disease, after applying it freely to the part, I prevented its removal by a piece of adhesive plaster put several times round the finger, which was allowed to remain for two days. On removing the plaster a visible change had taken place in the character of the surface of the excrescence, which now, in the place of being dry and hard, had become so soft and friable as to admit of being broken down by the slightest friction of the finger. The daily application of the creosote was, however, still continued until the remains of the wart had become of a horny consistence, after which, in about a fortnight, it desquamated, leaving the part beneath perfectly healthy.

"The creosote, in this case, caused no pain or uneasiness, or any symptom which indicated an escharotic action on the affected part, but seemed to act entirely by destroying that excessive and abnormal cell-development, which is the essential character of this form of disease.

"In these excrescences there is what pathologists call hypertrophy of the epidermis. The epidermic cells also retain their nuclei and power of cell-growth longer than the normal epidermic cells of the stratum Malpighii of the surrounding parts; and the transformation of these cells into non-nucleated particles or scales, takes place irregularly and at no certain distance from the surface, as in the healthy epidermis. After a time the capillaries become enlarged, but this seems to be only the effect of the excessive and abnormal development of the cells, which are dependent upon their contents for their supply of nutritive material.

"As only one instance of the beneficial effects of this substance would be totally insufficient to establish its claim to be a specific, I asked Mr. Ord, the house-surgeon of St. Thomas's Hospital, if he would try its effects on some of the out-patients, as, if it did no good, it could not possibly do harm, which he informs me he has done with a satisfactory result.

"I may further add, that it seems to me no unreasonable inference, that if creosote is capable of destroying excessive or abnormal cell-growth in the dermic tissue, it may also do the same in analogous diseases of the mucous tissues, and therefore that it may possibly be applied with advantage in nasal and uterine polypi. In these cases I would not recommend it unless it could be kept in contact with the diseased part for a considerable length of time. I have even recommended a professional friend of mine, who has at this time a case of epithelial cancer under his care, to make a trial of it in this disease.

"As this class of diseases, besides being distinguished by abnormal cell-growth of greater or less activity, is also attended with a disordered condition of the system, the local application of creosote would not of itself be likely to be of much service. In such cases it would require to be taken also internally, and probably to be persisted in for many months, according to the effect it might have upon the local disease or upon the general health. I may observe that I am by no means sanguine as to the beneficial effects of the remedy I am proposing in those diseases which are known by the term malignant. My expectations on this point are far from rising to an extravagant elevation. I merely think from what I have seen of its action that it is just worthy of a fair trial, especially as these diseases are at present incurable, and as the remedy which I propose for their cure or relief, very different to many others employed for the same purpose, is incapable of doing any harm, should it fail to do any good. It is impossible for me to say how far creosote may have been used in the diseases for which I have proposed to employ it. I have not read of any case of the kind where it has been employed, and no one of the medical men that I have interrogated upon the subject knows of any instance of its employment in the same complaint, and with the same physiological view, as that I have advanced. About a month since I went to a medical man's house to ask him if he could furnish me with any cases of warts, etc., upon which he could employ creosote. A person not in the profession was present, who, hearing the conversation, said he had taken a little boy to a druggist's some time before to have something applied to a wart, which he believed was creosote, and which cured it. This is all that I have heard of the employment of this substance in any of the above-named diseases."

(c) CONCERNING WOUNDS AND ULCERS.

ART. 76.—*The treatment of Chronic Ulcers by Opium internally.*
By Mr. SKEY, Surgeon to St. Bartholomew's Hospital.

(*Lancet*, Jan. 26, 1856.)

These remarks occur in a paper entitled " Reminiscences of Hospital Practice :"
"Abundant have been the examples of treatment of chronic ulcers of the legs and elsewhere by means of the internal use of opium. I know of no treatment at all comparable to this, so rapid, or so efficient. These cases have had many observers, who can bear testimony as to its value. Exactly in proportion to the amount administered is the regeneration of the defective structure. Years will probably yet elapse before this principle will be universally acknowledged;

before the medical community will admit that in opium we have an agent far more valuable than that derived from its *comparatively* worthless power as a sedative. It is notorious that the chronic ulcer—the disease of ten or even of twenty years' duration—is unattended with pain. To suppose that opium effects its local marvels by any sedative property in the drug, appears to be worthy only the advocacy of a senile female, or of an uninstructed youth. If we administer five grains of the soap and opium pill, night and morning, to a man advancing in life, who has been carrying about with him for ten years a large, callous ulcer, with an ash-colored base, surrounded by high walls of organized lymph, and in which there remains not a vestige of activity, good or bad, advancing or receding, the moisture from which is a hot ichor, becoming sanious under provocation,—if we examine carefully this surface at the expiration of forty-eight hours, we shall find it speckled with red points; these are future granulations, and, in ten days the whole base of the wound will be carpeted with them. And this is the mere result of suspended irritation?"

ART. 77.—*The dressing of Stumps under Water.* By M. LANGENBECK.

(*Medico-Chir. Review*, April, 1856.)

" By various apparatus, constructed in zinc or vulcanized caoutchouc, Professor Langenbeck contrives to keep the wounded part in constant contact with tepid water. The apparatus must not be resorted to where secondary hemorrhage is feared, and thus its application to stumps, after amputation, should be usually delayed for eighteen to twenty-four hours. In several cases it has, however, been resorted to even before the patient has recovered from the anæsthesia, this saving him from the pains after the operation and from the dressing. The part must be removed from the bath if the hemorrhage occurs. When applied immediately, the water should be at a temperature of from 10° to 13° C.; and if the water is not renewed it acquires in from three to twelve hours a temperature of from 15° to 31°. After the first day the latter is that which is most agreeable to the patient; and later, when the wound begins to clean and suppurate, a temperature of 34° to 35° is to be maintained. The patient's sensations usually form the best guide; and the temperature can be maintained pretty equable by covering the apparatus, or by adding warm or cold water from time, to time. In summer, with a temperature of 20° to 25°, the water rises in twelve hours to from 34° to 37°; and in winter, at 17° in the room, the water falls to 31° or 30° in the twelve hours. As a general rule, the water requires renewing only night and morning; and if there is a large wound, with abundant suppuration, it should be well washed with a chlorinated solution.

" The advantages of the procedure are thus summed up:—1. Diminution of pain subsequent to the operation. As long as the parts are kept under water, whatever the size of the wound, no pain is complained of, although this at once becomes severe when they are exposed ; general shivering then, too, coming on in a quarter of an hour. The author has never observed the shiverings, so frequently met with after large operations, when the water was at once applied. No dressings are required, the sutures are removed under water, and the greatest cleanliness is secured. 2. The traumatic and suppurative fever is much diminished in intensity. 3. The removal of the secreted fluids is favored, and their decomposition prevented. If the wounds are deep or sinuous, injections must be used, and the free issue of the discharges must be secured by the usual means. 4. Cicatrization is more prompt. 5. Professor Langenbeck believes the means to be operative in preventing purulent infection."

ART. 78.—*Treatment of Chancre.* By Dr. SIGMUND.

(*American Quart. Jour. of Med. Science,* Oct., 1855.)

From observations conducted on a large scale at the Vienna Hospital, Dr. Sigmund concludes—1. Chancre can only be treated locally during the first four days, and the further we recede from this, the greater the urgency of the general treatment. 2. The local treatment consists in cauterization, which effectually destroys all the chancrous exudation to the sound tissue. 3. The observation of more than a thousand cases during eleven years, assures Dr. Sigmund that secondary symptoms never occur when the chancre has been completely destroyed within the first four days. He is only aware of two doubtful cases in which cauterization on the fifth day even has not prevented accidents. The best caustic is the Vienna, composed of quicklime and two or three parts of caustic potass. Cauterization should also be practised even after the fifth day, for although the chances of preservation from secondary syphilis are diminished, they are not totally abolished; and we prevent the chancre being communicated to other parts of the same patient, or to other individuals. 4. The general treatment consists in the methodical employment of mercury, no other means curing so quickly and so surely. 5. In the exceptional cases in which secondary symptoms occur in spite of general treatment, they are not found in an aggravated form. 6. According to circumstances, the general treatment should be continued for six or twelve weeks. The levity with which the public and the profession at the present time regard venereal symptoms should be met by the strongest opposition. 7. Clinical observation shows that every chancre, well diagnosticated, and not carefully destroyed, leads to secondary symptoms, if general treatment has not been instituted. This will be admitted by all who establish a regular diagnosis, and look for secondary symptoms soon enough where they are first to be found, viz., in the lymphatic glands. 8. Positive diagnosis is alone attainable by inoculation or the production of secondary symptoms. 9. Secondary symptoms are usually observed about the sixth week after infection, and very rarely later than the twelfth; and we must not always depend upon the patient's assertion, but make ourselves a rigorous search for their early manifestation. If between the sixth and end of the twelfth week no secondary symptom has shown itself, and the local manifestation has disappeared, the patient may be pronounced cured—the few exceptions that occur notwithstanding. 10. The amount of mercury administered varies according to the indications offered by different patients. The dietetic and hygienic management, both during and after taking the mercury, is too much neglected.

(D) CONCERNING DISEASES OF THE BLOODVESSELS.

ART. 79.—*A case of extensive Arterial Obstruction.* By Mr. SAVORY, Demonstrator of Anatomy at St. Bartholomew's Hospital.

(*Lancet*, April 5. 1856.)

In this case the main arteries of both upper extremities and of the left side of the neck were completely obliterated. The case was read before the Royal Medical and Chirurgical Society.

CASE.—A. M. W—, æt. 22, was admitted into St. Bartholomew's Hospital on November 27th, 1854. No pulse could then be detected in any part of either arm. There was feeble pulsation in the right carotid; in the left, doubtful. A harsh systolic bruit was audible over the top of the sternum, which disappeared on tracing it downwards, and a feebler one was heard in the course of the right common carotid. She complained of general debility, of headache, vertigo, and obscure pains in various parts. She had been delicate ever since she was a child. There was satisfactory evidence to show that the pulse had ceased to beat for some years past. There was no distinct history of any previous attack to which her present condition could be referred. She remained in the hospital until she died—a period of thirteen months. During this time her strength gradually passed away. The sight of the left eye began to fail, and at length was nearly lost: an ulcer formed on the cornea, which yielded to tonic treatment. Subsequently, ulceration commenced in the integuments over the left parietal eminence, and, resisting all remedies, gradually extended, until the bone, and ultimately a portion of the brain, were destroyed. During the last few weeks of her life she was much distressed by impaired and disordered motion and sensation on the right side.

After death, the following condition of the arteries were revealed : The whole of the arteria innominata was much thickened, and it required considerable pressure to approximate its walls. The lining membrane was pale and smooth, but dull and opaque. The internal coat separated with the slightest force from the middle, and was almost as thick as the other two coats together. The middle and external coats were denser than natural, and slightly thickened. Owing to this morbid state of the tunics, a section of the vessel presented a remarkable appearance. The distinction between the coats was strikingly obvious. When the internal coat was stripped off from the middle, in a great part of the vessel irregular patches of an opaque yellowish deposit came off upon the outer surface of the inner coat, but some remained upon the inner surface of the middle. This deposit, to minute examination, presented all the characters of consolidated lymph intimately blended with the arterial tissues. It was probably in process of degeneration, for here and there many small globules of an oily nature could be detected. This morbid change extended into the right carotid and commencement of the subclavian artery. In the whole of the former vessel the same change, although to a less extent, was apparent: it was contracted and much thickened; there was no clot in the interior; the inner surface was not reddened. About an inch or less from their origin, the right subclavian, the left carotid, and the left subclavian arteries became suddenly contracted to one-fourth or one-fifth of their natural size. This change extended throughout these vessels: through the axillary, brachial, radial, and ulnar arteries on both sides, and the left external carotid artery. The contracted canal in their interior was completely blocked up and obliterated by a fibrous cord, which extended with scarcely any interruption throughout their entire length. Thus all the main arteries of both upper extremities and of the left side of the neck were reduced to solid cords. Other morbid appearances, of less moment, were described in the paper.

In his remarks upon the case the author observed that, from its history, the progress of the disease had probably been gradual, and unaccompanied by any acute or violent symptoms. He believed that the symptoms observed during life might almost all be referred to a deficient supply of blood to those parts of the body to which the obliterated arteries were distributed. The author then remarked upon the objections which the facts of this case opposed to Rokitansky's views on the subject, and discussed the question at some length. Lastly, he referred to the origin of the fibrous cord which filled up the interior of the contracted vessels. He believed it to be the remains of the blood which had coagulated in the canal, and not an exudation from the arterial tunics; and concluded by giving the grounds upon which this opinion was founded.

(E) CONCERNING DISEASES OF THE BONES AND JOINTS.

ART. 80.—On Myeloid and Myelo-cystoid Diseases of Bone.
By Mr. HENRY GRAY, Lecturer on Anatomy at St. George's Hospital.

(Lancet, March 15, 1856.)

In a paper read before the Medical and Chirurgical Society, on the 26th February, 1856, the author detailed the history of nine cases of tumors of this form removed during life, with a minute description of the results of his own microscopical examination of six of the tumors. The results at which he arrived were as follow:—That these tumors were not of a malignant nature, although in several of the instances given they had been so regarded both previous to and after removal by operation; that, on the contrary, their minute structure bore the closest analogy with the normal constituents of the marrow and other elements of bone in the early periods of life; that their growth is confined to the osseous texture, or its investing membranes, the periosteum and dura mater; that they occur at a period of life when the normal constituents of the medulla exist in the greatest amount, and are developed in those parts of the osseous system in which those structures exist in a most distinct and well-marked form (all the cases given took their origin in the epiphysal ends of long bones); that they are occasionally mixed with the other elements of bone in a rudimentary state, as fibrous tissue and cartilage, and even with bone itself; that they may probably occur in any bone; that since they are thus found to consist of an abnormal amount of some of the normal constituents of the medulla, the medulla cells, the name "myeloid" given to them by Mr. Paget is most appropriate, (the author proposes to add the term "cystic" to such of them as present a mixture of cysts with the structure above described, and regards their fibrous elements as most probably derived from the organization of lymph effused as a result of chronic inflammatory action, or from some abnormality in the development and growth of the fibrous element of bone;) that they occur in all the cases at present recorded at an early period of life, and that their growth is generally much less rapid than malignant disease, both which facts afford important diagnostic marks to distinguish them from malignant growths; that the absence of the malignant cachexia, or glandular lymphatic enlargements, and of disease in internal organs, combined with the facts that although these tumors attain occasionally a considerable size, yet they present no tendency to ulcerate or protrude externally, and generally retain some surrounding shell of bone within which they have grown, serve as additional aids to the surgeon in forming a diagnosis between myeloid and malignant growths; that they do not return when entirely removed; and that for all these reasons they are to be regarded as innocent tumors.

ART. 81.—*Cases of Fragilitas Ossium.* By (1) Mr. THOMAS WAKLEY, Surgeon to the Royal Free Hospital; and (2) Mr. HENRY THOMPSON, Surgeon to the Marylebone Infirmary.

(*Lancet*, Jan. 12, 1856.)

(1) *Mr. Wakley's case.*—J. T—, a cabman, æt. 42, was admitted into the ward on May 10th with rupture of the ligament of the patella of the right leg. The patient, a stout and robust man, states that he has generally enjoyed good health, and has never suffered from any injury in the leg before. His account of the accident is, that he was in the act of getting up to the seat of his cab, having placed his left leg on the wheel, and just raised his right leg, when he felt something give way in the knee, which he says felt as though a piece of cord had been cut through. He was unable to put the leg to the ground, and swelling immediately commenced above and below the knee. He was forthwith put in a cab, and conveyed to the hospital; when the house-surgeon found the patella about three inches above its natural situation.

June 30th (about seven weeks after the occurrence of the injury).—The leg has much the same appearance as the sound one, with the exception of a little swelling around the knee and two inches below it. The patient has, however, the power to raise the limb, and to flex and extend it; but he is unable to walk, as he cannot support the weight of his body on the affected limb.

July 7th.—The patient is up for the first time. An instrument has been made for him, consisting of three steel rods, connected at each end by a band of leather, one of which is fastened above and the other below the knee. With this instrument and a stick he is able to walk for a short time, but requires rest every five or ten minutes.

19th.—To-day whilst walking about the ward, the patient felt something give way in the right thigh, and on the house-surgeon coming to him he found the poor man had fractured his right femur at the middle third. There was no fall or other injury to cause the accident. The fracture occurred spontaneously while the man was walking about. He was put to bed, and Liston's straight splint applied. The fracture was a transverse one.

August 3d.—The limb was re-bandaged to-day, but it was found that there was no callus thrown out. He was ordered to remain quiet, and to take four ounces of port wine and three ounces of brandy daily, and milk.

17th.—The limb was put up in starched bandage to-day; a little callus has been thrown out around the fracture, but it is very soft.

September 8th.—The limb continues in a good position, and during the last day or two the patient has got out of bed, and sat in a chair. Pain at the lower end of the left tibia, and on examination it was found that there was some enlargement of the bone at the point of uneasiness. A cantharides blister to be applied over the enlargement.

9th.—Still complains of the pain. To remain in bed.

14th.—Patient is much better; no pain.

23d.—Fractured femur re-bandaged; callus still very soft.

October 18th.—Callus somewhat firmer. The fractured limb was this day put up in a short straight splint, reaching from the hip to three inches below the knee. The patient is ordered to get up to-morrow.

22d.—He has been able for the last three days to walk about on crutches, the leg being supported by a bandage slung from the neck.

24th.—Whilst walking about the ward, with the assistance of the nurse and another patient, he fractured the left fibula, about two inches from its head. There is a good deal of effusion about the seat of the fracture. He received no injury whatever to account for this third disaster.

December 31st.—The patient is now again sitting up in a chair, with both legs enveloped in gum and chalk bandages, but as yet unable to walk, or bear the weight of his body on his limbs.

The medical treatment of the case has been chiefly directed to the improvement and invigoration of the constitution generally. The man now takes large doses of cod-liver oil, combined with generous diet.

Mr. Wakley believes that the fragilitas ossium is due to one of two causes, viz., syphilis, or morbus mercurialis. The pains in the bones, the node on the left tibia, and the state of the mouth, showing the results of excessive salivation, all tend to the confirmation of this opinion. The patient states that he has always been a very temperate man, and positively asserts that there is no scrofulous or cancerous taint in his family.

(2) *Mr. Henry Thompson's case.*—Susan W—, æt. 58, had a scirrhous growth excised from her left breast five years ago in University College Hospital; and last June twelvemonth, it was found necessary to remove the axillary glands, which were attacked with cancer. Shortly after this second operation, she was admitted into the Marylebone Infirmary, with severe pains in her lower extremities, that rendered her unable to work: and upon the occasion of her being moved from one apartment of the institution into another, her right femur was fractured. This accident occurred about a year and four months from the present time. In August last, a second catastrophe occurred, the left femur breaking as the poor woman was turning herself in bed. The fractures have failed to unite, and consequently both limbs have contracted and have become painfully distorted. The pains still continue, but are allayed by belladonna plaster.

ART. 82.—*On Bone diseased by muscular overstraining.*
By Mr. SOLLY, Surgeon to St. Thomas's Hospital.

(*Lancet*, Nov. 3 and Dec. 8, 1855.)

These remarks, and the case upon which they are founded, appear in a clinical lecture on diseased bone:

"Sometimes, without any actual laceration of the surface of the bone taking place, the disease takes its rise from the tendinous attachment of a muscle, and extends to the ligaments and articulating surfaces in a joint. In some of these cases you find the bone neither carious nor necrosed, but the periosteum enormously thickened, and the bone in the immediate neighborhood softened. This is especially the case when the injury is through the medium of tendon, which performs the double office of a conductor of muscular power, and a ligament or guardian of a joint. Let me remind you of the origin and relation of the tendon of the popliteus muscle to the knee-joint. It arises in a deep pit on the outside of the outer condyle of the os femoris, a little above the articular margin of the bone; it descends obliquely behind the knee-joint, where it attains the space between the femur and the tibia; it is lined internally with the synovial membrane of the joint, and now plays the part of a true ligament. If, therefore, from any sudden or violent exertion on the part of this muscle its origin from the bone is injured and inflammation set up, you can readily understand how such inflammation may be extended to the knee-joint. This view is no mere theory. I will relate to you briefly a case, which many of the older students will remember as interesting me very much at the time. It would not yield to those measures which I have so frequently demonstrated to you are successful in arresting scrofulous disease of the cartilages; and though I was at last obliged to have recourse to amputation, I believe I delayed the operation, hoping against hope, some months after the case was considered hopeless by many who watched it with equal interest with myself."

CASE.—" E. B—, æt. 21, dark eyes and hair, rather strumous diathesis, was admitted under my care on April 11th, 1854. The knee is swollen and the shape altered, but apparently more from external than internal effusion. All motion gives her increased pain, which is not severe when at rest. It is much aggravated by pressure on the outer side, where there is a fistulous aperture, from which there is a slight discharge.

"History.—Two years previous to her admission she slipped and fell on the grass suddenly, when preparing to run a race, and immediately felt a severe smarting pain in the right knee; it caused her to limp for a few hours, but she did not leave the pic-nic party she was at, nor did she lay up until four days had elapsed.

"From this portion of the history we learn that the knee was not injured by a blow, but by a violent muscular exertion to save herself from falling after her foot had slipped upon the grass. The popliteus muscle would be called into play on such an occasion. The injury at this time could not have been very severe, for she did not lay by altogether until seventeen months after the receipt of this injury. If, therefore, she had rested it at once, I have no doubt that the serious mischief which afterwards ensued might have been prevented. About seven months ago the joint became enlarged and painful, and during the first month she used to lie upon a sofa during the daytime, and to walk up-stairs at night; at the end of that time, one evening when she was going up-stairs she experienced a sudden and severe pain in the knee, and felt as if something had given way in the joint. Since that night she has never been able to set her foot to the ground, and has lost all power of moving it, resting on it in the slightest degree, or any attempt to do so, giving her the most excruciating pain. At this time I believe that the connection between the tendon of the popliteus and the external semilunar cartilage was torn through.

"The surgeon who attended her placed the limb on a wooden splint, applied blisters from time to time, altogether amounting to eleven, eight leeches at six different times, cupped once, and used one seton. The pain during the last seven months has been very severe, sometimes worse at night, sometimes better; the general health does not appear to have suffered much. She has been well supported with wine, brandy, stout, and meat, all in moderation. Suppuration took place; the matter accumulated, and a swelling formed on the outer and back part of the joint. The surface broke, and a large quantity of pus escaped, and this opening has not healed.

"I shall not weary you by reading the daily notes, though they are well taken and interesting, if our time was not so short. Repeated abscesses formed in the neighborhood of the joint, and she had two or three attacks of hæmoptysis, and her sufferings at times were frightful; but still her health did not give way rapidly, and for ten months I combatted the disease. At the end of that time it was clear that she must sink into her grave if her limb were allowed to remain on. On the 28th of February I amputated it, under chloroform. I made a very long stump, as her friends were able to afford her an artificial leg. She rallied quickly after the operation, and left the hospital quite well on the 29th of April, little more than a twelvemonth after her admission.

"The examination of the knee-joint disclosed the following condition : the patella was adherent to the femur by slight bands. The greater part of the cartilage was healthy, but there were patches of ulceration, and from the patches these adhesive bands sprung. The cartilage was nearly entire, and sound over the front of the femur in a rotulator furrow, and also over the inner condyle, but it was gone over the whole of that portion of the outer condyle which articulates with the tibia. This bone was bare, soft, and eroded. The corresponding surface on the tibia was in a similar condition. The outer semilunar cartilage was softened and pulpy, and nearly absorbed. The tendon of the popliteus was brown, pulpy, soft, and disintegrated, and also the anterior crucial ligament; the posterior was discolored, but firm. The periosteum covering the lower and back part of the femur was thickened, but not so much so as that on the tibia, which was nearly one sixth of an inch in depth. The bone underneath was soft but not carious. There was a large abscess in the lower part of the popliteal and upper part of the posterior tibia spaces. The popliteus muscle was thickened and infiltrated with serum, and completely disorganized.

"The appearances just described are not those of an ordinary case of strumous ulceration of the cartilages. I must confess that I was glad to find that such was the case, as I believe it is only the second time that I have amputated a limb for disease of the knee-joint since I have been an officer of this hospital. In every other instance I have been able to procure anchylosis, though in one it required three years to accomplish it."

(F) CONCERNING ANÆSTHETICS.

ART. 83.—*Further remarks on the cause and prevention of Death from Chloroform.* By Dr. SNOW.

(*Medical Times and Gazette*, Feb. 2, 1856.)

In a paper read before the Medical Society of London, on the 26th of January, 1856, Dr. Snow said that he had pointed out, on a former occasion, as a result of experiments on animals, that, when the vapor of chloroform was sufficiently diluted with air, it produced its effects very gradually, and, if continued until death took place, the breathing ceased first, while the circulation went on until it was arrested for want of the respiration, as in asphyxia; while, on the other hand, if, at any moment, the vapor were not sufficiently diluted, it was absorbed from the lungs and circulated through the coronary arteries in such quantity as to stop the action of the heart by its direct influence. He considered that all the accidents which had happened during the exhibition of chloroform had occurred in the latter way, and never from the medical man mistaking the symptoms, and going on too long to administer chloroform sufficiently diluted with air. Dr. Black, of St. Bartholomew's Hospital, had, however, lately advanced the opinion that the patient did not die from the pathological effects of chloroform, but died simply of asphyxia, before they were brought under its influence, owing to the respiratory movements being arrested, or impeded by the pungency of the vapor, which had been administered in too concentrated a form at the commencement of the inhalation. He, Dr. Snow, considered this opinion incorrect for various reasons:

1. The process of dying by asphyxia occupied from four to nine minutes, after the access of air to the lungs was completely cut off; but no medical man could overlook the fact that his patient was not breathing, and persevere in preventing his doing so for this length of time.

2. In the greater number of cases of death from chloroform, the patient really inhaled the vapor, so as to be quite insensible from its effects, before the symptoms of danger set in. Out of 44 deaths from chloroform, 7 took place when the surgeon was just about to begin the operation; 12 occurred during its performance; in 8 cases the operation, being of short duration, was completed before it was discovered that the patient had expired; and, in the remaining 17 cases, the inhalation was discontinued, at some period of its progress, owing to the sudden occurrence of alarming symptoms.

3. In every case in which the state of the pulse had been noticed at the time of the accident, it was found to cease suddenly and abruptly. This was totally different from what occurred in asphyxia, where the pulse retained its strength for some time, and gradually diminished in frequency and force.

4. In twelve of the cases of death from chloroform, the face was observed to become suddenly pale at the moment when symptoms of danger set in. This symptom was indicative of cardiac syncope, and was incompatible with asphyxia; it had probably occurred in many cases where it was not recorded.

5. In several of the cases in which death occurred during the performance of the operation, attention was first called to the patient's danger by the sudden stopping of the hemorrhage: a symptom which also proved death by syncope, and not by asphyxia.

6. When animals are killed suddenly by chloroform, so as to imitate the accidents to the human subject, the blood is found to be of a florid color in the lungs immediately after death.

7. Except sometimes in the case of children and lunatics, it is not the custom to restrain a patient, so long as he is conscious. If he complains of pungency of the vapor, it is accommodated to his feelings; and, therefore, it is impossible that death should take place from the cause indicated by Dr. Black, unless in children and lunatics, to whom no accident from chloroform has yet happened.

8. The vapor of sulphuric ether was as pungent as that of chloroform, but accidents did not happen during its use.

A serious error, with regard to chloroform, was to suppose that the patient was safe so long as he had sufficient air for the purposes of respiration; the truth being, that the more air he breathed the greater was his danger, if the air were too highly charged with vapor. The air breathed by the patient should never contain more than about 5 per cent. of the vapor of chloroform; if it contained 8 or 10 per cent. it was liable to cause sudden death by suspending the action of the heart. He (Dr. Snow) recommended the use of an apparatus for regulating the quantity of vapor of chloroform in the air, but those who preferred to use a handkerchief, or sponge, might avoid the risk of danger, by diluting the chloroform with an equal measure of rectified spirit before using it. In case of accident, he considered the artificial respiration, very promptly and efficiently performed, afforded the best prospect of success.

ART. 84.—*On Death by Chloroform.*
By Dr. JOHN ADDINGTON SYMONDS, of Bristol.

(*Lancet*, March 22, 1856.)

It will be allowed by most observers, remarks Dr. Symonds, in a paper recently read before the Harveian Society, that in a very large proportion of deaths from chloroform, narcotism, in one form or other, is the first antecedent in time, and the most important in influence, when operating in its most favorable manner and degree. The chloroform having arrived at the encephalon, benumbs the central ganglia related to general sensibility, and in most cases involves also the ganglia of special sensation, as well as those of volition. But when the action becomes dangerous, it extends to the respiratory centre (medullary oblongata), and the patient dies in the way of coma. The order of events is, insensibility, interrupted breathing, and stoppage of the heart's pulsation; death. The series is identical with that which occurs in anæmic coma, or in congestive apoplexy. In such cases the intimation of peril is first given by the breathing, and if attended to, may save the patient. In another set of cases, death has been thought to take place in the way of asphyxia, or, to use Dr. Watson's more accurate term, apnœa; the fatal series beginning in the respiratory passages and cells, either because the air is too largely impregnated with chloroform to be chemically fit for respiration, or because the chloroform by its pungency, excites spasmodic closure of the glottis. "Each of these agencies," said the author, "may be an element, but I doubt its being unmixed with narcotism. The patient must have been stupefied in some degree, else in the struggles for breath there would be signs of consciousness in the unmistakable reference by the gestures to the cause of distress and danger. Still such cases may be conveniently classed under the category of apnœa, as an early and prominent fact. But in a third and more fearful, because more sudden and less remediable group, the chief character is the early cessation of the heart's action. The patient dies in the way of syncope. Dr. Snow, the most philosophical and skilful investigator of chloroform, after its immortal discoverer, Dr. Simpson, is of opinion that the heart is directly paralyzed by the poison in the blood. This view seems hardly admissible for two reasons:—First, in animals narcotized and killed by chloroform, the heart has been found capable of contraction, after all respiratory action had ceased; secondly, the supposition is superfluous; the direct action of the poison on the encephalon we know to be a fact—its direct action on the heart is only conjectured as probable. The former explains sufficiently the cases in question; therefore the latter is superfluous. But how does the former yield the requisite elucidation? Thus, we know that either by reason of a peculiar susceptibility, or by the suddenness and violence of an impression on the nervous centres, syncope—that is, stoppage of the heart's action—takes place in the way of shock. It is thus that the heart is paralyzed by the passionate emotion, by concussion of the brain, by crushing of limbs, by the instant apoplexy resulting from a large cerebral hemorrhage, which causes sudden and extensive compression, or from a smaller hemorrhage in the medulla oblongata, whether the fatal influence is transmitted through the sympathetic or the par vagum we need not stop to inquire. Analogous to such cases, in my opinion, is the occasionally sudden and overwhelming operation of chloroform on the nervous centres, and from these transmitted to the heart. The time is short for observing the phenomena in these deadly cases; but the pulse suddenly drops, the face shows a ghastly pallor, and there is a slight twitching of the features, a faint gurgling of the breath, and the patient swoons into death. In cases which have stopped short of this tragic ending, there has been vertigo, with fluttering of the heart, nausea, vomiting, extreme paleness of the face, and feebleness of the pulse, symptoms like those of slight concussion of the brain. In three instances I watched these phenomena with fearful interest, life having become almost extinct, without one sign of interrupted breathing, but with every indication of deadly faintness. That any narcotic agent may, even in small quantities, act variously on the nervous centres, is matter of daily observation. The normal operation of a quarter of a grain of morphia is to send the patient into a sound sleep. But in some individuals the hemispherical ganglia are so excited that delirium is the result; in other cases the patient suffers nausea, vertigo, faintness, and coldness, without any previous illness. These symptoms do not come on so suddenly as when they are induced by chloroform, and in the former case the quantity of the narcotic introduced into the system is not increasing every moment, as in the latter case; therefore these symptoms gradually subside. The danger of chloroform consists mainly in the suddenness with which it operates —the very property which renders it so valuable as an anœsthetic. Suddenness of action modifies the operation of all agencies on the encephalon. The gradual compression of a morbid growth produces phenomena very different from those which ensue on a hemorrhagic clot of the same dimensions; or, what is more to the point, blood exuding slowly from ruptured capillaries in the brain, gives rise to changes of function very different, in kind and in degree, from those which ensue on the same amount poured out suddenly from a larger vessel. And this, again, corresponds with Mr. Philip's experiments as corrective of the inference drawn from those of Legallois; for while the latter had concluded that the heart derived its contractile power from the cerebro-spinal axis, because destruction of the nervous centres was immediately followed by cessation of the heart's action, Mr. Philip proves that this effect did not occur if the injury was inflicted slowly instead of suddenly.

"That patients may die of chloroform in the way of syncope, is, I think, fully borne out by necroscopic observations. In several cases it is on record that blood was found in both ventricles, and in other cases that both were empty, neither of which conditions is significant of death by apnœa. Moreover, it appears that many have died in less than two minutes: from three to five minutes is the shortest time allowed to death by apnœa. Out of twenty-five cases in a table published in the 'Provincial Association Journal' (February 11th, 1853), I find that in nine cases it is expressly stated that death took place either within two minutes, or less, or 'instantly.' Stress has often been laid on the gorged condition of the lungs. This appearance in some of the cases is wanting, and when it is stated to have been present we do not find such evidence as would enable us to discriminate the amount due to the fact that the patient died suddenly and full of blood, from the amount assignable to death by apnœa. The heart has been occasionally found in a state of fatty degeneration of fibre; when thus structurally weak, its function is of course more likely to cease, whether the antecedent has been the interrupted breathing of coma, that of pure apnœa, or the shock from the nervous centres. To the danger of this, it has been the chief object of this brief paper to suggest some attention. To some of the members of this learned Society these remarks may appear so obvious that they ought not to occupy any of the time devoted to an evening meeting; but I cannot forget that men of the highest standing in the profession have seemed to ignore that mode of death from chloroform of which I have been speaking, and say authoritatively that the signals of impending danger are to be looked for only in the respiration. Chloroform is so priceless a boon to mankind, that we should all endeavor to ascertain, with the utmost exactness, the nature of the difficulties and perils which beset the use of it; and by so learning to prevent or overcome them, we may abate, if not altogether remove, the apprehensions which hinder recourse to this assuager of the anguish of disease, this spell against the terrors of surgery. I therefore venture to say to my brethren, that however important it may be to watch the breathing, we must not be content with doing this alone. Life rests on a tripod: each of.its three supports must be cared for; the narcotic surpriser of the encephalon may tell fatally on the heart, before the lungs have felt any disturbance of their function. It is our duty to insist on full recumbence, to watch the lips, the cheeks, and the pulse, and to be prepared to drop cold water on the face, and to apply galvanism when the indications of syncope are very manifest. I would even throw the head below the level of the body, as in extreme anæmia; for though the head has been for the time paralyzed through the brain, the latter organ must be immediately influenced in its turn by the failure of the circulation, so that the heart, which might otherwise have recovered from the first shock, has its action still further depressed by that very condition of the brain which the failure of its own function had deepened. So true is it that the healthful round of life may, by one interruption of the rotation, be converted into a vicious circle of disorder and death."

ART. 85.—*On some unnoticed effects of Chloroform.*
By Dr. C. HAPPOLDT.

(*Charlestown Med. Journal and Review*, Jan. 1856.)

Besides showing the large quantity of chloroform which may be introduced into the system without producing death, Dr. Happoldt is desirous of calling attention, in the following remarks, to some of its local effects on the nerves of special sense—whose seat of function is located in the passages through which the vapor passes on its way to the lungs—and to its remote effects produced on the organs supplied by the nerves which proceed from the lower segment of the spinal column. He says—

"Two cases recently came under my observation, which are interesting for the exhibition of these phenomena. The subjects of both were of the nervolymphatic temperament, and of sedentary habits. They had, during several months, resorted to the inhalation of chloroform for the purpose of procuring sleep, when this desired condition did not naturally occur at a seasonable hour. One or two ounces generally induced tranquil slumber, without being followed by any unpleasant consequence, except slight nausea, which usually disappeared after the morning meal.

"One of these patients had an attack of asthma, to which he had been previously subject; and being aware of the antispasmodic and anæsthetic properties of chloroform, he unadvisedly put himself under its influence, and continued the inhalations for forty hours; during which time he inhaled *twenty ounces of the fluid*. The asthma was relieved, and has not since returned—nine months having now elapsed—but he was left in an uncomfortable condition. The sense of smell was abolished, and that of taste perverted. The bladder and rectum lost their tonicity and excitability. When the former became distended, a concentrated effort of the will was necessary to effect urination. The latter remained for several months in a torpid condition, requiring the constant use of cathartics to effect the evacuation of its contents. The sexual appetite was for many weeks abolished, and the restoration of the functions of these organs was slowly accomplished. Saline substances were urgently craved for, and freely taken. Brandy was not disagreeable, and appeared to be of use in restoring the healthy conditions of the organs involved.

"The other patient supposes that he inhaled four fluid ounces without interruption, from the fact that the phial which had contained that quantity was empty on the following morning. He remained unconscious ten hours, and on awaking experienced no unpleasant symptoms. While breakfasting, he noticed the strange taste of the various dishes of which he partook ; but the taste of coffee was peculiarly unpleasant; and it was with difficulty that he could be persuaded that it was not the substances which he ate, but his sense of taste, which was at fault. During the day, whatever he ate appearing perverted in flavor, he became convinced that the cause of his altered sensations lay in his organ of taste. For more than a month neither fruits, wines, tea, nor coffee, could be taken with relish, and it was not until the expiration of two months that the sense of taste was restored.

"The sense of smell was, for nearly the same length of time, almost abolished. The nostrils were nearly closed by the swelling of the mucous membrane. The tongue became pale in color; and the mucous membrane of the mouth and throat was flaccid and swollen, as was that of the nares.

"Coincident with these phenomena, the penis was felt to be unusually flaccid, and there was no inclination to urinate. It was only after the bladder became considerably distended that urination was possible. There was no pain, but a strange sensation along the urethra while the urine was passing out. The specific gravity of this excretion was somewhat below the normal standard, and it contained a large proportion of the triple phosphates, and a trace of the crystals of uric acid. During two months there was no erection of the penis. The patient believed that the secretion of semen was not interfered with, from the sensation referred to the testes, and the desire which existed for sexual indulgence. The inability to perform the act he attributed solely to the paralysis of the perineal muscles.

"The rectum and intestines partook of a similar torpidity with the urinary organs; but the sphincter ani retained its contractile power. For a week there was no evacuation from the bowels, and no uneasiness was felt therefrom. The saline cathartics had very little effect. Calomel, rhubarb, aloes, and other more drastic substances, were found most efficacious. Nux vomica and strychnine, arnica, and iron, were resorted to, with no perceptible effect over the paralyzed organs. Brandy, which was most agreeable to the taste as a beverage, appeared to mitigate the symptoms, and was freely taken during their continuance.

"After the expiration of two months, the only remaining effect of the chloroform was constipation, which remains until this time (December 20th) five months since the last inhalation. This patient had never before suffered from constipation : now defecation seldom occurs without the aid of a cathartic."

(G) CONCERNING OPERATIONS.

ART. 86.—*Analysis of cases of Amputation of the Limbs, in the Radcliffe Infirmary, Oxford.* By Mr. HUSSEY, one of the Surgeons to the Infirmary.

(*Medical Times and Gazette*, April 26, 1856.)

The capital operations in the Radcliffe Infirmary are recorded in a register kept for the purpose, the entries being made from notes taken at the time of the operation. In this register and in the admission books are noted 164 cases of amputation from all causes, which are arranged in the paper in separate tables. Among the cases of disease, 91 were for diseases of joints ; 55 of these were in the thigh, of which 10 were fatal; 6 died from the immediate effects of the operation, and 4 did not recover sufficiently to be sent home. The mortality varied in the practice of the different surgeons. Of 20 cases in the leg, only 1 died ; of 6 cases in the upper arm, and 10 in the fore-arm, all recovered. Among those who recovered from the operation, 17 never permanently regained their former health ; 3 died from accidental illness ; in 1 the cause of death was not ascertained; 16 others died with phthisis, at various periods after the operation; the subsequent history of 5 was not known; the rest are all now in good health. The mortality was not affected by the duration of the disease, or the extent of disorganisation of the joint. The proportion of men who undergo amputation in early stages of disease is greater than that of women; in later stages the proportion of women is greatest. The operations for diseased joints in boys and girls under puberty are not successful; a larger proportion than in adults die from the effects of the operation, or do not recover their health after amputation. In 5 cases of malignant diseases, 2 died after operation; in 1 the disease returned within a year; the other two are living. In other diseases, necrosis, caries, gangrene, elephantiasis, old ulcerations, and inconvenient limbs, all the patients recovered. Of 6 cases of primary amputation of the thigh, only 1 recovered, and in that case the injuries were confined to the leg below the knee. In all the fatal cases, the operation was performed after very severe injury. All the operations on the leg (12 in number) succeeded. Of 15 on the upper arm, 3 died; and of 14 on the forearm, 1 died. Among the secondary operations, only 1 died, after amputation at the shoulder-joint for a burn. The operations were mostly done by circular incision. The chief veins of the limb were tied whenever they bled, without any bad consequences. The stumps were generally tied at the time of the operation. In several cases, where the stump was left open after the operation, there was secondary hemorrhage, and in all of them union was very slow. The healing of the wound, or the discharge of the patient, was retarded by so many accidental causes, that it was not easy to make a fair estimate of the time occupied in the recovery. The forearm generally healed rather sooner than the upper arm, and the upper arm rather sooner than the leg, the thigh being much the latest. After amputation for diseased joints, the stumps healed sooner than in other diseases. The greatest delay was after primary operations for accidents.

This paper was read before the Royal Medical and Chirurgical Society.

Art. 87.—*A word on Paracentesis.* By Mr. Birkett.

(*Assoc. Med. Journal*, April 26, 1856.)

A new mode of "tapping," or performing the ordinary operation of paracentesis abdominis, recently adopted by Mr. Birkett, deserves a word of notice. Every surgical practitioner must be aware how commonplace and uninteresting this operation has become, and how very like the analogous process as regards a beer-barrel; thus justifying in some measure the association of ideas with which the literal acceptation of the term, the process of "tapping," has come to be regarded by students and surgeons in operating theatres. Mr. Birkett proposes that the fluid should flow away by a piece of vulcanized India-rubber tube being slipped over a sort of flange on the canula, through which the trocar is passed; this piece of India-rubber tube fitted on to a further piece of tube of any convenient length, so as to carry the fluid away from the patient's bed. The finger and thumb are applied to the smaller piece of India-rubber tube, which is compressed firmly as the trocar is withdrawn, and this tube then fitted on to a longer piece of tube. The very unpleasant sound of a flowing stream of fluid is thus done away with; and where patients are not able to sit up to have the operation performed, it suits most admirably. It also prevents air from entering into the cavity.

SECT. II.—SPECIAL QUESTIONS IN SURGERY.

(A) CONCERNING THE HEAD AND NECK.

Art. 88.—*The general treatment of Scalp-wounds.* By Mr. Skey, Surgeon to St. Bartholomews's Hospital.

(*Lancet*, Jan. 26, 1856.)

These remarks occur in a paper entitled "Reminiscences of Hospital Practice:"—

"My wards have been singularly prolific of large wounds of the scalp occasioned by violence. Whether such wounds have been treated by plaster or by suture, erysipelas has too commonly followed on about the third or fourth day, extending more or less generally over the entire head and face. In the course of last winter I delivered a clinical lecture on these cases, advocating their treatment by means of quinine in full doses. I am fully confirmed in my opinion of the efficacy of this mode of meeting the difficulty by the enlarged experience of the last six or nine months, which has brought under my notice at least a dozen cases, additional to those I had previously treated on the tonic principle. The opposite treatment of such cases of traumatic erysipelas, by means of salines and aperients, may be equally efficacious for anything I can assert to the contrary. If it be equally efficacious, it is somewhat curious that the treatment by quinine, steel, and wine does so little injury."

ART. 89.—*On Gunshot-wounds of the Skull.* By M. STROMEYER.

(*Dublin Medical Press*, Jan. 30, 1856; and *American Quarterly Journal of Medical Science*, April, 1856.)

A very interesting and practical statement has been recently made by Stromeyer, as to his experiences of gunshot-wounds of the skull. He says that during three years he attended hospitals in Vienna, London, and Paris, during the times of Astley Cooper, he did not meet a single case in which the operation of trephining the skull had been successfully resorted to; while many severe wounds of the skull came under his observation which recovered without any operation. This weighed on his mind, till the chances of war placed recently a set of eight cases of gunshot fractures of the skull, with marked depression of bone, under his care, and all with brain symptoms—*the whole eight recovered by being let alone;* and notwithstanding the time-honored legends of Cooper, Dease, and Brodie, he is now satisfied this is the best practice! The plan he lays most value on is neither expectant nor operative, but, singularly enough, antiphlogistic, more particularly bleeding, if necessary, to anticipate inflammation of the membranes. Sir George Ballingall gives sixteen cases of wounds of skull which recovered quite unexpectedly after Talavera, by what he called "cold applications;" but Stromeyer says they recovered because Sir George was then flying before the enemy, and had not time to use his trephine. Stromeyer thinks, from what he has seen, that the chief danger consists in allowing atmospheric air to act on the brain substance, as it at once sets up a sort of decomposition or sloughing process, much more formidable than the "signs of compression" dwelt on by Astley Cooper, and that by using the trephine we go, as it were, into the very jaws of death.

ART. 90.—*Do eyes of different foci puzzle each other?* By Mr. CRITCHETT.

(*Medical Times and Gazette*, Dec. 1, 1855.)

A young woman presented herself, November 23d, among Mr. Critchett's outpatients, at the Royal Ophthalmic Hospital, on whom the operation for cataract had been performed on the right eye, the left being at the time perfectly sound. The cataract had been caused by an accident in childhood. Mr. Critchett remarked—"It has been laid down as a law, that in cases in which one eye is perfect, no attempt should be made to remove a cataract from the other, because by so doing you will get eyes of different foci, and your patient will be annoyed with double vision. Experience does not, however, confirm this dogma of à *priori* reasoning. In the woman before us I operated for cataract simply because the white opaque capsule was a deformity, and I subsequently operated for strabismus on the same eye with the same intent. The result you see. There is at present no visible imperfection in the patient's eyes. She has not much sight with the right, it is true; nor, indeed, could it be expected, seeing that light had been shut out for twenty-two years. The eyes do not, however, trouble each other, and there is no double vision. I am quite certain that, practically, eyes of different foci become in time accommodated to each other, and that, instead of confusing, the less perfect eye assists the other. It may be that, under circumstances where double vision would be likely to occur, the patient learns to disregard one of the impressions. A patient who has been operated upon for cataract in one eye, the other being perfect, will have better sight than if he were simply monocular."

Art. 91.—*The treatment of Chronic Entropium by Collodion.* By Mr. WILLIAM BATTEN.

(*Lancet*, Oct. 27, 1855.)

This mode of treatment was first employed by Mr. Batten in 1847, and again recently; and he now gives both the cases:

CASE 1.—Captain H— came under my care in October, 1847, suffering from various secondary symptoms of lues venerea. He had just left the military hospital at Plymouth, and had had, while there, severe inflammation of the eyes, which had resulted in entropium of both lower eyelids. For this especially he had come up to town to seek relief, but he had not been longer under the care of Mr. Alexander, and without any beneficial result being obtained, when the original disease reappeared with such gravity that I advised that the treatment of the entropium should be suspended for a time, and then proceeded to treat the syphilitic disease.

After a long course of treatment, the symptoms being of Protean variety, the patient at length perfectly recovered, the entropium of course still remaining. Collodion had then been but recently introduced, and as my patient was exceedingly anxious to avoid an operation, which he had been told was not always successful, I was induced, reflecting on the properties of the new agent, to give it a trial. The treatment was commenced in February, 1849. The mode of proceeding was this: by means of the thumb and finger the skin beneath the inverted tarsi was first corrugated transversely to the required extent; to this surface a sufficient layer of collodion was applied, and the fingers were then removed. The application was repeated three times a week at first, then twice, and lastly, once a week, for a period of four months, at the end of which time the patient was found to be perfectly cured, and has remained so ever since.

CASE 2.—Mrs. K—, æt. 40. This case was one of chronic entropium of the worst description, as it had existed since the patient was twelve years old, being a sequela of rubeola, and occupied the tarsi of both eyes. No treatment had been of the slightest avail, except that of plucking out the cilia, and this she had been obliged to have regularly done for her about every nine days, to obviate the aggravated inflammation which would otherwise ensue from the contact of the cilia with the globe of the eye.

Sixteen years ago the usual operation had been performed upon both eyes at Guy's Hospital, by Dr. Edenborough and Mr. Morgan, but without affording her any relief, of which, indeed, she had long given up all hope. Having proposed to her a trial of my treatment, to which she willingly assented, the application of the collodion was commenced on the 1st of May last, a small strip of zinc with a rounded extremity being used for the purpose. The application was regularly repeated on alternate days, the corrugation below being insured by the position of the finger, and that above chiefly by the open tarsus. The progress of the case from the commencement was highly satisfactory—marked, in fact, by one continued success. The eyelids, that had been so long inflamed and thickened, soon presented a better appearance; day by day the redness and swelling subsided; the inverted edges of the tarsi, with their growing cilia, by degrees emerged more and more outwards, until at length the full-grown eyelashes resumed their natural position. This was about the middle of June, and as the use of the collodion seemed now no longer necessary, it was discontinued, and an astringent collyrium prescribed, to be applied night and morning to the still disordered conjunctivæ. On the 14th of July, when I again saw the patient, I found no trace of the entropium, and she expressed herself, with much delight, as being perfectly free from a malady which she had so long deemed to be hopeless. The appearance of the conjunctivæ had much improved, and she now only complained of "a weakness" and occasional "itching of the eyes." On the 1st of August I again saw her. The eyelashes were well out, and the eyes were much "stronger;" but she still felt a good deal of the "itching," although the conjunctivæ had nearly regained their natural appearance. I prescribed a collyrium of acetate of lead in rose water, for occasional use, and dismissed the patient as cured.

Art. 92.—*Case of periodical Opacity of the Cornea.* By M. V. Rosas.
(*Wiener Medic. Wochenschrift*, No. 3, 1856.)

This case is very remarkable and very unintelligible, and the author has no satisfactory explanation to offer respecting it.

Case.—The patient was a young man, æt. 25, and he had been affected in the manner about to be described for eighteen months, when he placed himself under M. Rosas' care. The sight had been tried almost uninterruptedly for two days and two nights when the affection first made its appearance. When the patient wakes in the morning, and so long as he remains in the recumbent position, his vision is perfectly natural, and nothing unusual can be detected in the appearance of either eye; but immediately on getting up, or a few minutes afterwards, the cornea of the right eye becomes cloudy, and the vision obscure. This state continues, as a rule, for about two hours, and then slowly disappears. If the head be spouted with cold water, the eye may return to its natural condition in half an hour; or this return may be retarded if the patient is excited or irritated in any way. Examined during the time when the cornea was transparent, and the vision perfect, there was slight injection of the ocular and palpebral conjunctiva. The cornea to all appearance, was healthy, and so were the fluids in the anterior chamber. The iris was detached from the ciliary border in several points, except in its posterior or pigmentary layer, and this detachment is most marked towards the superior part of the globe. The pupil is of natural size, but oval in shape, and its position is carried somewhat downwardly and inwardly. The organ is not at all insensitive to light. Examined by the ophthalmoscope, the retina and choroid are seen to be very much injected. The left eye was at all times in a perfectly healthy state.

The treatment consisted principally in cold affusions to the head. They had the effect of shortening the duration of the daily disorder, but they had no effect in preventing the recurrence of that disorder. Quinine, opium, morphia, and iodide of potassium, were also tried, but without benefit. Mercurial inunction in the neighborhood of the eye, and the passage of an electrical current through the eye, were also tried, and equally without benefit.

Art. 93.—*Opacity of the Cornea treated by Operation.*
By (1) Mr. Haynes Walton, and (2) Mr. Taylor.

(*Medical Times and Gazette*, Aug. 18, 1855.)

The following cases are reported by Dr. M. Davis. They occurred in the Central London Ophthalmic Hospital, under the care of Mr. Walton and Mr. Taylor. A man, about 50 years of age, a patient of Dr. Taylor's had a quantity of lime thrown into his eye four years ago. The eye was immediately washed out, and it was supposed that all the foreign matter had been removed, but a dense white opacity remained, covering nearly two-thirds of the cornea, and completely concealing the pupil when in a state of medium contraction. Many ineffectual attempts had been made to remove or diminish the impediment to vision, by means of lotions and other local applications. On examining the eye minutely, it was seen that the opacity was smooth and uniformly covered by the epithelium; its upper edge, where it did not extend to the margin of the cornea, was shaded off gradually, and the surface generally appeared slightly more elevated than that of the clear part of the cornea. This elevation, taken in connection with the history of the case, led Dr. Taylor to suspect that the apparent cicatrix was formed by a portion of the lime which had not been removed at the time of the accident, and had become incorporated with the corneal tissues. He, therefore, with a fine iris-knife, carefully raised the epithelium in front of the pupil, and found that, by careful manipulation, the opacity could be chipped off in small flakes, and that in no part. towards the centre of the cornea, did it appear to have penetrated the anterior elastic lamina. After clearing the pupil, the operation was suspended for the time, partly on account of the severe pain which it occasioned, and partly to avoid the risk of inflammation. On a subsequent occasion, the remainder was removed, with the exception of a few small spots towards the margin of the cornea, which appeared to be due to interstitial inflammatory deposit.

The slight haziness which remained after the operation was speedily dissipated, and the man was dismissed with almost perfect vision. Chemical examination showed the opaque matter to consist of carbonate of lime.

In another case, also under the care of Dr. Taylor, the opacity was removed, partly by operation, and partly by the process of absorption, excited by mechanical irritation.

The patient, a female, 24 years of age, had been subject, till within the last six years to attacks of ulceration of the cornea. She now applied on account of a central milky opacity of the right cornea, shading the pupil and destroying useful vision in the eye. It had remained undiminished in size for six years, notwithstanding a great variety of local applications. Near the centre of the opacity were two small, dark brown spots, situated, apparently, in the substance of the cornea. These were, probably, the effects of a former long-continued use of nitrate of silver solution, while the cornea was ulcerated. The surface of the opacity was readily peeled off in small flakes, by a cautious use of the iris-knife, but the brown spots were found to be so deep-seated, that Dr. Taylor did not consider it prudent to interfere with them, especially as they would not impede vision. The result of this little operation, which has since been repeated, has been the rapid diminution of the opacity, and corresponding improvement in vision; and as absorption is still going on steadily, there is every prospect that the sight of the eye will be completely restored.

It might be objected that the following case ought not, in strictness, to be placed under the heading of this report, but it is given, not only on account of its great peculiarity, but because it is somewhat allied to the above.

T. P.—, æt. 38, a meteorological-instrument-maker, discovered about four years ago, that the left eye was misty. The mistiness increased slowly, and attributing the failing of sight to the injurious effects of his trade, he disregarded professional advice, till the right eye had given evidence of the same kind of obscurity that had attacked its fellow, and now he applied to Mr. Walton. The eye first diseased, the left, is virtually blind, for nothing can be seen with it, as in the centre of the cornea there is a brown oval opacity, placed transversely, large enough to cover the pupil, and dense enough to intercept light. It is of a sepia color, and shaded towards the extremities, not raised, and possessed of the same lustre as other parts of the surface of the cornea.

The right eye is affected in a similar manner, but in a less degree, and enough of the pupil is yet uncovered, that with a magnifying glass the coarser works of his trade can be executed. There have not been any subjective symptoms, and he himself is quite unaware that there are brown spots on his eyes.

Mr. Walton directed atropine to be used to the left eye, the effect of which was to dilate the pupil beyond the opacity, and thus to enable objects to be seen with that eye nearly as well as with the other.

The right eye was then treated in the same manner, and the vision was improved. The patient now expressed himself quite satisfied with the benefit received, and desired to cease attendance, but yielded to the request of Mr. Walton to attend another day, that he might ascertain how far the opacities were capable of being removed by operation. An attempt was made to scrape a portion of one away; but a clear surface beneath could not be obtained, as the disease had extended into the true texture of the cornea, and perhaps completely pervaded it.

Dr. Taylor, who had taken his microscope to the hospital to examine, in a fresh state, whatever might have been removed, found that the portion separated consisted of epithelium, some of which contained pigment granules.

ART. 94.—*On a case of Black Cataract.* By H. HAYNES WALTON, F.R.C.S., Surgeon to the Central Ophthalmic Hospital, Assistant-Surgeon to St. Mary's Hospital, and Lecturer on Anatomy.

This case is as follows:

CASE.—In October, 1855, Mr. Walton was sent for to see a gentleman, 75 years of age, who had lost the sight of both eyes for several years, and whose symptoms, objective and subjective, were as follows:

The cornea and sclerotica were healthy; the irides bright and in their natural planes. The pupils were of ordinary size, and acted but slightly, even when submitted to a bright light. The anterior chambers were large.

In the left eye there was an ordinary amber-colored cataract of advanced size; not, however, very opaque, and which it is unnecessary for me further to describe. With this eye he could see the outline of his hand, or any large body.

In the right eye, the pupil was not apparently clouded by any opacity, but was quite black; and when the left eye was shut he could but just discern light from darkness.

The history adds value to the case.

In the commencement of the year 1849, he was much troubled with muscae, and sight began to fail, the right eye being first affected. On the 15th of September, he felt a very decided impairment of vision, and on the 18th he could not read. He was now seen by a surgeon, who, after a few visits, called in Mr. Dalrymple, and the united opinion was to the effect that incipient cataract existed. At present he can see better with the left eye than when visited by Mr. Dalrymple.

"It appeared to me," writes Mr. Walton, "that there was a greater defect of sight in the left eye (that with the visible cataract), than the degree of opacity of the lens would account for; and this, together with the inactive pupil, and the very decided declaration of the patient, that he saw rather better at present than a year or two ago, induced me to suspect other disease in the eye besides cataract: but I shall not proceed further on this head.

"The remarkable blackness of the right pupil quickly attracted my attention. There was absent the gray-brown tint that is always seen in the healthy eye of an old person, which is due to the coloration of the lens; a natural change that is frequently mistaken for disease, and is, I fear, not sufficiently recognized by the majority of those who write on, or teach ophthalmic medicine. With the most careful examination, I could not detect a trace of color; the pupil was like that of a child, quite black.

"That the crystalline lens was present, I had full proof in the position of the iris, and the similarity in this respect between the eyes.

"That there was, therefore, before me some peculiar morbid condition, I was quite certain, for there was almost annihilation of sight in an eye to all appearance healthy, except that the pupil appeared darker than it should be, and I suspected that the lens or its capsule was black. My request to dilate the pupil, and examine the eye more in detail, was readily acceded to. A few days after, I applied a strong solution of atropine to both eyes, and obtained ample dilatation of both pupils. With the reflected light of the mirror of the ophthalmoscope, I saw in the right eye a cataract of a very deep brown color, uniform over its entire surface, being without striæ or markings of any kind. Even this was not made out except the instrument was used carefully. Since then, I have shown the cataract to one of my colleagues, by the means of sunshine concentrated through a powerful lens, and which affords a better light than the ophthalmoscope.

"From the opinion which Mr. Dalrymple is said to have given, one would naturally be inclined to think that there was at first nothing observable beyond what is seen in the early stage of cataract, but it would be unsafe to accept this, even as a probability. As Mr. Dalrymple's opinion was sought by a surgeon whose position should be guarantee of his proficiency in the diagnosis of eye disease, it is likely that the case was not therefore a straightforward one.

"I have met with very dark lenses, but nothing approaching to this, in the course of my professional career, nor do I know where any mention is made of a parallel condition of the lens where the eyeball was not disorganized, although I must confess to not having spent many hours in searching works that are not readily at hand.

"Very dark amber lenses are sometimes alluded to as being black; and it may be well to quote the short notices that have been made on black cataract by those of our countrymen whose opportunities for observation or extent of research have not been surpassed. Mr. Lawrence says—'I have never had an opportunity of seeing a cataract of a darker color than mahogany.' Mackenzie —'I have seen a few cases of lenticular cataract, in which the opacity was so dark, that without close examination the disease might have passed without detection.' Tyrell—'When the color is very dark the disease is not easily distinguished whilst the pupil is in the natural state, unless by careful and close inspection. The extreme cases of this kind are, I presume, those which have been denominated black cataract. I have not seen the lens after its extraction in any of these cases.' It would have added to the interest of this notice to produce the lens, which has undergone so remarkable a change, and were it certain that I am to be the operator, I should have delayed my communication till after extraction had been performed. Then also, would be ascertained the physiological state of the rest of the eye, and the admissibility of operation in such cases. However, this practical fact has been demonstrated, that the lens may become so dark, that a surgeon accustomed to treat diseases of the eye may not be able, without artificial means, to detect its presence. It is but probable enough, that similar cases have escaped detection, and been classed under the unexpressive term, amaurosis."

ART. 95.—*A case bearing upon the operation for Extracting the Lens.*
By M. Coursserant.

(*Archiv d' Ophthalmologie*, Sept. 1855.)

Everything which is calculated to throw light upon this operation ought to be collected with care, and for this reason we copy the following case :

Case.—The operation for extracting the lens was performed on the right eye of an old man, aged 82, who had lost the other eye on a previous occasion after the operation by depression. Eight days passed away without swelling of the eyelids or any other symptom to attract the attention of the surgeon, and everything appeared to be progressing favorably, but on separating the lids at the end of this time everything was found to be wrong—the flap of the cornea ununited, blood in the anterior chamber, false membranes across the pupil, the anterior surface of the iris of a greenish color, and so on. The eye, in short, was irreparably injured by inflammatory mischief, which mischief had progressed to this extent without giving any signs of its presence.

ART. 96.—*A peculiar form of Sclerotitis.*
By Dr. H. Taylor, Surgeon to the Liverpool Eye Infirmary.

(*Edinburgh Medical Journal*, May, 1856.)

"In the fifth fasciculus of his work on the 'Pathology of the Human Eye,' Mr. Dalrymple adverts to a form of inflammation originating primarily in the sclerotica, which he thinks has not been noticed in this country, or at least is not described in any of our systematic treatises on the diseases of the eye.

"The details which he gives of this affection are mainly derived from the review of an original paper by Dr. Sichel, of Paris, entitled, 'Upon a peculiar form of partial Inflammation of the Choroid, and of the Sub-conjunctival Cellular Tissue, and its Treatment.' My attention having been thus drawn to the subject, several cases in succession presented themselves, the symptoms of which closely resembled those described in Mr. Dalrymple's work. The disease appeared to be new to me, and peculiar in several respects. I have since met with other examples of it in different stages of development, and am now induced to collect and arrange my observations regarding it, as a contribution, however imperfect, to the sum of our knowledge of eye diseases.

"The disease seems to consist, as I think Mr. Dalrymple correctly observes, in a primary circumscribed inflammation of the sclerotica, which tends to spread *outwardly* to the sub-conjunctival cellular tissue, and *inwardly* to the structure of the choroid and corpus ciliare. He thinks that it is attended with the deposition of tubercular matter in the tissues above named, and at a more advanced stage of the disease the cornea is apt to become the seat of opacities, varying in size and density.

"The symptoms usually presented by the disease in a moderate state of development, are the following:—Several large and tortuous bloodvessels are observed advancing from the periphery of the eyeball towards the border of the cornea, usually the outer and superior portion, that which is directed towards the external canthus. At a short distance from the corneal margin, these vessels subdivide into a leash of smaller twigs, assuming a sort of circular or ovoid arrangement. Within the area thus marked off, one or more conical-shaped bodies are observed, separate from each other, of reddish color at the base, and white, or yellowish white, at the apex. They are firm in consistence, and evidently connected with the subjacent tissues, as they cannot be moved with the finger. The textures surrounding them are generally somewhat thickened and elevated, and the appearance presented is not unlike what we might suppose to arise from the deposition of some solid matter in the substance of the sclerotica and sub-conjunctival cellular tissue. The cornea is usually, although not always, the seat of some opacity. These opaque patches vary in form, extent, and density. They usually occupy the side of the cornea nearest to the thickened sclerotica, and are either separated from it by a clear strip of cornea, or, as more frequently happens, are united to it; presenting the appearance as if the opaque texture of the sclerotica had advanced upon the cornea. In some instances, where this union was only partially developed, minute red vessels could be distinguished, running apparently upon the internal surface of the cornea, and extending from the thickened portion of the sclerotica and corpus ciliare, towards the corneal opacity.

"*Pain* is usually slight in degree, sometimes it merely amounts to a sensation of tenderness on pressing the eyeball, or a feeling of stiffness on rolling it from side to side, or on exercising the eye much by artificial light.

"The movements of the *pupil* are usually sluggish, or almost wholly suspended, in the early stage of the disease; and at a more advanced period, it is apt to become irregular, and displaced from its central position towards the seat of the disease in the sclerotica.

"*Vision* is usually impaired in a greater or less degree; where opacities of any extent exist upon the cornea, it will, of course, be materially affected, but independently of this, it is generally imperfect, and liable to become more so when the eye is used for any length of time. There is an *increased flow of watery secretion* from the eyeball, which is promoted by anything which tends to augment the vascular congestion, as walking against a current of air, or exerting the eye in looking at minute objects.

"With regard to the *persons* most liable to attacks of this disease, it seems to affect females more frequently than males, usually young adults, and those especially of a strumous diathesis. One eye is usually attacked rather than both, although it may appear alternately in each; and when one is the seat of the disease, it may affect both sides of the eyeball simultaneously, or, commencing on one side of the cornea, may gradually travel round its entire circumference, disappearing in one spot as it is developed in another.

"One of the most characteristic features of the disease is its chronic obstinacy. It is slowly and insidiously developed. Commencing with a slight feeling of uneasiness in one corner of the eyeball, a little redness, which at first comes and goes, according to circumstances, and slight lachrymation, it gradually steals on, till at length the patient is aroused to a consciousness that there is something materially wrong with his eye, from observing an opaque spot upon the cornea, and finding that he can no longer use the organ as formerly. So much is this the case, that it is not uncommon to find that the commencement of the disease dates several months previous to the time when the patient first applied for medical advice.

*   *   *   *   *

"The only other disease with which this affection is likely to be confounded, and it is a mistake not likely to be made by any one familiar with the pathology of the eye, *is a pustular inflammation* of the conjunctiva. Both of these ophthalmiæ occur in young adults, and in both, we observe enlarged and tortuous bloodvessels, running towards, and subdividing round a common centre. In pustular ophthalmia, however, as its name implies, the point of attraction is a pustule, or vesicle, seated in the conjunctiva, and movable with this membrane; generally of a rounded figure, flattened upon the surface, and either filled with a semiopaque fluid, or, at a more advanced stage, forming a shallow ulcer. These appearances are very unlike the firm, immovable cone-shaped body, seated upon a dense thickened base, and described as a characteristic of the disease under consideration. Pustular ophthalmia, in addition, is rarely accompanied with dense opacities upon the cornea, or with any indication of inflammatory action in the tissues of the sclerotica, iris, or choroid."

ART. 97.—*On Rupture of the Inner Circle of the Iris.* By Mr. W. WHITE COOPER, Ophthalmic Surgeon to St. Mary's Hospital, &c.

(*Assoc. Med. Journal*, Oct. 19, 1855.)

Detachment of the iris from its ciliary border is a common result of external violence; but there is an injury occasionally caused by heavy blows upon the eye, which, with its consequences, are but slightly mentioned by the majority of ophthalmic writers. In many systematic works it is passed over altogether. This is rupture of the inner margin of the iris, an injury giving rise to wide and persistent dilatation of the pupil and serious disturbance of vision.

The following cases afford illustrations of this severe accident:

CASE 1.—In October, 1854, a man was admitted into St. Mary's Hospital, having received a very severe blow upon the right eye; the anterior chamber was full of blood, and no trace of the iris was visible. He was put to bed, and cold applications were ordered to be constantly applied to the injured eye; a brisk aperient was administered, and he was placed on low regimen.

I did not see him until the following day, by which time absorption of the effused blood had proceeded so vigorously, that the condition of the iris could be ascertained. It was then seen that this blood had issued from two fissures in the pupillary margin of the iris, which presented a jagged appearance. The pupil was widely dilated, perfectly motionless, and the sight was so far impaired, that large objects only could be discerned.

The eye was, however, free from inflammation, and the patient made no complaint of pain. Under these circumstances, as there happened to be a great demand for beds, the man was permitted to leave the hospital, under the promise of attending as an out-patient. This, however, he did not think proper to do; and it was only by accident that I subsequently obtained an opportunity of examining the eye. Its condition at the expiration of two months was as follows:

The pupil was still widely dilated, and the irregularity of the inner margin of the iris was very distinctly seen. Neither contraction nor dilatation of the iris could be excited; it remained perfectly motionless under every amount of light. The eye had speedily recovered from the accident, with the exception of the sight, which remained very dull, all objects appearing hazy and indistinct. The sight was improved by looking through a pin-hole aperture in a card. As there were no indications of inflammatory action, he was recommended to supply himself with a pierced diaphragm to limit the quantity of light entering the eye, and to avoid everything which could over-excite the organ.

CASE 2.—An officer of Dragoons, quartered in Dublin, early in October, 1854, was playing at racquets, when he received a violent blow from the ball on the left eye. For a time he was stunned, but on regaining his senses he found that sight had left the injured eye. He placed himself under the care of an eminent physician, and Mr. Wilde was also consulted, so that no skill was wanting in the early treatment of the case.

This gentleman was seen by me on the 16th of the following November, about six weeks after the accident. The condition of the eye was as follows:—The pupil was so enormously dilated, that the iris was reduced to a mere narrow strip, and was perfectly immovable under the strongest light. The lower portion of the margin presented two fissures, the edges of which being drawn asunder, gave a saw-like appearance to that part. The sight was very imperfect, large objects only being discernible; it was not improved by a pierced diaphragm.

Stimulating embrocations and instillation of tincture of aconite and of opium were tried, but without the slightest benefit.

I saw this gentleman from time to time, and six weeks after his first visit decided improvement in the sight displayed itself: by looking through a pin-hole aperture he was able to discern objects which had before been very indistinct. After the lapse of four months, an alteration became visible in the condition of the iris; a certain power of contraction had been regained, for there was a marked diminution in the size of the pupil, and an equally marked increase in the breadth of the iris. Still it could not be seen to act under the influence of light, there being no discernible alteration when the eye was alternately shaded and exposed.

In July, when I last saw the patient, a still further improvement had taken place, and now a faint contraction and dilatation could be excited. The sight was materially amended, for not only could he discern distant objects by means of the pierced diaphragm, but he could read and write with tolerable facility. There was, however, this drawback, that under the most favorable circumstances the vision of the two eyes was not equal; and as my patient could not constantly wear the diaphragm, he unconsciously acquired the habit of closing the injured eye when looking at any object.

CASE 3.—On the 14th of June, 1855, I was consulted respecting the case of a youth, aged seventeen years, who had received the following injury eleven weeks previously: a round and heavy pebble was thrown by a lad at another boy who had incensed him, but the missile unfortunately lighted full on the right eye of my patient, who happened accidentally to come between the two at that unlucky moment. He fell from the force of the blow, and was at once rendered blind of that eye. He was placed under medical care, and active measures were resorted to; but the sight was only restored to a very imperfect extent. He was therefore brought to town.

The nature of the case was unmistakable. The pupil presented the characteristic wide dilatation, and the lower margin had that serrated appearance which has already been described. In this case there were three fissures, so that the irregularities were very marked. The color of the iris was unchanged, and the eye was perfectly free from inflammation. On being desired to close the sound eye, it was ascertained that he could see large objects, but even these indistinctly. On placing a pin-hole aperture before the eye, he could recognize features, and read tolerably large type.

As the injury was extensive, I formed an unfavorable opinion as to the result of this case, and advised that instead of his being apprenticed to a printer (as was intended), some agricultural occupation, or other pursuit requiring little exertion of the sight, should be selected. The use of a pierced diaphragm was recommended.

Remarks.—"It is well known that clean incisions of the iris are seldom followed by inflammation, and an eye in which the iris has been ruptured by injury may be fortunate enough to escape: but when we consider the great violence done to the whole organ, the possibility of deep-seated effusion, and of subsequent insidious inflammation, such cases require to be closely watched. The effused blood which always veils the iris will speedily disappear under the influence of cold and of simple treatment, but strict antiphlogistic measures are to be enforced from the commencement; and if there should arise indications of inflammation, as pain deep in the eye, or about the brow, tenderness of the globe, and zonular redness of the sclerotic, mercury should be administered until the gums are rendered tender.

"In the cases under consideration, the dilatation of the pupil is as great as that produced by a strong solution of atropine (which is always attended with considerable confusion of sight); but the impairment of vision is for a long time after the accident far greater than can be accounted for by any such dilatation. This is not surprising, when the character of the injury is considered. A blow sufficiently violent to cause the rupture of the iris is likely to produce concussion of the retina, and separation of that membrane might even take place; again, chronic inflammation of the retina may be excited. If concussion merely, the effects will gradually pass away, and the improvement of vision through a pin-hole aperture will be the index by which amendment can be traced. If inflammation has been excited, the injury to vision may be permanent.

"So far as my experience has hitherto gone, injuries of the pupillary margin of the iris are little amenable to treatment. This will, no doubt, in a great degree depend upon the depth to which the fissure extends, and the consequent amount of laceration of the fibres which contract the pupil. If these are completely divided, the pupil will be widely expanded, and no application will cause its contraction; if only partially divided, a certain amount of contraction may be excited. The question will be anxiously asked—Is the eye likely to recover? for although after a time the organ becomes accustomed to the unnatural glare of light, the sight is under the most favorable circumstances seriously interfered with. A very cautious prognosis should be given. Time perhaps may improve the state of things; but if the laceration be extensive, it must be very doubtful whether the powers of reparation will be sufficient to bring the eye into a useful condition. The edges of the fissures are widely separated, and cannot be approximated by any means with which I am acquainted. The fissure may be likened to a cleft palate; but we are without the means which modern skill has supplied, of removing that defect by operation.

"But do we possess any means of remedying the inconvenience arising from this permanent mydriasis? Unquestionably! by artificially imitating the contracted pupil, the eye may be rendered useful, unless damaged by inflammation. This is best done by means of a spectacle-frame, fitted for the affected eye with an opaque plate, either of thin steel, horn, or blackened tortoiseshell, and having in the centre, to correspond with the pupil, an aperture, either circular, or as a transverse slit. The form and exact dimensions must be a matter of experiment. Various forms and sizes should be tried, and that selected which affords the best vision."

ART. 98.—*Congenital absence of the Nose, and a new Rhinoplastic operation.*
By M. MAISSONNEUVE.
(*Dublin Medical Press*, Dec. 19, 1855.)

Congenital absence of the nose is an exceedingly rare deformity, and it is questionable whether any case of the kind is on record.

CASE.—"Eugénie Marotte, aged seven months, was born strong and well formed, except that her face was completely devoid of any nasal prominence, and that in place of this natural projection there existed only a plain surface pierced with two little round openings scarcely one millimetre (0·03937 inch) in diameter, and three centimetres (1·1811 inches) distant from each other. In addition to giving the child a most grotesque appearance, this deformity occasioned her much inconvenience in the act of respiration, and therefore in that of sucking. In these two points of view, consequently, it was important to remedy this faulty conformation, and for this purpose her parents came to Paris to consult me.

"No similar instance having been known to science, the ordinary rhinoplastic processes were, of course, inapplicable to the case. I therefore devised the operation I shall now describe.

"On the 18th of May, 1855, the child having been previously placed under the influence of chloroform, I carried inwards from each of the nasal orifices, a transverse incision one centimetre (0·393708 inch) in length. Two vertical incisions, commencing from the inner extremity of the preceding, were now directed towards the free edge of the lower (sic) lip, near which they were brought together so as to form a V. From these latter incisions resulted a narrow flap comprising the entire thickness of the lip: it was dissected and horizontally raised to form the inferior septum of the nose.

"There then resulted a true artificial hare-lip, the edges of which I united by means of the twisted suture. But to obtain this union, it was necessary that the space comprised between the nasal opening should be shortened by the entire width of the flap detached to form the septum, and that consequently a projecting fold should be formed at the expense of the intermediate skin. This fold, supported by the artificial sub-septum, constituted a perfectly regular nasal prominence.

"In order to understand completely the mechanism of the operation, it is sufficient to repeat it on a piece of paper, when it will be immediately seen how satisfactory the result is.

"The final issue was not, however, obtained without some trouble. The infant, irritated with pain, did not cease during the first twenty-four hours crying, so to speak, and struggling: the consequence was, a partial disunion of the points of the upper suture. This, however, was attended with the incidental advantage of suggesting to me an improvement in the operation for hare-lip.

"This improvement consists in the subcutaneous division of the orbicular muscle at each side of the wound, in order to prevent its contractions from tearing open the cicatrix.

"Thanks to this improvement, union took place without difficulty, notwithstanding the uneasiness of the little patient; and at the time of her departure from Paris, the cure was complete.

"The nose was of a very regular shape, and the openings of the nostrils being ample, admitted of easy respiration."

Art. 99.—*Complete removal of the Temporal Bone by Caries.*
By Dr. Bigger.

(*Dublin Hospital Gazette*, Dec. 15, 1855.)

The two following cases are from the reports of the Dublin Pathological Society:

Case 1.—James Dignum, æt. 5, was brought to me on the 2d January, 1849, suffering from profuse otorrhœa, of a most fetid character, from the left ear: the right ear was sound. The fetor was that characteristic of diseased bone, and was unlike the aromatic odor which proceeds from discharges from the internal ear when the membrana tympani has been injured, and which is so well known to those accustomed to treat aural diseases. The mother of the child stated that the disease commenced by an attack of pain in the ear about eighteen months previously, and that this discharge commenced very shortly after, when the excessive pain ceased; that it had been treated by various practitioners without effect, and that caustic and blisters had been the principal means employed.

On clearing away the matter with a small glass syringe with a crooked jet, something sharp was found protruding into the meatus. The first impression was, that some foreign body had been introduced into the ear, but on further examination it proved clearly to be bone, and the fetor excited the idea that it must be some bone entering into the structure of the internal ear. Seized with a forceps it felt slightly loose, but as it could not be dislodged without using force, and not knowing what bone it was, it was left for fourteen days longer, during which period warm water injections, and poultices of bread and water, with powdered charcoal were used.

On the 16th of January, 1849, the bone yielded to very slight traction, and was drawn out easily and without hemorrhage. It was about an inch in length;

one end terminated in two prominences, not unlike the open beak of a bird; this was evidently the remains of the carotid canal, the internal wall of which had been completely absorbed, so as to permit the exit of the bone without injury to the artery; close to this was the internal meatus: the meatus externus was situated about one-third from the end of the bone on one side, and both it and the other cavities were full of cerumen. The surface of the entire bone was abraded and rough, as if the hard crust had been filed off, and the entire bone was more porous than in the normal state, but yet very hard. No bad effects resulted from the removal, and the poultices were continued till the 14th of February, when suppuration had nearly ceased, and the ear only exuded a little clear serum. On the 1st of March the child was perfectly well, and the ear externally quite normal: the internal meatus was narrowed, and gradually decreased until it ended in a fine point.

The pulsation of the carotids was equal on both sides, nor was there anything remarkable to be noticed in the jugulars. There was no paralysis in any of the muscles to which the portio dura of the seventh pair of nerves is distributed. It is hardly necessary to say that there was permanent deafness.

A month subsequent, this child had a sharp attack of scarlatina, succeeded by cellular dropsy in the face and limbs, from which it recovered under the use of bark and wine.

On the 16th May the child was last examined. He was then in perfect health; the ear was quite free from pain, and were it not for a slight serous discharge, perfectly well. The funnel-shaped cavity has become somewhat smaller. No cerumen.

Case 2.—Thomas Dowd, æt. 5, a strong, fat, yet strumous-looking child, the son of a mechanic, whose means were sufficient for every comfort, was brought to me on the 4th June, 1855, suffering from profuse otorrhœa of both ears. His cheeks bore marks of lunar caustic having been plentifully used, as they were blackened and blistered where it had overflowed with the fetid discharge.

The parents stated that the child had always been healthy and strong, with an inordinate appetite, and that the only thing which had ever ailed him had been occasional swelling of the glands of the neck, and some stiffness in the motions of the head, neither of which symptoms were constant. The running from the ears was first noticed in the summer of 1853, after a railroad journey, with some exposure, which caused inflammation and great pain in the ears, particularly the left, on the subsidence of which matter began to flow from it, and shortly afterwards from the other. This matter had not at first the horribly fetid smell which it lately exhaled. An English general practitioner treated the child, for the first six months, principally by syringing and blistering; he was then brought to Dublin and treated by an aurist, with constant applications of lunar caustic to the ears, and cod-liver oil internally; but not getting any better, regular advice was discontinued until the 2d of June, 1855, when a gush of blood from the left ear frightened the family. The child was immediately carried to the nearest apothecary's shop, who poured fluid caustic into the ear, and inserted a plug, recommending them to bring the child to me in the morning. On the 4th June the child was brought to me. I carefully removed the plug, which, although it had checked the hemorrhage, was not sufficient to restrain the discharge; there was no appearance of blood about the ear, but the smell from the copious discharge, was almost insupportable. From this peculiar smell I suspected diseased bone, and on clearing out the ear, I felt denuded bone, a very short distance from the meatus externus. The child's uneasiness and suffering prevented me from ascertaining whether it were loose or not, nor was I very anxious to interfere with it, through apprehension of again bringing on hemorrhage. I ordered digitalis to be administered in small doses, placed a small plug of matico leaves in the orifice, and directed that linseed-meal poultices and charcoal powder, in equal parts, should be applied.

June 12th.—Suppuration profuse. No further hemorrhage. Fetor decreased by the charcoal, but still indicative of caries. Having gained the confidence of the child by gentle treatment, I was enabled to feel that the bone was loose. I was afraid to remove it, suspecting that it might be a similar case to that of Dignum, and being impressed with anxiety about its deep vascular relations.

The same palliative treatment was pursued until the 24th of June, when a point of bone showed itself near the external meatus, and was drawn out gently without any hemorrhage.

The right ear, meanwhile, was pursuing the same course which had been run by its fellow; suppurating very freely, but without the occurrence of hemorrhage; and the mildest treatment being employed until the bone protruded, it was easily removed from its purulent bath by the aid of a forceps and gentle traction, on the 19th August, 1855, without either pain or hemorrhage.

The course of this case has been favorable from the period of the removal of the bones; all suppuration shortly ceased; a little glycerine was dropped in from time to time, and occasionally the openings were washed out with a solution of Bewley's iron alum, gr. x ad. ℥j.

On the 14th September, I closely examined the child. The ears were normal externally; a slight watery discharge, free from smell, is emitted; the apertures in both ears end half an inch from the external opening, by contracting into a fine funnel a little flattened from side to side.

September 25th.—No apparent ailment but deafness. Dr. Bigger then exhibited the bones which he had removed, and contrasted them with the healthy bone taken from a child of the same age. He said, no doubt could be entertained, notwithstanding the absorptive erosion of their surfaces, that they were petrous bones, and the same peculiarity was observable in both, that the portion of bone internal to the carotid canal had been absorbed, so as to prevent injury to the vessels when the diseased bone was removed. A large quantity of hard cerumen filled all the cavities. The great anatomical difficulty to be solved in those cases is the absence of paralysis in any of the muscles supplied by the *portio dura* of the seventh pair of nerves, as the internal auditory foramen was perfect in all the morbid specimens, and the parts through which the Fallopian canal wound its course were hard and uninjured; so much so, that it would have been impossible for the nerve, if following its ordinary course, to have escaped from the bone, as it was evident the carotid artery had done.

The wonderful provisions of nature in thus separating one of the hardest bones of the body from its deep and important connections with large sinuses, a great artery, most important nerves, and a very close proximity to the brain itself, are illustrated in these cases; as is also the value of an expectant practice in treating parts so much beyond our reach. A little meddling on the part of the surgeon might have obstructed the reparative processes which were safely proceeding to a happy result, and which he never could have so effectually forwarded, as by leaving the matter to be effected by nature's own handiwork.

ART. 100.—*Dislocation of the Lower Jaw reduced by a new method.* By Mr. W. COLLES.

(*Dublin Hospital Gazette*, July 15, 1855.)

The case was that of a young lady, æt. 25, whose lower jaw became completely dislocated during a prolonged yawn; and an unsuccessful attempt at reduction had been made before the patient applied to Mr. Colles. Mr. Colles proceeds—

"Before attempting reduction, I wished to ascertain the position in which I would have most command of the force to be used. Standing before her, I passed both thumbs into the mouth, but felt I would not have a position the most favorable for applying all my force, if necessary.

" I then stood behind her, and it at once struck me this was the position which afforded most advantages.

" Placing her head against my chest, I passed each thumb as far back on the corresponding side of the jaw as possible. By making a rotatory motion from the wrist, I found the bone to yield; by now adding a motion of drawing the hand in towards the chest, the left side first, then the right, slipped into their positions, and the patient closed the mouth, the rows of teeth falling into their relative positions, and she now could speak plainly

" I think there are many advantages to be derived from attempting reduction in this posture, viz.: the surgeon standing behind the patient, the head applied to his breast, and the thumbs turned inwards on the corresponding angles of the jaw, the fingers under the bone in front.

"In the first place, the head is much more secure than in the original process, where it is applied against a wall, because in the latter the surgeon may press down the bone, and the patient generally will draw the head in the same direction by moving the body forward in the chair.

"By standing behind the patient, while depressing and pushing back the thumbs, he is pressing forwards with the chest, and thus fixes the head more steadily and assists his manipulations; and even if the patient do move on the chair, a slight motion of his body will suffice to counteract this movement, and retain the head steadily fixed.

"Another advantage is, that he can use much more force, because when standing in front he can only use the muscles that depress the hands; whereas standing behind the patient he has the power of those muscles, and is assisted by the powerful class of muscles that rotate the thumbs inwardly; and, besides, in the former case his pressure is away from his body, whereas in the new position the pressure is more directly downwards and towards himself. The only disadvantage in this proceeding, if it can be considered one, is, that the mouth is stretched more than in the original plan."

ART. 101.—*On Congenital Deficiency of the Palate, and the means to be used for its relief.* By Mr. GEORGE POLLOCK, Assistant-Surgeon to St. George's Hospital.

(*Lancet*, Feb. 2, 1856.)

In this paper (which was read before the Royal Medical and Chirurgical Society on the 22d of January, 1856), the author states that his object is not so much the relation of a new operation for the closure of the imperfect hard palate (although various novel operative procedures are explained in the course of it), as to draw attention to the fact that few exceptions exist in which the fissures of the hard palate cannot be effectually and permanently relieved by operation—a fact, which for various reasons cited, appeared to have been much neglected by English surgeons. Mr. Pollock's paper was admirably illustrated by a great many models and drawings of the parts concerned, both previous to operation and during the different stages of the treatment of the cases related. The author divided the different conditions of deformity affecting the hard palate into six groups. 1. The first and most extensive fissure extending through the soft and hard palate—and then dividing in front, passes through the alveolar ridge, making a gap on each side of the incisor teeth. 2. The second extends, through the soft and hard palate, and through the alveolar ridge also, by a single gap only, on one side of the incisor teeth. The author had always found congenital fissure of the upper lip associated with fissure, either double or single of the alveolar ridge; and that when the latter is double, the former was so also. 3. The third passes through the soft and hard palate, and terminates in front immediately behind the alveolar ridge. In this variety there is often great irregularity of the upper incisors. This group of cases is also accompanied by congenital fissure of the lip. 4. The fourth extends through the soft and about three-fourths of the hard palate. 5. The fifth extends through the soft palate and the palate bones only. 6. The last exists as an opening in the hard palate, and the soft may be entire. Upon this classification Mr. Pollock laid down the principle, that the more extensive the deformity, the more extensive the surface of the soft tissues, and greater, therefore, the facility of bringing the edges of the fissure together, and the greater the hope of ultimate success. He gave various admeasurements of the parts, in different degrees of deformity, all tending to prove that the lesser the fissure in the bony palate, the more natural will be the curve of the arch, a condition which is found to add to rather than diminish the difficulties of the operation; for although in such cases the soft parts may be readily separated from the bone, yet they will rarely be sufficiently broad or free to meet in the median line without traction, or a resort to some other operative measures; whereas, in the greater degrees of deformity, the sides of the fissure run upwards, in a direction almost perpendicular, and thus afford a larger surface from which to obtain soft parts. Several cases were next related from the author's own practice, and from that of the late Mr. Avery, to whom Mr. Pollock paid a well-merited tribute of respect and regard. In the relation of the cases, and the sequel of the paper, the following points were insisted upon :—The line of the first incision of the edges of the cleft ran along the line of union between the mucous membrane of the mouth and that of the nose. It is made with a knife, consisting of a flat piece of steel, bent at a right angle, about a quarter of an inch from the extremity, the cutting edge of which is about an eighth of an inch broad in the centre, and rounded off narrower to each end ; a much broader knife, of the same character, is used to detach the soft parts from the bone, an operation requiring great care, to avoid lacerating and bruising them. Knives bent at various angles are required for various parts of the mouth, and one was recommended, the blade of which should be acted on by a screw; they should be strong and firm, and as broad as can conveniently be used. The edges, when detached, should never be brought together by sutures, unless they fall and meet together without traction. The author advocated the introduction of a suture through each of the curtains of the newly detached palate, as preferable to the use of forceps, when manipulating them. The ends of the sutures are brought out of the mouth, and tied in a knot, so that there may be no fear of their being withdrawn, and thus the flaps can be raised or moved about without fear of bruising or lacerating the edges, one of the most frequent causes of failure of union. When the flaps or curtains do not meet of their own weight in the mesial line, a curved knife is introduced through the palate, near the last molar tooth on each side, and pushed upwards and inwards between the bone and soft parts, until its point is seen in the fissure, when the blade is moved slightly backwards and forwards. Lateral incisions may also be required. The author strongly insists on the propriety of not attempting too much at once, and for these reasons: the separation of a large surface greatly interferes with its nutrition ; both anterior and posterior palatine arteries would be divided at the same time, and sloughing rendered thereby probable ; the length of the operation, and consequent fatigue and pain to the patient. The author prefers to operate upon the hard palate first, because the anterior palatine artery being usually divided in that procedure, the flaps obtain ample nourishment from the posterior palatine vessels; and again, firm union of the new-formed palate is usually followed by a sensible diminution in the breadth of the fissure of the soft palate. Again, it is the more tedious and painful operation of the two. In operating on the soft palate, the author advocates a novel mode of dividing the levator palati muscle. The flap being put on the stretch by the traction of the suture above mentioned, a sharp-pointed, double-edged knife is run through the side of the palate, on the inner side of the hamilar process, which can be readily felt through the soft parts. The point being kept in a direction upwards and inwards is soon seen to have passed through the soft palate, and projecting into the gap of the fissure above the line of the levator. The handle is next raised, and a sweeping cut made along the posterior surface of the soft palate. The knife, being withdrawn, leaves but a small opening in the mucous membrane, and the levator is found to be freely divided. If this proceeding do not sufficiently liberate the curtain, the incision may be carried down to the free margin of the soft palate. Sutures should never exert the slightest traction or pressure. Their removal, of course, will depend on the circumstances of the case ; but usually the first may be removed on the third or fourth day. After the operation, fluid or pulpy food should be given liberally ; it is very important to insist on this, as the patient will otherwise be deterred by the pain of swallowing. Whiteness and coating of the tongue after operation are not to be considered indications for the administration of physic : nor are various conditions of the tongue and fauces previous to operation, and which are due to the absence of the hard palate, to be regarded as indications of defective general health ; the latter, however, should always be perfect at the time of operation. The operator upon the hard palate is not to be discouraged by failure in gaining union at first, for parts which were thin and scanty are often rendered thicker and more vascular by separation from their attachments. When attempts are made to close an aperture in the palate, caused either by malformation or disease, after paring the edges and separating the soft tissues from their attachments, lateral incisions are frequently necessary; and great general support may be given to the sutures used below the wound, by passing a broad suture through the lateral incisions, and thus including both flaps within its embrace. And this is not its only effect; it prevents the healing of the lateral incisions until the opening has had time to unite. Its use is preferable to that of sponge or lint introduced into the wounds. As chloroform is not applicable to these operations, a degree of self-command and endurance is required, which cannot be expected in an individual under the age of seventeen or eighteen, at which period, also, the development of the parts affected may be presumed to be nearly completed. Mr. Pollock suggests, in conclusion, that although in all cases in which operative procedure has been attended with success, a great improvement has invariably been noticed in the speech and articulation, yet much remains to be done by education. Efforts must be made to change the acquired habit of pronunciation for a new method of articulation, which may be best and easiest effected by the patient repeating words after a teacher, or reading aloud, subject to correction. Difficulties in this respect will, however, often be found to depend upon the fissure in the alveolar ridge, or irregularities of the teeth.

ART. 102.—*Case of Pharyngotomy.*
By Mr. Cock, Surgeon to Guy's Hospital.
(*Medical Times and Gazette*, Feb. 9 and 23, 1856.)

Cases of this kind are of such unfrequent occurrence that any new case is of considerable interest.

CASE.—Mr. T. G., æt. 22, a highly respectable tradesman at Dartford, was brought to Mr. Cock's residence on Thursday, January 17th, by Mr. Martin, surgeon, of Dartford.

It appeared that for some time he had been wearing a false central incisor tooth fixed to a gold plate, which extended some distance on either side. The foreign body, which was subsequently removed from the pharynx, may be thus described:—The plate formed the segment of a circle corresponding with the hard palate behind the incisor cuspidati and bicuspides teeth. The one extremity terminated in a slender clasp, with two points as sharp as needles, and encircling the bicuspis tooth; the other extremity formed a single sharp point. The anterior edge of the plate presented three acute angular projections, which corresponded with the inter-dental spaces; and from this margin also the false tooth formed a prominent projection. The extreme length of the plate—in other words the *sector* of the circle—was an inch and five-eighths; while a line drawn from the edge of the tooth to the sector measured exactly one inch.

This plate had been swallowed by the patient during sleep, about two o'clock, A. M.; and Mr. Martin, finding that it had stuck in the gullet, and could neither be seen nor felt from the mouth, brought him up to Mr. Cock for further advice.

There could be no doubt that the foreign body had lodged in the cervical portion of the swallow, but its exact situation was not very clearly indicated. The pain and irritation together with tenderness on pressure, all of which were very considerable, were referred to the top of the œsophagus, just below the larynx; but no projection indicating the precise locality of the plate could be detected from the exterior. He was able to swallow fluids, although in very small quantities and with great difficulty. His breathing was not impeded, but he had an irritating laryngeal cough.

Under these circumstances, Mr. Cock judged it most expedient to delay any active measures for extraction, until the patient had recovered from the immediate effects of the accident and the fatigue and excitement of his journey. He was, therefore, advised to go into the hospital, in order that every available means might be used; and he willingly agreed to this arrangement. In the course of the afternoon he was visited by Mr. Cock, who passed a bougie into the pharynx, and found a total obstruction about the lower edge of the larynx, in fact just at the junction of the pharynx and œsophagus. A pair of strongly curved forceps detected the plate, but it could neither be grasped nor moved from its position. As his respiration was unimpeded, and the pain quite bearable when kept at rest, it was determined to postpone further measures until the next day. A full dose of opium was given, as much fluid nourishment as he could get down was ordered, and he was furnished with ice to suck at his leisure.

On Friday, January 18th, Mr. Cock saw him with Mr. Hilton. He was calm and tranquil, and had not suffered acutely except when pressure was made from the exterior, or when he attempted to swallow. It appeared very doubtful whether any fluid which he took into his mouth found its way into the œsophagus. Attempts were made with several instruments to grasp or dislodge the plate, but they all proved abortive, and it was found impossible to pass any instrument between the foreign body and the walls of the gullet, so as to get it below the obstruction. Mr. Cock, at length, succeeded in introducing a flexible catheter, No. 5, which appears to have found its way between the horns of the clasp which formed one end of the plate. As a means of conveying fluid into the stomach had now been obtained, it was suggested that the action of vomiting might possibly alter the position of the plate, and render it more accessible from the mouth. A pint of milk was accordingly conveyed into his stomach, and then half a drachm of sulphate of zinc and a scruple of powdered ipecacuanha administered. Strange to say, not even a sense of nausea was produced, and the emetics were retained without producing the slightest constitutional effects. A mode of administering nourishment had, however, been obtained, and we could, therefore, afford to wait and take the chance of any favorable contingency. On Saturday, January 19th, Mr. Cock made another attempt. Since the previous day he had twice fed the patient with milk, wine, and beef-tea; but the catheter was passed with great difficulty, and there was only one particular spot on the left side where it could be made to penetrate into the œsophagus. He was unable to swallow a drop of fluid by natural efforts, but derived great comfort from sucking ice. Mr. Cock attempted to pass a looped wire round the plate, and also manipulated with a flexible tube, from the extremity of which a pair of forceps could be projected, but no success could be obtained, and further proceedings were laid aside for the present. On Sunday, January 20th, no attempts were made, but the patient was fed three times through the catheter; the introduction of the instrument becoming more and more difficult each time. On Monday, January 21st, Mr. Cock again met his colleagues. It was now imperative that some decisive step to remove the foreign body should be taken, as the flexible catheter could no longer be passed, and the patient was beginning to feel seriously the effects of want of nourishment and rest. The position of the plate was pretty clearly ascertained. It was impacted either at the commencement of the œsophagus or else just above (where the œsophagus and the pharynx join). It was determined to cut down and open the gullet. Mr. Hilton assisted Mr. Cock in the operation.

The patient was placed on his back, with his head and shoulders slightly elevated. Chloroform was given, and he was soon quietly under its influence. An incision of about four inches in length, was carried from the upper edge of the thyroid cartilage, nearly as far down as the sterno-clavicular joint; on the left side of which the platysma and cervical fascia were divided, bringing into view the carotid sheath and the omo-hyoideus muscle, which was thick and fleshy where it crossed the wound. This latter was divided, together with some filaments of the descendens lingualis nerve, and two or three small arteries, which were immediately tied to prevent as much as possible infiltration of blood into the cellular tissue. A little further dissection laid bare distinctly the common carotid artery, the inner connections of which were easily separated with the handle of the knife and the finger. It was considered to be an important object to separate completely the carotid artery from its internal attachments; and this having been accomplished, the vessel, together with the sterno-mastoid muscle was drawn outwards and retained by retractors, and thus rescued from injury or molestation, while the further steps of the operation were carried on, the object of which was to reach the upper portion of the œsophagus.

The thyroid body was now exposed by dividing a few of the external fibres of the sterno-hyoid and sterno-thyroid muscles, and the dissection was continued along the outer surface of the gland backwards towards the spine. The tissues were separated partly by the handle of the knife, partly by the blade. An artery, probably a branch of the superior thyroideal, was divided where it crossed the upper part of the wound, bled freely, and was secured with some difficulty. A larger vessel, probably the inferior thyroideal, was seen running across lower down, but escaped without injury. The larynx and trachea were gently drawn over towards the right side, so as to widen the large wound which gaped along the side of the neck.

The œsophagus was reached by following round the surface of the thyroid body, which completely covered and concealed the trachea.

About two inches of the gullet could now be traced with the finger, but no projection indicating the presence of the foreign body could be felt. It therefore seemed tolerably certain that the plate had not descended into the œsophagus, and must be lodged in the lower part of the pharynx. With some difficulty, by tilting the larynx a little forwards and over to the left, the finger was passed behind it, that is, between the pharynx and the vertebræ, and the body was now obscurely felt exactly behind the cricoid cartilage, protected as it were by the inferior course of the thyroid. The point of the knife was now brought to bear on what appeared to be the most prominent part, which proved to be the single tooth, and the grating sensation of the blade indicated that the pharynx was opened, and the foreign body reached.

The white tooth, in fact, became visible at the bottom of the wound; and, being grasped with a pair of forceps, the opening into the pharynx was dilated upwards and downwards with a blunt-pointed bistoury. After a little manipulation, one end of the plate was disentangled from its attachments and brought out of the wound, but the entire body was not extricated until a further slight division of the walls of the pharynx had been made. This, however, was soon accomplished with the assistance of Mr. Hilton, who cut along the edge of the gold plate, while Mr. Cock gently withdrew it with one hand, and protected the parts with the fingers of the other. The patient was carried to bed, and cold water applied to the wound, no means being used to bring the edges together. On recovering from the effects of the chloroform, he seemed to have suffered but little from the operation, expressed himself as comfortable and free from pain, and returned eagerly to his former occupation of sucking ice. An enema of beef-tea and wine was thrown up, as he had no nourishment since the previous day. In the evening, he complained of great exhaustion, or rather sense of starvation, and Mr. Cock gave him nourishment through the catheter, and a full dose of opium.

January 22d.—Was free from all untoward symptoms, and only complaining of an empty stomach. He was fed with milk and beef-tea three times. Sucking ice was a great luxury, although he believed that none of it passed into the œsophagus, and as far as could be ascertained, no water found its way out by the wound. On the third day, January 24th, Mr. Cock introduced the common œsophagus feeding-tube, which passed readily, without pain or obstruction. He has since been regularly fed by his dresser, Mr. Dyer, at first, three times, but afterwards, at his own request, four times in the twenty-four hours. He is always ready, indeed eager, for his meals, and receives them with great enjoyment. His diet consisted of beef-tea, brandy and egg, arrow-root, with milk or wine. Notwithstanding this nourishment, of which he swallowed about four pints in the twenty-four hours, he was evidently losing flesh and strength. Accordingly, Mr. Cock ordered as much pounded meat to be mixed with the beef-tea as could be made to pass through the tube, and directed an ounce to an ounce and a half of cod-liver oil to be given at each meal. He takes an opiate every night, but the quantity is undergoing gradual diminution.

February 5th.—The increase of nutriment, or the oil, or both, have produced a decided improvement in his appearance, and he expresses himself as feeling stronger and better. His spirits have all along been good and hopeful.

The wound has looked healthy from the first, and has now contracted to half its original size. Since the operation nothing has been swallowed by natural deglutition, and he is very unwilling to make the attempt, as it causes considerable pain, and a sensation as if the wound was being rent open. He does not appear to swallow his saliva.

Had the foreign body been lodged in the upper part of the œsophagus, its extraction would probably have been more easily accomplished; but the protection which was afforded by the cricoid cartilage in front, and the posterior edge and inferior course of the thyroid, which, as it were, overlapped it at the side, rendered the access to it difficult and tedious, and materially complicated the operation.

— In the "Medical Times and Gazette" of February 23d, we learn that about a month was occupied in the closure of the wound, and that all the nourishment was administered by means of the stomach-pump during the first three weeks.

Art. 103.—*Cases of Laryngotomy.*
By Mr. HENRY THOMPSON, Surgeon to the St. Marylebone Infirmary.

(Lancet, Oct. 27, 1855.)

The following cases are worth recording, inasmuch as they bear on the question of employing laryngotomy in place of tracheotomy in circumstances of impending death by asphyxia from laryngeal occlusion; a question which, during the last few years, has been receiving a practical solution in the successful substitution, in many instances, of the simple and easy operation for that which is not unfrequently both dangerous and difficult of performance.

CASE 1.—I was called, at four o'clock in the morning of the 27th of September, by Mr. Joseph, of Manchester Street, to see a patient, to whom he had been summoned two hours previously. I found a man, of about forty years of age, lying on his back in bed, with extended neck and livid countenance, gasping for breath. An attack of acute laryngitis had supervened on an ordinary cold in the course of the previous day, had been vigorously treated by applications of ammonia, &c., but was now threatening to prove fatal by asphyxia. There was no time for delay, and with Mr. Joseph's concurrence and assistance, I proceeded at once to make an opening into the larynx. Having made a short incision through the skin in a vertical direction, over the crico-thyroid membrane, I found it necessary to tie a small artery, which spouted freely on dividing the tissues beneath. The membrane itself was then incised to an extent sufficient to admit a full-sized double trachea-tube, which was inserted and adjusted without the slightest difficulty. The relief was instantaneous. A few very forcible inspirations and expirations followed, the lividity vanished, and the patient was soon in a sound and comfortable sleep. A piece of muslin was folded three or four times and laid on the orifice of the tube, to modify the temperature of the inspired air.

I saw him once a day on the three following days, during which he was recovering rapidly. The tube did not cause the slightest pain or irritation. Meantime, Mr. Joseph's assistant removed the inner tube twice a day, in order to detach the adhering viscid mucus, and returned it each time well oiled within and without. I have often had occasion to observe before that this application tends to retard the accumulation considerably.

On October 1st, the fourth day after the operation, finding that the patient could speak well when the tube was closed, and that there was scarcely any tenderness about the larynx, I removed the apparatus, approximated the edges of the small wound, and applied water dressing.

On the 8th of October the wound had entirely closed, and on the 10th the patient walked out, and, with the exception of debility, had recovered from his attack.

CASE 2.—On June 2d, 1854, I accidentally met in the Strand a well-known physician, who had just been summoned to a case of urgent asphyxia, and who requested me immediately to accompany him. We found a little boy, three years of age, livid and almost insensible, struggling violently for breath. There was evidently no time to be lost. Not being provided with the necessary appliances, I ran into the shop of Weiss, the instrument maker, fortunately only a few doors off, and instantly obtained them. Opening first, the crico-thyroid membrane, I found it necessary subsequently to divide the cricoid cartilage and upper ring of the trachea, in order to introduce the tube. Before, however, this could be accomplished, he had almost, if not quite, ceased to breathe, a significantly long interval having been noted during the last two inspirations; and it was not until we had performed artificial respiration, in part by applying the mouth to the tube, but chiefly by performing repeated acts of pressure upon the abdomen and ribs, that the natural action of the lungs was established. We had the satisfaction, however, of leaving him, in the course of half an hour, completely relieved, and enjoying comfortable sleep.

June 3d.—We saw the patient together. He was breathing comfortably, taking nourishment freely, and in all respects improving. A good deal of mucus was passing through the tube.

I subsequently learned that, contrary to express orders, the tube was removed for a short time, by the attendants of the child, on the 5th inst., and that in this condition he suddenly died of asphyxia, in less than ten minutes after taking, with considerable relish, a basin of beef-tea. No post-mortem was permitted.

These cases are practically valuable, inasmuch as they present additional evidence in favor of an opinion, the accuracy of which is becoming more and more apparent—namely, that a tube may be introduced into the interior of the larynx, and be retained there for some time, without exciting irritation of the organ, even in the presence of acute laryngitis; and that it is therefore unnecessary to resort to the severer method of tracheotomy, on the assumed ground that it is calculated to occasion less disturbance to an already diseased larynx.

(B) CONCERNING THE CHEST, ABDOMEN, AND PELVIS.

ART. 104.—*Case of Subclavian Aneurism in which a new mode of treatment was adopted.* By Mr. FERGUSSON, Surgeon to King's College Hospital.

(*Lancet,* Sept. 1, 1855.)

Mr. Fergusson presented to his class on the 4th of August, 1855, a most interesting case—one of a series, thinks the surgical reporter to the "Lancet"—where a very remarkable cure has been effected in well-marked subclavian aneurism, by a new and specific method of manipulation which he has adopted. We may state here that we saw the case about a year and a half ago, also, when the man was previously under treatment. Some short period before that time Mr. Fergusson conceived the plan of stopping the circulation in the aneurism by pressing the sides of the aneurismal sac together, with their intervening fibrinous deposit; and in this case, from the phenomena attending the manipulation, there appeared to us very little doubt that the object held in view by Mr. Fergusson had been attained—viz.: the clots of fibrin in layers in the aneurismal sac had been displaced, and spreading from the subclavian into the axillary and brachial, a new sort of Brasdor's operation, at the distal side of the subclavian, had been the result. In other words, we believe that Mr. Fergusson, without ligature, had attained all the advantages of the last-named operative proceeding; for not only had a blocking up of the axillary and brachial been followed by a partial stoppage of the current through the enlarged aneurism of the subclavian, but even with very marked, but not so satisfactory, results as regarded the pulse in the radial at the wrist, which became completely stopped for a time, with symptoms of paralysis in the arm, all resulting from the displacement of the fibrinous clots.

The aneurism in the present case was situated in the subclavian, in the usual site of subclavian aneurism—namely, between the scaleni muscles, and to us seemed almost to invite some modification of the Dublin surgeons' plan by compression on the first rib. The plan by compression, we need hardly observe, is in general applied to the artery above the aneurism, between the latter and the heart. Crampton, however, in 1816, showed that the obliteration of an artery can be effected without rupture or ligature of its coats, as generally conceived, simply by this blocking-up process. The early volumes of the "Lancet" contain cases also cured by Brasdor's operation; it seems, however, more applicable to carotid than subclavian aneurism.

Mr. Fergusson related to his class on the 11th, at some length, the details of a previous case of subclavian aneurism, of the same character as the present, in which his ideas on this subject were first matured. In both cases the method of cure by deligation at the tracheal side of the scaleni, as well as Brasdor's operation at the distal end of the aneurism, were inadmissible; yet it was gratifying to find the present plan, by firm pressure of the thumb on the aneurism, so as to displace some of the fibrinous clots, followed up by local pressure, succeeded in obtaining most striking and in many respects curious but satisfactory results. Intimately associated as the subclavian is at the right side with the vertebrals and carotid, the method of displacing fibrinous coagula is not without danger. A patient under such circumstances will fall down, perhaps, in a fit from want of circulation in one side of the "circle of Willis," formed by these arteries; yet, as the cause is so apparent, the danger may not be very alarming. Some instances of cure of aneurism of even the innominata have been given by American surgeons, in which recourse was had to ligature, on Brasdor's plan, of the subclavian; the result here ought to be equally dangerous. Hodgson gives us cases also in which a plug of effused lymph had nearly obliterated the subclavian: while Gendrin has imitated all the phenomena of arteritis and blocking up of aneurisms, by injecting irritant substances into a portion of artery contained between two ligatures. In Mr. Fergusson's new mode of operation, we believe an entirely novel idea is acted on—namely, the displacement of the lamellated fibrin of the aneurism, on which no operation has been performed, and so directing the clots of fibrin that they shall block up the distal end of the artery so diseased. As Mr. Fergusson has expressed an intention of bringing the entire subject under the notice of the Medical and Chirurgical Society, we purposely abstain from giving the cases in detail. The method of treating aneurism by compression, originating with Desault and Hunter, and recently revived with such excellent results by the Dublin surgeons, will gain an immense accession of interest, if it should prove that the fibrinous deposit of the sac of the aneurism may be thus as it were utilized in bringing about the results hitherto gained in a different mode by Brasdor's operation at the distal end of the aneurism. Considerable caution will be at first necessary, as observed by Mr Fergusson, in selecting cases which are fitted for the present method, as premature or ill-judged experiments in the shape of direct pressure or manipulation on the sac of aneurism not requiring it, one of which we mentioned recently as brought into Guy's, where direct and prolonged pressure had been made in the popliteal space before the patient came into hospital, would be certain to be followed by severe inflammation of the sac and other dangerous results. The spontaneous cure of aneurism is not unknown in practice; it may take place, it must not be forgotten, by a coagulation of the contents or increase of the quantity of lamellated blood in the sac, the cavity becoming filled, and the circulation conveyed to the parts beyond the disease by the collateral vessels; or, again, in some rare cases the aneurismal tumor may be doubled up and press upon the portion of artery leading directly to the aneurism; or in a third fashion, as in a remarkable case given by Mr. Liston, where the patient had well-marked subclavian aneurism, which subsided and disapppeared—an aneurism of the innominata pressing on and obliterating the aneurism of the subclavian!

Whatever may prove to be the correct pathological explanation of the phenomena in Mr. Fergusson's present cases, we deem it our duty to state here briefly that the cure seems complete and unequivocal without any ligature of vessels, nor is there any reason to believe the case was one of spontaneous cure of subclavian aneurism, as in the case given by Mr. Liston. It is now two years since the man came first under observation; he has been, on and off, under treatment all that time in King's College Hospital and at home in the country; but happening to be in town at the time, Mr. Fergusson took advantage of the opportunity to exhibit the case to his class.

ART. 105.—On Abdominal Emphysema.
By Mr. ERICHSEN, Surgeon to University College Hospital.
(Lancet, Dec. 15, 1855.)

" Emphysema of the subcutaneous cellular tissue of the trunk is looked upon as one of the most certain signs of thoracic injury, and its occurence from other causes than wounds of the lungs or pleura is scarcely, if it all, recognised by writers on surgery. My object in this communication is to show that it may arise without any injury of the chest, by the escape of flatus from a ruptured or wounded intestine into the subperitoneal cellular tissue, and thence into the more superficial cellular planes of the trunk; and it may thus become important, or possibly the sole evidence of serious abdominal injury. So far as I have been able to ascertain, the remarks on this subject in surgical writings are of a very incidental character, and not commensurate with the importance of this lesion as a diagnostic sign of intestinal injury. Haller alludes to it as occurring in a case of abdominal injury; and Morgagni states that in a case of stab of the abdomen, perforating the colon, 'a beginning emphysema was brought on.'

"The only practitioner who, to my knowledge, has treated of 'abdominal emphysema' as a special symptom, is Dr. O'Ferrall, of St. Vincent's Hospital, Dublin. That gentleman, in March, 1854, published, in the 'Dublin Hospital Gazette,' a very valuable practical lecture on 'Abdominal Emphysema, consequent upon Diseases of the Intestines, especially Malignant disease of the Rectum, Hernia, and Ileo-cæcal Abscess;' but in that communication he makes no mention of this condition as a consequence of abdominal injuries.

" The two following cases will illustrate the importance of this symptom in the diagnosis of intestinal injury :

"CASE 1.—A man, about 30 years of age, was admitted into the hospital, under my care, in February, 1854, having been squeezed between the buffers of two railway-carriages about half an hour previously. He had been struck on the pit of the stomach and the small of the back. On examination, no bruise of skin or fracture of ribs or spine, or positive sign of injury, could be detected; but the patient was collapsed, and complained of pain in the abdomen. There was some retching, but no vomiting. From the nature and the seat of the injury, and the severity and the continuance of the collapse, there could be little doubt that he had sustained rupture of some one or other of the abdominal organs; but no positive signs existed to indicate which one in particular had suffered. He was, accordingly, kept quiet in bed, opiates administered, and the urine, which was untinged by blood, drawn off. On the following day, some emphysematous crackling was noticed in the subcutaneous cellular tissue of the right flank; and this gradually crept upwards and forwards, so as to occupy a considerable extent of the side of the abdomen and lower and back part of the chest, as high as the scapula. These parts presented the ordinary characters of emphysema, being somewhat tumefied, doughy, and crackling on pressure. There was no discoloration of the integuments. The state of depression continued, notwithstanding the administration of stimulants, and the patient died about forty hours after the accident.

"On examination after death, it was found that the anterior margin and the under surface of the liver were lacerated to some extent, and that a considerable quantity of blood had been extravasated into the peritoneal cavity. The intestines at first presented no appearance of being injured; but, on closer inspection, it was found that the posterior part of the duodenum, at about the juncture of the descending and transverse portion, was ruptured to the extent of an inch behind the peritoneum; the laceration in no way implicated that part of the duodenum which was invested by serous membrane. No extravasation had taken place into the peritoneal cavity; but a considerable effusion of thin, bilious-looking intestinal matter had been extravasated into the subperitoneal cellular tissue in the loin, for some distance around the ruptured gut and the flatus from this had found its way through the cellular planes until it had reached the subcutaneous cellular tissue, when it had given rise to the emphysema which had been noticed during life. There was no injury to any of the organs within, or to the parietes of the chest: no fracture of any ribs.

"The practical interest of this case lies in the fact of the emphysema being the only sign of intestinal injury. There was no wound penetrating the abdominal cavity, nor injury to the lungs or ribs; hence the air which became extravasated into and widely diffused through the cellular tissue could have come from no other source than the ruptured gut. The peculiar and very unusual situation of this injury in the only portion of the small intestine that is uncovered by peritoneum prevented the occurrence of the more ordinary signs of intestinal injury, viz., feculent or tympanitic extravasation into the cavity of the peritoneum.

"In such a case as this the suspicion would naturally arise on the occurrence of emphysema, that the chest had been injured; but the first appearance of the effused air in the abdominal rather than the thoracic wall, the absence of pneumothorax and of all stethoscopic indications of thoracic lesion, would enable the surgeon to make a satisfactory diagnosis as to the seat of the injury that furnished the air.

"CASE 2.—A young man was admitted under my care last December with a pistol-bullet wound in the abdomen. The ball had entered close to the navel, and had traversed the body, being extracted from under the skin to the left of and close to the lumbar spine. From the course the bullet had taken, there could be little doubt that the intestines had been traversed, but there was no positive sign of the occurrence of such an injury by the escape of fæces or flatus through the external aperture. A few hours after admission, however, emphysema began to show itself in the left flank. This gradually extended forwards and upwards, so as to occupy a very considerable extent of surface on the left side of the body. The emphysematous swelling presented the usual doughy crepitation so characteristic of this morbid condition, differing in no way from what is observed about the chest or neck in cases in which the cellular tissue of these regions is inflated from a wound of some part of the respiratory organs. The patient died about twenty-four hours after admission. On examining the body, it was found that the small intestine had been traversed, and the upper part of the rectum wounded by the bullet. It was from the wound in the rectum that the flatus had escaped through the meso-rectum into the cellular tissue of the loin, and thence into that of the trunk generally.

"In this case the occurrence of emphysema, though interesting as a pathological phenomenon, was less important as a diagnostic sign than in the former instance, the direction of the bullet leaving little doubt that the bowel had been wounded; though of this, as in the former instance, the occurrence of emphysema was the only positive evidence.

"There are but two morbid conditions with which 'abdominal emphysema' can be confounded—viz., thoracic emphysema, and the putrefactive emphysema from gangrene of the cellular tissue.

"From thoracic emphysema it may be distinguished by the absence of all sign of injury about the chest, by its spreading more slowly, and probably by its being seated, or at all events commencing, in a lower part of the trunk—rather the abdominal than the thoracic wall.

"From the putrefactive emphysema of the cellular tissue, consequent on low cellulitis or gangrene, the distinction would necessarily be easy, in the absence of all precursory inflammation, and of all concomitant signs of suppurative slough.

"The mechanism of 'abdominal emphysema' appears to be simple. When the wound in the intestine is so situated, as in both the instances related, that it communicates directly with the subperitoneal cellular tissue, the flatus, by the compression to which all the abdominal contents are subjected during expiration, will be forced into the contiguous cellular tissue, and a fresh portion being pumped in at each respiratory movement, the inflation will gradually extend through the different planes of cellular tissue until the more subcutaneous layers are reached.

"There is another way in which this 'abdominal emphysema' might occur—viz.: by the escape of flatus into the peritoneal cavity from the wounded intestine, and thence into the subcutaneous cellular tissue at the edges of an oblique wound through the abdominal wall. That would appear to have been the way in which it occurred in the case related by Morgagni, as quoted by Mr. Travers ('Injuries of the Intestines,' pp. 26 and 27):—'The transverse and oblique muscles were perforated with a wound that would admit two fingers, and between them the air had entered, so that a beginning emphysema was brought on. This air had got out of the colon, which was wounded, into the cavity of the belly, and had distended it; nor had air alone come forth, but excrement also.'

"When the emphysema happens in this way from a previously existing tympany, the mechanism of its occurrence would appear to resemble that of a thoracic emphysema, resulting from a previously formed pneumothorax."

ART. 106.—*Case of Diaphragmatic Hernia.*
By Dr. C. W. CHANCELLOR.

(*American Quarterly Journal of Med. Science*, Oct. 1855.)

The site of the hernia in this case is in some degree peculiar.

CASE.—"On Monday, September 3d, 1855, I was called to see J.'P—, æt. 6; delicate frame; light complexion; strumous habit. His mother informed me that the boy had been unwell, to her knowledge, from the Friday morning previous, complaining of pain in the left shoulder and side, with occasional vomiting, and had had no evacuation from the bowels since Wednesday, August 29th, for which calomel and oil had been given, and retained without producing any effect. He had taken no food, except a piece of bread, which was immediately ejected. Water could be retained only in small quantities. His appearance at this time was quite natural, with but little expression of suffering; he still complained of pain in the left side, which was slightly increased by pressure under the margin of the ribs of that side; there was no pain elicited on pressure elsewhere. His abdomen was very much distended and tympanitic throughout its whole extent; skin hot and dry; tongue furred and coated with a light brown deposit; pulse accelerated, but otherwise normal; respiration slightly hurried but easy, no cough, and but little thirst.

"On questioning the mother of the boy she stated, 'that on the day previous to his complaining, he had in a scuffle with a play-fellow been thrown across a plank, on the abdomen;' but there was no external evidence of injury. I ordered an active purge to be followed by a purgative enemata.

"Tuesday, September 4th, the enemata had produced quite a large evacuation but there was no improvement in the general condition, showing that the discharge had only come from that part of the intestinal canal below the point of obstruction. Thinking the case to be one of invagination, I proceeded to treat it *secundum artem*. The countenance daily grew more anxious and dejected, and all the symptoms more aggravated, until death furnished relief. His mental faculties remained unimpaired throughout the disease, and intelligent—I might say precocious—answers were given to questions, until the hour of death, notwithstanding a large amount of opiates had been used to palliate suffering and quiet the stomach, which had become very irritable; but at no time was there stercoraceous vomiting. Nothing was ejected but the articles swallowed, mixed with the mucus of the stomach. About twelve hours before death, which occurred on the 8th of September, nine days from the period of attack, the pulse became slower and softer, and the surface covered with a profuse perspiration: the extremities retained a pleasant temperature.

"Having examined all of importance connected with the onset and progress of the case, we will now proceed to the pathological condition furnished by a *post-mortem* examination, which was conducted in the presence of several distinguished professional friends, fifteen hours after death.

"The only marked abnormal appearances externally, were a slight general emaciation and great discoloration of the integuments of the abdomen. On opening the cavity of the abdomen, the bowels, viewed *in situ*, as may be inferred from the foregoing, were very much distended. The stomach and liver were in a healthy condition, the latter natural in size and color, and the gall-bladder well filled with bile. The bloodvessels of the intestines were considerably injected. Continuing our examination, by tracing up the colon from the ileo-cæcal pouch, we discovered that the large intestine was perforated just at the upper part of the angle which it makes in forming the transverse colon. The perforation was about seven-eighths of an inch in length, sufficiently large to permit the escape of the contents of the intestine, which had been poured out into the peritoneal cavity: about two and a half inches to the left of this perforation a knuckle of the transverse colon, and also of the jejunum near its junction with the duodenum, had passed through an artificial opening in the middle of the left leaflet of the diaphragm, and were tightly constricted. The contents of the bowels, finding an obstacle to its progress in every direction, had pushed the diaphragm high up, considerably diminishing the thoracic cavity. The diaphragm was then cut loose from its attachments with the ensiform cartilage and ribs, and the viscera of the thorax exposed. Two or three inches of the colon and jejunum were found to be included within the cavity of the chest in a gangrenous state, and adherent to the inferior lobe of the left lung, which latter was also attached firmly to the upper surface of the diaphragm."

ART. 107.—*A case of Wound of the Diaphragm.* By Dr. P. FRAZER.

(*Lancet*, Jan. 19, 1856.)

Commenting upon this case, Dr. Frazer asks, Was this one of the cases in which the bold and original suggestion of Mr. Guthrie, to cut down and relieve the incarcerated organ, should have been tried? Will the excessive thirst and vomiting help us in future cases to a diagnosis? Or will the sight of the aperture or apertures assist us? And to these queries, Mr. Guthrie (who communicates the case to the "Lancet") answers:—"I am not aware that more could have been done with propriety, unless perhaps the posterior wound had been more enlarged, so as to allow of no retention of fluid; but this would not have rendered any important aid in saving the life of the patient, the occurrence of the hernia not being suspected previous to the man's death. The operation I have recommended, of making an incision through the wall of the abdomen, for the purpose of dividing the structure of the diaphragm, and of withdrawing the parts protruded into the thorax, can, I fear, only be attempted with a hope of success in what may be termed secondary cases—where the sufferer has recovered, with a hole in his diaphragm, through which, after a time, portions of the viscera of the abdomen ascend into the thorax, and become incarcerated in the first instance, and subsequently strangulated, from distension of the hollow viscera."

CASE.—M. O'G—, æt. 18, private in the 30th regiment, was struck by a Minié bullet, while in the act of retiring into the trenches, after the failure of the attack on the Redan on the 8th of September. The bullet entered midway between the angle of the ninth rib and the spine, and made its exit one inch outwards from the left nipple. On his arrival at the hospital a few hours only after the infliction of the wound, he labored under considerable dyspnœa, had hæmoptysis, and some emphysema was present around the posterior wound, through which air and frothy fluid freely passed during respiration. The pulse was 70, feeble and irregular; skin cool and clammy. Ordered warm tea and a little wine.

September 9th.—The dyspnœa was greatly relieved.

10th.—The pulse rose to 80, still feeble, and very irregular; number of inspirations, 28.

12th.—Pulse 100, very feeble; emphysema continues; no hæmoptysis; no morbid murmurs heard in the lungs. Low diet strictly enjoined.

13th and 14th.—The patient is very easy and composed.

15th.—Early this morning he was seized with severe vomiting whenever anything was swallowed. I found him pulseless; number of respirations 40 per minute; countenance haggard and anxious; enormous aqua-sanguineous discharge was going on from the posterior wound. The thirst was now excessive, and his plaintive moanings at not having as much cold water as he desired were painful to hear. He drank a large quantity a few minutes before death, and expired at 10 P.M.

Post-mortem examination.—On opening the thorax, and pursuing the investigation from the wound of entrance, the ninth left rib was found fractured; the bullet must then have grazed and injured more or less of the muscular portion of the diaphragm, then passed through the base of the lower lobe of the left lung, making its exit at and fracturing the fourth left rib. The lung was pressed upwards (but not backwards, as in cases of effusion), and occupied only half the cavity; recent adhesions existed between the two lobes, also between the pleura pulmonalis and costalis. Half a pint of bloody fluid lay in the posterior part of the cavity. Around the track of the wound in the substance of the lung there was considerable congestion, which gradually shaded off into healthy structure. No attempt at reparation in the wounded parts. An unusual appearance was seen at the base of the cavity, and, resting upon the diaphragm, a shining elastic swelling occupying the whole of the lower half of the cavity. This was found to consist of the stomach, duodenum, and a portion of omentum. The finger could not be passed from the thorax into the abdomen, and, on farther exploration, recent adhesions were observed between the diaphragm and extruded parts. There must have been considerable strangulation, although the opening was nearly two inches in diameter, and of a circular form. The mucous membrane of the stomach was intensely red and swollen, peeling off easily. The stomach was perfectly empty.

ART. 108.—*On the employment of Nitric Acid in Piles and Prolapsus Ani.*
By Mr. HENRY SMITH.
(*Medical Times and Gazette*, Dec. 8, 1855.)

"In the summer of last year," says Mr. Smith, "I published in the ' Medical Times and Gazette,' some cases, which proved the great utility of the nitric acid, as a local application, in some forms of hæmorrhoids, which demand a surgical operation for their cure. Since that time, I have had repeated opportunities of testing the value of this mode of treatment, and have found that the nitric acid is not only a speedy and efficacious destroyer of hæmorrhoidal excrescences, but that it will cure a condition of the lower bowel, which, existing in an exaggerated degree, generally demands, even for its relief, some severe operation.

"I refer to prolapsus ani, and not to those more simple forms which frequently coexist with internal piles, and which more or less depend upon them ; but to the state which exists, when the tissues are so much relaxed, that a considerable portion of the lower bowel is in a continual state of prolapsus, occasioning to the patient the greatest misery, from which he has not the courage to get himself freed, under the dread of a surgical operation with the knife or the ligature."

CASE.—" A. B—, æt. 70, was sent to me on August 25th. The aspect of this patient was very careworn, and he looked much older than he really was.

"On examination, I found that there was a swelling outside the anus, consisting externally of thickened integument, and within of the mucous membrane of the rectum, highly vascular, thickened, and relaxed, the whole forming a very large and prominent tumor.

"The patient stated that he had suffered from prolapsus of the gut for twenty years, and that latterly the protrusion had increased so much that he could not return it, consequently there was constant prolapse, and he was always in pain ; but what caused him most misery, and drove him to obtain further surgical advice was, the circumstance of his not having any control whatever over his rectum. The fæces escaped quite involuntarily.

"I had not before tried the nitric acid in a case of anything like the same severity, but my previous experience of its effect in slighter cases determined me to use it in this instance. Accordingly, having carefully cleansed and dried the protruded part by means of lint (a very necessary preliminary), I applied the strong nitric acid, by means of a piece of wood, freely over the whole protruded mucous membrane. Oil was abundantly smeared over the parts, which were then returned within the anus.

"I am bound to admit that the patient suffered great pain for a time, but it was mainly whilst I was returning the parts—a work of difficulty. He was ordered to keep quite quiet.

"'gust 30th.—The bowels have been moved since the application, and the ...ates that he had at the time more control over his rectum ; and on exam... ..., I found that the protrusion was already much lessened in magnitude

—that the mucous membrane, which had been touched by the acid, was corrugated and hardened; and that the parts were altogether in a more healthy condition. I therefore applied the acid a second time, using the same precautions and means as before.

"A few days after this, a friend of mine saw the patient during my absence from town. He told this gentleman that he was 'better than he had been' for twenty years.' The acid was applied a third time.

"October 9th.—This patient came to see me. His countenance indicated a mind at ease and renovated health. He informed me that he was well, and on examination I could not discover a trace of the protrusion.

"The above is the worst case for which I have tried the nitric acid as yet, and I must confess that the result was far beyond my expectations, although I hoped for an ultimate amelioration of the distressing symptoms, from my experience of the action of the acid in less severe cases; but more especially by the result of a case to which I had been previously called by Mr. Thomas Bennett, of Oxford Street. Here a gentleman, between 20 and 30, had had for some time such severe prolapsus, that he was compelled to wear a pessary; at times he could not return the immense protrusion; and on an occasion of this kind Mr. Bennett requested my assistance. In this instance I smeared the whole of the protruded mucous membrane well over with solid nitrate of silver, and then by degrees, and with great difficulty, returned the immense mass within the anus. This gentleman shortly afterwards left London; but I was informed that he was enabled after this operation to dispense with his pessary.

"Doubtless, there are many cases of prolapsus of the rectum which nitric acid will not remove; and I would not affirm that the treatment by this remedy is superior to the use of the scissors or of the ligature; but some patients will not submit to either of the latter operations, who will readily allow the surgeon to apply a remedy, which, if cautiously used, is not productive of danger, nor of more than temporary pain, and which will, in numerous instances of hæmorrhoids, and in some cases even of severe prolapsus of the rectum, effect an excellent cure."

ART. 109.—*On the Treatment of Fistula in Ano, without division of the sphincter.* By Mr. HIRD.

(*Lancet*, Oct. 27, 1855.)

After alluding to the painful and hazardous operations practised by surgeons for the cure of fistula, until a more correct view was taken of the disease by Percivall Pott, under whose influence and example the barbarous treatment at that time had recourse to was renounced by the profession in this country, the author gives a minute description of the anatomical structure of the lower part of the rectum, and of the tissues which fill up the ischio-rectal fossæ, and observes that many obscure collections of matter can only be diagnosed by those who are familiar with the complicated fascial and muscular boundaries of the space surrounding the extremity of the gut. Mr. Hird then describes the varieties of spontaneous abscess which affect this region, and gives the result of several cases of fistula which had not entered the rectum or laid bare its walls, in which no operation was performed, and strongly opposes the assertion made by Mr. Syme and many other surgeons who have written on this disease, "that all remedial measures, except the knife, are ineffectual." As a preventive treatment against the formation of fistula, he urges the necessity of freely laying open all abscesses in the neighborhood of the rectum, before the walls of the bowel are laid bare. The incision should be directed from before backwards, and not transversely, so that the discharge may have no mechanical difficulties to overcome in its exit. When the abscess does not close by the ordinary process of granulation, Mr. Hird advises the use of mild injections of nitrate of silver (four grains to the ounce), and the application of well-adjusted pressure on the part. In two cases of eight and ten years' standing, in which this treatment was not successful, he effected a cure by means of a platinum wire heated by electricity, and connected with the poles of a galvanic battery, similar to the one used by Mr. Marshall for applying electro-cautery to fistulous openings in the cheek, and advises the use of this agent before resorting to division of the septum. In cases of complete fistula, the author has no confidence in any treatment except that of laying the cavity of the abscess and of the rectum into one, by dividing the sphincters. This, he says, might be accomplished either by means of the knife, the ligature, or electric heat. Although the knife is the favorite instrument of the majority of surgeons, he prefers the use of the ligature in all cases where the hæmorrhoidal veins are unusually large, or when the patient has a dread of the knife. He considers also that this method of operating possesses advantages over the knife in many special cases, and, if judiciously applied, and only tightened by means of the fistula-tourniquet, to a degree of tension sufficient to accomplish the division of the septum, is not so painful as the operation with the knife, less so in the after-treatment, and frequently accomplishes a cure in a shorter space of time. Hemorrhage and the dread of a cutting operation are avoided by this plan. Mr. Hird's experience does not confirm the opinion of Sir B. Brodie, that all fistulæ have an internal orifice leading into the rectum; neither do his observations verify the opinion of many writers, that fistulæ are most frequently found in phthisical patients; but, on the contrary, these observations are in harmony with the views of Andral and Louis, both of whom demonstrate, by statistical inquiries, that these affections, occurring simultaneously in the same individual, are merely the result of accident, and that they do not stand to each other in the relation of cause and effect.

This paper was read before the Medical Society of London.

ART. 110.—*Statistics of* 258 *cases of Intestinal Obstruction.* By Dr S. F. HAVEN, Jun.

(*American Quarterly Journal of Medical Science,* Oct. 1855.)

The concluding passages of the paper, and a table which comprehends nearly all the items of several other tables, excepting the symptoms, will serve to show the results of Dr. Haven's long and careful inquiry. The table is as follows:—

	Whole number.	Males.	Females.	Unknown.	Average age.	Operated on.	Not operated on.	Artificial anus.	Recovered.	Died.	Gastrotomy.	Recovered.	Died.	Total recovered.	Total died.	Small intestine.	Large intestine.	Both.	Unknown.	Total.
Cancerous stricture,	24	15	9		51	8	16	7	6	1	1	1		7	16	1	23			24
Non-cancerous stricture,	46	18	28		43	11	35	10	6	4	1		1	6	40	2	44			45
Intususception,	59	34	10	15	18	3	56				3	3		13	46	23	1	23	2	59
Intususception with polypi,	4	2	2		46		4									4				4
Total of intramural,	133	69	49	15	39½	22	111	17	12	5	5	4	5	26	106	30	78	23	2	133
Bands and adhesions,	39	21	17	1	32	6	33		1		5		1	1	38	34	4	1		39
Twists and displacements,	18	16	2		35	1	17								18	3	15			18
Diverticula,	10	9	1		30		10				1		1		10	10				10
External tumors or abscesses,	5	2	2		31	1	4								5	3	2			5
Mesocolic and mesenteric hernia,	6	3	1	1	29		6								6	5	1			6
Omental hernia,	3				55½		3								3	5				3
Obturator hernia,	11	6	10	1	67	2	9				2*	1*		3	8	9			2	11
Diaphragmatic hernia,	8		2		41		8	1	1				8		8	1	7			8
Total of extramural,	100	61	35	4	39	10	90	1	1	1	9*	1	8	4	96	68	29		2	100
Intramural,	15	11	4		26	1	14	1				1			15	6	7	1	2	15
Unknown,	10	6	4		47	6	4	5	5		1	1		6	4	2	5		3	10
Total,	258	147	92	19	38	39	219	24	18	6	15*	6*	9	39	219	106	119	24	9	258

* In one out of these cases an incision was made below Poupart's ligament.

Dr. Haven then proceeds to make the following remarks:

"We have now gone through with the different species of obstruction found in our 258 cases. It only remains to consider them in the aggregate, and draw such inferences as may prominently suggest themselves.

"We find that intramural obstructions exceed the other two in number by 18, and the extramural alone by 33; while the obstructions from foreign bodies are to the other two in the proportion of 1 to 15½. Intussusception occurs more frequently than any other species; non-cancerous obstructions, and those from external bands and adhesions, stand nearly on a par; while all the other varieties are considerably below in point of number, cancerous obstructions holding the next rank. Omental hernia is found the least often of all.

"The proportion of males to females proves to be about as 1 to 1¾.

"Thirty-nine out of the whole number were operated upon. Twenty-four had an artificial anus formed in the side, two-thirds of whom recovered. This would seem to be an argument in favor of operating when the diagnosis is tolerably clear; but there are so many things to cause hesitation and delay, that the right moment is rarely taken advantage of. On the other hand, gastrotomy was performed 14 times, and but 5 recovered. The first or these five occurred in a case of cancer of the sigmoid flexure. Three inches of the diseased intestine were cut away, the arteries of the mesocolon tied, the extremities of the divided bowel united with glover's suture, and the abdomen sewed up. Ten days after a copious evacuation took place, and in eighteen days the patient was pronounced well. Twelve months after, however, he died from an extension of the disease. In the next three cases, the abdomen was opened and an intussusception withdrawn.* In the last case, the seat and kind of obstruction were not mentioned. Our statistics, then, do not offer much inducement for the operation of gastrotomy. It is surprising, however, what inroads upon the abdominal cavity may sometimes be made without causing death, as is shown in the first case above mentioned, and in many experiments upon animals.†

"Notwithstanding the unsuccessful results of gastrotomy, the following question has occurred to us as deserving some attention. If a diagnosis could be made out in cases of simple twist, or of simple strangulation of knuckles of intestine through loops, rings, openings, or under bands, how far should we be justified in performing abdominal section? Evidently, in cases of twists, the answer would depend much upon the relative frequency of peritonitis; and in those of knuckles it would depend upon the frequency of peritonitis, adhesions, thickening, disorganization, &c., preventing a withdrawal of the incarcerated portion. In view of this, we have drawn up the following table of 34 cases:—

	Knuckles.	Twists.	Total.
No. of cases where there was no peritonitis and where it seems probable that the intestine might have been withdrawn or untwisted	7	6	13
No. of cases rather more doubtful, but where no mention was made of peritonitis or other obstructing cause	10	0	10
No. of cases where peritonitis was mentioned .	4	3	7
No. of cases where the intestine could not be withdrawn	4	0	4
Total . . .	25	9	34

"Considering that a large portion, if not all, of the 10 more doubtful cases, in the second line of figures, may have properly belonged in the first line, and that peritonitis in all the 7 cases may not have existed two or three days before death, there remain but 4 cases out of the 34 where we are certain that no operation could have been performed. In one instance, peritonitis was spoken of as very

* These must be regarded as remarkable and exceptional cases, as it is well known that in intussusception the adhesions are generally too strong to permit withdrawal.

† "Brunner sewed a wound one inch and a half long, in the small intestine of a dog, with a glover's suture. The dog soon recovered; but it is difficult to say what he would not have recovered from, as, subsequently, milk was injected into his thorax, his femoral artery was tied, his spleen was extirpated, his pancreas cut away, and, finally, he was compelled to swallow a scruple of opium—and all without serious consequences, as he made his escape three months after the last attempt upon his life."—*Brit. and For. Med. Rev.*, Jan. 1847.

slight; and, in another, it resulted form perforation. Indeed, it does not appear, from the preceding tables, that peritonitis is of very frequent occurrence in any class of intestinal obstruction.

"We will leave these figures to speak for themselves, and let others judge of their value when brought to a practical bearing.

"In intramural obstructions, the large intestine was affected more than twice as often as the small, while in the extramural it was just the reverse; thus rendering the aggregate nearly equal in this respect. The average duration of attack seems to be very much shorter in the intramural obstructions than in the extramural, that of the whole being about three weeks.

"Rokitansky, perhaps the ablest writer on this subject, states that obstructions occurring from the causes enumerated under the different heads of bands and adhesions, diverticula, mesocolic and omental hernia, are most frequent in females, from the liability which the internal sexual organs in women have to contract adhesions. Our tables, however, do not go to confirm this opinion, but rather show a proportion to the contrary. In diverticula, especially, there occurs but one woman to nine men. Rokitansky also observes that intussusception affects equally the large and small intestines; but here, too, our statistics seem inclined to disagree, and give the preference to the small intestine.

"In regard to the symptoms—constipation, vomiting, and abdominal pain and distension are the most prominent. Diarrhœa occasionally happens. Bloody stools, tenesmus, and convulsions are peculiar to intussusception, and generally to infants.

"Retention and suppression of urine occurred about equally in obstructions of the large and small intestine, most frequently in those of the ileum and rectum.

"In the latter case, probably, the retention was most generally due to the vicinity of the obstruction to the bladder, and in the former, the diminution or suppression may have been occasioned by the high seat of stricture, and the consequent early interruption of nutrition.

"Early prostration occurs decidedly more often than gradual.

"Acute peritonitis is not mentioned as often as we might at first be led to expect; a circumstance exceedingly favorable in the question of operation.

"Gangrene is found most frequently in intussusception and obturator hernia. We have not made any statistics of it in the other classes, though it may have been mentioned.

"Strangulation is said sometimes to occur from an adherence of the appendix cæci in consequence of inflammation within that organ. In none of the eight cases of obstruction from such an adhesion was this inflammation mentioned. Since completing the list, however, we have met with one case of this sort, reported in the proceedings of the Boston Medical Improvement Society.

"Three other forms of intestinal obstruction are mentioned by Sir Astley Cooper: hernia at the ischiatic notch, at the foramen Winslowii, and perineal hernia; but as no instances of these were found in our list of cases, we have made no recognition of them in the preceding pages.

"It is much to be regretted that medical men have not taken more pains, in reporting their cases of obstruction, to give the symptoms in full, and, particularly, to give them in their order of occurrence. Thus, it is especially desirable, as a diagnostic sign, to know whether stercoraceous vomiting commenced early or late. If the former, we should be led to place the seat of obstruction high up, but low down if the latter. The nine instances mentioned of early fecal vomiting, though good evidence, as far as they go, are by no means numerous enough to admit of drawing any solid deductions from them. Retention of urine is another interesting symptom rather rarely noted in our list, but which would be exceedingly useful in localizing the strictured part."

ART. 111.—*On some points in the Surgery of Hernia.*
By Mr. NATHANIEL WARD, Assistant-Surgeon to the London Hospital.

(*Lancet*, Jan. 19, Feb. 9, and March 8, 1856.)

· Mr. Ward founds the remarks he has to make in these papers upon cases which for the most part have occurred in the London Hospital during the last four years and a quarter. Sixty-nine of these cases have been already grouped together and commented upon in a pamphlet which we noticed in a former volume; and thirty-one have occurred from the middle of May, 1854, to October, 1855, making 100 cases in all.

Of the 100 cases alluded to, 4 were umbilical, 63 femoral, and 33 inguinal. The aggregate mortality amounted to 33. Three deaths occurred amongst the umbilical, 19 amongst the femoral, and 11 amongst the inguinal class. The peritoneal sac was opened in all the cases of umbilical hernia; of the 63 femoral, it was *not* opened in 42, and opened in 21. The average period of strangulation in the former amounted to 37 hours and a fraction, and of age to 52 years: in the latter that of strangulation to 57 hours, and of age to 56 years. Amongst the 42 cases of unopened sac, of the 32 that recovered the average age was 47; and of the 10 that died the average age was 66. Of the 21 cases of *opened sac*, 12 recovered, the average age being 54, and 9 died, the average age being 59. Of the 63 collectively, 9 occurred in the male, and 54 in the female; 43 were on the right, and 20 on the left side. Of the 34 cases of inguinal hernia, the sac was not opened in 10, and opened in 24. The average period of strangulation in the former was 28½ hours; in 18 of the latter, 30 hours. Of the cases collectively, 25 occurred on the right, 9 on the left side: all took place in the male subject.

"On glancing over this analysis," says Mr. Ward, "we are struck in the first place with the fact of the operation without opening the sac having been performed much more frequently in cases of femoral than of inguinal hernia. The greater applicability of Petit's operation to the one class than to the other, appears to be attributable to the fact of the neck of a femoral sac not undergoing hypertrophy so frequently as the neck of an inguinal sac. In the latter, the pad of the truss bears directly on the narrowest portion of the sac, which is usually situated at or near the immediate neighborhood of the outer ring, and this narrow portion receives a counter pressure from the pubis. In the former or femoral, the pad bears mainly on the body of the sac and not on the neck; we consequently find more thickening in the structure of the neck of inguinal than of a femoral sac, a less amount of capability of yielding, and a similar calibre. The neck of an inguinal sac offers, therefore, a greater impediment to the reduction of a strangulated bowel than the neck of a femoral, and necessitates the more frequent opening of the sac. I of course exclude from this remark quite recent cases of inguinal hernia, and also those cases of large, irreducible inguinal herniæ in which the pressure from within has ultimately gained the better of the resistance from without, and in which a recent additional protrusion has been followed by symptoms of strangulation; for both to the one set and to the other, the operation without opening the sac is peculiarly appropriate. I limit the remark to those cases of inguinal protrusion of intermediate duration which, most frequently demand surgical attention, and in which the contents have been reduced, and retained in the abdomen by a truss, which temporarily occludes or diminishes the calibre of the neck of the sac, and by the irregular and inconstant pressure it exerts, leads to the thickening of its walls. In the second place, we observe, *that in the forty-two cases of femoral hernia in which the sac was unopened*, the period during which symptoms of strangulation had lasted prior to the operation was less *by 20 hours* than the period of strangulation *in the cases in which the sac was opened*, and that the age was less by four years. I should have also mentioned in the analysis that the average day of recovery in the unopened series was the 23d, the average age also being less by nineteen years than in the unopened cases that died; in the opened series the 31st day. In 2 of the former class the wound had healed on the 5th day; in one case the recovery had taken place on the 6th, 8th, 9th, 10th, and 12th day respectively. The shortest period in which a case of unopened sac had recovered was the 10th day; and after this the 21st day was the next earliest period. Now, it is admitted on all hands, that the chances and rapidity of recovery after operation, both in cases in which the sac has been opened and in those in which it has not, materially depends on the length of time the bowel has been subjected to mechanical obstructions and its consequences. Post-mortem evidence also corroborates the conclusion, that the amount of intestinal lesion, and the risk of abdominal inflammation, bear a direct proportion to the period and intensity of strangulation. Based on this conclusion, the propriety of an early operation has become prominent to the mind of every thoughtful surgeon of the present day, and his great anxiety is to relieve a strangulated rupture before its organic capabilities have been seriously interfered with, well knowing that procrastination, even for a few hours, will now and then lead to a fatal result, in consequence of gangrene of the gut, collapse, peritonitis, or other fatal complication.

"For a formation, consequently, of an unbiassed estimate of the causes that determined the relative result after the peritoneal and extra-peritoneal operations, in this series of cases, the period of strangulation should of necessity constitute a primary feature in the calculation. Considering, then, the short period in which the gut had been strangulated in the series in which Petit's operation had been had recourse to, the less advanced age of the patients, and the comparatively healthy state of the bowel, it becomes a question of interest to determine, whether in *these very cases of unopened sac*, the addition of a peritoneal incision, the exposure and the manipulation of the gut would have influenced injuriously, to any great extent, the ultimate event. The expression of opinion on this matter cannot be considered as decisive. It is quite clear, however, that had the sac been opened, in this series, something would have been done not required by the exigencies of the case; and to repair that additional something which could be looked on in no other light than as the infliction of an injury, a prolonged effort at restoration would have been required on the part of the system. The progress to recovery would in consequence, no doubt, have been retarded, without, however, the certain addition of enteric or peritonitic symptoms, which I think no one could deny would be more likely to ensue from prolonged mechanical obstruction to the intestinal circulation, than from an exposure of the bowel and incision of the serous membrane. My own opinion is, that the risk of leaving the bowel unrelieved *for a long period—say* 30 *hours*—and then *operating without opening the sac*, would be greater than relieving *the bowel at a comparatively early period of strangulation—say* 20 *hours—and opening the sac.* I should even not be surprised to find that if ten cases of strangulated hernia, in which the symptoms of obstruction had been of short duration, and exactly similar in every respect, were operated on without opening the sac, and ten of a like nature by opening it, all the operations being performed by the same surgeon, in the same manner, and with an equal amount of skill, that the results as to recoveries and deaths would be alike. I should think, however, that the period of recovery would be longer, and the attendant casualties during and after the operation would be greater in those instances in which the sac had been opened. than in those in which it had not been opened. I would refer, therefore, the more favorable termination, as established by this analysis, in cases of unopened sac, mainly to the early period of operation, and the less advanced age of the patients, without in any way denying that the limited nature of that operation, *though not usually of vital importance*, contributed essentially to safety and the rapidity of the cure. We have direct evidence on the very point of early herniotomy, in which the sac was opened, in a very interesting *résumé* of a series of cases that have occurred at St. George's Hospital, published by Mr. Prescott Hewitt in the 'Medical Times and Gazette' of September 23d, in the last year.

"Mr. Hewitt states, that the rule at St. George's Hospital is the reverse of that adopted at the London Hospital, being, in fact, to open the sac freely. The mortality amongst 75 cases, in which this plan was adopted, amounted to only 19; the operation having been performed, as we glean from the context, as early as practicable, with every amount of attention to a previous cautious use of the taxis, and a subsequent non-purgative treatment. This result I think a very good proof, as far as it goes, that opening the sac, although it may retard the progress to recovery, is by no means of that serious or fatal character entertained by many of the advocates of the extra-peritoneal operation. Mr. Hewitt 'considers, however, that if cases of hernia were seen at a much earlier period than they commonly are at our hospitals, and if protracted efforts at reduction were more generally given up, that the rule of not opening the sac would find many more advocates than at present.' In this remark I perfectly agree; and for the sake of surgery, and the relief of suffering, should be glad to see this view practically acted up to.

"Independently of these 100 cases that have been operated on during the last four years and three quarters, 254 other cases of hernia have been admitted, the patients suffering more or less from symptoms of strangulation, but who have been relieved by general or local measures—the use of the warm bath, chloroform and opium, the taxis, and application of cold. The taxis has been found, with few exceptions, of eminent service, and has frequently done away with the necessity for an operation, which, prior to its application, seemed imperatively called for; and I can call to mind several cases in which it succeeded when no impulse could be detected in the body of the tense tumor. This reduction of bowel into the abdomen by manipulation requires, of course, in its use extreme care, delicacy, and tact, and will frequently succeed in the hands of one understanding the principle of the proceeding, whereas it will fail over and over again, and do considerable mischief even if it should succeed, when applied by one either ignorant of or indifferent to it. I think it may be serviceable to append the following description of the professional way of applying the taxis; for to attempt to define or put in practice the frequently successful method adopted by patients themselves would be almost impossible, inasmuch as the proceeding they have recourse to appears peculiar, and at times complicated and ridiculous, and is followed by most serious consequences. My friend, Mr. Hovell, gave me an opportunity, a short time ago, of seeing an elderly woman, who had had a right femoral hernia for many years, and on being seized, as she frequently had been on former occasions, with symptoms of strangulated bowel, applied the taxis herself during the night. It was successful, as far as referred to the reduction of the gut, but so much force had been used, that when I visited the patient, she had great prostration with marked mitigation of the symptoms of strangulation. Concluding that she would probably sink during an operation, and that the bowel had been ruptured, we decided on not interfering. In a few hours, an after-death inspection confirmed the qualified diagnosis that we had made. The following is the plan to be recommended in the use of the taxis:— Draw the body of the tumor gently down with one hand, and with the thumb and two or three fingers of the other steadily compress the neck of the hernia, with the view of causing the contained fluid to pass into the intestine above the swelling. When gurgling is heard, or when, from the sensible diminution in the size and tension of the hernia, there is reason to infer that the passage of fluid has commenced, then, at the same time, keep up gentle pressure on the body of the tumor without pressing it upwards, and the possibility is that the contents of, and then the hernia itself, will be reduced. If the body of the tumor is not drawn somewhat downwards and kept so, the part of the gut (and the neck around it) just below the lower orifice of the protrusion will be forced up, and doubled a little on itself against the borders of the opening, and injury to the intestine and a failure in reduction be the probable consequence. If this plan be found not to succeed after one carefully-conducted trial, it will rarely be found to answer after many, and an indication is then given for the performance of an operation, as delay will but complicate the case, and further endanger the life of the patient. It may seem absurd to assert or insist on so obvious a truism, but the gloomy part of the records of surgery bears such painful testimony to the neglect of this precept, that the propriety of operating early, without persisting in the taxis, cannot be too strongly enforced and too clearly illustrated."

ART. 112.—*Cases of Urethrotomy.*
By Dr. JAMES WALLACE, Surgeon to the Greenock Infirmary.

(*Glasgow Med. Journal,* April, 1856.)

In an able paper on the treatment of stricture in the urethra, we find two cases which are well calculated to illustrate the expediency of Mr. Syme's practice of urethrotomy under certain circumstances.

CASE 1.—E. C—, a nailmaker, æt. 30, was admitted into the wards under my care on the 3d of February, 1853. He was of dissipated habits, and had a pale, sickly appearance. He stated that he had labored under gonorrhœa on three occasions—first in 1839, then in 1843, and afterwards in 1851; but that he had enjoyed comparatively good health till 1847, when he became affected with difficulty in making water, which had several times amounted to absolute retention, and for the relief of which he had frequently been under medical treatment. This, however, was followed by little benefit, and that only for a short time; the disease in the intervals becoming more troublesome and less submissive to the ordinary modes of management. A swelling, moreover, had, eight days previous to admission, formed in the perinæum, in consequence, as he supposed, of straining during micturition, which had since been more than usually frequent and painful; the stream at the same being remarkably small. On examination, a very tight stricture was found to exist about two inches in front of the bulb, towards which, and commencing from the point of obstruction, the corpus spongiosum was expanded for the length of an inch and a half into the form of an oval tumor, having a semi-cartilaginous consistence, and a short diameter of about three quarters of an inch.

On the 5th, 8th, and 11th, systematic attempts were made to pass a catheter, but without success. On the 5th and 8th, however, a No. 2 was introduced half way through the stricture, which appeared to be coextensive with the tumor, and was felt to be very rough and hard; and on the 12th, a No. 6 was found to have slipped into the bladder, after having, on the day previous, been fixed with its point pressing against the impediment. The instrument was then withdrawn, and its place supplied by a No. 7, which was retained till the 14th. But two days afterwards a No. 5 only could be introduced, and on the 23d none larger than a No. 4, although on the 18th the urethra admitted a No. 8. Nor did any improvement follow, for on the 25th and 26th the patient was unable to make water without the use of a catheter—a No. 7 being passed only with difficulty, and without obviating contraction, which was so great on the 28th, as well as on the 1st of March, as to prevent the insertion of an instrument of the smallest size. The swelling, moreover, was unchanged, and micturition as frequent and in as small a stream as formerly; and although, on the 2d, a No. 8 could be introduced, it was felt so firmly grasped as to lead to the belief that the urethra would again resist as capriciously as before.

Treatment by dilatation having thus signally failed, I resolved to perform the operation of urethrotomy, as recommended by Mr. Syme. Accordingly, on the 4th of March, I placed the patient fully under the influence of chloroform, and, after passing a staff grooved on its convex side, divided the corpus spongiosum through a little more than the whole extent of the tumefied portion. The staff was then withdrawn, and a No. 8 catheter introduced and retained in the usual way for the space of two days, the section being attended with the loss of scarcely more than an ounce of blood, and followed by no immediate disturbance further than a slight feverishness, which commenced with a rigor on the 5th, and terminated thirty-six hours afterwards. At that time the urine was flowing equally by the opening in the perineum and the meatus; but on the 12th, no instrument having been employed in the interval, it was found to escape more freely by the latter than the former; and a fortnight afterwards, catheters, rising gradually from No. 8 to No. 12, having been passed every third or fourth day, the swelling was entirely reduced, and the lips of the incision closed to about the diameter of an ordinary-sized quill, micturition at the same time being not more frequent than natural. After this, unfortunately, the patient became affected with dysentery, which continued more or less during the whole of April, and retarded very materially the healing of the aperture. Cicatrization, notwithstanding, was complete by the 3d of May, at which date, as well as on the 2d, 9th, and 16th of the month preceding, a No. 12 was passed with the most perfect ease. The general health, at the same time, was so far established as to enable me to discharge the patient three days afterwards, with an injunction to return to the dispensary once a fortnight, in order to have a full-sized instrument introduced. With this, however, he complied only twice or thrice, and I lost sight of him entirely till the 23d of May last, when I accidentally met him dressed in the uniform of the —— Militia. At my request he called at the hospital, where, in the presence of Mr. Macintyre, the house-surgeon, I passed successively, and without the slightest difficulty, a No. 8 and No. 12. He informed me, that after leaving my care he had enjoyed excellent health, and that he had never had the least indication of a return of the contraction; the stream of urine having kept always full, although no catheter had been passed in the interval, and although he had frequently indulged to excess in the use of ardent spirits. So well, in fact, did he consider himself, that, after enlisting, he never thought, though anxious to get off, of calling the attention of the surgeon to the cicatrix, which was so smooth and close as to be visible only on the strictest scrutiny.

CASE 2.—G. D—, a sailor, formerly in the navy, but now in the merchant service, æt 37, admitted 2d February, 1853. Eight years ago, in consequence, as he supposes, of a gonorrhœa which he had contracted twelve months previously, became affected with the ordinary manifestations of stricture, complicated with perineal fistula, for the relief of which he was transferred from his ship to the Haslar Hospital, where repeated attempts were made to pass a catheter, but without success. After one of these trials, he had a severe attack of inflammation of both testicles, on the subsidence of which—the original disease being considered as not likely to yield to further treatment—he was discharged from the service as well as the hospital. The opening in the perinæum, however, closed up, but be has since, in addition to the other symptoms, frequently suffered from acute retention, which was usually relieved by the reformation of the fistula either in the old or some other situation. Being of dissipated habits, and engaged in the merchant service since leaving the navy, he scarcely ever had an opportunity of obtaining access to medical skill when he stood most urgently in want of it; so that his existence, to use his own expression, has been truly miserable. On the present occasion, however, he did not labor under such a disadvantage, his complaint becoming aggravated shortly after his return from sea a fortnight ago, when, in consequence of drinking to excess, he became affected with swelling and pain in the perinæum, which gave way ten days afterwards in three places, but without alleviating, as formerly, the difficulty of micturition.

On examination, the perinæum feels indurated, and is slightly pained on pressure; an opening sufficient to admit a probe—which can be passed two inches in the direction of the membranous portion of the urethra—existing nearly half an inch to the left of the raphe, and one in front of the anus; while, on the opposite side of the mesial line, and almost on the same level, are the cicatrices of two others, which closed in little more than twenty-four hours after they were last formed. On attempting to introduce a catheter, a stricture is detected about half an inch behind the meatus, and allowing to be passed—and that, moreover, only after considerable manipulation—no instrument larger than a No. 3, which is again caught about the bulb, where the obstruction is so great as to resist even a No. 1. The urine is passed very often and with great straining, and escapes from the fistula as well as the meatus in a small dribbling stream. The patient, besides is remarkably irritable, and suffers much from spasm during attempts at catheterism.

Such being the nature of the case, I began on the 4th to dilate the stricture systematically, and succeeded in passing a No. 5 through the anterior. On the 8th and 10th the operation was repeated, the catheter on the last of these occasions being fixed with its point pressing against the deep-seated impediment, and retained for twelve hours—an expedient which produced no apparent benefit, in consequence of the irritability of the patient being so great as to lead him frequently to withdraw the instrument. For three weeks after this, catheters gradually increasing in size from No. 5 to No. 12, were every third day introduced through the anterior obstruction, and attempts made at the same time with others of smaller calibre to pass the one at the bulb. In this way the stricture behind the meatus was completely overcome, and the patient enabled to keep his water for four or five hours at a stretch, the stream being much fuller and the aperture in the perinæum entirely closed. This, however, was followed by the re-opening of one of the old fistulæ on the right side of the raphe, from which, also, there was an escape of urine during micturition, but only in drops. At last, on the 1st of March, while the patient was fully under the influence of chloroform, a No. 7 was introduced into the bladder; the posterior stricture being found to be very rough and hard, and to embrace the catheter very tightly. The instrument was then kept in for twenty-four hours, and a further attempt made to pass it on the 4th, but without success, the bulbous portion of the urethra resisting so spasmodically as to admit not even a No. 1. On the induction, however, of a state of anæsthesia it again yielded, and to such an extent that a No. 9 could be got in, though not without difficulty.

Both strictures having been thus dilated, I was desirous of watching, for a short time, the progress of the case under no interference at all; for, as I regarded the deep-seated one as peculiarly adapted for Syme's operation, I thought it necessary to ascertain, before having recourse to division, whether the other would again contract so as also to require the use of the knife. But this I learned in a way different from what I wished, for the patient, in consequence of the great relief afforded by the measures already employed, believed that the disease was entirely removed, and, with the precipitancy common to his class, insisted, notwithstanding the existence of the perineal fistula, on being discharged from the hospital. On the 7th, accordingly, I had to let him go, but with great reluctance. Four days afterwards, however, he came to the dispensary for the purpose of having a catheter passed, but on that occasion, none could be insinuated through even the anterior obstruction, which became relaxed only on the exhibition of chloroform, when a No. 8 was got in, but only to be effectually opposed at the bulb, where the resistance was so strong that a No. 1 could not be introduced. Nor did matters improve after this: for on his appearing again on the 15th, the penis, anterior to the scrotum, as well as the adjoining portion of the latter, was considerably swollen and pained, pus being observed to escape freely from the meatus when pressure was made on the corpus spongiosum a little behind the seat of stricture. In this situation, moreover, fluctuation was distinctly perceptible, so that there was unequivocal evidence of a perforation of the urethra. The patient being now under the necessity of coming into the house, a common director was passed through the first stricture, and an incision made through the skin and fascia, the latter of which was found separated on both sides from the body of the penis. Vent having been thus given to about an ounce of healthy purulent matter, another incision, an inch in length, and extending from a little before the constricted portion to the point of rupture, was made through the corpus spongiosum itself. After this the cellular inflammation rapidly abated, and without anything of an untoward nature following, except an attack of orchitis on both sides, which was, however, easily subdued by appropriate treatment. Cicatrization, besides, advanced so favorably that by the end of the month the opening made in the urethra was entirely closed, no urine having escaped from it since the 24th. At that date, as well as on the 29th, a No. 9 was passed down to the bulbous portion of the canal, and for five weeks afterwards, repeated attempts, aided and unaided by chloroform, were made to overcome the obstruction in that situation, but without success, till the 7th of May, when a No. 7 was got in with some difficulty, and while the patient was under the influence of the anæsthetic.

The stricture being then found as gristly as ever, and the perineal fistula still patent, and micturition, at the same time, frequent and unaccompanied with straining, I resolved to delay no longer performing urethrotomy, as I had originally intended. On the 10th, accordingly, after the patient had been rendered insensible by chloroform, a staff, grooved on its convex side, was passed into the bladder, and an incision, two and a half inches long, made through the skin and fascia in the mesial line of the perinæum, its lower angle being about an inch in front of the anus. The finger placed in the wound now detected the deep portion of the urethra separated from the subjacent parts, the interspace being in communication with the fistulous openings, and extending for some way anterior to the bulb. This itself was considerably enlarged and extremely condensed, and the canal, in that situation, as well as for a few lines in front, remarkably constricted. The whole of the bulb, therefore, and a small portion of the corpus spongiosum anterior to it were divided; the incision which was made from behind forwards, being about an inch in length, and attended by the loss of no more than two ounces of blood. The staff being then withdrawn, a No. 9 catheter was introduced into the bladder, and kept in for forty-eight hours,

two days after which it was again passed, and in four days more a No. 10. At
this time the urine was found to escape equally from the meatus and the aperture made in the perinæum, but a month afterwards it was observed to flow
principally from the former, the incision being closed to an opening existing in
the centre of the cicatrix, and having a diameter of about the eighth of an inch.
During the interval, a No. 10 had been passed every fourth or fifth day, and
nothing unfavorable had occurred except a slight attack of hemorrhage, which
set in on the 21st of May. This, however, did not appear to proceed from the
divided surfaces of the corpus spongiosum, but rather from between the latter
and the fascia at the place where they were separated from one another in front
of the bulb. It amounted, moreover, to no more than six ounces, and was easily
checked by a compress and bandage, gallic acid being given, at the same time,
internally, for greater security. Nor did any other complication afterwards arise
to interrupt the progress of the case, the only source of anxiety being the slow-
ness with which cicatrization advanced for a month after the middle of June.
During that time a No. 11 was passed every fifth or sixth day, but during the
next four weeks no instrument whatever was used, in consequence of the point
of the catheter being found to slip readily through the opening in the urethra
into the space below the membranous portion. The incision, at the same time,
was occasionally touched with the nitrate of silver, and with so much benefit,
that by the middle of August it was contracted to an aperture capable of admitting merely the point of a small probe, and allowing the urine to escape
during micturition only in drops. The original fistula, besides, was completely
closed, and the local uneasiness entirely removed, the canal being in such a state
that a No. 11 could be passed with the most perfect ease. The general health,
likewise, was so good, that I would then have had no hesitation in discharging the
patient, but for the nature of his occupation, which would necessitate his leaving
the place before I could have the means of judging as to the probable perma-
nence of the cure. For this reason, as well as because he made himself
generally useful in the house, he was allowed, although the incision had been
wholly closed since the beginning of September, to remain till the 27th of the
following month. During the interval, a No. 11 had been passed every fortnight,
but after that only one opportunity was afforded of repeating the operation.
This occurred about two weeks after the patient left the hospital. He was then
about to proceed to sea, in consequence of which I gave him a No. 9 metallic
catheter, and taught him how to use it himself. This he was enjoined to do
every four weeks at least; but in a letter which he sent me, and dated Moul-
mein, May 24th, 1854, he stated that he attempted only once to introduce the
instrument, and was afraid to pass it much beyond the seat of the anterior obstruction. Micturition, however, was easy and in a full stream, the general
health, at the same time, being better than it had been for ten years previous.

ART. 113.—*The rationale of Dilatation in the cure of Stricture.*
By Mr. HENRY THOMPSON, Surgeon to the Marylebone Infirmary.

(*Lancet*, Feb. 16, 1856.)

"It may be assumed that the safest, simplest, and most widely applicable
mode of treatment for stricture of the urethra is that which consists in the employment of gradually progressing dilatation—dilatation by itself, uncomplicated
by any associated action of lacerating, sacrifying, or cauterizing. No axiom in
surgery has been better established, or perhaps more commonly received, than
this. And it is worthy of remark, especially in relation to caustic applications,
that whatever agent is employed, the amount of its influence cannot be estimated altogether apart and separate from that which arises from dilatation. The
introduction of any instrument into a stricture exerts a certain influence upon the
obstruction, altogether independent of the action of any caustic matter which
may be introduced with it. It is impossible to avail ourselves of any force existing in the latter without exerting also the influence of the former. We may
use dilatation alone, or dilatation plus the action of some chemical body, but
we cannot employ the chemical agent dissociated from the dilating action by

which its application is accompanied. What, then, is the rationale of the operation of this agent, which we commonly speak of under the term dilatation?

"The universally acknowledged influence of dilatation—that is to say, of pressure exerted upon the internal surface of a portion of urethra preternaturally thickened and contracted, has frequently formed a topic for discussion amongst physiologists. Some have regarded the action of the sound or catheter upon the stricture into which it is introduced as merely mechanical, believing that the hard and unyielding instrument enlarges a passage, the walls of which are composed of extensible materials, just in the same manner as a tight glove, or a small hat, may be stretched to suit the wearer's proportions. On the other hand, most have felt the necessity of attributing to the act of pressure some power of producing absorption, and consequent removal of the organized materials of the obstruction, and such reject the notion of dissipating a permanent stricture by the mere mechanical action as untenable, or at least improbable.

"I have long sought to obtain, by observation, some clue to the rationale of the action of dilatation as a means of cure in stricture; and I think, by regarding closely certain phenomena which accompany its employment, we may obtain some little light upon the subject, at all events a hint or two which may be useful in practice.

"The first effect of passing an instrument gently through a narrow stricture (and let me be understood as speaking in general terms, and not of exceptional cases), such an one, for example, as will only admit an instrument of the size of about No. 1 or 2, without occasioning much pain or irritation, is that an immediate increase in the size of the stream is usually noted by the patient on the first succeeding act of micturition: but, in the course of a few hours afterwards, the stream is observed to be narrower than it was before the instrument was introduced; there may be even a temporary inability to micturate—in other words, an attack of retention may supervene. Subsequently the stream gradually regains its previous size and force, and in a day or two probably exhibits a degree of enlargement as the final result of the catheterism employed. The increase, however, is rarely quite equal to that which appeared at the first act of micturition following the operation.

"Now the first or immediate improvement must have been clearly due to the mechanical action of the dilating body on the stricture. No one will for an instant imagine that absorption or any allied vital action could have taken place so rapidly as to produce that effect. It was, doubtless, mechanical only. The next result observed, or that of diminution of the stream, may be regarded as the consequence of some temporary congestion, together with some spasm, possibly, in the parts, arising from the slight degree of irritation necessarily occasioned by the pressure of the foreign body introduced, a phenomena which may be designated by the term *reaction;* and this reaction will correspond, other things being equal, with the degree of pressure exerted, and with the amount of sensibility possessed by the urethra. The third and final result is that of gradual increase in the size of the stream, indicating the stage of subsiding reaction, during which congestion disappears, and at the same time the removal by absorption of some portion of the original deposit forming the stricture, appears to take place, perhaps, in some degree, as a consequence of the action, whatever it may be, which is dissipating the recent congestion. The rapidity with which these actions follow one another, and the extent to which they are developed, vary greatly in different individuals. It is the existence of undue sensibility in the urethra, or its disposition to exhibit the phenomena of reaction with rapidity and intensity, which in a great measure constitutes that condition of a stricture which we commonly understand as 'irritable,' and the extent of which irritability correspondingly prolongs or retards the progress of cure. It is during the last stage, that of subsiding reaction, that the *vital* or *permanent* dilating effect (as distinguished from that which is merely mechanical and transient) is obtained. It is then that the true benefit to be obtained from the employment of dilatation is realized.

"Granting that these observations are correct, we at once have explained some phenomena which all must have encountered, who are frequently called upon to pass instruments in stricture. All such know practically that nothing is gained by shortening unduly the interval of time which must elapse between each consecutive application of the catheter; but that, on the contrary, considerable irritation is often thus induced, and the progress of the case is rather impeded than advanced; in other words, that the surgeon is making more haste than good speed—a principle which has long been insisted upon as important by the most experienced teachers of surgery.

"At this point let us call to mind what is the essential nature of organic stricture. It is the presence of a deposit of organized material in and around the urethra, occasioned by inflammatory action originally set up in the mucous membrane. Bearing this in mind, it should be a cardinal principle of treatment to avoid producing any action which might in any way tend to excite renewed inflammation. A repetition of the catheterism should never be made until what has been termed the period of reaction has subsided, and the disturbing effects of it have disappeared. If we pass an instrument during that period, we increase or prolong reaction without attaining the permanent benefit of the process which would have succeeded it. It is not possible to achieve progress at that moment. We may pass instruments day after day; but if on each occasion this is done before the period of reaction has disappeared, we shall not only fail to advance, but we shall probably intensify that condition, or convert it into one of inflammation, and thus increase an evil, which the same application, were it less frequently employed, would effectually obviate. The golden rule which must guide us in applying dilatation, both in regard of the extent to which it is to be carried at the time, and of the proper length of the interval which is to elapse between each repetition of it, is to apply just so much dilating power as is compatible with a minimum degree of irritation; to exercise just so much mechanical pressure as can be exerted without producing pain or uneasiness, much less any obvious signs of inflammation; and not to reapply the instrument during the period of reaction—that is, until any excitement produced by the previous catheterism has completely subsided. The fulfilment of these indications will conduce most safely and certainly, and in the long run the most quickly, to a successful result.

"From this point of view, we may at once perceive how it is that rudely or rapidly conducted dilatation, although apparently successful for a time, is certain ultimately to increase the evil which it was intended to avert. Thus it is that a patient with long-standing stricture will frequently observe that his complaint has become notably more obstinate and confirmed after each succeeding course of treatment—that is to say, the contraction reappears with greater rapidity and force than it has done before. He has probably been treated by a too rapid succession of instruments, or by some irritating agent which, at the same time that it opened the passage for awhile, has induced fresh inflammation, and therefore fresh deposit in or around the existing stricture, a result which is destined with absolute certainty to assert itself at some future period more obstinately than before.

"It is probably due, in a great measure, to a disregard of the vital actions resulting from its employment, that dilatation has been pronounced by some surgeons inadequate to afford a complete and lasting cure of any stricture, and has been by many unquestionably under-estimated as a therapeutic agent. And thus it is that complicated machines, in almost inexhaustible variety, have been designed for the purpose of scarifying, cutting through, and even of cutting out the urethral obstruction. The construction of these appears, for the most part, to be based on the idea that the urethra is a tube possessing merely mechanical properties, an obstruction of which is therefore to be treated by the application of merely mechanical powers. If, however, dilatation be employed by steps sufficiently gradual, and with special care not to excite any degree of inflammatory action, the result will generally be exceedingly satisfactory, not merely in mild cases, but in those of no ordinary severity. But if, while opening the contraction by dilatation, we at the same time irritate unnecessarily or inflame the parts acted upon, we shall at least only afford temporary relief to the complaint at the expense of its future augmentation. Employed in this way, dilatation is assuredly no cure for stricture.

"It would be easy for me to demonstrate, by the recital of numerous illustrative cases, that the rationale of the action of dilatation upon stricture here offered, and the principles deduced from it, result from an extended observation of the physiological phenomena which arise in connection with catheterism, but I forbear to occupy space in this manner. The foregoing remarks form a brief record of the facts which the details of many cases would but present in a manner necessarily less forcible and trite. I am daily more convinced that simple dilatation, regarded in relation to the vital action with which its employment is associated, is a safer and much more powerful remedy than when it is applied as a mere mechanical agent, irrespective of the indications which a regard to its physiological action affords; and that the cases are exceptional which are not amenable to its influence, provided it be judiciously employed and maintained for a sufficiently long period of time. The exceptional cases are, for the most part, those in which the urethral sensibility is so great, that the reaction following simple dilatation is sufficiently violent to render this mode of treatment extremely tedious and uncertain; or in which extensive and long-standing deposit around the canal has taken place, and manifests a retractility so obstinate and confirmed, that nothing short of free division of the abnormal tissue appears capable of effecting a complete cure."

ART. 114.—*Mode of testing the Translucency of Hydrocele.* By Dr. W. FRAZER.

(*Dublin Hospital Gazette,* Nov. 1, 1855.)

Dr. W. Frazer directs attention to what he believes to be one of the best methods of employing the valuable test of translucency in hydrocele, a test which is practically so important as a differential diagnostic in discriminating between mere serous effusions in the cavity of the tunica vaginalis and various affections of the testicle, or scrotal hernias. Of course, every one is aware that the test is not free from objection; thus, it is almost or entirely useless in those instances in which the effused fluid is of very dark color, or is mixed with blood, &c., and also whenever the tissues of the tunica vaginalis are of unusual thickness, or are the seat of cartilaginous or osseous deposit, or when they are coated internally by the products of previous inflammatory action. Independently of these exceptional cases, however, there are a number to be met with in practice, in which the test is of value.

"As ordinarily employed, by placing a candle at one side of the tumor, and excluding the passage of the light laterally by means of the hand, it is, at best, a clumsy proceeding, and liable to errors. I have found the stethoscope much more useful, as a means of excluding the diffused light, and by applying the eye to its expanded bell-shaped portion—the ear-piece being firmly placed upon the scrotum, held in a tense condition—we can even map out the state of the parts with tolerable accuracy, if the contained fluid be of ordinary character, and detect the position of the testicle by the opacity it produces, especially when it occupies any unusual locality, as the front or sides of the scrotum, or is adherent from inflammation after previous tappings. We can employ either a lighted candle or bright sunlight, as our best means of obtaining the requisite illumination; but even in diffused daylight I have succeeded very well in the manner I mention."

ART. 115.—*On the influence of Circumcision in preventing Syphilis.* By Mr. JONATHAN HUTCHINSON, Surgeon to the Metropolitan Free Hospital, &c.

(*Medical Times and Gazette,* Dec. 1, 1855.)

The Metropolitan Free Hospital being situate in a locality in which many Jews reside, its out-patients' rooms furnish a good field for estimating the relative prevalence of different diseases amongst them and others. The following statement of my past year's experience as to venereal diseases, appears to have some importance, and I am induced to communicate it at the present time with especial reference to a paper which appeared in the "Medical Times and Gazette" of the 17th, from my friend, Mr. Cooper Forster, recommending the more general practice of circumcision as preventive of certain diseases of childhood. My Jew patients have, I believe, been in proportion of nearly one-third to the others. The subjoined table shows the proportion of the two classes of venereal disease.

	Total of Venereal Cases.	Gonorrhœa.	Syphilis.	Proportion of Gonorrhœa to Syphilis.
Not Jews . .	272	107	165	0·6 to 1
Jews . .	58	47	11	4·3 to 1

Thus we find that, notwithstanding a gross proportion of nearly one-third to others, the cases of syphilis presented by Jews are only as one to fifteen. That this difference is not to be accounted for, either by their superior chastity, or by their unwillingness to seek medical aid for such diseases, is conclusively proved by the fact that they furnish very nearly half the cases of gonorrhœa. The circumcised Jew is then very much less liable to contract syphilis than an uncircumcised person. This conclusion has, I believe, been long entertained by many surgeons of experience, but I am not aware that it has ever before been made the subject of demonstration. No one who is acquainted with the effects of circumcision in rendering the delicate mucous membrane of the glans hard and skin-like, will be at a loss for the explanation of the circumstance.

Taking then this fact as established, it suggests itself as probable that circumcision was by divine command made obligatory upon the Jews, not solely as a religious ordinance, but also with a view to the protection of health. Among them promiscuous intercourse was certainly not regarded in the heinous light which it is under the present dispensation, while polygamy and concubinage were openly permitted. One is led to ask, witnessing the frightful ravages of syphilis in the present day, whether it might not be worth while for Christians also to adopt the practice. Such a proposition, if intended only to protect the sensualist from the merited consequence of loathsome vice, would, it is to be hoped, be dismissed at once by every right-thinking man. But the matter is much wider. In syphilis the innocent suffer with the guilty, and the wife and the children often have to bear the penalty of the sin of the husband and father. During the period from which the statistics just adduced have been obtained, I have had under care at the hospital a total of 252 children, under the age of five years. Of these 179 have been of Christian parentage and 73 of Jewish. Among the former have occurred 27 cases of congenital syphilis, while among the latter there have been but 3. Thus it would appear that but one twenty-fourth of the surgical diseases of Jewish children acknowledge a syphilitic cause, while no less than one-sixth of those of Christians are of such origin. In this calculation I omit altogether the numerous diseases which are, in all probability, remotely dependent on syphilis, and comprise those only which present the disease in a well-marked form. The same inferences are pointed out by counting the proportion of syphilis cases in women. Of a total of 97 women who have, during the year, come under treatment for one or other form of venereal diseases, 92 have been Christians and 5 Jews. Of the 91 of the former, no fewer than 61 have suffered from syphilis, and at least two-thirds of these have been married women, who, there was every reason to believe, had contracted the disease from their husbands without any fault of their own.

With regard to its being the duty of the surgeon invariably to remove the prepuce of infants born with congenital phymosis, which Mr. Foster, in the paper referred to, so ably points out, I have long held a similar opinion with his own.

ART. 116.—*On the non-mercurial treatment of certain forms of Syphilis.*
By Mr. HENRY LEE.

(*Medical Times and Gazette*, Nov. 17, 1855.)

In a paper, read before the Medical Society of London, Mr. Lee began by stating that the opinions of men of eminence should not form rules of practice, except those opinions could be corroborated by well-ascertained facts; and in alluding to the treatment of syphilis, he showed how diametrically opposed had been the opinions of the mercurialists and non-mercurialists. He (Mr. Lee) thought that the different kinds of syphilitic affection, from which these authors originally took their opinions, might account for the different treatment which they seem to have been inclined to adopt, without discrimination, in all cases. He considered, for his part, that there are distinct morbid actions produced by the application of the syphilitic poison, which actions might be divided into four classes. These had been mentioned in a former paper, and required distinct methods of treatment. The first class referred to the syphilitic ulcer, presenting adhesive characters, the globules of the pus exhibiting a smooth outline; the second included those cases in which the secretion from the infected part consisted of well-formed pus from an early period; the third class was that in which the local disease extended to the lymphatic vessels, and in which the glands consequently suppurated; and the fourth where the contact of the syphilitic matter produced mortification or phagedæna of the part to which it was applied. The author had proved, on a former occasion, the truth of the proposition enunciated in the third class, supporting his opinion by forty-nine cases, in which suppurating bubo was a symptom. As he had failed at that period to convince some of his hearers, he had again put this proposition to the test of experience, and had caused statistical tables to be drawn up, including all the patients treated at the Lock Hospital. These tables are extremely elaborate, and, from their analysis, Mr. Lee concludes that those sores which affect the patient's constitution are not often accompanied by inflammation of the absorbents; and that when they are, this inflammation may be traced to some accidental complication. Hence the author lays it down as a practical rule, that when a primary ulcer has clearly given rise to an inflammatory bubo, there will be no infection of the patient's system from that disease; and inasmuch as the local disease will, in general, heal as soon without mercury as with it, and will not be more likely in the one case than in the other to be followed by secondary symptoms, such a mode of treatment is, as a rule, unnecessary, if not injurious. Mr. Lee, in referring to some of the other classes above mentioned, came to the conclusion that there are three of them which do not require mercury:

1. Those accompanied by lymphatic inflammation.

2. Those in which the inflammation produced by the contact of the poison terminates in mortification, which latter may be either superficial or deep.

3. Those in which the poison gives rise from the commencement to suppurative inflammation.

ART. 117.—*On Gonorrhœa and Gleet.* By Mr. ACTON.

(*Lancet*, Dec. 22, 1855.)

The following remarks are from a series of papers on the modern treatment of diseases of the generative and urinary organs in Paris as compared with the treatment in London.

"I think," says Mr. Acton, "surgeons may now congratulate themselves that these complaints have ceased to be the *opprobrium medicorum.* Ever since the attention of the profession has been called more immediately to these diseases, the treatment of the complaints have ceased to be empirical, and we now pretty well know the cause of the relapses, as well as the reason why gonorrhœa and gleet have been so difficult of cure. Amongst the out-patients, M. Ricord employs cubebs in powder, which he gives in large doses, but in private practice he usually prescribes copaiba capsules, together with his favorite injection, consisting of ten grains of the subnitrate of bismuth to six ounces of water.

"Private practice in London offers great opportunities for the treatment of this complaint, and I find when the acute inflammatory stage of gonorrhœa has passed, or before it has gained ground, few cases fail to be immediately benefited by taking capsules together with a lead injection. I still, however, continue to lay great stress on the necessity of showing patients how to employ an injection; but as I have, in my treatise on these complaints, dwelt at great length on this subject, it is superfluous to recapitulate my observations. The modern improvements consist in carefully investigating the cases that do not immediately improve under the treatment spoken of above. If the patient be desired to pass urine in a large test-glass, the urine will be found to deposit, on cooling, more or less of a thick, tenacious, jelly-like mucus. In some cases this is easily shaken up, and mixes for a moment with the urine. In more severe cases the deposit is tenacious, or holds together at the bottom of the glass. In addition to these signs, which to the practical surgeon are of great importance, we not unfrequently find pain in passing urine, as well as a frequency in doing so. This pain is occasionally referred to the neck of the bladder, end of the penis, or may be felt in the perinæum. In other instances the patient complains that there is a heaviness in the perinæum, and some uneasiness along the spermatic cord. Pain, however, is not necessarily present. I am at the present moment attending a gentleman from the country, who had for three months been taking capsules and employing nitrate of silver injections without success. Suspecting the affection of the neck of the bladder, I requested him to pass urine, which, even before cooling, showed an appearance similar to what is often witnessed—viz., at passing it is not clear; in a few minutes we notice a cloud suspended for the moment in the clear transparent fluid. As the fluid cools, this falls to the bottom, and in the instance cited formed a quivering, jelly-like body, with a little pus on the surface, which is readily mixed with the urine on slight motion: not so the mucus. In other instances, where there is less secretion from the bladder, the pus is entangled in the mucus, and we see it suspended in the jelly-like mass a little way from the bottom.

"The occurrence of any of the symptoms alluded to above during the treatment of gonorrhœa, should induce a surgeon to test the urine and examine it carefully; for, as a general rule, it would be well to lay aside injections and copaiba, as in this stage both are worse than useless. The complaint has become complicated by irritation of the neck of the bladder, or prostate, and unless timely treatment be employed, the patient will suffer from some subacute affection of the bladder, which it will be difficult to cure. Two faults, equally great, may be committed at this stage of the complaint; if feeble treatment be prescribed, the disease goes on unchecked; if nitrate of silver be employed, and active treatment put in force, acute symptoms set in, and the patient is liable to affection of the testicles, or great irritation of the bladder.

"A case, strongly exemplifying the difficulties a surgeon occasionally encounters, has occurred to me since returning from Paris. A pleasant, agreeable fellow, who had lately left a northern city, came to consult me for an affection of the testicle. I found the left epididymis enlarged, as well as the testis slightly, without pain along the cord. My patient told me that there was a slight discharge from the meatus, which he considered as of little or no consequence. These symptoms had been somewhat augmented by recent connection. The history he gave was as follows: the complaint had existed some months, getting sometimes better, sometimes worse, until he had become weary of it and its treatment; as long as he was tolerably quiet, he remained much in the same state as when I saw him; but as he was obliged to travel. every now and then accessions came on, and he wished something to be done. I saw the difficulties which the case presented; but not at all deterred by them, I applied pressure on the testicle, ordering an injection and capsules. The pressure at once relieved the testicle; but frequent desire to pass urine coming on, I at once desisted from the capsules and injections, and prescribed opiate suppositories. In a few hours the more urgent symptoms were relieved, and the patient was doing well, when, in the next twenty-four hours, pain came on in the testicle. (I may mention, that the bandage on the testis had been getting loose.) I now removed the pressure, and the pain in the testicle at once became tranquillized, but the organ relapsed into the former state of enlargement. During the next few days I continued the suppositories, together with the internal use of the tincture of hyoscyamus, and liquor potassæ; and, lastly, laying aside these, I ordered the patient to take the extract of spruce for some days, which I find acts best on these subacute affections of the bladder.

"I mention the case as one strongly (though fortunately rarely occurring) marking the course disease will run when it has once obtained the mastery; for, as we cure one complication, another occurs. Yet such instances by no means deter me from again recurring to the former treatment as soon as the irritation has ceased. Thus in the present case, I had recourse to bandaging the testis; and, at a later period, employed copaiba and injections to cure the discharge. If this course be not pursued, the patient is a long time in getting well, and, unfortunately, permanent mischief too often results.

"Inattention to the symptoms spoken of above have caused great blame to be thrown on injections, which are indispensable in the treatment of these subacute cases of gonorrhœa. I am constantly meeting with instances in which (to a minor degree, it is true) gonorrhœa is allowed to run on, and the patient's stomach becomes enfeebled by large and long-continued doses of copaiba, without any amendment of the discharge. Let me advise the surgeon, in all such cases, to lay aside the oil, and examine the urine, when he will find it in the condition I speak of. Under these circumstances, copaiba appears to have no action whatever, whereas the turpentines have particularly the extract of the spruce fir,—an infusion of the young shoots is to be preferred; but as in London we find a difficulty in procuring the tops of the branches, I now recommend in all such cases the inspissated extract of the spruce fir, a substance introduced from Norway in small jars, for the purpose of making spruce beer, and which may be procured at most of the Italian warehouses. I formerly gave the spruce drink, but patients complained that it was not easily obtained, and was a flatulent remedy, so now I order it as follows:

> ℞ Ess. Abietis Nigr. (spruce fir), inspiss., Ʒij;
>   Mag. Carb., q. s.
> M. ft. pil. xxx.
> Cap. i vel ij, bis vel ter in die.

"Under the influence of this remedy and opium suppositories the mucus in he urine ceases. As soon as this occurs the spruce may be laid aside as well as the suppositories.

"Formerly I was in the habit of prescribing opiate enemata; but it is often difficult to induce patients to undertake their administration, and the suppository is preferred. In private practice the young surgeon will find that the feelings of the patient must be studied as far as is compatible with reason, and this reminds me of another hint, which may not be thrown away upon the novice who wishes to succeed. I allude to the vehicle in which the opium is conveyed. I was in the habit of using Spanish soap until complaints were made that it was difficult to introduce the suppository from the pill becoming soft. I therefore prescribe it now as follows, with the butter of the cacaonut:

> ℞ Pulv. Opii. gr. j;
>   Butty. Cacaonis, gr. x.
> M. ft. suppositorium.
> Hac. nocte utend.

There are contrivances for passing soft suppositories; but patients dislike them, and they are difficult to be manipulated, and I find if the pill is firm it can be readily passed up the anus.

"Gleet.

"As the disease of the urinary organs become better known, the profession lays aside specifics, and studies the indications which each case presents. One of the most important which the surgeon will have to attend to in gleet consists in ascertaining the cause of the chronic discharge. I presume, after what has been said in the above article, he will not now fail to look for a mucous deposit thrown down when the urine stands. Supposing that such deposit is not found to exist, and that gleet has been troubling the patient some time, the most important proceeding consists in passing a bougie to ascertain the condition of the canal of the urethra. It is now a well ascertained fact that long-standing inflammation of the urethra will produce thickening of its walls, as well as an irritable granular condition of certain portions of the canal, resulting in stricture attended, by a purulent secretion from the surface. Now, in this state of things, all the medicine in the Pharmacopœia taken by the stomach will fail in curing the local complaint. Experience havingt aught us these facts, the first step is to ascertain if in any given case this morbid condition of mucous membrane exists. Formerly the common bougie was employed, but more recently Ricord employs a bougie terminating in a bluntly pointed knob. It is made of gum-elastic, which renders it very pliable. The instrument, previously oiled, is passed along the canal until it meets with resistance; gentle force should be employed in the attempt to pass the obstruction. If the instrument does not pass, smaller sizes are used until the stricture is passed. The instrument is then withdrawn gently, and a stricture is thus detected by the instrument being held firmly from behind by the contraction. In slight cases of stricture, and in the spongy condition of the urethra we are now speaking of, no plan can succeed as will as this. Moreover, by measuring the distance on the instrument, we are enabled to judge of the exact length of the change of structure of the canal. The form of gleet depending on this condition of the passage becomes one of the most tractable the surgeon has to treat, and it readily yields to the introduction of the bougie two or three times a week. In my treatise I have at great length dwelt on the necessity of continuing the employment of injections with dilatation, and shall therefore not further allude to the subject on this occasion.

"Before closing my remarks, I would call the attention of the profession to these facts as explaining the apparent contradiction that has existed on the employment of injections, which by some have been as strongly recommended as they have been reprobated by others. The indiscriminate employment of these useful adjuncts to treatment must be laid aside; but I can assure my readers that no ill consequence will attend their employment should the simple precaution be taken of testing the urine, and laying the stimulating liquid aside as soon as traces are discovered of its acting on the bladder. These are the modern acquisitions of science."

(C) CONCERNING THE UPPER EXTREMITY.

ART. 118.—*Ununited fracture of the Humerus cured by resection.*
By Mr. SPENCE, Surgeon to the Royal Infirmary, Edinburgh.

(*Edinburgh Medical Journal*, Nov. 1855.)

We take the following interesting case from the case-book of the "Edinburgh Medical Journal:"

CASE —On the 11th November, 1852, A. Johnston, æt. 22, had his arm caught in a threshing mill, by which the humerus was broken at two points; there was one fracture two inches below the cervical neck of the bone, and another at the junction of the middle and inferior thirds of the bone. He was seen by Mr. Falconer of Loanhead, who adjusted the fractures, and put up the limb in pasteboard splints. I saw him in the beginning of February, 1853, at the request of Mr. Falconer, as the lower fracture had not united. On examining the arm, I found the upper fracture firmly united; the lower one, however, was quite movable. but there was no overlapping of the ends of the bone, nor any deformity when the limb hung by the side.

As the injury was comparatively recent, I advised a further trial of the splints, with pads, so as to keep the parts in accurate contact, the use of nutritious diet, and exercise in the open air. This plan was persisted in till the end of March, 1853, when I again examined the arm. There was no attempt at union, and the ends of the bone were felt as if atrophied. I tried to excite action by introducing, by subcutaneous puncture, a strong sharp needle, or rather narrow knife, down to and between the ends of the bone. so as to break up the fibrous structure between them, and to scrape their surfaces. The splints were then carefully reapplied, and the arms firmly supported. At the end of six weeks, I found that no change had been produced.

In September, 1853, I passed a seton between the ends of the bones, and retained it for some days, till suppuration occurred; but even this gave rise to very little local excitement, scarcely any inflammatory swelling supervening. What little there was, passed off very quickly on the seton's being withdrawn, and no benefit resulted from its use.

I had previously proposed resection of the ends of the bone, but at the same time thought it right to explain that it was attended with more risk than the methods hitherto adopted, and the young man's friends were at first opposed to its performance. After some months had passed, however, the patient was so anxious to give it a trial, that his friends consented, and I performed the operation in April, 1854.

I made a longitudinal incision on the outer side of the arm, about three inches in length, its centre corresponding to the seat of fracture. The arm was then bent at the false joint, so as to render prominent the ends of the bone, and the incision was carried down to them. I had determined to separate the bone as little as possible from the surrounding parts, and therefore merely cleared the lower end of the upper portion sufficiently to enable me to saw through about half its thickness, and completed the section with a pair of strong bone-pliers. I then did the same to the end of the lower fragment, and snipped off some irregular portions. There was very little bleeding, and no vessel required ligature. The incision was closed with four points of suture, dry lint applied, and the arm placed in a rectangular splint, so adjusted as to allow the wound to be dressed without moving the limb. No constitutional disturbance followed the operation; the pulse never rose above 80, he suffered almost no pain, and the wound united entirely by the first intention. Indeed so little swelling or irritation appeared at first, that I was afraid this operation also would fail, but at the end of ten days there was firm limited swelling at the seat of fracture, and the patient stated that he felt the sensation of constant pricking pains in the part. At the end of six weeks from the operation, there was hard swelling, involving the ends of the fractured bone, and it seemed firmly consolidated. I therefore sent him home to the country, but directed him to keep on the splints for some time.

I saw him several times, and I allowed him gradually to use the arm; but in November, 1854, I found that from using too much liberty with the arm, it had bent considerably at the united part, showing that it had not quite consolidated. I therefore fractured it fairly across, and readjusted it. This was attended with more pain and swelling than had yet occurred after any operation; but in two months afterwards, when I removed the splints, I found firm osseous union, and he can now use the arm with perfect freedom.

ART. 119.—*A new operation in Anchylosed Elbow.*
By Mr. BUTCHER, Surgeon to Mercer's Hospital, Dublin.
(*Dublin Quarterly Journal of Medicine*, Nov. 1855.)

"There is a condition of the elbow free from disease, the result of injury, when it has become fixed by bony anchylosis in the straight position, that requires special notice. I at once cede the point that, by many, such an inconvenience might be borne with rather than running risk by submitting to a severe operation; but, on the other hand, there are some upon whom the effect would be to deprive them of the means of earning their bread, and, having no resources, would, of necessity, consign them to be inmates of a poor-house for the rest of their days. Here, I think, surgery legitimately offers her powers to relieve. In such a condition of parts I would not excise the joint, but would execute the following operation. I have frequently performed it on the dead body, and a dexterous hand may readily accomplish it in the living. The arm being placed in the same position as that for resection, an incision should be made, about an inch in length, behind the internal condyle, and the ulnar nerve freed from its bed, and drawn forwards with a blunt hook; a second incision should pass outwards to the most prominent part of the external condyle, at right angles with the first, dividing the integuments and ligamentous expansion covering the olecranon. The fine blade of the saw which I use for resection being detached, it should be passed from the extremity of the transverse incision, that is, from without inwards, in front of the condyles and the joint, its flat surface being applied to them; the blade, being sharp at the point, can be readily made to pass along this direction, and by drawing the integuments a little in front of the internal condyle it will appear through the perpendicular incision, or that made in the first instance; the serrated edge may then be turned backwards, the blade connected with its frame, a few movements will sever all resisting parts from before backward, corresponding to the line of the transverse incision through the soft parts; the limb should then be bent at less than a right angle, and any vessels requiring ligatures must be secured. The after treatment should be exactly in accordance with the rules laid down when speaking of resection. An operation accomplished after this plan is not, I conceive, nearly so serious a measure as excision of the joint: the brachial artery need not be considered in danger, except through undue rashness, and the hopes of a more perfect motion may rationally be expected, when no muscular attachments are divided."

Art. 120.—*A new mode of Excising the Wrist-joint.*
By Mr. Butcher, Surgeon to Mercer's Hospital, Dublin.

(*Dublin Quarterly Journal of Medicine,* Nov. 1855.)

After describing some other modes of operating, Mr. Butcher proceeds:
"The operation which I think best suited to those cases is the one which I put in practice myself; it meets every objection which has been urged against the measure; and to which I have already alluded. Mr. Stanley's operation is somewhat similar, but mine is superior, inasmuch as the tendons of the muscles of the thumb are not divided or disturbed from the soft tissues which immediately surround them, and are thereby protected from sloughing and death, so that all the motions of the member in its integrity can be preserved. No doubt, after excision of the wrist-joint and carpus, much motion cannot be expected; a firm fibro-ligamentous structure fills up the place of the removed bones, and fuses the surrounding textures into its dense tissue, and mats all together. But, according to my views, the hand may be retained nearly as useful as ever; the fingers being kept semi-flexed during the process of repair, they retain this position, and the thumb, being preserved perfect in its motions, readily approximates either of the fingers, so that the hand can be applied to its most delicate uses, such as writing, sewing, &c.; as well as to the most severe and commonplace, using implements for husbandry, grasping bodies, &c. I can best enforce this position by reference to a few cases conjointly bearing on the subject."

Case.—Terence Farrell, æt. 53, a large, powerful, muscular man, by occupation a laborer, was admitted into Mercer's Hospital, February 14th, 1853. He stated that three weeks before, he was finishing some task-work, violently laboring with a shovel; that he blistered and bruised the palmar aspect of the middle phalanx of the ring finger of his right hand; it was exceedingly painful, yet he continued to work; the pain increased, and also the tenderness and swelling, and for five days he suffered great torture; he stuped and poulticed the part at night, at the same time that he endeavored to work by day to support his family. The "blister" gave way, and the finger became exquisitely sensitive, and the man was forced to give up his employment, and sought relief from a medical attendant. Now the part was not incised at first; however, it was some time afterwards cut open when the "blister" had given way.—this was eight days after its first commencement. This superficial cutting did not arrest the mischief, which gradually went on until three weeks had expired, when the patient was sent to hospital to be placed under my care. At this time the hand was enormously swollen, each finger tense, engorged, and more than double its natural size, the thumb alone being exempt from the surrounding mischief. The palm of the hand was hard as a board, tense and unyielding, while its dorsum was puffed up and ready to burst from distension by fluids; but the inflammation did not stop here,—it had passed up the forearm with alarming rapidity to nearly as high as the elbow, seizing with impunity on both aspects of the limb. The engorgement and tension were beyond anything which I had before witnessed, and the deep purple-red discoloration of the parts most alarming. The œdema was so abundant as to totally obliterate the proportions of the forearm, and convert it into a shapeless mass, twice and a half the size of its normal configuration; the pain produced by pressure on any part was severe, and the pitting deep and lasting, the compressed part slowly regaining the surface. The annular ligaments before and behind were sunken, depressed, as if a tight band had been girt around the limb and strangled its vitality. The man upon admission was stricken by the lowest fever; though originally a powerful man, of gigantic proportions, he was totally prostrated and feeble as a child; his pulse was rapid, small, and feeble; his gait tottering; his tongue dry, hard, and brown. Great and constant suffering, perpetual watchfulness and want of sleep, imperfect nourishment from privations by want, stamped the type of the constitutional disturbance purely asthenic. I determined at once upon freely incising the parts, but before attempting to do so, had copious draughts of wine administered. The beneficial effect of the stimulant was soon manifest by the enlarged circulation, the heat disseminated over the body, and the increased confidence arising from resuscitated nervous energy. Two hours after his admission this great and desirable change was brought about, and then I did not hesitate to slit up freely the palmar fascia through its entire extent, observing the cautions which I have elsewhere alluded to.* I likewise freed the fascia over the muscles of the little finger fully to two inches in extent, and also over the anterior surface of the extremity of the metacarpal bone of the index finger; thus the three compartments of the hand, created by the dipping in of the fascia, were each laid open, and all tension taken away. I also laid freely open the fibrous sheath binding down the tendons of the ring finger, as much pain was still referred to this region. The hand being changed into the prone position, I freely incised its dorsum, from which the rush of blood and serum was most copious; and likewise cut through the fascia over the metacarpal bone of the little finger on the same aspect. So much for the hand; the forearm next required attention. Parallel to, and midway between the radial and ulnar arteries, I slit the fascia of the forearm to fully three inches in extent; the evidence of tension relieved was manifest from the edges flying open, leaving a gaping wound, from which gushed out serum and blood; the limb was then plunged in a vessel of warm water, and permitted to bleed until the loaded capillaries were allowed time to disgorge themselves. At the same time attention was bestowed upon the pulse to insure no ill effects from over-bleeding. Afterwards the entire forearm and hand were enveloped in a linseed-meal poultice; and lastly, the most powerful adjunct, *position*, was favorably insured, by placing the limb partially flexed, and supported on an inclined plane of pillows, the hand being higher than the chest or centre of circulation; stimulants and opiates were liberally given.

February 15th.—Slept, and great relief from the burning tension of the limb, yet apparently little local amendment; no doubt the coloration of the arm is changed; it is paler, and its volume is slightly lessened; stupes and poultices to be continued; chops, wine, porter, and opiates, freely.

17th.—Pulse slightly intermitting; tongue red, but not dry; slight hiccough; tension greatly lessened on the anterior aspect of limb; rugæ formed; nevertheless had to incise the fascia on the posterior surface of the forearm, above the wrist, to two inches in extent; imperfect suppuration in the wounds first made; local treatment as before, and constitutional strictly stimulant.

19th.—Much as at last report; pulse occasionally intermitting; tongue red, yet moist. He is able to take animal food; no sickness or tenderness of abdomen; stimulants and opiates as before; stopped poulticing, and applied pledgets of old linen steeped in a solution of chloride of soda, as a wash, made warm,—the fingers and forearm were covered by them; a thin layer of cotton wadding was next put on, and outside all a sheet of oiled silk to prevent evaporation; the limb was again steadied in its elevated position.

21st.—Improved in every respect; pulse has lost its intermission, and gives a full beat; hiccough gone; matter streaming from the wounds; redness, swelling, and tension of the hand and forearm nearly gone; applied dressings as at last report; chops, eggs, spirits, and opiates, as before.

23d.—Constitutional symptoms greatly improved; stopped the chloride of soda dressings, the wounds being now healthy, and all increased inflammatory action so totally subdued. I rolled the limb, bandaging each finger separately, padding

* See "Dublin Medical Press," July, 1852, "On Wounds of the Palmar Arch, and of the Arteries in the vicinity of the Wrist-Joint.

the hand carefully, and interposing over the wounds lint smeared with zinc ointment; gentle bandage support as far as the elbow; the same position enforced, and the same amount of stimulants, &c., given.

26th.—Had to make a small opening over the posterior surface of the ulna in its lower third.

March 2d.—Another abscess formed about an inch above the wrist, which had to be laid open; continue stimulants, opium, &c.

6th.—Permitted to get up and move about the garden, the limb being supported in a sling.

7th.—Had to lay open another small abscess over the end of the radius.

12th.—Had to open an abscess on the posterior surface of the hand in the cleft between the thumb and index finger, close to their junction with the metacarpal bones; and, to free effectually the parts, had to slit up the thin fascia covering the radial artery in this locality. In every other respect matters rapidly improving; the fingers are a good deal stiffened, but semi-flexed, and the motions of the thumb are perfect.

22d.—All sinuses and abscesses obliterated, and wounds healed; and on the 7th of April the patient was dismissed cured, his hand useful for all practical purposes.

ART. 121.—*Importance of saving the soft parts in operations about the ends of the Fingers.* By Mr. BUTCHER, Surgeon to Mercer's Hospital, Dublin.

(*Dublin Quarterly Journal of Medicine,* Nov. 1855.)

" When speaking of excision of the wrist-joint," says Mr. Butcher, " I have laid great stress upon the advantages accruing from the motions of the thumb being preserved perfect: for the fulfilment of many of its offices it is essential that its length be retained, or nearly so; for instance, in using the pen, pencil, &c. &c.

" Now, when caries or necrosis attacks either of the phalanges or metacarpal bones, or when, from accident, they are disruptured, broken up, irremediably shattered, it is with me a rule to take away the dead or crushed bone, and preserve the soft parts as nearly as possible in their natural configuration, sedulously leaving the flexor and extensor tendons, so that they may contract new attachments to the denser tissue deposited as a substitute for the bone removed."

CASE 1.—T. B. æt. 22 years, admitted to Mercer's Hospital, March 4th, 1854. When oiling a steam-engine, the crank which steadies the shaft broke, and struck the thumb of his right hand, and crushed it against the framework: the third, fourth, and fifth fingers were all considerably lacerated, but the first phalanx of the thumb was smashed in pieces, and split to its ends, while the integuments covering the unguinal phalanx were torn and spoiled a good deal. I saw the patient immediately after being brought to hospital, at 5 P. M.; having carefully examined the lesion, discovered that the flexor and extensor tendons were not torn through, though the broken bone was so extensively comminuted; I had to extend the wound, which lay over the base and outer edge of the broken phalanx, forwards, and through this wound removed the entire bone, leaving the unguinal phalanx with the flexor and extensor tendons attached. At the same time, and through the same wound, I pared off with a strong knife the cartilage of incrustation, covering the ends of the preserved phalanx, as well as that upon the exposed surface of the metacarpal bone. I put a few stitches in the wound, and fixed the finger at its full extension on a splint, and then dressed the torn integuments of the hand. The entire forearm and hand were then steadied upon a splint by a few turns of a bandage. The finger operated upon was cold, particularly at its extremity; to preserve its vitality and create reaction, I wrapped it in lint soaked in oil of turpentine, and then enveloped it and the entire hand in carded wool. The patient was afterwards conveyed to bed, and warm stimulants given, with an opiate.

10 P. M.—Pain had almost subsided, and the finger was of natural temperature: ordered to continue the turpentine dressing and to repeat the anodyne.

March 5.—He slept quietly, and upon waking had no starting or pain in the hand;

finger fully preserves its vitality, being 90½° in temperature, while the hand is exalted to 108. To be dressed in the same way as before, and half a grain of muriate of morphia to be taken every fourth hour to allay all nervous irritability.

8th.—Full temperature in the finger, and now perfect sensibility restored to the unguinal phalanx; the wound looks most satisfactory, and the minor lacerations present a healthy aspect.

11th.—The finger was nearly healed, and the patient had the power of slightly flexing it; and on the 12th he left the hospital to attend as an external. This he regularly did for about a month, when the cure was complete. A firm, dense tissue occupied the site of the removed phalanx, and even at this time the power of flexing the unguinal phalanx was nearly complete.

The wound was now healed, and I lost sight of the man for two months, when he called at the hospital to show himself. The distance between the unguinal phalanx and the metacarpal bone was half an inch less than that of the left thumb; in other words, the substituted tissue was less by that quantity than the excised bone; however, this was scarcely appreciable; and though the new structure was not as hard as bone, yet it furnished sufficient resistance for almost the perfect development and exercise of the muscles of the thumb, even when opposed by great resistance; and all the minor and rapid actions were perfect as ever; the man could use his pen with as much dexterity as before the operation. There are two points which I would strenuously urge as conspiring to the favorable issue of this case : *first*, the restraining of the unguinal phalanx from the end of the metacarpal bone, until the exuded fibrine thrown down in the bed from which the phalanx had been taken acquired sufficient consistence to resist any great amount of shortening; and, *secondly*, when this object was accomplished, removing restraint, and favoring gentle passive motion.

· CASE. 2.—John Robinson, æt. 60, a house-smith, admitted to Mercer's Hospital towards the end of July, 1855. *History* —Six months before his admission he bruised the top of his left thumb when at work; severe inflammation followed, and he went through all the routine of poulticing, stuping, leeching, &c., but with no benefit; after three months' suffering, an abscess formed on the dorsum behind the nail, and burst, from which matter was constantly flowing; some small bits of bone next came away; this was all very tedious; for months he was idle, being unable to work; a fortnight before his coming to hospital, he attempted some gentle employment, where the hand was not severely engaged, yet after following it for two days, ho had to desist; increased and violent pain attacked the finger, inflammation ran along the absorbents, and the glands in the axilla became enlarged; this state lasted for two days, when he came to the hospital: then the finger was greatly swollen, the irritated lymphatics were conspicuously present along the entire extremity, and the swollen glands in the armpit painful and exceedingly sensitive to the touch. The patient was greatly prostrated for want of rest and food, his appetite having altogether failed; after some days' suitable treatment this local accession of inflammation was subdued, and the healthy state of the lymphatics and glands restored. When the local and constitutional disturbance was quieted, then came the question of the best mode of dealing with the finger. Upon moving the phalanges in opposite directions, the grating of diseased bone was quite audible; two apertures existed, one behind the nail, the other at the point of the finger, a little below it; on passing a probe into either, the dead bone could be felt. On ascertaining these points, I decided on resection of the diseased bone, and saving the soft parts; the way in which I accomplished this object was the following:

August 10th, 1855.—The man was seated in a chair, and the arm and hand steadily supported in the position of pronation; I made an elliptical incision, corresponding to the phalangeal articulation; the arms of the ellipse embraced the anterior extremity of the first phalanx, while its most convex part lay a little behind the matrix; the flap being dissected back, I opened the joint, and then passed a very narrow sharp-pointed knife along the first phalanx, without perforating in front, and keeping its edge to the surface of the bone, liberated it from the soft parts, and with a dressing forceps then drew it back; I next cleared the projecting end of the second phalanx, and with one of my own fine saws removed its cartilage, with a thin slice of the bone, cutting from before backwards; the vessels divided were far larger than could have been expected, and three of them required ligatures. All bleeding being checked, I brought down the flap and secured it with a few points of suture, and then wrapped strips of lint wetted in cold water around all; they not only kept the parts cool, but likewise afforded a gentle support; the hand and forearm were then steadied on a splint, and the man put to bed.

· I did not use chloroform in this case, as the man had an exceedingly feeble heart, besides visible pulsation in all the main arteries, or, in other words, open aortic valves; before the operation a large stimulant was given, and after it wine and opium administered.

10 P. M.—Suffering no pain of any amount; the finger being a little cold, enveloped the hand in cotton wadding: to repeat the opiate.

12th.—Suffering no pain; slept; heat of finger perfectly restored.

15th.—Wound suppurating healthily through the opening of the old sinus included in the flap, while the edges of the wound are united by first intention.

24th.—The wounds inflicted by the knife all healed; only a few drops of matter discharge through the old opening; the part bears handling wonderfully well.

September 5th.—The old sinus entirely obliterated, and now its external aperture is on the point of being healed; he is able to move the finger freely, and allow it to be handled without pain.

7th.—On this morning the patient was dismissed from hospital, the parts being perfectly healed.

22d.—On this day the man called to hospital, as I directed, to show me his hand. His thumb is perfectly firm and capable of holding, with the index finger, the numerous small instruments which his trade requires; had the phalanx been amputated, the finger would be too short for this purpose, and thus the poor fellow, as he feelingly asserts himself, would be prevented earning his bread, which he is now enabled to do as well as ever, by this preservative operation in surgery.

The same arguments which have been used to establish the principle of saving the thumb as long as possible will also apply, though in somewhat a minor degree to the index finger. When the second and third phalanges are diseased, the bones should be exsected by a longitudinal incision, and the soft parts retained as long as possible; in this way the finger may be saved efficient for many useful purposes; the operation is particularly applicable to scriveners, a class of people that earn their livelihood by writing.

Instances are also given where great good resulted from attention to the same point of practice in regard to the other fingers.

(D) CONCERNING THE LOWER EXTREMITY.

ART. 122.—*Two cases of Amputation at the Hip-joint.*
By Mr. HUMPHREY, Surgeon to Addenbrooke's Hospital, Cambridge.

(Assoc. Med. Journ., Jan. 19, 1856.)

These cases were both successful.

CASE 1. — Burd, aged about 35 years, met with a severe compound fracture of the right thigh, near the middle, from a wheel passing over it. Mr. Welsh, of Saffron Walden, who saw him soon after the accident, did not think that the main vessels were injured, but considered the injury of so severe a nature that he recommended amputation. The man would not submit to this. The limb was accordingly done up with splints and bandages. For the first three or four days, though restless, he was thought to be doing well. Soon after this it became apparent that mortification had set in. The entire limb below the fracture sloughed, and was separated by the efforts of nature, with little assistance from the surgeon. All this took place without much constitutional disturbance. Unfortunately, the sloughing of the skin extended up the limb higher than the fracture, so that a large uncovered surface was left.

On November 28th, 1854, about six weeks after the accident, I went over to Chesterford to see the patient, at the request of Mr. Welch, who was of opinion that amputation at the hip joint would be necessary. The bare broken extremity of the bone projected half an inch from the end of the stump: it was surrounded by a great granulating mass, overlying the muscles and other soft parts, which was bounded by the cicatrizing edge of the integuments. The latter for the most part, did not reach within six inches of the end of the stump. The man, though not unhealthy in appearance, was blanched, and had a quick pulse. He took a large quantity of nutriment, meat, wine. porter, &c., digested it well, and seemed to thrive upon it. The granulations looked healthy. The stump was large in comparison with the corresponding part of the other thigh, but was not tender and he could move it at the hip.

The discharge was considerable. It was scarcely to be expected that the health would long hold out under such circumstances. There was little hope of cicatrization proceeding over this extensive surface, so as to close the stump: already it was advancing less actively than it had done. The patient was anxious that something should be attempted to secure the healing of the part and willing to submit to any measure that we should propose. I agreed with Mr. Welch that it would be the best plan to remove the part at the hip-joint, as this was the surest means of obtaining a sufficient covering of integument. Moreover, the operation in that situation could be performed more quickly than through the upper part of the thigh bone; and the risk from hemorrhage, which constituted one of the great dangers in the feeble state of the patient, would be diminished proportionately, or nearly so. Accordingly, on December 17th, I went to the patient's house, and removed the stump at the hip joint. Dr. Webster administered the chloroform; and Mr. Welch, Mr. Bailey, and Mr. Carver, rendered such efficient assistance, that very little, not above four or six ounces, of blood was lost. We placed the patient with his hips projecting beyond the edge of the table. The horse-shoe tourniquet was applied, with one pad upon the external iliac artery; the other upon the back of the ilium, so as not to be in the way of the incisions. This, being tightened and held in its place prevented the flow of blood through the artery. The stump was raised a little; the point of the knife was inserted an inch below the spine of the ilium, passed across the hip-joint, and protruded at a little below and to the side of the anus. The inner flap was then cut by carrying, the knife downwards and inwards. Mr. Welch followed the knife with his fingers, grasped the artery between the fingers and thumb, and raised the flap. The hip-joint had been opened, and the head of the thigh-bone exposed by this first cut. A little further division of the capsule enabled Mr. Carver, by rotating the stump, to throw the head of the femur from its socket; enough to expose the ligametum teres, which was divided, and the bone completely dislocated. The hinder part of the capsule, and the tendons running to the digital fossa, were then cut, so as to allow the knife to pass behind the great trochanter, when the flap from the buttock was quickly formed. During this time, one gentleman with a sponge pressed upon the lower part of the anterior flap, so as to prevent bleeding from the obturator and other arteries; while another, kneeling in front of the patient followed the knife with a sponge behind the trochanter, so as to compress the gluteal and ischiatic vessels. In this way the hemorrhage was almost entirely prevented, and we were able to proceed at leisure to tie the vessels, taking those upon either flap which first bled as they were uncovered. The femoral was about the fifth tied; the sciatic bled briskly when uncovered; the gluteal less than I expected. We took great pains to secure the vessels in the immediate neighborhood of the acetabulum, the neglect of which has been the cause of fatal hemorrhage in other cases. Forty-three ligatures were applied. The patient was now rather faint, so we covered up the wounds for half an hour, when he became warm, and his pulse good: and, as there was no bleeding, the edges of the flaps were approximated by sutures. A pad was placed under the hinder flap, and secured there by a bandage passed round the pelvis.

Two hours after the operation his pulse was good. There was some disposition to sickness, attributable probably to the chloroform; this continued for two days, and subsided gradually. The progress of the case, under the management of Mr. Welch, was most satisfactory. Partial union took place by first intention.

Some dirty fetid pus, tinged with blood, was discharged after a few days: this soon ceased, and nothing occurred to interfere with the speedy and complete union of the flaps. I heard a few weeks ago that he was quite well and strong.

CASE 2.—Richard Fuller, æt. 27, a healthy man, blanched and thinned by confinement and disease, was admitted into the hospital June 23d, 1855, with an ulcer as large as a cheese-plate on the outer side of the left thigh; its upper edge being four or five inches below the trochanter. It was flat, with a coarsely granular surface, which presented a red color, interspersed with small whitish spots. The discharge was thin and bloody; the edge smooth, not everted or raised, but decidedly indurated. At the middle was a deep depression, extending down to or into the thigh bone. Sixteen years previously he suffered a severe injury at this part by a thrashing machine; the skin being, he said, torn up a great way, and the ulcer left was a very long time in healing. It appears however to have done so quite soundly. A year ago he thought he hurt the cicatrix, by chafing it with a sack of beans he was carrying. At any rate, about that time a sore commenced, which had been gradually increasing up to the time of his admission. There was no enlargement of the inguinal glands.

The ulcer presented the general characters of a cancerous or epithelial disease, and the cursory examination made upon his admission left on my mind no doubt of that being its nature. On the morning of the 25th, I found him agonized by most painful and severe cramps in the thigh, which had come on during the night and were evidently caused by the giving way of the bone at the part where the ulcer extended down to it. Upon the gentlest handling of the limb the muscles were thrown into action, and he shrieked out with pain. We determined, therefore, at once to remove the limb, through the upper part of the thigh bone, and to extend the operation if it should seem desirable. As the ulcer reached high up on the fore part of the thigh, and the cicatrix higher still, it was necessary to make the incisions very close to the pelvis, especially in front. The pad of the horse-shoe tourniquet was placed above Poupart's ligament. Thrusting the knife from the outer side, a little below the great trochanter, I cut a short flap from the fore-part, and then made a longer one behind, sawed through the bone, and tied the vessels. We next examined the thigh-bone. At the middle it was quite destroyed; its place being occupied for about two inches by a firm white cancerous mass. A section of the bone showed the disease extending some distance up the interior. It was not certain at what part the disease ceased; for in places, above its apparent termination, were spots in which a white soft substance has been infiltrated between the separated laminæ of the bone. In its whole length the wall of the shaft seemed to be more porous and vascular than natural; a condition which is not uncommonly met with when part of a bone is the seat of cancer. In the knee-joint we found the cartilage removed, in an irregular and remarkable manner, from the inner side of the outer condyle. The bone thus exposed, though smooth and covered by synovial membrane, looked dark. It was evident, therefore, that no part of the thigh-bone which had been removed was in a very sound state; and my colleagues, Mr. Lestourgeon and Mr. Hammond, agreed with me that it would be the best plan to take out the remainder, now that it could be so easily done. Accordingly, with a long scalpel I carried the incision along the front of the bone to the joint, cut through the fore part and sides of the capsule, and, grasping the end of the bone with the strong forceps made for such purposes, turned the head out of the socket. Having divided the ligamentum teres and hinder part of the capsule, I carried the amputating knife behind the bone, and cut outwards through the posterior flap already made, so as to reduce it to proper dimensions. There was some difficulty in securing the gluteal artery. By the time the operation was done, the man was very faint; for a time pulseless. However, he gradually revived. We took great pains to secure the vessels sufficiently, and waited some minutes to see if there was any bleeding. The flaps were united by sutures, and supported by a bandage, with a pad on the lower one.

No unfavorable symptom occurred till the fifth day after the operation, when hemorrhage took place. The blood flowed quickly, but stopped when Mr. Carver, the house-surgeon, who was quickly upon the spot, compressed the femoral artery. Mr. Lestourgeon and Mr. Hammond were summoned in my absence.

They opened the stump and found a good deal of blood and pus. The bleeding had then ceased; and, being unable to discover its source, they left the stump open, with some lint in it. The patient was very faint, and the prospect by no means bright. However the next morning he had rallied. Suppuration took place; the lint came away after a time; no further bleeding and no other unfavorable symptom occurred; the wound slowly healed, and the patient was discharged cured in September.

January 11th, 1856.—The Rev. Mr. Mortlock, in whose parish he lives, writes me word that he is in full health and activity.

ART. 123.—*An improvement of " Butcher's Splint for Fractures of the Thigh-Bone."* By Mr. BUTCHER, Surgeon to Mercer's Hospital.

(*Dublin Quarterly Journal of Medicine*, Feb. 1856.)

"Since the period when I wrote my Memoir 'On the Treatment of Fractures of the Femur,' published in the Dublin Quarterly Journal of Medicine for February, 1853, I have had frequent opportunities of employing the splint which I then recommended, and testing its efficacy in numerous instances, both in hospital and private practice, additional to the weight of evidence cited in the original paper. Complicated and varied have been the conditions and positions of the fractures in which it has been used, yet efficient has it been found in every requirement and emergency to achieve similar successes. It is absolutely essential to follow the minute directions which I have laid down for its perfect adjustment. Indeed, the splint is so well known now, and its advantages admitted by the profession, that I only advert to it, to make mention of a simple alteration which I have made in the mode of liberating the cylinder at the end of the screw from the transverse piece of wood in which it rests. By the former arrangement a nut and washer steadied it below, and after the splint was applied; and when it was found requisite to change the apparatus, the limb and splint had to be lifted ' en masse' from the bed, and that to a considerable height, to allow the application of a turnscrew to the binding nut beneath. Now this entailed much unnecessary disturbance of the limb, and constrained exertion and stooping on the part of the surgeon. To obviate, then, these inconveniences, the arrangement is as follows:—

" The cylinder has cut in its circumference, about the centre, a groove a line and a half in depth, and two in width; through the side of the transverse piece of wood corresponding to this point, a screw is brought to bear, which prevents any upward or downward motion, while it admits freely all circular movement; thus it follows by a few turns the cylinder may be steadied or left at liberty in its socket. Though trifling this new arrangement may appear to some, yet by those practically engaged at their profession—by men, who, from experience, are cognizant of the difficulties encountered in the management of fractures of the thigh bone, any additional improvement in changing the apparatus that shall conduce to the maintenance of a more steady and quiescent position of the limb will, I have no doubt, be duly appreciated, and hailed with satisfaction."

ART. 124.—*Two suggestions respecting Excision of the Knee-Joint.* By JONATHAN HUTCHINSON, Esq., Surgeon to the Metropolitan Free Hospital.

(*Medical Times and Gazette*, March 15, 1856.)

"In an excision of the knee-joint which I had occasion to perform the other day," writes Mr. Hutchinson, " it was my intention to have adopted two precautionary expedients, which, as far as I am aware, have not hitherto been either practised or suggested. On cutting away its condyles the femur was, however, found so extensively diseased, that amputation was necessary, and I consequently lost the opportunity hoped for of testing the practical value of the measures referred to. Under these circumstances I am induced, although untried, to bring them before the attention of surgeons, being more especially encouraged to do so by the high opinion as to their importance, which has been expressed to me by several authorities to whom they have been mentioned. The first is the *division of the hamstring tendons,* by which I should hope to prevent that repeated displacement of the bones which is often so very difficult to obviate in the after-treatment, and is the source, when it occurs, of so much suffering to the patient. By thus putting the tibia completely at rest there could be no doubt but that apposition would be easily obtained and preserved, and that all risk of non-union would be done away with. The second is the *making of an opening into the popliteal space.* An excision of the knee-joint differs from all other operations of its class, in that it provides no direct escape for the matter secreted in the subsequent stage of suppuration. In several cases which I have seen, the greatest inconvenience was produced by the bagging of the pus into the depending part of the large wound. It often burrows among the muscles, and requires counter-openings, in various directions, for its removal. All this I would endeavor to prevent by making a free depending opening by the side of the tendon of the popliteus, at the time of the operation. A circumstance strongly indicating the desirability of such a practice, and which, in fact, first suggested it to me is, that in several of the cases which have done best after excision of the knee, a sinus into the popliteal space existed prior to the operation."

ART. 125.—*Three cases of Excision of the Knee-joint.*
By Mr. HUMPHREY, Surgeon to Addenbrooke's Hospital, Cambridge.
(*Assoc. Med. Journ.* Feb. 9, 1856.)

Among other remarks upon these cases, Mr. Humphrey says, " The object of the operation being to lead to a solid union between the tibia and femur—in short, to reduce them to one bone—there cannot be any great advantage gained by leaving the patella. The attempt to do so must render the operation more difficult, as it did in Case 1. Moreover, it seems probable that the presence of the patella after the operation, by covering in the front of the wound, and preventing the free escape of purulent matter and other fluids, may do harm."

The cases are these:

CASE 1.—Eliza Hobbs, æt. 20, a light-complexioned, not very healthy-looking person, had suffered from disease of the left knee for more than six years. The synovial membrane was the first affected, and subsequently the other structures of the joint. She was under my care in the hospital three years ago, when the disease was so severe that we feared amputation might be necessary. However, it gradually fell into a quiet state, and she went to her home to wait the effect of time. She returned in October, 1854, with her general health improved. But the lower limb was useless, indeed burdensome; for though the disease in the knee had ceased, and the swelling had subsided, the joint was left in so mutilated and impaired a state that she could not bear upon the limb, or move the leg upon the thigh, or even lift it from the bed. Passive movements could be effected in a limited range, but these gave pain. The patella was fixed; the whole extremity flabby, though not much smaller than the other. There was little hope of the limb being brought into a useful state by any ordinary treatment, because some displacement of the ends of the bones had taken place, causing deformity of the limb. The inner condyle of the femur projected on the inside of the knee, and could be felt to be knotty from bony deposit upon it. The leg was inclined outwards from the knee to the ankle, forming an obtuse angle with the thigh. It was also a little bent and rotated outwards. I contemplated amputation, but the girl was very anxious that some attempt should be made to save the limb. My cousin, Mr. Frederick Humphrey, now practising at Brighton, was going round the hospital with me and saw this patient. He told me that he had seen good results from excision of the knee, and recommended me to try it in this case. Having thought over the matter, I proposed the operation to my colleagues, who agreed in thinking it worth while to give the operation a trial in a case of this kind, although they, like myself, were not much prepossessed in its favor.

October 27th.—I made a transverse incision over the patella, more than half round the joint, and short cuts upwards and downwards at right angles to it at either end; reflected the flaps thus made, and cut into the knee-joint, dividing the lateral ligaments. The patella had acquired close connections with the outer condyle; and in the endeavor to separate it, and press it on the outside of the joint, with a view of saving it, the ligamentum patellæ was torn up from the head of the tibia. I thought it best, therefore, to remove the bone. The joint was then bent, the adhesions between the bones, which were of fibrous nature, and the crucial ligaments being at the same time divided with the scalpel. The ends of the bones being now sufficiently uncovered, I sawed about three-quarters of an inch off the condyles of the femur, and a thinner slice from the tibia. Placing the cut surfaces together, I found that the leg was inclined a little outwards. This was rectified by sawing off another thin oblique slice from the inner part of the cut surfaces of the bones. Some of the articular arteries required ligatures. Finally, the limb was bandaged upon a straight splint, with a pad under the head of the tibia to raise it; and proper apposition was secured by the pressure of broad lateral splints.

No unfavorable symptom followed. Not the slightest fever, and scarcely any inflammation at the knee. The discharge found its way through the bandages, which I seldom disturbed—not more than once in a fortnight or three weeks. In January, the wound being healed all but one small orifice, and the union of the bones being tolerably firm, the limb was encased in a gum-chalk bandage, and the patient went home. In September she returned, the part having been painful and inflamed. There was a sinus extending three or four inches up the fore part of the thigh. This I laid open in its whole length, but could discover no evidence of diseased or exposed bone. The wound healed up, and she again went home. There was pretty firm osseous union between the bones, and every probability of her being able to walk upon the limb.

CASE 2.—Edward Wells, æt. 47, was admitted April 19th, 1855. He was a native of Barbadoes, and a sailor. He broke his right patella transversely by a fall upon the deck six months ago, the knee coming in contact with an iron ring. He was taken ashore and treated in the hospital of Rio Janeiro. In three weeks, as his vessel was about to sail, he got up with crutch and stick, and went on board. No medical treatment could be there obtained, and he continued to go about with a crutch. Subsequently, he sought relief in various places; but finding none, and the limb being useless, he came into the hospital for the purpose of having it removed. The fragments of the patella were four inches apart. The lower one was a little nearer to the tuber tibiæ than natural; the upper one lying above the condyles of the femur. There appeared to be no direct connecting medium at all, the articular surface of the femur lying immediately under the skin. He could bend the leg, but had no power whatever to extend it; consequently, walked with a crutch and stick, scarcely using the right leg. Examining the left patella, I found that it also had been broken across, the fragments being movable upon one another, though in close contact. This was caused by a fall on the slippery deck, fourteen years ago. The knee was cupped and bound up for a fortnight; after which he went about, the joint feeling only weak for a time. Of late years he had felt no inconvenience from it, and was not aware that the knee-cap had ever been broken.

I had an apparatus constructed for the purpose of fixing the limb in a straight position, hoping that he would be able to walk with this assistance, and that gradually the part might acquire more strength. However, the upper fragment of the patella and the adjacent part of the thigh was so tender, that it would bear no pressure, and he became very impatient for some more decided treatment. Accordingly I proposed to excise the joint, which, being agreed to by my colleagues, and assented to very willingly by the patient, was done on May 4th.

It being desirable to remove the fragments of the patella, which could be of no use if left, and which might interfere with the after treatment, I determined to make crucial incisions, instead of those practised on the former occasion. The first was transverse, more than half way round the joint, over the interval between the tibia and fibula. This was crossed by a longitudinal cut from the upper edge of the superior fragment of the patella to the lower edge of the inferior. The four angular flaps thus marked out were reflected, and the two fragments of the patella were dissected away. In doing this, I found that both the latter were quite shut out from the cavity of the joint. The hinder and lower surfaces of the upper one were connected by tough fibrous tissue to the fore part of the femur, above the condyles, and there was no tissue at all constituting a direct medium of communication between the fragments. It would have been hopeless, therefore, to have made any attempts by treatment to enable the quadriceps to act upon the tendo patellæ. Having removed the fat from the front of the joint, and divided the lateral and crucial ligaments, I sawed off nearly three-quarters of an inch of the condyles of the femur, and a thin slice of the upper end of the tibia. The bones were secured in good position by splints behind and on either side, well padded, as in the last case.

No unfavorable symptoms followed. Suppuration took place; and after a time, the discharge gradually diminished. On June 19th, the wound was nearly healed, and there was pretty firm union between the bones, though he could not raise the limb from the bed. On September 21st, the wound had long been soundly healed, and the bones firmly united. He could raise the limb from the bed, and bear some weight upon it; could move about very well with crutches, and there was every probability of his being soon able to walk without them. On this day he left the hospital, and I have heard no more of him.

CASE. 3.—William Childs, æt. 12, a pale, but not unhealthy child, was admitted with the knee bent to a right angle. Indented cicatrices of sinuses, which had evidently extended deeply, told of former serious disease. At the present, all acute symptoms had passed away; there was no swelling, and no pain; but the joint had been destroyed; no movement could be effected, and the limb was rendered quite useless by the contraction. I first determined to try whether the joint could be brought into better position without any operation. Accordingly, when he was under the influence of chloroform, extension was commenced steadily and carefully. I found that the joint yielded without much difficulty; and having straightened it, we fixed it upon a splint bound to its hinder part. Having been kept thus for several weeks, it was done up in gum-chalk bandage, and he was allowed to bear upon it a little. The progress, however, was not satisfactory. The joint gained no strength. The limb was quite unable to bear the weight of the body. No movement could be effected. There was some swelling and tenderness. The contraction began to recur, and it was evident that the limb would remain a useless one, unless some more decided treatment were adopted. It appeared a favorable case for excision, which I performed August 31st, 1855. The external incisions were crucial, as in the last case. The patella was firmly anchylosed to the femur, and was accordingly left. The tibia and femur were united by firm fibrous tissue, which was partly divided by the knife, partly torn in flexing the joint. A small portion of each bone was removed, and the limb placed in a straight position, supported by splints.

The operation was not followed by any febrile disturbance or bad symptom. Suppuration took place in the usual manner, and subsided as the healing of the wound went on. The latter process was completed in little more than a month, and in about two months there was firm union between the bones. A gum-chalk bandage was applied, and he went home.

ART. 126.—*Two Cases of Excision of the Knee-joint.*
By Mr. PETER BROTHERSTON, of Alloa.

(*Edinburgh Medical Journal,* April, 1856.)

These cases are as follows:

CASE 1.—Robert Strang, æt. 10, son of a collier residing in Clackmannan, has had strumous disease of the left knee-joint for two years. The leg is slightly flexed, the joint very much enlarged, and an ulcerated opening, about half an inch in diameter, over the inside of the joint. A probe, introduced into this opening, and pushed backwards, enters the joint. He has continual pain, aggravated on motion, and the discharge is very considerable. The boy is pale and emaciated, and has a quick pulse, of about 120. Having stated to the parents that an effort should be made to save the leg, and explaining to them the nature of the operation for excision of the knee-joint, they at once consented to have the operation performed without delay. I wrote to my friend, Dr. James Gillespie, of Edinburgh, requesting his assistance in this case, he having assisted the late Dr. Richard Mackenzie in his previous cases at the Royal Infirmary; and, accordingly, on the 19th May, 1854, I performed the operation as follows: the boy being put under the influence of chloroform, I made a free incision across the front of the knee-joint, below the patella, from a little above the posterior edge of the inner tuberosity of the tibia, across to the posterior edge of the outer tuberosity; and having divided the lateral and crucial ligaments, I proceeded to separate the connection round the condyles of the femur, which being done, about three quarters of an inch of the condyles were sawn off. A slice of about one-third of an inch in thickness was then taken from the head of the tibia, and the cartilage was removed from the inner surface of the patella by means of a gouge. Four arteries required ligature. The ends of the bones were then placed in accurate apposition, and the wound was closed with seven sutures. A splint, covered with lint, was applied to the ham, and the whole secured with a bandage

It is needless to give a detailed account of this case; but I may remark, that in seven months complete anchyloses of the bones had taken place, and the boy could walk with freedom. There were two or three sores in the neighborhood of the incision; but they were superficial, and unconnected with the bone.

Case 2.—The progress and cure of the case just related was anxiously watched by a gentleman in Alloa, whose son, eleven years of age, was laboring under acute synovitis and ulceration of the cartilages of the right knee. From seeing the boy Strang progress so favorably, he asked me if a similar operation might not save his son's limb; and on being told that the case was a remarkably favorable one for the operation, he at once consented to have it done. I may state there was urgent necessity for this operation, or amputation being immediately performed. The extreme paroxysms of pain which came on whenever the boy attempted to sleep, caused by the ulceration of the cartilage being brought in contact with the opposing bone during sleep, when the natural control of the limb was lost, and his state of nervous debility, showed that he could not have borne up longer under the source of irritation. There was no other external ulceration, except a sinuous opening in the ham, which discharged a quantity of matter. I was assisted again by my friend, Dr. James Gillespie, and the operation was performed on the 12th January, 1855, in every way similar to the former case.

There was a considerable quantity of pus in the joint, and distinct ulceration of the cartilage on the condyles of the femur and head of the tibia. The incision nearly all healed by the first intention, and everything went on favorably till about the beginning of March, when an abscess begun to form on the outside of the thigh, a little above the seat of the operation. This I opened on the 28th of March, and shortly afterwards the abscess gradually closed, and finally healed altogether. It is now eleven months since the operation was performed, and the limb is fairly anchylosed. All swelling has disappeared, and the limb is as straight as its fellow, and only an inch shorter. The patella is found slightly movable, a little above its former seat, and he can walk with a firm, decided step, without a crutch, although he uses one at present, by my orders, to save the limb.

I may mention here the great benefit I found from the use of sandbags, recommended me by Dr. Richard Mackenzie, laid on each side of the leg, along the sides of the joint, and fastened with two bits of tape, one above and another below the knee. They served admirably to keep the bones in accurate apposition, and, from their weight, keep the leg *in situ*, especially preventing its movement during sleep.

Art. 127.—*On the real origin of Varicose Veins in the lower extremities.*
By M. Verneuil.

(*American Quart. Jour. of Med. Science*, Jan. 1856.)

M. Verneuil lately read a paper before the Academy of Medicine of Paris, on the above subject, in which he endeavored to make out the following points:
1. Whenever varicose veins, which have sprung up spontaneously, are ob-

served on the lower extremity, there are deep veins similarly affected in the corresponding part of the same limb.

2. The converse, however does not hold, for the inter- or intra-muscular veins may be found dilated, without any change having taken place in the superficial vessels. But when the deep veins alone are found in an exposed state, it is almost certain that sooner or later the superficial ones will in their turn swell, become tortuous, and very apparent under the skin.

3. The varicose state of the veins of the lower extremity, as it is usually seen, does not primarily arise from the subcutaneous vessels (the internal saphena not excepted), but generally from the dilatation of the deep veins, and most often from the muscular veins of the calf of the leg! The deep veins are first affected with valvular inefficiency and dilatation, and these two lesions then spread to the super-aponeurotic branches of the second and third order.

4. This succession of phenomena is not only made manifest by simple dissection, but also by a careful study of the special arrangement of the venous system of the lower extremity.

5. These facts, which may be looked upon as a new discovery, throw much light on the whole subject of varicose veins of the lower extremities. The etiology and symptoms of the affection are thus elucidated, and this circumstance allows of a more rational choice of therapeutical means.

6. The mechanism of relapses will henceforth be more easily understood; for it must be confessed that the obstinate return of the complaint, which experience shows to be so frequent, has been explained more by a train of reasoning than by direct demonstration.

ART. 128.—*On Amputation of the Ankle-joint.*
By Mr. PEMBERTON, Surgeon to the General Hospital at Birmingham.

(*Assoc. Med. Journal*, April 19 and 26, 1856.)

After referring to other modes of operating, Mr. Pemberton describes the mode adopted by himself: " A semilunar incision is made across the front of the joint, commencing at the centre of the extremity of either the external or internal malleolus, according as the right or left foot is operated on, and terminating at a corresponding point on the opposite side. The convexity of this incision is directed to the toes, and it should only divide the integuments. From the malleolus, at which the knife terminated its course, a second incision is carried downwards deeply and forcibly through everything to the bone, across the sole of the foot, in a direction exactly in a line corresponding to the malleolar projections, and terminating at the commencement of the first. The foot being firmly grasped by the left hand, a sweep of the knife divides the remaining tissues, including the external, anterior, and internal ligaments of the ankle-joint, and exposes the articular surface of the astragalus. The flap is now dissected from the os calcis from above downwards, attention being directed to separate the soft parts from the bone in the middle line first, until the insertion of the tendo Achillis is fairly divided. This accomplished, the lateral attachments to the os calcis are easily separated, a strong grasp of the foot enabling the operator unaided to give the requisite degree of tension to the parts he is dividing in any direction at pleasure. During all this, the edge of the knife must be directed so as to cut on the bone, and the hollow of the calcaneum on the inner side must be borne in mind in reference to the preservation of the posterior tibial artery. Lastly, one turn of the knife is carried round the extremities of the tibia and fibula, and their malleolar projections are sawn off sufficiently high to include the removal of the intermediate cartilaginous surface.

" In a recent case, in which I performed this operation, I changed the order and direction in which I had been in the habit of detaching the flap from the os calcis, following more particularly the method which I believe Mr. Syme himself adopts—namely, that of dissecting it from below upwards.

" I certainly found no difficulty in pursuing this method; but I cannot say that I found any additional facility, so as to lead me to adopt it again. An awkwardness appearing to arise from having to turn the patient partially on the side, in order to twist the sole of the foot uppermost.

"It will be noticed that in the method of operating described, the foot had been disarticulated before the malleolar projections have been removed. Mr. Birkett ('Lancet,' 1854, vol. ii, p. 456), after having completed the dissection of his flaps, applies the saw to the extremities of the tibia and fibula, and removes them, together with the thin slice of the articular extremity of the tibia, without opening the cavity of the joint. This modification appears to me to be particularly applicable to those cases in which there is reason to suspect the existence of disease in the extremity of the tibia. Two sutures should be inserted to retain the flaps in contact; a single strip of adhesive plaster, a piece of wetted lint, and a light roller, completing the dressing.

"On the second day, I am in the habit of removing the sutures and the dressings, in order to allay the swelling, which always arises in the lightest dressed stumps; and which, if allowed to continue unrelieved for even another day, is certain to produce irritation. Subsequently, so far as the stump is concerned, there is but one point to keep in view, in order to avoid unpleasant complications. Let there be no pressure applied to the flap. Let it simply be retained in apposition by the gentlest means possible. This can easily be done, as the flap is most tractable, and not at all like the unyielding mass that is necessarily obtained in a Chopart's amputation.

"By attending to this, all danger of bagging of matter, so far as my experience has taught me, will be avoided, and the healing process will go on with wonderful rapidity. I have never once had occasion to relieve any collection of matter in the pad of the heel, or indeed in any other part of the stump formed in this operation. In no instance have I obtained or desired 'union by first intention.' Care has, however, been taken to obtain an accurate apposition of flaps in the first instance without straining, so as to admit of a free escape of discharge; at the same time that every endeavor must be made to prevent the least gaping of the wound, in order that the line of granular union may not exceed the width of a few lines."

Mr. Pemberton then relates four cases in illustration of what he has previously advanced, and he concludes his paper by giving a table of the operations performed in the General Hospital at Birmingham since 1851. The table is this:

Age.	Sex.	Primary.	Secondary.	Time.	Result.
24	F.	...	Secondary.	6 weeks.	Cured.
29	F.	....	Secondary.	6 weeks.	Cured.
12	M.	....	Secondary.	10 weeks.	Cured.
33	F.	....	Secondary.	9 weeks.	Cured.
26	M.	....	Secondary.	3 months.	Cured.
13	M.	...	Secondary.	5 weeks.	Cured.
27	M.	Primary.	....	17 days.	Died.
19	M.	Primary.	....	8 weeks.	Cured.
18	F.	....	Secondary.	6 weeks.	Cured.
1	F.	....	Secondary.	7 weeks.	Cured.
18	M.	....	Secondary.	6 weeks.	Cured.
39	M.	....	Secondary.	3 months.	Cured.
14	M.	....	Secondary.	7 weeks.	Cured.
24	M.	....	Secondary.	8 weeks.	Nearly well.

ART. 129.—*On Amputation of the Foot at the Ankle-joint.*
By Mr. HENRY THOMPSON, Surgeon to the St. Marylebone Infirmary.

(*Medical Times and Gazette*, Feb. 23, 1856.)

At a meeting of the Medical Society of London, held on February 16th, Mr. Thompson read a paper on this subject, illustrating his remarks by a patient upon whom he performed this operation a short time previously. The following gives a concise view of the chief points to which he directed the attention of the Society, commencing with a brief outline of the history of the patient. A girl, æt 10, had suffered from caries of the tarsus and metatarsus, during rather more than four years, for the greater part of which time she had resided at Margate for her health. The disease becoming confirmed and spreading, Mr. Thompson decided to remove the foot at the ankle-joint. A considerable portion of the flaps healed by the first intention, and the wound was soundly cicatrized, and the stump firm, in six weeks from the date of the operation." Mr. Thompson attributed the excellent result of this operation to the adoption of a certain mode of performing it, which involved the following as its chief points, the neglect of which is liable to produce tedious suppuration, a sloughing or unsoundness of the flap :—1st The division of the posterior tibial artery should be made as low down as possible in the flap; a point admitted on all hands. 2d. Care must be taken not to inflict injury upon the heel flap, either by the knife, or by the forcibly handling it during the operation. 3d. The lower incision, with which the operation commences, should take its origin not at the centre of the lower margin of the malleolus externus, but somewhat behind that point, should be carried obliquely backwards, to the posterior part of the heel, and be concluded at a corresponding point below the inner malleolus. The heel-flap is thus far less hollow in form than that which is ordinarily made. The objections to the cup-shaped heel-flap are, the impossibility, from its form, of union occurring between it and the upper part of the wound by the first intention; its liability to become a receptable for blood or purulent matter, and to lose part of its substance by sloughing. The author stated, that he had adopted this plan with a most rapidly successful result, on the recommendation of Mr. Syme, who appears to have been led, by the result of his experience, to carry the lower incision further back than he did at the period when he first performed the operation. It was not to be lost sight of, moreover, that the operation was easier of performance by this method. The paper was illustrated by diagrams of the foot, showing the lines of incision described.

ART. 130.—*Sequel to a case of Luxation downwards and backwards of the third internal Metatarsal Bone.* By Mr. JOLLIFFE TUFNELL, Surgeon to the City of Dublin Hospital.

(*Dublin Quarterly Journal of Medical Science,* Nov. 1855.)

This case is related in a former volume, XIX. The sequel is thus related:

"From July, 1852, to the same month of the present year, I saw no more of the case. I now heard that he had re-enlisted, and was serving in one of the smartest infantry regiments in the service. I was certainly surprised, and doubted the correctness of the statement, but the man having been sent on duty to Ireland, he called upon me to exhibit his foot, and show the alteration that had taken place. Its form had now considerably changed. It had become almost natural in appearance. The relative measurements of the injured member, as compared with its state six months after the accident, were the following. The length of the foot had increased half an inch. The breadth round the basis of the toes three-quarters of an inch, and its girth round the instep had also similarly increased, the whole foot, in fact, having become developed and spread out. The most striking changes, obvious to the eye, were the removal of the sharp angular prominence formed by the anterior edge of the tarsal bones, and the absence of the projection formerly caused by the head of the metatarsal bone of the great toe in the sole. The heel, too, had become flattened and wider by half an inch.

"The full use of the extremity was now regained; he could walk and run with scarcely any perceptible halt. The statement which he gave of the progress of his case was this. For nine months after the accident he used crutches for comfort, although he *could* walk supported by a stick. During the succeeding eighteen months he was crippled, but took exercise daily for some hours, hobbling along with a stick, using the douche night and morning, and having the foot regularly rubbed. He now threw away the stick, and drilled himself into walking alone, increasing the distance until he could go four or five miles at a stretch. In October, 1854, he felt so far recovered that he thought he could re-enlist, which he did, joining his depot at Chatham, going through the ordinary drill, and marching in heavy marching order for two miles.

"I saw him in July following, that is, three years and a half from the time that the accident occurred. He now could walk perfectly well, run and jump with both feet, but he could not hop on the injured leg; the instant he was directed to do so, he made the effort, then hesitated and declined, feeling as he said, the wish, but being unable to move. He wore very thick and clumsy-looking boots, which he said he did purposely, for he found in them both confidence and support, whilst with a light shoe, or in his stockings, he could do comparatively little, for he then threw the weight of his body on the outer border of the foot.

"I have been thus particular in describing the progress of this case, because I consider it probable that any *similar* dislocation will, as in this instance, remain unreduced,* and the knowledge of its favorable termination may be useful in reference to future prognosis. Nowhere, I think, could the efforts of nature, in her power of removing impediments by absorption, be more beautifully exemplified than here, whilst at the same time I have no doubt that recovery was greatly assisted by the steady perseverance of the patient in following the directions given him to use the tepid or cold douche twice a day, followed by hand-rubbing the foot, and taking as much exercise as he could without producing heat or pain."

ART. 131.—*On certain Affections of the Feet.* By M. NELATON.

(*Gazette des Hôpitaux*, Nos. 97, 98; and *Medical Times and Gazette*, March 15, 1856.)

M. Nelaton recently ("Gaz. des Hôp." No. xcviii), called the attention of his class to a singular deviation of the toes, especially of the great toe, not infrequently met with in the aged, but undescribed in books. It is principally met with in persons pursuing laborious occupations, and in the indigent who are ill-shod. It offers different characters. In some the great toe is carried outward to such a degree that the projection of the first metatarsus is covered only with the integuments, in place of corresponding to the surface of the phalanx. Instead of being carried to the side of the other toes, the great toe may mount above them and form a right angle with the first metatarsus. At other times the toe may pass below in place of above, and become lodged in the furrow corresponding to the metatarso-phalangean articulations. M. Nélaton believes that the deviation arises from retraction of the extensor muscle of the great toe, and before the deviation takes place the tendon of the extensor presents a corded appearance. At the same time there is retraction of the extensor tendon of the four neighboring toes, which do not become luxated outwards, but are curved upon themselves. Not only is this disposition of parts a great impediment to walking, but it may give rise to irritation and perforation of the integuments by the metatarsal bone. When the patient is not much advanced in age, and the luxation is incomplete, the tendon of the extensor tendon of the great toe should be divided subcutaneously, and the ends kept apart while cicatrizing. In the case of the present old man such an operation would be useless. The extremities of the bone being deformed, and the phalangeal surface obliterated, the reduction of the toe would be impossible, and all that can be done is to order him a shoe suited to the deformity.

Another affection, which from time to time is witnessed at the Paris *clinique*, and known under the title of *perforating disease of the foot*, forms the subject of a thesis by M. Leplat ("Gaz. Hôp." No. cxvii), who witnessed eight examples during his *internat*. The course of the affection is as follows:—There is (1), usually at the commencement, a horny production found at the sole of the foot, and over the most projecting parts; (2), an ulcer forms, surrounded on all sides

* Because the proximal end of the metatarsal bone of the great toe becomes immovably fixed behind the tuberosity of the internal cuneiform bone, wedged in the cavity which exists between it and the cuboid bone, locked in the hollow of the tarsal arch.

by a circle of very thick epidermis, and from which is discharged a sero-sangui-
nolent, ichorous fluid; (3), inflammation of the serous bursæ, the tendinous and
articular synovial membranes, and of the periosteum; (4), osteitis, caries and
necrosis.   M. Leplat has found the most common seat to be—at the sole of the
foot, over the prominent line of the metatarso-phalangean articulations, the pulp
of the toes and the heel.   It has been also met with, exceptionally, at the dorsal
surface of the toes, and at the upper and posterior part of the heel, giving rise to
the exfoliation of the tendo-Achillis.   He believes it to be quite local in its
nature, and to arise from prolonged compression between two resistant bodies,
first between the shoe and the bone, and later between the bone and the plantar
induration.   As a consequence of this compression, the dermis undergoes mortification, a molecular destruction of its elements taking place, resembling that
which is observable in many ulcers, as after contusion, or in the production of a
varicose ulcer.   It seems to be met with especially in persons whose occupations keep them much on their feet, and one only of the author's eight cases
occurred in a woman.   Still, in a case observed by M. Nélaton, he was unable
to refer the origin of the affection to any known cause, and it was hereditary in
the family.   M. Vesignié, who has met with several of these cases, regards the
affection as a variety of psoriasis palmaria.   Some have attributed its origin to
sweating of the feet, others regard it as papillary hypertrophy of the plantar
region, while others, again, consider it as the effect of a certain diathesis, as the
syphilitic.   M. Leplat has not been able to trace any of his cases to any of these
causes, and yet cannot but allow that some special predisposition must exist,
seeing the great rarity of the affection as compared with the general prevalence
of mechanical causes it has been attributed to.   Moreover, it is sometimes unpre-
ceded by any induration, while its rapid progress in some cases, and its multiplication at various points in others, forbid its being explained by a mere local
cause.   When abrasion of the diseased tissues is performed, the affection usually reappears in the cicatricial tissue.

PART III.

MIDWIFERY AND DISEASES OF WOMEN AND CHILDREN.

(A) CONCERNING PREGNANCY AND PARTURITION.

ART. 132.—*A sign of Pregnancy.*
By Dr. OLDHAM, Obstetric Physician to Guy's Hospital.

(*Medical Times and Gazette*, Jan. 26, 1856.)

In a case some little time ago, under care in one of the medical wards of Guy's Hospital, in which a consultation was held to determine whether a large tumor in the abdomen of a young unmarried woman were a pregnant uterus or not, Dr. Oldham took the opportunity of showing to the students that a certain power of contraction was possessed by the tumor which marked its true character. The patient's abdomen being well exposed, the outline of the tumor was seen to be less defined before manual examination than it became afterwards. The hand being applied, the tumor at first felt soft and ill-circumscribed, rapidly, however, assuming under pressure a tense rounded form, becoming firm and resisting. The alteration from flaccidity to tension was very marked, and might, as Dr. Oldham observed, be taken as a trustworthy characteristic of a pregnant uterus, since there was no other tumor which possessed any power of altering its form when irritated by palpation.

ART. 133.—*The influence of Pregnancy in controlling or retarding the development of certain diseases.* By Dr. MONTGOMERY, Professor of Midwifery in the King and Queen's College of Physicians, Dublin.

(*Dublin Quarterly Journal of Medical Science*, Nov. 1855.)

After alluding to the probability that women who bear children generally enjoy more health and are less disposed to disease than those who lead a life of celibacy, or who, being married, are childless—that pregnancy is in some measure a protection against disease, and that pregnant women suffer severely when attacked by disease—Dr. Montgomery proceeds to say—" I think also I have seen sufficient to satisfy me that pregnancy does, at least occasionally, exercise another kind of influence over disease in the system, namely, of preventing its development during that state, although the infection may have been caught; as is proved by the disease showing itself immediately after delivery, as in the following cases :

" Mrs. W., when in the ninth month of pregnancy, was much about her brother, who was dangerously ill of malignant scarlatina; she seemed to have escaped the danger completely, but the day after her delivery she was covered with the disease, of which she died in a few days; between the time of her exposure to the infection and her delivery, there had intervened three weeks, during which she appeared to be quite well.

" When Mrs F. was in the eighth month of pregnancy, her husband had typhus fever, in which she assiduously attended him; after his recovery, she went to her father's house, some fifty miles from town, where she was delivered in due time, and immediately afterwards was seized with typhus fever, of which she died in eight days: between five and six weeks had elapsed between Mr. F.'s illness and her labor, and during that interval, she seemed in perfect health.

"In the month of November, 1854, I attended a young lady in her first confinement; previous to which she had both the lower extremities much enlarged by anasarca, but she appeared, in other respects, quite well, with one exception, which was that she had such *soreness* of the abdomen, she found a difficulty in lying on either side: and when I passed my hand over the abdomen, she complained that the pressure hurt her everywhere.

"On the 12th, she was confined, after a favorable labor, but the abdominal tenderness remained, and there was a peculiar doughy feel of the whole abdomen; next day this was equally felt, but with little or no pain or fever, and a perfectly quiet pulse.

"On the 14th, I found the insteps of both feet, but particularly the left, covered with well-developed erysipelas; her mother, who seemed very anxious about her, was present when I examined the feet, and on our reaching the drawing-room said, 'Doctor, isn't that very like erysipelas?' I said, 'Yes, certainly, there was no doubt about it.' 'Dear me, sir, do you think she could have taken it from her husband?' She then, for the first time, informed me, that some weeks before leaving home, to come to town for her confinement, her husband had a severe attack of erysipelas, during which she had assiduously nurse-tended him. Immediately on the appearance of the erysipelas on the feet, the abdominal symptoms began to decline, and, after two or three days, ceased to exist. I cannot but believe that this lady caught the infection from her husband during her close attendance on him, that it remained in abeyance until gestation was over, and was then developed. She recovered well.

"It is, I believe, a matter of common observation, that when women who have been laboring under certain forms of disease happen to conceive, the morbid affection previously existing is oftentimes either greatly mitigated, checked, or even altogether suspended for a time, as has been frequently observed in persons affected with phthisis; though I must add, that the influence of pregnancy in cases of phthisis is a question on which a variety of discordant opinions has been given by high authorities. Andral's[*] conclusion, from his latest observations, is, 'that in the great majority of cases the symptoms of phthisis are suspended, or at least remain stationary during the course of pregnancy.' Louis[†] says he is not 'in a condition to determine whether pregnancy is, or is not capable of retarding the progress of phthisis,' but he suggests that the fact might be, that several of the symptoms become somewhat more obscure during pregnancy, without any check being in reality given to the advance of the disease. My own experience would lead me to the conclusion, that if a woman predisposed to phthisis, but in whom the disease has not actually become developed, prove pregnant, she is likely to be benefited thereby; and I think I have seen life thus prolonged, for years, in several instances; but, on the other hand, if pregnancy takes place in a woman already actually in consumption, or if this disease supervene on pregnancy, the fatal issue is as likely to be accelerated as postponed, or, perhaps, even more so.

"Several years since, I had a patient under my care affected with white swelling of the elbow-joint, which had gone to a great length, and was very little benefited by treatment, when all of a sudden a very rapid amendment was observed. On questioning the lady, I found that she had reason to think herself about six weeks pregnant, which was the fact; from that time, the cure advanced uninterruptedly, so that before the end of her gestation the arm was perfectly well, and has continued so ever since, she having, in the interval, borne several children."

ART. 134.—*On the frequency of Laceration of the Perinæum in Primiparæ.* By T. SNOW BECK, M.D., Londin., F.R.S., Physician to the Samaritan Free Hospital for Women and Children, &c.

(*Medical Times and Gazette,* Feb. 23, 1856.)

"About four or five years ago, it was stated, during a discussion at the Medical Society of London, that laceration of the perinæum often occurred during

[*] "Clinique Médicale," tom. iv, p. 367.
[†] "Researches on Phthisis," Walshe's Translation, pp. 279, 280.

first confinements, and was seldom followed by consequences of any importance. A statement of this kind was so contrary to the received opinions, that I recollect appealing to different practical accoucheurs at the time, who all declared that they had never met with a case during several years of extensive practice. And I should have also said, if I had given an opinion, that no such accident had ever occurred in my own practice. But as I was then engaged in testing the correctness of an opinion which had been put prominently forward about that time, i. e., that laceration of the orifice of the uterus not unfrequently happened during labor, and was followed by ulceration, entailing nearly all the ills which woman was heir to,—I determined, also, to ascertain carefully the condition of the perinæum after each labor which came under my own observation.

"A few days after the discussion at the Medical Society, I was called upon to attend a young lady, æt. 23, in her confinement with her first child. She was of middle stature, sanguine temperament, and broad conformation, and had enjoyed uninterrupted good health during her pregnancy. The labor pains came on naturally, the vagina was lax and lubricated with a free secretion of mucus, the vulva and perinæum were soft and distensible. The waters broke after the orifice of the uterus was freely dilated, and the head came down and presented naturally at the orifice of the vagina. The pains were sufficient but not violent, and the head was expelled with apparently less suffering than usual, and while the perinæum was carefully guarded. Not any evidence of laceration was perceived, either from unusual suffering by the mother, or from any sensation of the hand whilst guarding the perinæum. In a short time the shoulders and body were expelled by another parturient effort; and the placenta was found detached and readily removed. I felt so assured that nothing unusual had taken place, that I scarcely considered it necessary to make an examination after the placenta had been taken away. I was therefore greatly surprised to find on examination, that the perinæum was lacerated through its whole extent, the lacerated portion presenting the sharp defined edges of a recent breach of surface. No perceptible laceration, however, could be detected at the orifice of the uterus after the most careful examination with the finger. At the visit in the evening I mentioned that some tearing had occurred, and that it was necessary to ascertain the extent; when by placing the patient on her side, the parts were carefully examined by the eye. This confirmed the previous diagnosis, and showed that the laceration had taken place a little to the left side of the fourchette, and had extended to the rectum, exposing the circular fibres of the sphincter ani. The parts were flaccid, and the sides of the laceration in apposition—no unusual soreness was complained of. The knees of the patient were tied together, in order to prevent too much movement of the body, and the nurse directed to wash the part with warm water twice or thrice daily. On the third day the laceration was again examined, and I was surprised to find that union by the first intention had taken place through the whole extent. No further incouvenience followed, and when I took my leave the perinæum was as perfect as if no laceration had ever occurred.

"The next case was somewhat different. The lady was rather tall, about 25 years of age, fair, soft skin, and had been 'rather poorly' during her pregnancy. There was but little secretion from the vagina, yet the parts were cool and dilatable. After the pains had continued for twenty-four hours, and the patient become much exhausted, I thought it desirable, as the hand was pressing on the perinæum, to apply the short forceps and complete the labor. No difficulty was experienced in this procedure, the child being readily extracted with one hand, while with the other the perinæum was supported. No laceration had taken place immediately before the expulsion of the head. After a little time, another pain expelled the body, but the placenta did not immediately follow, and was brought away by traction at the cord, combined with gentle pressure over the body of the uterus. By the examination which was then instituted, not the least laceration of the orifice of the uterus could be detected; but, as in the former case, the perinæum was torn through its whole extent. The following day I examined the parts with the eye, and found that such was undeniably the case. The same treatment was followed, but no union by the first intention took place. For some few days the laceration presented the same appearance, but subsequently granulations formed, the sides united at the posterior part, and gradually union followed through the whole extent; thus forming nearly as good a perinæum as before the accident.

"It will be unnecessary to detail each case, suffice it that I have before me the notes of one hundred and twelve cases of primiparæ, observed within the last five years, of which seventy-five, or two-thirds, had laceration of the perinæum through the whole extent; while in thirty-seven, or just one-third, no laceration took place. Unless this result had been fortified by notes made as soon as I returned home, and by the examination of the parts by the eye, as well as by the touch, I might have considered that some error had crept into these observations; but, with the precautions taken, I feel assured of the accuracy of the result, however contrary it may be to previous opinions.

"The laceration apparently took place just as the head was extruded. The perinæum was perfect immediately before the head was expelled, and was lacerated after the birth of the child. In a few instances, by keeping the finger on the centre of the perinæum, it was felt to give way, to allow the head to pass; but in the great majority no indication of laceration was perceived until after the completion of parturition. In the interval between the extrusion of the head and the expulsion of the body, the parts were so much on the stretch, that it was impossible to determine with certainty whether laceration had occurred or not; but as the shoulders passed without the least difficulty through an opening of sufficient size, it appears most probable that the laceration did not take place at this period, but had occurred previously.

"Of the seventy-five cases in which laceration occurred, fifteen of these, or twenty per cent., healed by the first intention, and the perinæum was as perfect as before the confinement; while fifty-three, or seventy-five per cent., healed by granulation, and produced a more or less perfect perinæum. In not one instance has any inconvenience followed,—such as prolapsus of the uterus, bearing-down pains, &c.—and in only one case was there any trouble attending the accident. This case was amongst the first observed, and while my mind was still imbued with the serious consequences which followed laceration of the perinæum. It did not heal by the first intention, and the granulations were small, and showed little inclination to unite into those of the opposite side. I became anxious, applied different remedies, and, finally, the quilled suture. Nothing which was applied appeared to produce any effect, and the operation of the sutures was decidedly injurious. In the first instance it frightened the patient; was a source of constant annoyance; produced irritation of the part; and, from the pressure of the silk inducing ulceration of the deeper structures, became loose, and was obliged to be removed. The laceration, however, gradually healed, leaving not more than a quarter of an inch of the rupture unclosed. In this case, the effect of the ligatures were such as to deter me from applying them on any subsequent occasion. In all the cases I have observed, neither the patient nor the nurse was aware that anything had occurred more than usual. The patient said she felt very sore, could not sit up in bed for some few days in consequence, and when she began to sit up out of bed, required a pillow, or some soft substance to sit upon. But these were considered as nothing more than usual on such occasions.

"Little need be said of the thirty-seven cases wherein laceration did not occur, except that some, at least, were such as might, à priori, have been supposed likely to suffer from this accident. The patients were spare, and rather above the average size; the perinæum small in extent, firm, and somewhat unyielding. But in women with this conformation, scarcely one suffered from laceration, and then only when the size of the child was disproportioned to that of the pelvis of the mother; but when the perinæum was broad, thick, and soft, scarcely one escaped being torn through.

"It, of course, will remain for further observation to determine whether these cases, taken indiscriminately from the practice of one physician, fairly represent the average occurrence of this accident in women confined with their first child. If it does, then laceration of the perinæum becomes the rule in such cases, instead of the exception; but even if it does not, it yet shows that this accident is of much more frequent occurrence than has been supposed. These cases further show that when laceration does occur, this will heal perfectly by ordinary attention, rest, and cleanliness. Such, at least, must be admitted from the result of the seventy-five cases, every one of which has healed with little trouble, and none have been followed by any annoying consequences. From these facts we may, I think, advance a step further, and conclude that, in cases where the laceration has extended through the sphincter ani, there is great probability that the laceration will heal, in many cases, by the natural process; and that time should be given for this purpose, before any operative procedure is had recourse to.

" The majority of those females who form the subject of these observations, have been confined with the second, and several with the third child; but in no instance has laceration again taken place, and in only one was there a slight tearing, during the birth of a large child, which soon healed. It would then appear that the cicatrix which follows a lacerated perinæum is less liable to give way during parturition than the natural structure of the part.

" It is an acknowledged fact that severe laceration of the perinæum, involving the sphincter ani, has not unfrequently occurred without the accident having been discovered until some time subsequently, by the inability of the patient to retain the motions, and other distressing consequences. And it is also known that tearing of the perinæum, up to the sphincter, has taken place, and has not subsequently healed. But we have no information as to the circumstances which have interfered with the healing process, which these present cases appear to show usually takes place. My own experience would lead me to conclude that many cases may, and do occur, without the medical attendant being aware of the accident. For although my attention was specially directed to this point, yet several occurred wherein the laceration was not perceived until a careful examination of the parts had been made after the labor was completed. Had this examination, which is unusual, not been instituted, the accident might not have been discovered, either at the time, or subsequently, by reason of the strong tendency which appears to exist for the healing of any tearing or other injury to the generative organs of the female, when the process of parturition has been completed.

ART. 135.—*On Ruptured Perinæum.*
By Mr. J. BAKER BROWN, Obstetric Surgeon to St. Mary's Hospital.
(*Medical Times and Gazette*, Nov. 3 and 10, 1855.)

The object of this paper (which was read before the Medical Society of London) was to add further confirmation to the truth of the four propositions laid down in Mr. Brown's previous papers on this subject, viz.,—

1. That the oldest and worst forms of ruptured perinæum can be cured by the operation already described.

2. That the worst forms can be cured by operation immediately after the lesion.

3. That the new perinæum is not torn by, or prejudicial to, subsequent parturition.

4. That those forms of rupture where the sphincter is not torn through, should be cured, to prevent prolapsus uteri, &c.

Another object of this paper is to add a fifth proposition, viz.,—

5. That the operation may even be performed three or four days after the accident, although the parts may be in a sloughy condition.

He adduces instances illustrating all *five* propositions, and relates seven severe cases upon which he had operated, all of which terminated successfully. He then proceeds to offer a tabular statement of all the cases he had yet published, including those read before the society, tabulating the statement as to age, duration of rupture, nature of rupture, character of operation, and result, with summary remarks. From this statement, it is seen that twenty-eight of the cases were completely successful, two were *partially so*, and *one died*. Of the two *partially* successful, the first was entirely attributable to the entire unmanageableness of the patient after the operation, refusing the absolute quiet so essential to success; and further, to the patient leaving the hospital before anything could be done to remedy the recto-vaginal opening, which might easily have been done, had the patient submitted to treatment. The second was the most serious case he had

seen, with a greater loss of the recto-vaginal septum, and yet so satisfactory was
the result, that the patient left the hospital with control over the bowels, and with
every prospect of having a permanent and sound perinæum; but as she refused
to remain sufficiently long in the hospital for the united surfaces to gain sufficient strength, and as, on her return home, contrary to Mr. Brown's injunctions to
remain quiet, in a recumbent posture, she got up every day and took violent
walking exercise, a gradual giving way of a great portion of the united surfaces
resulted.   The case of *death* was interesting from the fact that the subsequent
history (which he, Mr. Brown, had ascertained from his friend and colleague,
Mr. Coulson) proved that a slight wound, even from cutting her finger, in one
instance, took three or four months to heal, assisted by a residence at the sea-
side; and that was, of course, unknown to him at the time of the operation.   Of
the twenty-eight successful cases, he observes, that in twenty-one cases there
was complete rupture of the perinæum, with the loss of the sphincter ani; and
in the remaining seven there was either prolapsus of the uterus, bladder, or rectum, all of which affections were completely cured by the operation. He remarks
also, that five of these patients had been delivered subsequently to the operation,
and with no injury to the perinæum but what was easily remedied by suture;
and that of the thirty-one cases, in thirteen of them the cause of rupture was the
use of instruments.   He (Mr. Brown) then proceeds to place before the society
a tabular statement of the operations performed by the late M. Roux, of Paris—
tabulated in the same way as he (Mr. Brown) had done with his own.   M.
Roux's cases were fifteen in number: of these he returned twelve as successful, two as unsuccessful, and one death.   But of the twelve returned as successful, he (Mr. Brown) observes, that in six of them M. Roux stated that a recto-
vaginal fistula remained.   It could not, therefore, be said that the operation was
successful; and if those six were added to the three confessedly unsuccessful, it
would give nine out of fifteen, or nearly two-thirds of the whole, as unsuccessful. He observes that M. Roux used the quill-suture in them all; but there was
no mention of a division of the sphincter ani in any one of them, a fact to which
he (Mr. Brown) attributed the large number of failures.   The author briefly sums
up by recapitulating the points to be observed, in the following few words—
quill-suture, division of sphincter, free use of opium, generous diet, and frequent
catheterism.

Art. 136.—*Case of birth through the centre of a lacerated Perinæum.*
By Dr. J. F. Lamb.

(*American Quarterly Journal of Medical Science*, April, 1856.)

This case is as follows:

"Case.—In June, 1821, I was called to attend a primiparous woman, whose
age was about thirty years.   The pelvis was well formed, and the presenting
part was found to be the head: ascertained ultimately to be the occiput to the
right sacro-iliac symphysis.   The labor was progressing favorably, though for
some hours the parts seemed unyielding, and I found it impossible to correct the
presentation.   As the head advanced, and the pains became strong, my attention
was directed to the perinæum, which became violently stretched, and I presume
in an unguarded moment, when the support was not where it should have been,
the infant seemed really to have jumped through the perinæum !   Being then a
mere novice in obstetrical practice, at the instant I did not understand the nature
of the accident.   A single pain had expelled the child, which was of ordinary
size, and full of life.   My first business was to secure and divide the cord, and
then to ascertain the nature and extent of the injury, which was directly manifest.   The funis umbilicalis was carefully withdrawn from its unnatural channel,
and brought out through the vagina.   The placenta was detached and expelled
without delay or difficulty—when, upon a more careful examination, I found
the rent in the perinæum very nearly central; the fourchette and the sphincter
ani were uninjured, and the accident was attended with very little hemorrhage.
A stitch appeared to me to be unnecessary.   Having a reliable nurse, I satisfied
myself by placing the patient comfortably on her back, with the thighs in close

apposition. and impressing on both patient and nurse the absolute necessity of maintaining that position for several days.

"On examination at the close of the fourth day, I was pleased to find the edges of the wound adhering with firmness. The patient made a very good recovery, and, indeed, the whole case was attended with so little trouble, that she was scarcely aware that anything very unusual had happened.

"The union was firm and perfect, and this patient subsequently gave birth to several children without the recurrence of accident."

ART. 137.—On the use of Chloroform in Midwifery.
By Dr. Murphy, Professor of Midwifery in Univ. College, London.

(Lancet, Feb. 2, 1856.)

In a paper read before the Medical Society of London, on a recent occasion, Dr. Murphy directed attention to three points as worthy of reflection. First. The progressive effect of chloroform on the nervous system, from which he derived the safety of its application. Secondly. The difference that exists in its effect on different constitutions, showing the importance of a guarded use of it. Third. The remarkable disparity in the amount of suffering from the pains of labor, which women experience when going through what is called "a natural labor," which proves the infinite value of this agent, not only in assuaging an amount of agony which overcomes the fortitude of women of the strongest resolution, but also in promoting their more rapid recovery. He mentioned as the result of his own observation, that the nerves of sensation were first affected, and that pain may be relieved before chloroform acts on the brain, or impairs consciousness. The brain then becomes engaged, and mental power disturbed, causing giddiness, rambling, and ultimately sopor. At the same time, or nearly so, the reflex nerves manifest its influence. He did not wish to pass what he might call the first stage, the relief of pain, because he thought it quite sufficient for ordinary obstetric purposes. The profound stertorous sleep required for surgical operations he did not think necessary in midwifery. He described the effect of chloroform on a patient when used in this way, and for this purpose preferred inhalation by the mouth alone as being safer. Such use of this anæsthetic might be considered inefficient. because the patient still suffers some pain. He (Dr. Murphy) found it quite the contrary, because the pain is as nothing compared with what she otherwise would have endured, and her recovery is always rapid. She does not suffer from the exhaustion which follows a severe labor, rendering the patient restless, and obliging the practitioner to employ opium to procure sleep.

He looked upon chloroform, in this respect, as the most valuable assistant in the management of labor that has ever been discovered. The author alluded to the difference in the effect of chloroform on different constitutions. All women are not equally susceptible to its influence. With some, a few inhalations are sufficient to control all pain, and even put them to sleep; while others continue to inhale for a long time before they experience any relief. In these instances caution is necessary, which is very easily exercised if chloroform is given in the gradual manner stated. It is necessary to watch its action on the reflex nerves, and to withdraw the vapor when they become affected. He (Dr. Murphy) thought the respiration and action of the uterus especially should be attended to. It is of importance to watch for stertor during the sleep of the patient, and not to mistake the cause of the short and feeble pains. The uterus is not paralyzed, as has been supposed, but the aid which it receives from the reflex muscles is diminished. In this, as in the former case, the sound sleep which follows labor perfectly restores the patient. The third variety is rarely met with, and is very perplexing. He related a case where chloroform seemed to increase the pains, although in the intervals the patient was in a profound sleep. When stertor was observed he withdrew the vapor. The patient was safely delivered, slept for some time, awoke, and had no recollection of anything that occurred from the time she inhaled the chloroform. He attributed this effect to a kind of dream. What in other patients would cause incoherent rambling here exaggerated the one idea, pain. The remarkable difference in the amount of suffering which women experience when going through natural labor proved the value of chloroform most clearly. Some suffer comparatively little; at no period of labor are the pains beyond their power of endurance; chloroform is not therefore called for. But there are cases of a very opposite character, in which the patient is acutely sensitive, where even slight pains cause great distress, and where the more powerful pains become so intolerable, and cause such an amount of suffering, that the action of the uterus is often suspended. It is in such instances that the value of chloroform shines the most conspicuously, and it is here that the practitioner will find its aid most clearly unquestionable. He concluded by apologizing for an imperfect paper. He avoided entering upon, or replying to, the objections offered to its use, not only because he had already fully examined them, but he was unwilling to make this valuable agent a kind of battle-field for the collision of strong and decided opinions. It was in the power of every one to arrive at a just conclusion from his own experience. He entreated those who would follow this rational mode of investigation not to be led away from it by "post hoc ergo propter hoc" arguments; not to believe that all the well-known casualties of labor are caused by chloroform, because this agent happens to be administered; not to take second-hand histories of its effect, but as the members of a highly scientific profession are bound to do, to take nothing for granted, but examine and judge for themselves. He thought that there was nothing singular in the reception it has as yet met with in this great metropolis. It took fifteen years before gaslight triumphed in London. The light shone conspicuously wherever it was introduced, but it only made more manifest the prejudices and apprehensions of the public. It was declared to be most offensive, most dangerous; houses were blown to atoms by explosions of the gas, and the event was recorded with all the avidity of a death from chloroform. Still it continued to be used by its advocates; they gradually increased; at length its use became general, explosions were only recorded as unfortunate accidents, and now gaslight has obtained its triumph. It gives not only light, but heat, it supplies the place of coals as well as candles, and every house in London considers this noisome and most dangerous agent an indispensable requisite. He (Dr. Murphy) anticipated from chloroform the same career. It is now under its trial, but as it becomes better understood will be more generally used, and ultimately become indispensable in the lying-in apartment.

ART. 138.—*Cases of Cæsarian Section.* By (1) M. WIECKEL; and (2) Dr. MERINAR.

1. *Med. Zeitung.* Aug. 1855.
2. *Charlestown Med. Jour. and Rev.*, March, 1856.

(1) *Dr. Merinar's case.*—The subject of this case was a servant girl, æt. 27, upon whom the operation had been performed twice previously (v. "Abstract," xxi.) There was no difficulty in the operation, and a living male child was the result of it; but the mother sank five days afterwards, apparently from peritonitis. The operation was performed on the 22d October, 1855.

(2) *M. Wieckel's case.*—In this case, also, the operation had been performed twice previously, (v. "Abstract," xxi,) and each time in consequence of rupture of the uterus, and the passage of the child into the abdominal cavity. On this occasion the rupture took place while the patient was engaged in lifting a great weight, and on examination, the child could be distinctly felt through the abdominal parietes. The operation was performed, under chloroform, on the 14th April, 1855, and a female child of about five months and a half was extracted without any difficulty. The process of recovery was not interrupted by a single untoward event, the wound healing by the first intention, and the mother being able to resume her domestic duties in about fifteen days.

In our previous account of this case M. Wieckel's name is spelt as Winckel, and the patient's name which is spelt Lieper, ought to have been Sieper.

ART. 139.—*On the expediency of Symphyseotomy.* By Dr. KEILLER.

(*Edinburgh Medical Journal*, Aug. 1855.)

Dr. Keiller recently reported to the Obstetrical Society of Edinburgh the results of a series of experiments which he had performed with the view of ascertaining the nature and extent of motion in the sacro-iliac and pubic articulations, and of determining the expediency of the operation of symphyseotomy. The experiments were performed on female subjects, several of whom had borne children, and in three of the cases an advanced state of pregnancy existed.

Dr. Keiller admitted that a certain degree of separation and motion occasionally took place in the pelvic joints, and that a small amount of space might be obtained by forcible separation of the pubic articulation, either by nature or operative procedure, but denied that the space so gained was in the direction where it was usually required in deformed pelves, viz., in the antero-posterior diameter of the brim.

Dr. Keiller demonstrated that, on dividing the inter-pubic fibro-cartilage, great retraction of its fibres took place in front, where its structure was comparatively thick, thus giving rise to the idea that considerable separation of the bones had taken place, which was not actually the case, a point easily ascertained by examining the posterior aspect of the joint, where the bones, after the operation, would be still found almost in close apposition. This apparently great separation of the articulation in front had no doubt frequently misled those who believed that by division of the symphysis real space was gained.

Dr. Keiller stated that he could not in any other way account for the conclusions arrived at by Dr. Duncan, who, in his recent communication to the society on this subject, had affirmed that, in experimenting on the pelvis of a subject, he had succeeded in readily procuring about two inches of space between the pubic bones, by simply dividing the symphysis, and without applying any force to increase the amount of separation.

Dr. Keiller had now performed the experiment of dividing the symphysis pubis on a great number of subjects, and had carefully noted the comparative measurements, and had arrived at conclusions widely different from those come to by Dr. Duncan.

At the same meeting, Dr. Simpson exhibited three recent pelves illustrative of this subject, and mentioned the results of his experiments with them. He agreed with Dr. Keiller that the extent of separation and motion was by no means so great as had been stated by Dr. Duncan. Dr. Simpson considered the Sigaultian operation inexpedient and dangerous, and thought that it would not again be revived from its present obsolete position.

Dr. Duncan made a few remarks on the preparations, and adhered to the opinions he had formerly expressed as to the mobility of the articulations in pregnancy, and as to the propriety of the question of adopting the Sigaultian operation in particular cases being reconsidered.

ART. 140.—*Cases of Labor where the heads of Twins were locked in the Pelvis.* By (1) Dr. SIDEY and (2) Dr. MATTHEWS DUNCAN.

(*Edinburgh Medical Journal*, Oct. 1855.)

The two following cases were read before the Edinburgh Obstetrical Society. In the first both children were born alive.

(1) *Dr. Sidey's case.*—Mrs. B—, her fifth confinement, and her second of twins; saw her during the day, when the pains were slow and weak, the presentation being high, and of the breech. I left word that when the pains became stronger I was to be sent for. In the evening they became so, and when I arrived the breech was just expelled; having relieved the cord from pressure on the head turning into the hollow of the sacrum, a hard tumor came pressing down under the arch of the pubis during a severe pain, preventing the presenting head being extracted. Upon examining carefully, I found this tumor nothing else than the head of a second child, jamming itself firmly on the first, and had some trouble in relieving the now locked heads; taking advantage of the interval of pains, and keeping up the head of the second child during the pain, I succeeded in extracting the head of the first child, and the second followed. The twins were of the usual size; mother and twins did well.

(2) *Dr. Duncan's case*—Mrs. F—, æt. 21, was taken in acute labor of her second child at noon, after being for some hours affected with lingering pains.

The body of a child was born at two P.M. Matters continued in this state, under very strong pains, till nearly five P M., when Dr. Rosa first saw the woman.

Dr. Duncan saw the case soon after, and found that while the body of the first child was born, its head was prevented from entering the pelvis by the head of the second child, which was lodged in the hollow of the sacrum, having the neck of the first lying between it and the region of the thyroid foramen of the left side of the mother. The occiput of the second child was directed to the right side of the mother; that of the first child was in nearly an opposite direction. During a pain, both heads descended, but especially the second, which then pressed strongly into the outlet of the bony pelvis. It appeared to Dr. Duncan that both children might have been delivered entire. But a different plan was followed.

The child half born was certainly dead; and the second child was so also (as far as could be made out). The vagina was much stretched, and as if dragged upwards, and the uterine tumor tender to the touch. The woman had been long in this distressing state, and was urgent for relief. Dr. Duncan, therefore, resolved to deliver quickly, and as easily and safely as possible for the mother.

With a bistoury he decapitated the first child, already certainly long dead. After this, a few pains were observed. The heads continued in the same relative position, and both were propelled downwards during the contractions, but without any decided progress. The forceps were then applied to the head of the second child, which was thus delivered almost without any traction. The head of the first child was then easily removed by seizing the stump of the cervical spine with a Lyon's forceps, and extracting it. The placenta was soon afterwards delivered (6·15 P.M). The woman made a very good recovery. The twins were large, well-formed children.

ART. 141.—*A case of spontaneous Restoration of the Retroverted Uterus.* By Dr. RAMSBOTHAM, Obstetric Physician to the London Hospital.

(*Medical Times and Gazette*, Dec. 1855.)

In the "Medical Times and Gazette" for October 23d, 1852, will be found eight cases of retroversion of the gravid uterus, treated by Dr. Ramsbotham, which go far to prove the truth of the position laid down by Denman, in opposition to the doctrine inculcated by William Hunter, Baudelocque, and others,—that if the bladder be kept duly empty, the womb will in the great majority of instances, spontaneously regain its natural position, without the employment of any manual operation, beyond the frequent introduction of the catheter.

Since some members of the profession, however, may still incline to the opinion that the use of active means is absolutely required for its restoration, and, as consequently forcible attempts to push the fundus upwards may very likely be had recourse to unnecessarily, he thinks the publication of every case that tends to confirm our reliance on the passive mode of treatment useful.

CASE.—A. G., of Hannibal Road, Stepney, æt. 41, married twenty-one years, having had nine children and suffered two miscarriages,—the last at two months, in January of this year,—applied to me among the out-patients at the London Hospital, on Saturday, the 29th of last September. She stated that she had not menstruated since the middle of June, that seven days before, while lifting a heavy pailful of water out of the water-butt, she felt a sudden pain at the lower part of the abdomen; this was followed by some difficulty in passing urine, though it did not amount to an absolute stoppage. On the next Tuesday, however, after riding from Stepney to Pimlico in an omnibus, which shook her exceedingly, she found she was quite unable to expel the least quantity from the bladder. On her return home, the urine was drawn off by the catheter, and the same instrument was used again on Wednesday, but not by the same gentleman. From that day till I saw her on the Saturday, the catheter had not again been had recourse to, nor had she passed any urine voluntarily, though some had dribbled away at different times, or come in gushes. The bowels had not acted since Tuesday. She did not know whether she was pregnant or not; but inclined to the latter opinion.

She appeared to be in great pain, and her countenance was indicative of much distress. Independently of the agony of a distended bladder, she complained of a violent forcing and bearing down, and a tearing and dragging sensation at the groins.

The history and symptoms led me immediately to suspect that the uterus was gravid and retroverted. I found the bladder largely filling the lower half of the abdominal cavity, its fundus rising as high as the umbilicus; introduced the catheter without delay, and drew off the enormous quantity of ninety-two ounces of dark colored, but not offensive urine. On making a careful examination, my suspicions were confirmed; for the hollow of the sacrum was occupied by a hard tumor, which was, indeed, the fundus and body of the uterus; while the mouth of that organ was canted upwards and forwards, behind or rather above the symphysis pubis. The anterior face of the vagina was considerably stretched, and there was general tenderness of the whole pelvic structures.

I admitted her into the hospital and ordered her to bed; fomentations were applied, and she took 30 minims of laudanum. My resident assistant was directed to draw off the urine every eight hours, and to administer some castor-oil the next morning. The medicine acted satisfactorily on the bowels in the course of the day; the bladder was kept empty as described; she was confined scrupulously to the recumbent position; no attempt was made to replace the uterus artificially; nor was any fresh vaginal examination even instituted; and in three days she was able to void her urine of her own accord satisfactorily. The anxiety of countenance had then disappeared, and she expressed herself as feeling quite well. On examination per vaginam, the fundus uteri was now no longer to be felt in the pelvic cavity, the os uteri was in its natural situation, and none of the previous tenderness remained. I kept her in the hospital merely for the sake of precaution, to prevent a recurrence of the accident, for a fortnight. During this interval she was confined to bed; was enjoined to pass water frequently; and, when she attempted to do so, to place herself on her hands and knees. She left the house on October 13th, and is going on in pregnancy, not having experienced any return of the symptoms. She tells me that she quickened last week.

No case could more strongly prove the value of rest and the recumbent posture, together with a diligent attention to the bladder, under such circumstances, than this does. I scarcely expected that the uterus would have righted itself so speedily, after having been three days partially, and four completely, retroverted, with its fundus pressed so low down towards the perinæum as this was: and I was prepared to use some mechanical efforts to restore it, if it had continued in this abnormal position for two or three days longer.

ART. 142.—*Case of complete Inversion of the Uterus at the time of labor.* By Dr. MONTGOMERY, Professor of Midwifery in the King's and Queen's College of Physicians.

(*Dublin Hospital Gazette*, April, 1856.)

This case is remarkable on account of the absence of the ordinary symptoms of the accident, and its value is enhanced by the comments which accompany it.

"CASE.—On the 10th of September, 1854, Mr. M— called on me to request that I would immediately visit his wife, whom he stated to be dangerously ill after her confinement. I accompanied him at once, and on my arrival at the patient's house, at 9 o'clock, A. M, found a physician-accoucheur, of experience and discretion, in attendance, who subsequently gave me the following account of what had occurred before my arrival:

"'He had been sent for to see Mrs. M— about 11 o'clock, P. M., of the evening before, when he found her in labor of her fourth child, with the head presenting. She was 28 years of age, healthy, and her former labors had been quite favorable. The liquor amnii had been discharged about twenty-four hours previously, without pain; for some time after the doctor's seeing her, the pains which had recently set in were pretty active, and as the pelvis was a roomy one he expected that the labor would terminate in two or three hours. It was not, however, till about half-past seven o'clock that the child, a female, was born. During the night, two half-drachm doses of ergot had been given, with little apparent effect, and it was not till after a pretty large dose of laudanum and peppermint was administered that the pains became really efficient. There was no hemorrhage, but as the placenta did not seem likely to come away speedily, the womb being sluggish and not disposed to contract, the nursetender was directed to make pressure over the uterus, while the doctor drew down the cord. In about ten or fifteen minutes the placenta came away, followed, on the instant, by a *large round tumor which passed completely out of the vagina*, and was, for an instant, supposed to be the head of a second child, which it equalled in size.

"'It was, however, soon ascertained to be the uterus completely inverted, no os being to be felt. The tumor was at once returned within the vagina without much difficulty, but pressure on the fundus failed to effect its restoration to its proper place. There was some hemorrhage, both on the sudden descent of the uterus, and after its return, *but not much.* The patient felt a pressing desire to make water, and a distressing sense of pressure on the bladder, and becoming anxious, it was deemed advisable to have further advice. Although alarmed, from the knowledge that there was something wrong, she presented little change in countenance, or pulse, no faintness, and but little hemorrhage. Her recovery, after the replacement of the uterus, went on most favorably, and at the end of a month she was as well as after any previous confinement.' 'February, 1856, she has been in good health ever since, and now considers herself two or three months pregnant.'

"Such are the accounts I received of this case at the time of the accident, and since, and I am now to state what I was myself present at. I was at the patient's bedside at 9 o'clock, delivery having taken place at half-past 7 o'clock. I found her looking tranquil, her pulse good, firm, and quiet, and although she was anxious about herself, believing that there was some cause of alarm, there was not the least approach to that kind of overwhelming nervous distress which so often accompanies so serious an accident. She complained of nothing except the sense of pressure on the bladder; there were very smart periodical pains, which, however, she rather made light of, as she regarded them only as afterpains, such as she had had after former labors, which indeed they perfectly resembled; there was very little hemorrhage.

"On examining the abdomen, there was to be felt *a considerable tumor in the supra-pubic region*, and taking this fact with the other conditions above mentioned, I confess I felt almost certain that it could not be a case of inversion, the symptoms were so widely different from those which almost universal experience would lead us to expect. An examination *per vaginam*, however, soon removed all doubt. I found that passage, indeed I may say the whole pelvic cavity, filled up with a firm fleshy tumor, *which was perfectly insensible;* and on passing the finger along it upwards, it was found to terminate in a *cul de sac* all around, and about an inch within the margin of the os uteri; so that the inversion, or, perhaps, more properly, the eversion of the organ was as complete as I believe it ever is in *the first instance.**

"In proceeding to effect the reduction, I, in the first place, put the patient fully under the influence of chloroform; I then introduced my hand, and grasping the tumor, I compressed it as strongly as I could from the lateral circumference towards the centre, and at the same time pushed it upwards and forwards towards the umbilicus; for several minutes this proceeding seemed quite without effect, but at length I felt the tumor begin to yield, receding and gliding, as it were, by a spontaneous movement *of the whole tumor* upwards, and not of the lowest part of the fundus re-entering itself; and then, all at once, it suddenly almost sprung away from my hand, and was restored to its proper place. I pressed my hand into its cavity, up to the fundus, and kept it there for a few minutes, and before withdrawing it I took the precaution of making sure that there was no dimpling in, or cupping of the fundus, by feeling the hand so retained with my other hand through the parietes of the abdomen. The resistance to the replacement of the inverted organ was so great that I do not think I should ever have suc-

* When the displacement has been for some weeks or months in existence, the tissue of the organ having gradually contracted and greatly diminished in bulk, the *cul de sac* vanishes.

ceeded had I not put the patient to sleep, and subdued its contractile efforts by the administration of chloroform. I cannot but consider myself very fortunate indeed in having succeeded in restoring this uterus fully an hour and a half after its complete inversion, during which interval, moreover, active contractions had not ceased to occur. Dr. Merriman says that under such circumstances, unless the inversion be reduced in a few minutes after the accident has happened, all attempts to return it will be ineffectual. And Denman tells us that although present at the moment when the accident occurred, in a patient of his own, and only waiting until he had separated the placenta, he could not possibly effect the replacement of the organ."

"Inversion of the uterus at the time of delivery," adds Dr. Montgomery, "is like the spontaneous evolution of the child, an accident of such rare occurrence, especially in private practice, that few, even of those most extensively engaged in practice, have ever seen a case of it; and still fewer have been actually present at the moment it took place. I have spoken with several practitioners on this subject, and, like myself, until lately, none of them had ever met with it in private practice; one gentleman said that, in forty years, he had been called in once to a case of the kind; but found the lady dead when he arrived; another gentleman had seen it once in thirty years. The late Dr. Douglas told me, within a year or two before his death, that he had just then met with it for the first time, in private; and he assured me that it had taken place after he had left the lady apparently safe and well. Denman says, expressly, that it was an accident of very rare occurrence during the whole of his life; and Dr. Ramsbotham, whose practice and experience were equally extended, says he never saw a case immediately after inversion.

"The inevitable consequence of this rarity is, of course, that no one man can, even during a long life, acquire much actual personal experience of the accident, its symptoms, or its management; and hence, these are, by very many, comparatively, but imperfectly understood; and in some important respects, most inaccurately described by many of those who have undertaken to write instructions for the guidance of others; not having witnessed, or treated the accident themselves, they are obliged to borrow from the descriptions of others equally without experience, and so the statements of one writer are copied by another, without the possibility of accurate correction. For example, one of the diagnostic marks of an inverted uterus is commonly stated by authors of credit to be its sensibility, by which it may be distinguished from a polypus, which is quite insensible. Thus, Mr. Newnham, after mentioning several circumstances connected with recent complete inversion, says, 'the pain is very severe, and the tumor is exquisitely sensible.' Dr. Merriman, says, 'the inverted uterus is sensible to the touch.' So, also, the late Professor Burns stated unreservedly, in all the editions of his very valuable work, previous to the ninth, in which he modified his former assertion, and mentions that I had shown him an inverted uterus which was quite insensible. The case thus referred to was that of an aged woman who had the uterus inverted by a polypus which sprung, by a broad attachment, from the fundus of the organ.

"This case of Mrs. M. may be regarded as one of many instances met with in practice, in which the severity of the symptoms is not at all in proportion to the gravity of the accident which may have produced them; in this case, for instance, the inversion was complete, and the symptoms insignificant.

"One of the most remarkable illustrations of this remark, to be found in the annals of medicine or surgery, as well as the most extraordinary instance of recovery from a desperate injury, is the case which occurred to Mr. Cooke, at Coventry, in 1835, in which the completely inverted uterus, with the Fallopian tubes and one ovary, was, on the third day after delivery, taken away, either by the woman herself, or, by the attendant midwife, without any injurious consequences, or, indeed, the occurrence of a single bad symptom; no hemorrhage of any importance, no exhaustion, no peritonitis, and convalescence nearly as quick as after an ordinary confinement. When I was in Birmingham, in 1840, I saw the uterus of this woman in the museum there, and at that time I was informed that she was alive and well. A case, much resembling the above, was brought before the Medical Section of the Congress at Florence by M. Rossi, in which a midwife partly tore, and partly cut away, a recently inverted uterus; the woman, notwithstanding, recovered in about thirty days. Wrisberg's case of the same kind is well known.

"The production of this accident is, I think, too generally ascribed to injudicious traction of the cord to bring down the placenta; and the inevitable consequence of this presumption is, that whenever it is found to have occurred, it is taken for granted, that the attendant practitioner must be to blame, as having thus caused it, when, in truth, all that depended on him may have been done with all proper care and skill, and the accident have arisen from causes over which he had no control; at the same time, undue pressure over the fundus uteri, and strong traction by the cord, are likely to be productive of so many untoward, or even fatal consequences, that no prohibition of their adoption can be too strongly enforced, and, I may add, that the last two cases of inversion, of which I am aware as having happened in this city, were, I believe, justly attributed to the combined action of these agencies; but, if this displacement were easily produced by the mismanagement alluded to, instead of being, as it confessedly is, very rare, it would assuredly be of very frequent occurrence indeed, considering that the objectionable plan of interference is so constantly that of midwives, and, too often, of better educated practitioners.

"I think we have quite sufficient grounds for believing, with Merriman, that 'there can be no doubt that a spontaneous inversion has sometimes occurred;' or, to use the words of Dr. Blundell, that 'the whole uterus may be pushed down, and this independently of anything done by the obstetrician.' Ruysch states that the accident may happen, and did so in his own practice, when no undue force was used; and, after animadverting on the impropriety of forcible extraction of the placenta, as the general cause of this accident, he adds, 'aliquando tamen, ortum ducit a conatibus post partum remanentibus.'

"Rokitansky describes a condition of the uterus immediately after delivery, which might readily lead to inversion: it consists in a paralysis of the placental portion of the uterus, occurring at the same time that the surrounding parts go through the ordinary processes of reduction; the part alluded to is thus, he says, 'forced into the cavity of the uterus by the contraction of the surrounding tissue, so as to project in the shape of a conical tumor, and a slight indentation is noticed at the corresponding point of the external surface.' And he adds an observation, the truth of which I had occasion to verify, I may say anticipate, several years ago. 'The close resemblance of the paralyzed segment of the uterus to a fibrous polypus may easily induce a mistake in the diagnosis, and nothing but a minute examination of the tissue can solve the question. The affection always causes hemorrhage, which lasts for several weeks after childbirth, and proves fatal by the consequent exhaustion.'

"The following case was an instance of this occurrence. In July, 1831, I was summoned, at four o'clock in the morning, to see a lady who had been delivered at ten o'clock the previous night. The placenta was still retained, although she had had, all through the night, rather severe expulsive pains; she had lost a good deal of blood. On examination, I found the serous surface of the placenta lying upon, and pressed against, the internal surface of the os uteri, but although the uterine contraction continued, I could not get it down by traction of the cord. On passing my hand into the uterus, I found the placenta was adhering to a globular tumor, which seemed to be as large as a good sized orange, and which, at the moment, I had no doubt was a fibrous tumor projecting from the inner surface of the uterus. To this tumor the placenta was morbidly adherent, and was only separated therefrom with difficulty. Having, however, accomplished this, and turned my hand freely in the uterus, to secure its complete contraction, the tumor, which was evidently the 'placental portion' of the uterus partially inverted, completely disappeared, and the lady afterwards recovered well. Denman relates a case very much resembling this.

"With regard to those cases, in which inversion has been supposed to have occurred *spontaneously*, after the departure of the medical attendant, I think we may take for granted, that in not a few of them the displacement had *commenced* while he was present, though without his knowledge; perhaps with very slight manifestations of its occurrence, or it may have remained unnoticed from want of sufficient observation, and proper examination on his part. In the *Gazette des*

Hôpitaux, for 7th February last, there is a case reported in which partial inversion of the uterus was only discovered on the 6th December, in a patient who is stated to have been *safely delivered* on the 13th November; but, from the whole details of the case, it appears almost evident that the inversion occurred at the time of labor, but was not then noticed.

"There is obviously this danger in supposing, as so many do, that this accident is always attended and announced by a particular train of urgent symptoms; that if such symptoms are not observed, the attendant may be induced to conclude, what he would naturally so much desire, that no such accident could have happened, and so the patient is left to die, or linger out a life of misery. The instances in which this happened are numerous indeed; one such is above referred to, and another we may quote from Dr. Merriman, in which it is stated that 'the placenta came away without any difficulty, and certainly without any suspicion of injury to the uterus;' but, between six and seven months afterwards, it was discovered that the uterus was inverted.

"Now, when we succeed in effecting the replacement of a completely inverted uterus, how is its restoration really accomplished? Is it, as is generally stated in books, by re-inverting first the dependent fundus, or, in the words of Sir C. M. Clarke, 'by making pressure on the lower part only of the tumor, so as to cause this part to be received into that above it,' and so on, gradually up to the angle where the cervix is flexed on itself? Judging from what happened in this case of Mrs. M., and from the accounts given by others of what happened in their cases, I think the above is not the mode of reduction; but that, as we compress the bulk of the tumor, and try to press the fundus back into itself, and push it upwards, *the flexure at the cervix* yields, and presently the fundus seems to escape upwards by springing as it were from our hand; so that the part which was the last inverted is the first restored. This springing away from the hand is expressly mentioned by more than one writer of authority, and is, I presume, produced by the contraction of the orbicular fibres of the partially restored cervix lifting up quickly the globe of the fundus.

"I have now only to observe, that however small is the number of cases of inverted uterus met with in practice, it would be still smaller if it were the universal rule carefully to examine every recently-delivered woman, both through the abdominal parietes, to ascertain the size and form of the uterus, and also *per vaginam,* to be satisfied that there was no tumor protruding into that canal; nothing can excuse the neglect of this simple proceeding, and if it were *invariably* adopted, I think, with Mr. Newnham, that 'chronic inversion of the uterus would be known only by description.'"

ART. 143.—*Remains of a Fœtus expelled periodically.*
By Dr. BARAVILLI.

(*Presse Méd. Belge,* Feb. 3, 1856; and *Dublin Medical Press,* Feb. 26, 1856.)

Among several clinical observations read before the Academy of Sciences of the Institute of Bologna, by Dr. Baravilli, the following case appears to us to be calculated to interest our readers.

The subject of the observation was a robust woman, æt. 38, who did not become pregnant until eighteen years after marriage; in the fifth month of pregnancy she experienced a powerful emotion, subsequently to which a small quantity of liquor amnii was discharged, and soon after the umbilical cord of a fœtus appeared externally. Some days later, having been attacked with slight uterine contractions, she saw, to her great surprise, the thigh and leg of a little fœtus escape from the vagina. No pain, nor any inconvenience other than that caused by a colored and fetid discharge, followed this sort of partial delivery. But what was most remarkable was, that she subsequently expelled from the womb once a month, precisely at the menstrual period, at one time the tibia and fibula, at another two ribs, at another the ilium or the second femur, some of the bones of the head, &c., and all without experiencing the least derangement of her health, or being obliged to suspend her domestic duties.

The author promised to communicate hereafter the further state of this woman's health, as well as the mode of issue of the remaining portions of the fœtus still retained in the womb. The case, however, abridged and incomplete as it is, is not less interesting to the obstetrician than to the physiologist.

The most important practical·deduction to be made from this observation is, that it is not always advisable to have recourse to obstetrical operations in cases in which a dead fœtus or a [premature] placenta is retained in the womb, for circumstances have often occurred—and do still daily occur—which exhibit clearly the utility of prudent expectation.

(B) CONCERNING DISEASES OF WOMEN.

ART. 144.—*Derangement of the Liver as a cause of Uterine Disease.*
By Dr. MACKENZIE.

(*Lancet*, Dec. 15, 1855.)

This paper was read before the Medical Society of London, on the 8th December, 1855. In it the author began by drawing attention to the importance of studying the constitutional origin of uterine diseases, believing them to be far more frequently dependent upon constitutional than local causes. In a series of papers published by him in 1852, he had dwelt upon the origin of uterine disease from disturbed states of the nervous system, when the exciting cause makes its impression upon the nervous centres, such as settled grief or anxiety, and impoverished or unhealthy states of the blood. He now proposed to resume the subject by considering another mode in which the nervous system might be unfavorably impressed, and uterine disease equally result—viz., from severe or persistent disease or derangement of any of the more important organs of the body; and as none illustrated the principle more fully than the liver, both from its extensive sympathies, and great liability to disorder, he had selected it as the subject of this evening's paper. Having indicated the general influence exercised by the liver upon all the processes of health and disease, he referred to its special influence upon the uterus, founded upon the intimate sympathy subsisting between these organs, &c., and showed from statistical data, how frequently derangements of these organs coexist. Contrary, however, to prevailing opinions, the facts he had collected clearly proved that the hepatic disease generally preceded, and probably occasioned, the uterine, when both coexisted. He believed that it might do so in the three following ways: first, through the medium of the direct sympathy subsisting between the uterus and the liver; secondly, through the derangement of the assimilative processes, which invariably results from chronic hepatic disturbance; and, thirdly, through the debility of the nervous system, which sooner or later inevitably follows upon long-continued derangement of any important organ of the body.

From the first of this series of causes could be deduced many uterine affections of a variable and casual character, such as hysteralgia, leucorrhœa, and menstrual irregularity; from the second, many functional and structural lesions of the uterus of a more fixed and persistent character, such as congestion and inflammatory conditions, indurations, hypertrophies, fibrous growths, certain forms of leucorrhœa, and rheumatic hysteralgia; from the third, a predisposition to uterine disease generally, the precise character and nature of which would vary with the nature of the exciting and other occasional causes. In connection with this part of the subject, attention was directed to the generally depressed state of the nervous system which accompanies the majority of uterine affections, and this, from various facts referred to by the author, was regarded by him as being rather due to the coincident hepatic than uterine complaint. The latter had, however, received greater attention, because, whilst the liver was an organ of dull sensibility. the uterus, on the other hand, had extensive sympathies with the sensorial parts of the nervous system, and its functional and structural conditions admitted of the closest scrutiny. The author then proceeded to show how the pathological history of the more common uterine affections supported the views he had submitted to the society, and concluded by adverting to the practical conclusions to be drawn from them. The treatment of these cases should, in his opinion, be conducted with reference to three principal indications

—first, to restore the tone and functional activity of the liver by the persevering employment of small, undebilitating doses of mercury, keeping strictly within the tonic and stimulating range of the remedy; secondly, to improve the assimilative functions generally, by careful attention to dietetic and hygienic measures, together with various therapeutical means, which were cursorily alluded to; thirdly, to restore the tone and vigor of the nervous system, which had been impaired by the long continuance of hepatic derangement. The general means adapted to this purpose were treated of, and the author took occasion to lay before the society some observations upon the remedial powers of amorphous phosphorus in certain affections of the uterine organs, attended with weakness and irritability of the nervous system. He had given it a large and extensive trial in these cases, and in some had found it remarkably beneficial. It could be given in doses averaging from ten to thirty grains, and, although insoluble, it readily diffused itself in water or any aqueous vehicle, and could be conveniently given in that way. It appeared to act as a direct tonic or stimulant upon the uterine system, and when properly prepared could be given without any risk or danger. He had given it with much success in certain cases of amenorrhœa, hysteria, and passive menorrhagia. He had known pregnancy to supervene upon its employment after a lengthened period of sterility subsequently to marriage, and had found it useful in correcting the tendency to miscarriage when dependent upon morbid weakness or irritability of the uterine organs. Under these circumstances, he thought it worthy of a more extended trial, and recommended it confidently to the notice of the members of the society.

ART. 145.—*Singular case of Vicarious Menstruation.* By Dr. BORING.

(*New York Journal of Medicine*, Jan. 1856.)

This case is as follows:

CASE.—A negro woman, about thirty-five years of age, of apparently good constitution, and, with the exception about to be mentioned, of general good health.

She began menstruating at the age of fifteen, and continued regular in this respect until about three years since. Eight years ago, when about twenty-seven years of age, she was attacked with violent pain in the foot, which was succeeded by an abscess, which was lanced, but did not heal. Ulceration succeeded, which continued to move upwards until the leg was involved and became the seat of its permanent location. About three years since, the catamenial discharge began manifestly to decline, and so continued until it ceased altogether, when she was seized with severe shooting pains, passing from the sacro-lumbar, to the uterine region, and to the ovaries At the approach of her next menstrual period, she noticed a slow oozing of blood from the ulcer on the leg (I give her own account of the matter), which continued about the usual time of that discharge and ceased. At subsequent *periods*, the same discharge sometimes occurred, while at others, instead, small sacks of blood were formed contiguous to the ulcer, which were obliged to be opened, and the blood discharged, before relief could be obtained.

In June last, the ulceration of the leg had become so extensive and threatening, as to require, in the judgment of Dr. —— (whose patient she then was), amputation.

Since the operation, the ulcer being removed, there has been no regular monthly periodic discharge of the blood, but, at each monthly period, sacks, such as were above described, formed round the stump of the amputated limb, and required to be lanced for the relief of the patient. I have seen these sacks, and in fact opened them, and can entertain no doubt as to their true nature. So uniform are these singular occurrences in their periodic character, as to have induced this woman to keep a lancet for the purpose, and thus *surgically* to perform the work of menstruation. It should be observed, that she continues without any vaginal discharge, and that the determination of blood to the stump of the amputated limb, together with the formation of these sacks of blood, occur periodically, and observe *strictly* the menstrual periods, as to the time of their recurrence and duration.

ART. 146.—*On the treatment of Uterine Deviations.* By Dr. TILT.
(*Medical Times and Gazette,* Jan. 26, 1856.)

Dr. Tilt has been led to believe that, in general, uterine deviations are unattended by symptoms, and are, therefore, only accidentally detected; and that the cases of uterine deviations practitioners are called upon to treat are all complex problems, problems embracing various elements, each one of which has more particularly struck various medical men, and guided their practice. The result has been, that one of the indications of such cases being often alone attended to, partial relief has alone been effected. The radical cure, he says, will be more frequent when all the bearings of the case are taken into consideration. Dr. Tilt also remarked. that women who had suffered much from uterine deviations are likewise affected with inflammatory congestions, erosions, or ulcerations of the neck of the womb. The pathologist then infers that the pains experienced, depend upon those inflammatory lesions, at all events the indication is clear,—to heal all ulcerations by the surgical modes of treatment on which Dr. Tilt has dwelt in his work on 'Diseases of Women,' and to subdue inflammation; for, by so doing. the uterine deformity will in some cases be entirely removed, though in others the patient's sufferings will be only diminished. It is also equally true that in other patients the inflammatory affection of the neck of the womb may be cured, and yet they may still continue to suffer. Dr. Tilt further observed, that uterine deviations are often complicated by neuralgia; the indication then is to treat such cases by the means found useful in neuralgic affections. Thus he has removed, or much alleviated, the sufferings of many affected with uterine deviations by the use of sedative injections into the bowels. Dr. Tilt, was, moreover, satisfied that much may be done to relieve the neuralgic symptoms of deviation by hydropathic treatment, and observed, that uterine deviations were complicated, and often determined by excessive relaxation of the vagina; detailing a somewhat novel plan of restoring to the vagina the tone which in health enabled it to serve the womb as a column of support. IIe further observed, that uterine deviations were generally most painful in married women in whom the abdominal walls had been greatly distended by gestation, and it rightly occurred to observers that if they could artificially restore to the abdominal walls the tone they had lost by being once dis'ended, the patient's sufferings would be appeased. Dr. Tilt also spoke, in words of commendation, of Mme. Caplin's and M. Bourgeaud's elastic abdominal bandages. Dr. Tilt further stated, that when the vagina is irremediably dilated, that not being able to contract it by astringents, it was judicious to fill up the distended portion of the vagina, in order to fix the womb, and relieve the patient's sufferings, and for this he recommended the india-rubber air pessary now generally employed in Paris, in preference to Dr. Simpson's stemmed pessary, to which he objected, as the risk was too great. The fourteen deaths which are known to have occurred in Paris, America, England, and even Scotland, from the imprudent use of the intra-uterine pessary, ought, Dr. Tilt says, to deter practitioners from its use, when we consider that the victims were in the prime of life, and that life was in nowise compromised by the uterine deviations. Some of those cases were most worthily reported by the operators themselves; some, however, were only accidentally brought to light; so it may be fairly supposed that all the fatal cases that have occurred are not known. In the most prudent hands the stemmed pessary has, in some cases, perforated the womb; in others, it has produced flooding to a dangerous extent, or agonizing colics, or metritis, or peri-uterine inflammation, or ovaritis and inflammation of the broad ligaments, or peritonitis, or metro-peritonitis. But the patients were saved! True. Taught the dangers of active treatment, they seek surgical interference as little as possible; but will not the life of many of them be curtailed by the sequela of peritonitis and other pelvic inflammations? Having thus critically commented on the various modes of treating uterine deviations, Dr. Tilt concluded by the following practical remarks:—

1. Treat all ulcerations, and remove all inflammatory affections of the womb, and seek to restore its lost tone to the vagina, by the systematic use of astringents, for by so doing the deviation may be corrected, and the nervous sufferings

abated; but, if the vagina be much dilated, support and steady the womb by an air pessary, for it is also true that, in some cases, the inflammatory swelling of the womb disappears when it is steadied by a pessary.

2. Remove all hard swelling of the womb by cold-water douches, vaginal and rectal, and also by a judicious internal exhibition of mercury and iodine.

3. Attack the neuralgia, as such, by narcotic rectal injections, and by hydropathic measures.

4. Apply pressure to the womb, outwardly, by hypogastric bandages; internally, by well-adapted air-pessaries.

5. With regard to the prevention of uterine displacements, the first thought is, to advise a patient not to exert herself too soon after parturition; the next is, to bear in mind the great frequency of inflammation in the pelvic tissues, and its agency in producing uterine deviations, so as especially to direct our antiphlogistic treatment to the inguinal regions when they are painful, and when swelling or fulness can be detected there, after painful menstruation, miscarriage, or parturition.

ART. 147.—*Prolapsus Uteri treated by the local application of Tannin.*
By Dr. C. A. BUDD.

(*Philadelphia Medical Examiner*, March, 1856.)

The plan which is here carried out, and which was originally recommended by Prof. B. F. Barker, of New York, is as follows :—From a double thickness of lint a triangular portion is cut out, of a sufficient size to fill the capacity of the vagina when rolled up so as to form a cone, and near the apex of this cone is attached a piece of string to facilitate withdrawal. The patient being placed upon her back, with the hips slightly elevated, the uterus is replaced in situ, and the lint, soaked in a saturated solution of tannin, is applied with its apex downward and its base immediately in contact with the os tincæ. This is repeated once in twenty-four hours, for a period of time in accordance with the extent of the displacement. I have usually found a daily application for a period of about a month to be sufficient to perfect a cure. During this time and subsequently, constipation must be rigidly guarded against, and the state of the general health attended to. The vagina soon begins to acquire its wonted tonicity and contractility, and the lint is consequently obliged gradually to be lessened in quantity; the strain being taken off the round ligaments, also allows them to return to their normal condition. The following cases exemplify the admirable effects of this plan of treatment.

CASE 1.—Mrs. G., æt. 24, the mother of two children, the youngest fifteen months of age, had always enjoyed good health until the birth of her last child. The placenta in this last accouchement (I having attended her in both) was retained over three hours, in consequence of irregular uterine contractions. She has been complaining ever since of pain in the lumbo-sacral region, with bearing-down pains in the hypogastrium; great constipation, with vesical and rectal tenesmus; and a sensation of faintness after an evacuation, leucorrhœa, &c. &c. Upon examination, I found the cervix protruding at the vulva, extensive ulceration extending into the canal of the cervix, inflammation of the posterior wall of the uterus, and enlargement of the organ itself, its long diameter measuring 4½ inches. After three months treatment, these conditions, save the prolapsus, were all removed, the applications to the cervix having been made weekly, and without the aid of a speculum, and the uterus at this time measuring less than three inches, in its long axis. The treatment, consisting of the lint and tannin, was soon after commenced; and in about three weeks' time she was enabled to resume her ordinary duties. She is now four months pregnant with her third child, all treatment having been suspended about six months ago.

CASE 2.—Mrs. S., æt. 20, the mother of one child aged two years, applied to me in July, 1854, suffering from all the symptoms of uterine prolapsus. She had aborted with a three months fœtus about a month previous, but had been complaining for two years before. An examination revealed incipient prolapsus, the cervix lying on the floor of the perinæum, and slight epithelial abrasion of its mucous surface. Two applications of nitrate of silver removed this; and the use, for ten days, of the lint and tannin, effected a perfect cure.

CASE 3.—Mrs. G., æt. 54. A widow, the mother of five children, the youngest sixteen years of age. Had ceased menstruating about ten years previous. She stated to me that upon using the slightest exertion, such as lifting or straining at defecation, her womb would entirely protrude from the vulva. She had used a variety of abdominal supporters, and had attempted on several occasions to wear pessaries of different kinds, and at that time was wearing constantly a **T** bandage. Upon examination I found the uterus just within the vulva; and, requesting her to lift a chair, the whole organ was protruded, dragging with it the posterior wall of the bladder; it was perfectly healthy in appearance, though somewhat atrophied. I commenced the treatment with the lint and tannin, interdicting active exercise, and in six weeks ceased making any applications. She gradually resumed her ordinary duties, and is now (some two years since) perfectly recovered, and is considered a very active old lady. She has not had the slightest disposition to a return of the displacement, and enjoys excellent health.

I have here given an example of the three different degrees of prolapsus,—incipient, partial. and complete—illustrating the curability of this treatment in each. I could, if it were desirable, cite many others which have been under my observation, and which have resulted, without a single exception, in a perfect and complete restoration.

ART. 148.—*A new Pessary.* By Dr. G. J. ZIEGLER, of Philadelphia.

(*American Quarterly Journal of Medical Science*, Oct. 1855.)

This instrument is composed of two substances, viz.: a metallic base or frame, and a shield or envelop of organic matter. The first consists of steel wire, though that of common iron, or other suitable metal, will probably answer sufficiently well. This is covered with gutta percha, the quantity of which, however, should be as small as is consistent with efficiency, so as not to unduly increase the bulk or weight of the instrument. In general form it resembles the so-called horseshoe pessary of Dr. Hodge, though materially differing therefrom in some particular features. It is oblong, and so curved longitudinally as to be best adapted to the curve of the vaginal canal, the axes of the inferior and superior straits, and the arc of the pelvic circle. In breadth it gradually diminishes from the base or pubic upwards to the uterine extremity, so as to lessen the lateral distension at the upper part of the vagina. The uterine extremity is slightly rounded. The pubic end is considerably curved inwards, downwards, and upwards on the same plane as the outer limbs, so as to form, when in situ, a bridge or opening for the urethra and neck of the bladder.

The size, curves, and thickness of component materials may be varied according to circumstances.

The whole is so simple in shape, material, and manufacture, as to be readily constructed by any one of ordinary ingenuity.

The theoretic value of the instrument, thus presented, rests upon the simplicity and economy of its component materials, facility of construction, general flexibility, small bulk, light weight, cheapness, peculiar shape, the ease with which it may be introduced and removed, its ready adaptation to the form of the parts it is designed to occupy and the mechanical changes incidental to the functional operations of the pelvic viscera, as well as those induced by the general movements of the body. Its practical value, however, must be determined by experience.

ART. 149.—*A new Utero-raginal Plug.* By Mr. CLEVELAND.

(*Lancet*, Feb. 2, 1856.)

At a recent meeting of the Medical Society of London, Mr. Cleveland exhibited an instrument he had invented to be used as a mechanical plug in certain cases of hemorrhage from the uterus, as well as a means of applying cold in more immediate proximity to that organ. The principle of its construction is as follows:—A common vulcanized india-rubber air-ball, of about three inches in diameter, sold at the shops as a child's toy, is fastened to one end of a thin metallic pipe, six inches long. At the other end of the pipe is a stop cock, with shoulder fitted to receive the nozzle of a large syringe. The air is to be pressed out of the ball, and kept excluded by turning the tap, when it (the ball) may be folded into a small and compact mass, and introduced into the upper part of the vagina. The syringe is now to be applied, the tap turned, and ice-cold water or a freezing mixture injected into the ball until it is distended to a sufficient size, when the tap may be again turned and the syringe removed. The ball, being strong and elastic, will admit of considerable distension. The apparatus may be used with air instead of water. Mr. Cleveland thought some of the advantages of this instrument over the ordinary means employed would consist in its easy and rapid introduction and removal, its greater efficiency as a plug on account of the equable expansion to which it could be subjected, while the application of cold, the non-absorption of blood, the cleanliness and inexpensiveness of it were worthy of consideration. As regards the latter point, Mr. Cleveland stated that the syringe could be used for other purposes, and the cost of a new air-ball was a mere trifle.

ART. 150.—*On Peri-uterine Inflammation.* By M. GALLARD.

(*Gaz. des Hôpitaux,* Nov. 1 and 3, 1855; and *Assoc. Med. Journal,* Jan. 12, 1856.)

In a monograph, entitled "Inflammation of the Cellular Tissue surrounding the Uterus, or Peri-uterine Phlegmon," M. Gallard has collected fifty-three cases of this disease, the observation of which has led him to some interesting results regarding its causes, progress, diagnosis, and treatment.

Peri-uterine inflammation occurs between the ages of fifteen and fifty; most frequently at the middle period between these ages, and generally during menstruation. Abortion and delivery seem equally to predispose to it. Obstetric manipulations, and exposure to cold or fatigue after delivery, do not appear to have any special influence. Nor is previous delivery an essential cause; for the disease has occurred several times in females who have never been pregnant.

The swelling is most frequently posterior to the neck of the uterus; sometimes it is central, sometimes it inclines to one or the other side; sometimes the entire posterior semicircumference of the neck is attacked. Inflammation of the anterior part of the uterus is much more rare; and when it is present, the whole circumference of the neck is liable to participate in the disease. In some cases, the inflammation seizes on only one or the other side, apparently without preference. On examination through the abdominal walls and the vagina, the uterus is ascertained to preserve its normal form and direction. By introducing the index and middle finger of the same hand, one into the vagina, and the other into the rectum, it will be found that the tumor is situated in the recto-vaginal septum, and that it is neither a growth from the posterior part of the body of the uterus, nor retroflexed uterus. When retroflexion of the uterus causes the body to form with the neck an angle identical with that which is formed by a tumor in the vicinity of the neck, a correct diagnosis can be arrived at only by the use of the hysterometer (or graduated uterine sound). The same instrument may also be necessary to establish the diagnosis between peri-uterine phlegmon and fibrous tumors: the latter often projecting into the cavity of the uterus and rendering it irregular, which never occurs in phlegmon. The diagnosis between peri-uterine phlegmon and metritis is perhaps more difficult; but in the latter disease, the uterus remains movable, and the pain is much greater when the uterus or its neck are pressed on than when the neighboring tissues are examined; while the contrary is the case in phlegmon.

The prognosis is not unfavorable, as is shown by the want of opportunity afforded of studying the disease by post-mortem inspection. The usual termination of the malady is by resolution: this is very rapid in first attacks, and especially so if the case has come early under treatment. The disease is very liable to return, and the patients recover less rapidly. After repeated attacks, there is a tendency to induration, and to a chronic form of the disease. Suppuration is very rare. M. Gallard observed it in only three cases out of fifty-three; while resolution occurred in twenty-seven.

The treatment consists principally in bloodletting, mild purgatives, baths, enemata, and emollient injections, during the acute stage and in first attacks. The bloodletting, whether general, or by cupping or leeches to the hypogastrium, or by leeches to the neck of the uterus, ought to be moderate, on account of the anæmic state which often accompanies the disease. M. Gallard advises that the patients should not be kept on a very low diet, and that food should be given as soon as the fever begins to abate. When the pain is very severe and persistent, some laudanum may be added to the injections and enemata. If the phlegmon tends to pass to a chronic condition, M. Gallard advises the use of iodine and iodide of potassium, both internally and in the form of friction. When this is not sufficient, he advises friction with croton oil or tartar emetic, the cautery, small setons, or other counter-irritants. To combat the chloro-anæmic state, tonics and peparations of iron may be useful. The most important preventive measure to be employed by females who are liable to this disease is rest in bed, or at least avoidance of all fatigue, and especially of all excess during the menstrual periods.

Art. 151.—On Puerperal Fever.
By Dr. MURPHY, Professor of Midwifery in University College.

(Lancet Dec. 22, 1855.)

At a recent meeting of the Medical Society of London, Dr. Murphy dwelt at some length upon the importance of defining more accurately the true character of this disease. He objected to the terms "puerperal peritonitis," "uterine phlebitis," "arthritis," &c., as correct expressions of what he would prefer to call a puerperal plague. The name puerperal fever is the most commonly used, and therefore the best understood. He denied that it was puerperal peritonitis, because it did not agree with that inflammation, either in the mode of the attack, in the symptoms, in its morbid appearances, or in the influence of remedial agents. He pointed out the sudden manner of the attack without any obvious cause, the cases where the symptoms of puerperal peritonitis were absent, and yet the patient died of this disease, and presented all the usual morbid appearances in the peritoneum. He compared the morbid changes observed in peritonitis from ruptured uterus with those described in puerperal fever, and pointed out the difference; and, lastly, directed attention to the great difference in the effect of the treatment most commonly pursued for peritonitis, stating that depletion has been used successfully in cases of puerperal fever to such an extent as fifty ounces of blood, in cases the parallel of which in peritonitis will not bear bleeding at all.

Mercury has failed utterly in arresting this disease, and opium is equally useless unless in combination with the most powerful stimulants. He therefore thought it quite incorrect to call puerperal fever "puerperal peritonitis." It seemed to him equally an error to name the disease "acute uterine phlebitis," admitting the greater difficulty of distinguishing each because both were blood diseases. He thought true uterine phlebitis a rare disease; that the most eminent pathologists have agreed that the lining membrane of the veins is scarcely susceptible of inflammation; that the uterine veins consist only of a lining membrane, and do not inflame: if they did so easily, uterine phlebitis would be the result of every severe labor, especially with putrid children. He quoted some cases of true uterine phlebitis and puerperal fever with the veins chiefly engaged, in order to point out the difference. He considered the depositions of pus so frequently found as the evidence of depraved or poisoned blood, and quoted a case of Mr. M'Whinnie's, from the 'Transactions' of the Royal Medical and Chirurgical Society, as an illustration of his argument. Assuming puerperal fever to be the result of a poison, he stated that we did not as yet know what that poison was, but the nearest approach we could make to it was its close resemblance to the poison of putrid animal matter. In illustration he mentioned the effect of the effluvia from Mont Fanen on the Maternité at Paris. He referred to a case of severe labor, in which, having to remove a putrid placenta, his arm afterward exhibited a malignant pustule, which was very like the pustules sometimes found amongst the meat-slaughterers in the south of France from putrid meat. He mentioned a case of putrid uterus, which produced all the symptoms of so-called puerperal peritonitis, although in the Dublin Lying-in Hospital, where the patient was, there had not been a single case of this fever for a year before or for a year and a half afterwards. He referred to Mr. Henry Lee's researches, and to Weal, in support of his opinion, that the uterine veins do not easily inflame, and concluded by making a marked distinction between pus and putrid matter. He denied that healthy pus was a poison; its properties were to preserve the circulation from contamination; decomposed animal matter had the contrary effect, because it destroyed those healthy properties of the blood; it had less power of coagulation, was easily dissolved into pus, and in such cases pus, or what is called pus, is found everywhere, infiltrating the uterus, in the liver, spleen, lungs, and even the heart, and all this without inflammation. He therefore objected to the term "uterine phlebitis," as used to express that form of puerperal fever, but did not wish to be understood to assert that a specific inflammation could not form a part of this epidemic, but it appeared to him that we might as well adopt Broussais' doctrine, and call typhus fever "gastroenteritis," as name puerperal fever by these local inflammations.

(c) CONCERNING THE DISEASES OF CHILDREN.

ART. 152.—*The "Algidité Progressive" of the newly born.*
By M. HERVIEUX.

(*Archiv Gén. de Méd.*, Nov. 1855.)

The conclusions to which M. Hervieux arrives are these:

1. Under certain circumstances newly born infants are seen to pass into a state which may be designated as "Algidité Progressive," a state which may be confounded with scleroma, but which is different from that affection.

2. This state is marked, not only by progressive failure of the animal heat, but by a simultaneous failure of the circulation and respiration.

3. The majority of the infants thus affected are pale, discolored, and often shrivelled like little old men, their movements are feeble, their cry is scarcely audible, and their sensibility almost wanting.

4. The three principal causes are congenital feebleness on the one hand, and on the other hand insufficient food and an improper confinement to the horizontal position.

4. Maternal care, and, in hospitals, a sufficient number of kind nurses, are the only remedies.

This resumé, traced by the author himself, suffices to show that this state is no new malady. On the contrary, it is one which is well known to those who have seen much of the diseases of children. At the same time, the affection has never before been so carefully described, and least of all in the progressive cooling of the system which distinguishes it.

ART. 153.—*Chronic internal Hydrocephalus treated by injection of Iodine.* By Dr. J. M. WINN, Physician to the Metropolitan Dispensary.

(*Lancet*, Nov. 3, 1855.)

The following case, in Dr. Winn's opinion, is calculated to show that iodine may be injected into the brain without causing any poisonous effect, and that the strength of the injection may be so regulated as to produce an amount of stimulation sufficient to restore the balance between the secreting and absorbing functions, without causing destructive inflammation of the cerebral tissue. In a case in which Dr. Winn merely tapped the brain, without employing any injection, the fluid began to reaccumlate in the head on the third day; whereas, in the present instance, where the injection was employed, there was no perceptible increase of fluid on the tenth day after the operation.

CASE.—The patient was a little girl, fifteen months old, who was afflicted with one of the most enormously distended heads from dropsical effusion I ever witnessed. Although the child's mother attributed the disease to a fall that it had sustained five weeks after birth, and which was followed by convulsions, she admits that the infant had a peculiar expression of the eyes, and was subject to startings of the limbs soon after it was born. I have, therefore, no doubt that the disease was congenital. The fall probably accelerated the effusion, as the head began to enlarge rapidly after the accident; its dimensions had gradually increased up to the day when I operated, at which time it measured twenty-four inches and a half in circumference. The bones of the head had acquired considerable thickness, and were united at the lambdoidal suture, and partly so at the inferior portions of the coronal suture. The anterior fontanelle measured about four inches in each direction. The child had an anæmial appearance, the natural consequence of having been confined in one of the closest and dirtiest courts in Spitalfields; in other respects it was tolerably healthy, and its bodily functions were duly and properly performed. Its perceptions and memory were fairly developed.

On the third of October, with the concurrence and assistance of Mr. Childs, I tapped the head, and after evacuating seventy-two ounces of a straw-colored serum, two ounces of a solution of tincture of iodine (fourteen minims to two ounces), previously raised to the temperature of the body, were slowly injected into the brain, where it was allowed to remain. A hydrocele-trocar was used, and the head punctured in the coronal suture, about two inches below the lower angle of the anterior fontanelle. Although compression of the cranium was maintained during the time the fluid was escaping, it was impossible, owing to the strength and resiliency of the cranial bones to prevent a quantity of air from entering the skull. After the operation the head was firmly bandaged, a pad having been previously placed over the superior fontanelle, in consequence of its having become much depressed during the evacuation of the fluid. The child bore the operation well, and did not appear to suffer much pain.

October 4th.—Lies in a tranquil and comatose state; convulsed occasionally during the night; skull tympanitic; bowels and kidneys have not acted; skin warm; took the breast once: has also swallowed half a cupful of arrow-root, flavored with port wine. I ordered calomel, two grains, to be taken immediately.

5th.—Bowels have acted freely; conjunctivæ suffused, and discharging abundance of mucus; pupils sensible to light. It has unfortunately happened that the mother's sister committed suicide in the course of the night: and in consequence of the shock which her nervous system sustained on hearing of her relation's death, I deemed it advisable to order the child to be kept from the breast during the next twelve hours. I prescribed milk and beef-tea.

6th.—The child sucks freely, and looks better; eyes less suffused. The head, although still tympanitic, has become so far reduced in size that I found it necessary to tighten the bandage. Bowels open.

7th.—Not so well; surface cold: legs rigidly extended; refuses the breast, but swallows whatever is placed in its mouth; eyes have become more suffused. To take chlorate of potass, two grains and a half, every four hours.

8th.—Has rallied from the partial collapse of yesterday; skin warm; took the breast once; takes a sufficiency of nourishment; muscular rigidity has subsided; bowels confined; urine scanty. There is not the slightest sign of a return of the dropsical effusion. To take a calomel purge, and to repeat the chlorate of potass mixture.

9th.—Sucked once only; muscular tremors of the right arm: has passed one copious and dark-colored motion. To take mercury with chalk, one grain, every six hours, and sesquicarbonate of ammonia, one grain, every four hours; to omit the chlorate of potash.

10th.—No material change; has taken a considerable quantity of beef-tea and milk; bowels confined. Ordered to take castor oil, and to continue the mercury with chalk every eight hours.

11th.—Has lost ground again; feet spasmodically adducted; bowels freely opened by the oil; takes food less freely. On removing the bandages from the head, it was found that the protuberances of the frontal bone were slightly inflamed and ulcerated to a small extent on the right side. After bathing the head the roller was carefully readjusted.

12th.—Some slight improvement; appeared to recognize her brother for the first time; takes food more freely; eyeballs spasmodically depressed.

13th.—Gradually sank, and died at half-past six a. m.

Being exceedingly anxious to obtain an examination of the head, I called on the parents the following day, and, to my annoyance, found them violently opposed to an inspection of the body. It was not until after half an hour's earnest talking that I succeeded in obtaining their consent, and then only on condition that I was not to use either a saw or hammer.

Autopsy, twenty-seven hours after death.—Owing to the strength and partial ossification of the bones, and to my being restricted to the use of a knife, the sphere of observation was greatly limited. I succeeded, however, in determining the following interesting facts : The head had not enlarged in the slightest degree since the operation. The cavity of the arachnoid contained a large quantity of inodorous gas, and about six ounces of serum. The arachnoid itself was quite healthy. The brain, which was lying collapsed at the base of the skull, was much more vascular than natural, but its consistence was normal. The marks of the convolutions were quite distinct. The lateral ventricles were empty, and enormously dilated; their lining membrane was thickened, but smooth. On one side a small pellucid cyst, the size of a grape, was attached to the inner wall of the lateral ventricle by a small vascular pedicle. The cerebellum, the cerebral nerves, and other structures at the base of the brain, were in a natural condition. No fluid was discovered in the spinal canal. The opening made by the trocar through the right lateral ventricle had evidently become wider since the operation ; the edges of the aperture, nevertheless, presented a smooth and healthy appearance.

ART. 154.—*Case of Chronic Hydrocephalus cured by spontaneous evacuation of the fluid.* By Mr. L. W. SEDGEWICK.

(*Medical Times and Gazette*, March 15, 1856.)

In an early volume of the "Medico-Chirurgical Transactions," Dr. Barron relates a case of chronic hydrocephalus, in which, during the latter stage, a bloody fluid oozed from the mouth and nostrils, and where, after death, there was found to be an aperture between the cranium and nose ; but we do not remember a case like this of Mr. Sedgewick's.

CASE.—The patient, who was two-years old, had always had a large head, a heavy countenance, and a sallow complexion. His father was healthy, his mother scrofulous; they had lost one or more children previously from hydrocephalus. For some months his appetite had been capricious, his bowels irregular, and his abdomen large. He had been gradually getting more listless for a week back; he laid his head down frequently, and complained of pain in it. He slept badly, frequently starting up with a scream. There was little heat of skin, a quick but feeble pulse, thirst, rather sluggish pupils, no appetite, relaxed slimy motions, large and hard abdomen; his whole aspect betokened scrofula. He took salines, and Hydrargyrum cum Creta, and had occasional blisters behind the neck ; the pulse and general symptoms did not warrant depletion. Gradually there became more and more evidence of compression of the brain; the head increased in size, the anterior fontanelle got very wide, the pupil was dilated, there was occasional stertor, considerable insensibility to external impressions, pulse slower, and respiration oppressed. At the end of five weeks coma was imminent, almost present, and I looked for speedy dissolution; but one morning about six weeks after the commencement of the more decided symptoms, I found him much better. There was renewed intelligence in the face, and more vigor in the limbs; the pupil was more sensible to light, and the appetite considerably improved. During the night there had been a very considerable flow of clear fluid from the nostrils, often so rapid as to run in a thin stream, and so copious as to soak the pillow for a considerable distance. The mother was catching the drops on a handkerchief, while I was there; the eyes were suffused with tears. After the first twenty-four hours, the drain of fluid from the nose was not so copious; but it continued, in gradually diminishing quantity, for some days. During this time, the head symptoms had been rapidly subsiding, and in a very short time, he had attained his usual state of health.

A twelvemonth afterwards, the same series of head symptoms presented themselves—the dilated pupil, the disturbed sleep, the stupor, the coma. All things indicated extreme effusion of fluid within the cranium, and all things foretold a fatal termination; even with the recollection of the extraordinary cure of the last attack, I could not hope for recovery. He was treated in the usual way, but for some weeks with no result; when, again, just as death seemed closest at hand, did the same wonderful change in the symptoms appear, coincidently with a positive flood of fluid from the nostrils. All indications of disordered brain speedily subsided, and, under the use of cod-liver oil, the child got fat and quite well.

There is little needed in the way of comment upon this case; there could be no mistaking its character; the symptoms were plain to read, and the nature of the relief furnishes sufficient demonstration of the offending cause. That there was fluid within the cranium, compressing and gradually overcoming the brain, was evident; but it was not quite so easy to determine the exact site of the disease. Whether the fluid was contained in the sac of the arachnoid, in the subarachnoidean space, or in a cyst, it is impossible to say; I am inclined to believe that it was in the arachnoid sac.

ART. 155.—*A Peculiar Form of Insanity in Children.*
By M. DELASIAUVE.

(*Journ. of Psychol. Med.* Jan. 1856.)

M. Delasiauve brought this subject under the notice of the Societe Medico-psychologique, February 26th. This affection M. Delasiauve described as having for its fundamental character a disturbance of the intellectual faculties, manifested more or less by confusion of ideas, but was always complicated with ecstatic phenomena, the paroxysms of which varied in duration, and in some cases returned at short intervals. The patients remained several hours of the day as if wrapt in a sort of mystical contemplation. Often the attention was fixedly directed to one spot, from which not even the most vivid impressions could arouse them. In other cases the attention was alternately directed to different points. The limbs and body were placed in the most grotesque attitudes and positions; sometimes the head was bent in forced directions, sometimes the arms and legs remained elevated and extended. In some of these cases there was seen slow and measured jactitation, after the fashion of Punchinello. Of the eight or nine cases seen by M. Delasiauve almost all were cured within a limited period, in some cases with relapse. Bathing, sulphate of quinine, and attention to hygiene, were followed by successful results.

Although these cases were important, they did not, in the opinion of M. Delasiauve, deserve a special nomenclature, as a new form of mental disease. The phenomena of these cases do not belong to mania, nor specially to early age. They are met with in those forms of partial insanity attended with convulsions, such as catalepsy and epilepsy. The ecstatic state corresponds to a slight degree of cerebral erethism, whereby the intellect, acting through volition, is subordinated to the automatic-organic system. Hence, if this view be correct, ecstasy may take place whenever from moral or physical causes the normal activity of the nervous centres is increased, and favors the production of spasm. The preference of these attacks shown towards early age, may be explained by the greater impressionability of that time of life. In some instances this special predisposition is referable to onanism, or intimidation, which either depress or concentrate the nervous sensibility. Several of the patients were addicted to the solitary vice, nearly all had been the subject of cruelty or unjust rigor, or had been frightened by exaggerated representations of their offences, and by fear of the wrath of God.

M. Moreau had met with instances of this form of affection, and regarded them as cases of epilepsy, attended with a degree of stupor, offering some resemblance to ecstasy.

M. Belhomme inquired if M. Delasiauve considered that an analogy existed between ecstasy and catalepsy?

M. Delasiauve in reply, stated that he recognized in ecstasy a state of muscular immobility without contraction, accompanying a particular cerebral disorder, while in catalepsy there was abolition of feeling with tetanic rigidity. The difference is one rather of degree than of kind. Ecstasy seems to be a slighter degree of this cataleptic state.

M. Alfred Maury, mentioned an epidemic melancholy which had prevailed among the inhabitants of a district in Siberia, some years ago, under the influence of a Buddhist prediction. In this disorder the sufferers uttered a sad monotonous chant, concluding with a paroxysm or excitement, which was followed by insanity or restoration. The moral and physical condition of this people resembled that of childhood.

M. Buchez did not consider that either of the speakers had elucidated the phenomena related by M. Delasiauve. He would ask whether ecstasy occurring in the insane and epileptic is of the same nature as ecstasy occurring in the previously healthy and in those persons who can induce the ecstatic condition by profound meditation? He further asked, whether ecstasy and catalepsy are physiologically the same? whether they might exist separately? whether they have the same organic seal?

M. Baillarger had seen cases of melancholy stupor pass into ecstasy. He objected to the use of the word "physiological" to express conditions referred to in this discussion, and which he considered as strictly pathological. For instance, if ecstasy be a suspension of the intellectual powers, how can it be said to be a physiological state?

M. Alfred Maury compared the state of ecstasy to the passing delirium of fever, which, frequently recurring, may pass into insanity.

M. Buchez considered that there was a great analogy, but not an identity between the ecstasy occurring in health and that occurring in disease. M. Buchez further illustrated his opinions by reference to the state of internal abstraction or contemplation under which musical composers, without the presence of a musical instrument, veritably hear the pieces they compose; and a painter sees in imagination the persons he transfers to his canvas.

M. Ferrus asked if a person in a state of ecstasy was, medico-legally-speaking, responsible for his acts? M. Ferrus promised to lay before the Society the particulars of some cases bearing upon this point.

ART. 156.—*On the Pneumonic Catarrh of Infants.*
By M. TROUSSEAU.

(*Dublin Hospital Gazette*, July 5, 1855.)

Diseases of the lungs present very different characters in infants, according as the children happen to be newly born, at the breast, or growing up. The lung of the newly born infant becomes hard and impervious to air, hepatized, as in the third stage of pneumonia in adults. This state of impermeability of the lung has been described as a *return to the fœtal state.* In a physiological point of view, however, I must declare this to be quite erroneous.

From the first month after birth to the fourteenth, infants are subject to a pulmonary inflammation, called lobular or infantile pneumonia. In this disease the pulmonary catarrh is the chief complaint; the pneumonia is secondary; so in place of calling it catarrhal pneumonia, a name given to it by several practitioners, I prefer the more logical and expressive name of pneumonic catarrh.

Pneumonia is an acute affection, which either resolves quickly or kills rapidly. There is, as it were, a great battle, the issue of which is soon decided on one side or the other. Catarrh (bronchitis), on the contrary, is a series of skirmishes; the attack diminishes one day to be augmented on the morrow, and the child whose lungs are repeatedly attacked, either in the same or different parts, generally succumbs.

Pneumonic catarrh is most frequently caused by a simple cold, a slight febrile attack, or coryza. The mother of the child, although the most affectionate and anxious, sees no cause of uneasiness. Suddenly the fever is lighted up, great oppression comes on, and the child presents soon most alarming symptoms. The face becomes congested in a remarkable manner, the cheeks and lips are livid, the skin is hot and very dry, the dilatation of the alæ of the nose very considerable and almost constant; the epigastrium is retracted towards the vertebral column, the diaphragmatic belt becomes more marked, forming what is called the *peripneumonic fissure*. Orthopnœa increases; the pulse gains an extreme frequency, rising to 120, 140, or 160 in the minute. Percussion is a mode of exploration both difficult and uncertain in the diseases of infancy. If, however, the hand be applied flat upon the thorax of the child while crying, it will feel the vibration of the voice much more distinctly upon the diseased than upon the healthy side. When about to auscultate the chest, care must be taken not to alarm the infant; it should be placed upon its nurse's knees, and then the physician can apply his ear to the posterior and lateral regions. A subcrepitant râle is most frequently heard, sometimes preceded by a mucous or sibilant râle; it is not rare to hear crepitation as fine as in the adult. Bronchial breathing is heard during inspiration, but chiefly during expiration; but it has neither that dryness nor clearness which we observe in the adult; it is heard most frequently not altogether at the base, but at the superior part of the inferior lobe of the lung. The presence of the souffle can perhaps be determined in four or five different parts of the chest. The signs furnished by auscultation are very changeable; thus you may not find to-morrow, in a certain part, the souffle which you heard this evening. This arises from the principal bronchial tube leading to this part of the lung being blocked up with mucus, and thus the air is directed to other parts. In many cases we know but too well that the disease is both of long duration and liable to frequent relapses. A pneumonic catarrh remains fifteen days, a month, six months, or even more. During the course of hooping-cough, you may have acute attacks of it five or six times; never entirely ceasing, the malady becomes chronic, an important differential character from pneumonia of adults.

The anatomical lesions are well marked; besides the inflammation and tumefaction of the bronchial mucous membrane, we see a number of small indurated lobules, between which the tissue of the lung is healthy. The surface of the organ presents a marbled appearance. Independent of these indurated lobules, which invade sometimes a portion of a lobe, sometimes the whole lobe, we remark other lobules, of a violet-red color, indicating a pneumonic inflammation of the first degree, whilst here and there these masses are harder, and form projections, when the lung is collapsed. The microscope discerns globules of pus in these red lobules. In fine, we find lobules of a yellowish color in the third stage of inflammation.

Pneumonic catarrh is followed by a special lesion, viz., pulmonary abscess, little cavities filled with pus, which in a single lung sometimes amount to the number of 100, 200, or even 500. It has been supposed that these pulmonary abscesses are nothing more than the dilated vesicles of exaggerated emphysema; but I think that the anfractuosities which are seen in these cavities arise from a number of vesicles much broken up. It is a difficult point often to determine between pulmonary phthisis when the vesicles are filled with pus, and the third stage of pneumonia.

ART. 157.—*On Congenital Phymosis.* By Mr. J. COOPER FORSTER, Surgeon to the Royal Infirmary for Children.

(*Medical Times and Gazette*, Nov. 17, 1855.)

Every surgeon must have been frequently struck with the anomalous diseases of a purely sympathetic character to which children are liable; diseases arising simply from irritation, yet assuming frequently a very serious aspect; every one, indeed, must have observed how the irritation of a tooth, or undigested matter in the bowels, gives rise to the most apparently cephalic symptoms, and the mere removal of the former is the means of immediately restoring the child to its natural health. In frames so delicate and susceptible we are not surprised to find such results arising from such trifling causes; and of a like nature is the subject of this communication, which has reference to a cause of disease as trifling as the above mentioned, as easily removable, though requiring most frequently surgical interference.

."The subject is that of urinary irritation arising from long pressure, or from congenital phymosis. Cases of this affection are rarely to be seen in hospitals, except among the out-patients, but are of very frequent occurrence. I find no special remarks concerning them in our own literature, and therefore, having during the last few years seen many instances, I have deemed the subject worthy of a few observations.

" It is not my intention to report several cases all having more or less the same symptoms, but to relate the most common features of one as a type of the class.

" A boy is brought for advice, varying in age generally from two to ten years or more (adults even may apply, as they are by no means free from the same symptoms arising from the same cause), and the mother complains that for some time the child has wetted the bed, he has frequent desire to pass his water, and seems to suffer a little pain in the act of micturition ; the urine also, instead of passing freely, frequently distends the prepuce, and trickles away through the constricted opening in a very slow and irregular manner: the little patient also frequently seizes the penis, as if it itched, and elongates the prepuce. These, and other symptoms, resemble calculus in the bladder, though, as a diagnostic difference, I have never known any blood passed by these children, and they do not suffer any inconvenience from riding or jumping ; the urine also is quite natural, and in all respects they are in perfect health. If the surgeon is content with the description given by the mother, alkalies or iron are administered, sometimes with temporary relief, but more frequently with no benefit. If the penis be examined, as should always be done in such cases, the boy is found suffering from a lengthy, puckered, and contracted condition of prepuce, any attempt to withdraw which over the glans, is attended with much pain to the patient, and therefore a view of the glans, in most cases, is quite impossible. The orifice of the urethra is sometimes, with a good deal of trouble, to be brought into view, though more frequently the constriction of the prepuce is so great as totally to prevent even that part being exposed. In those cases where the whole of the prepuce is distended with urine each time the child passes his water, there is also frequently some ulceration on its under surface. As the cause of the disorder appears to arise from nature having been too prolific in the supply of skin at the extremity of the penis, every nurse should be directed carefully to wash away the secretion that may form, which may easily be done by withdrawing the prepuce from the glans ; and if that simple expedient were adopted in early infancy, no inconvenience would, I believe, ever result. Where the symptoms are such as I have described, there is no doubt that the operation of circumcision is the surest means of relief ; indeed, I think if this operation was more frequently performed upon young children, even when suffering from much less severe symptoms than I have described (if the above-named precautions have not been adopted by the nurse), it would do much to prevent the occurrence of many of the diseases and troubles that occur in after-life. Of the advantages of circumcision to adults every surgeon must be fully aware. Who has not seen the annoyances of retained secretion, syphilitic sores under the prepuce, the swelling accompanying gonorrhœa, &c., as the result of congenital phymosis ? And I have no hesitation also in saying, that it is the exception to see a case of cancer of the extremity of the penis, where the patient has not also been the subject of this malformation. No doubt the most natural state of the penis is with a covered glans, but, at the same time, the prepuce becomes a source of evil where the glans cannot be uncovered for the purposes of ablution.

" With a part so plentifully supplied with nerves, it is not to be wondered at that any undue irritation at the extremity of the penis should give rise to symptoms connected with the bladder, and therefore the constant contact of the prepuce with the orifice of the urethra, sufficiently accounts for the frequent desire to micturate complained of by these children. The irritation and itching have their origin in the masses of filthy secretion poured out by the glandulæ

Tysoni, which secretion is seen lying in a ridge behind the corona, becoming inspissated, and having no means of escape, frequently causes a superficial ulceration in the part in which it is lodged, though occasionally there is such perfect union between the prepuce and glans as to leave little space for its collection. These few remarks would scarcely be complete without a description of the mode of performing the operation of circumcision which I have found most useful. After the chloroform has been administered, the prepuce, close to the extremity of the glans, should be seized transversely with a pair of dressing forceps, and all the loose skin removed with a knife; the skin of the penis immediately retracts to a level with the corona, or not quite so far back; the prepuce resting on the glans, not being elastic like the skin, is then to be slit up with a sharp-pointed bistoury (on a director or not, as the surgeon deems fit), and the part on each side turned back. A piece of lint placed around the cut edges, which are now closely in contact, is all that is required; sutures are quite unnecessary, no bleeding occurs, and in the course of a few days the whole unites, and leaves a very elegant organ for after use. During the performance of what I may call the second part of the operation, adhesions may be found more or less uniting the prepuce to the glans, and occasionally entire agglutination of the two parts is seen. The separation is easily accomplished. I need hardly give the caution not to slit up the urethra, which I have known accidentally done."

REPORTS

ON THE

PROGRESS OF THE MEDICAL SCIENCES.

January—June, 1856.

THE intention of the following Reports is to pass in review the principal additions to each department of Medical Science, which have been placed on record during the preceding six months. It is not contemplated that they should be confined exclusively to the notice of what is new; any fact or doctrine which may be considered practically useful, will, although not strictly novel, be regarded as worthy of commemoration. It must be obvious to all who are aware of the immense mass of information which is almost daily put forth by the medical press of this and other countries, that the notice of every subject would be an impossibility. It therefore devolves upon the writers of each Report, to select only such articles for retrospection as may possess superior recommendations, either of an intrinsic character, or in relation to the main end and aim of all medical knowledge,—the alleviation of suffering and disease.

I.

REPORT ON PRACTICAL MEDICINE, ETC.

Cell Therapeutics. By WILLIAM ADDISON, M.D., F.R.S.
(8vo. Churchill, 1856, pp. 84.)

IT is well known that granulations and pus are both forms of nucleated cell-growth, and common in disease and in processes of repair. All cells have a property of selective absorption, and the main point of Dr. Addison's argument is, that the opening of bloodvessels for the junction of new ones without bleeding—ulceration and sloughing—the discharge of poisons from the blood—scarlet fever and small-pox—and sundry changes of texture observable in organic or parenchymatous diseases, are phenomena referable to the absorptive properties of nucleated cells. For instance—

"Of an abscess in a gland of the groin from ulceration in the foot, the argument is, that a poison, entering the circulation by absorbent *vessels*, is arrested and discharged by the *cells* of the gland in the thigh. The phenomena being inflammation, abscess, and purulent discharge. An *indiscriminate* absorption by vessels, may thus be supposed, rectified by the *discriminate* activity—the metabolic processes—of cells."

The following extracts will put our readers in possession of the main object of Dr. Addison's work :

"1. Reparation in the human structure is not limited to wounds and fractures from mechanical violence. It extends to injuries of the blood, and to disease in the parenchymatous organs. It is accomplished by a new or perternatural cell-growth, in the common vascular tissue—and of this growth there are two prominent forms,—the one a vascular form, 'Granulation,' the other a deciduous form, termed 'Pus.'

"2. The cells of granulation and pus exhibit peculiar relations to the surrounding parts,—a property of selective absorption. Those of granulations open bloodvessels for the junction of new ones, and are elements of repair in virtue of a capacity, in the cells or cell-contents, of metamorphosis into fibrous tissue. Those of pus are elements of repair, in virtue of the deciduous mode of cell-growth. The same sort of vital activity which causes leaves to fall in autumn, discharges sloughs from sores, and poisons from the blood without bleeding.

"3. During the formation of granulations and pus, the natural bloodvessels undergo a species of retrograde metamorphosis, for the fibrous coat of the vessels becomes the seat of new cell-growth. A state of growth in which we know in the embryo, bloodvessels bleed upon the lightest touch, and multiply with great rapidity.

"4. The formation of granulations and pus are accompanied by phenomena termed 'Inflammation.' That is to say, inflammation is the sign or signal of a change commencing in the coats of the bloodvessels, and thereby is distinguished from congestion,—in which there is no morphological change in the coats of the vessels."

"In support of these conclusions, the following reflections occur. In mechanical injuries the process of repair has at first a pathological aspect. We say inflammation arises. On the other hand, in gout, small-pox, scarlet fever, and measles, inflammation vindicates its therapeutical purport by the limitations it observes, by the order and regularity of its times and stages, and by the recovery

of the person concomitantly with a discharge of morbid secretion or preternatural cells at the sites of inflammation. Cell therapeutics, after mechanical injury, has then a mixed pathological and physiological aspect. The pathological
part is the first part. The injury has been inflicted and there is need of reparation. This is responded to by new cell-growth in the vascular tissue, the primi-
tive form of growth of that tissue. The new growth requires for its support new
bloodvessels, and new bloodvessels appear. But these new vessels cannot
carry on the circulation without joining to openings in the older vessels. The
openings are made by the absorptive property which all cell-growths possess.
And thus the new growth establishes itself at the expense of the existing vascular tissue. The proper healing or repairing part of the process cannot be said to
have commenced while these operations are in progress—while cell-growth and
new bloodvessels are increasing. It is only when these have accomplished
their part—when cell-growth is beginning to give place to fibrous connective tissue, and new bloodvessels are diminishing in number—that regularity and success entitle the phenomenon to rank as the process of repair.

"In like manner, in blood-distempers the phenomena have a mingled pathological and physiological aspect. In small-pox, the pustules arise with inflammation. These are pathological to the vascular tissue; they alter the form and
properties of the bloodvessels. But the new cell-growth performs a therapeutical act as respects the blood, the cells of the pustules transferring injurious matter from the circulation to the solid texture for discharge.

"Cell-growth in the vascular tissue or inflammation—whichever term we employ—is at all times and from whatever cause arising, a thing of mingled good
and evil, even when accomplishing the process of repair with success. And we
may agree, when the good purpose is evident and in course of fulfilment, to call it
the process of repair, and when the evil predominates, a disease. This would
be a consistent and intelligible distinction. But, to call inflammation when it
observes a regular order, strict limitations, fixed periods, and is followed by cure,
as in small-pox, scarlet fever, measles, and gout—*a disease*, when the distemper is
in the blood—and inflammation and suppuration in burns and compound fractures, often greatly more protracted, more dangerous and exhausting to the patient, *the process of repair*, as though they had nothing in common with each
other, seems 'an inappropriate form of mental apprehension to apply to the facts
which cannot give rise to any exact or substantial knowledge.' Whereas, if the
evidence produced shows that forms of inflammation—described by Mr. Hunter
as adhesive, suppurative, and ulcerative—and the process of repair, are both re-
solvable into forms of new cell-growth in the common vascular tissue; that
granulation, suppuration, and ulceration in burns, compound fractures, necrosis
of bone, tubercular consumption, &c., separate the dead from the living parts,
sever bonds of union, interrupt the continuity of bloodvessels and create new
ones without bleeding;—that vesicles, pustules, or abscess, are appointed means
for the discharge of poisons from the blood, then the subject assumes altogether
a physiological aspect, and therapeutical operations are based upon the properties of cells."

"New cell-growth in the vascular tissue is, we contend, the natural provision
which severs and opens bloodvessels without hemorrhage. Granulation, the
natural provision for the repair of solutions of continuity; and pus, for the throwing off of sloughs and poisons. If granulations are wanted, and they appear,
they belong to the category of therapeutics. If they be in excess, so much of
them as is in excess belongs to pathology, the rest are physiological. If pus be
required to loosen and discharge a slough, and pus appears and performs the
task, it belongs to the category of therapeutics; but if pus, having performed its
office, continues to form and be discharged when it is not wanted, we treat it as
we would any other pathological growth—not by encouragement, but repression.
And thus it is that inflammation has two bearings."[*]

" 'Granulations' and 'Pus' have the most general type of organized structure
—they are forms of nucleated cell-growth; we find them possessing the essential elements of glandular organs. In their *elementary composition*, and in the *acts*
to which they are subservient, there is sufficient to excite an earnest attention.

* See the subject more fully treated in " Healthy and Diseased Structure," p. 68, &c.

The sore occasioned by a common blister is an *excreting* surface; there is a copious discharge of cells from it, yet the influence of the blistering fly may be traced, extending by *absorption*, to the urinary organs. In other cases the influence of medicines and poisons may be communicated to distant organs, if the medicine be brought into contact with the granulations of a wound, although from these granulations there may at the time be a copious discharge of pus. An abscess is both an excreting and an absorbing surface. It may be regarded as a kind of new organ developed in the body. In the formation of an abscess there is purulent accumulation or cell-growth, which forms the principal part of the swelling; and there is also at the same time absorption of the vascular tissue. Sores give rise to different kinds of pus, and we can make no doubt that the different parts of which the blood is composed, will come away more in one kind of pus than in another. The poison of small-pox comes away in the matter of the pustules. Each pustule acts as a temporary new organ for the excretion of the abnormal material from the blood. And when the pustules have performed their task, they fade away and disappear, as do many forms of temporary cell-growth during the development of the germ. There is no natural organ for the elimination of small-pox poison from the blood, therefore the common vascular tissue of the outer integument takes on the excretory function, and cells of the most general type eliminate the poison.

" A common issue is established as a drain to the blood. But there can be no drain except in conjunction with cell-growth. A sore having been made, and granulations established, the peas are inserted to prevent them healing. These foreign bodies, in contact with the granulations, fulfil the conditions we have supposed in tubercular consumption, in necrosis of bone, carbuncles, diseased joints, &c.; they are hindrances to the process of repair; they alter the destination of the young and growing cells, so that instead of becoming fixed in the granulations and proceeding to a fibrous transformation, they are checked, become deciduous, and fall away as cells, at the same time carrying out from the system the materials they have taken for their own growth from the blood. Such an operation as this upon any great scale must impoverish the blood. But in a smaller degree, and under particular circumstances—those, for example, in which an issue is required—the circulating fluid, by such an action, may be relieved of excrementitious matter, as it is by the several natural actions of the same kind. The granulations of the issue becoming a preternatural excretory organ."

For the distinction Dr. Addison points out between the common vascular tissue —bloodvessels and connective tissue—and the parenchymatous elements of the different organs, and upon which he grounds his argument for the therapeutical action of granulations and pus in organic diseases, we must refer to the work itself, which we do, with a hearty recommendation to the perusal and attention of our readers.

Observations on the Life, Disease, and Death of John Hunter, in elucidation of the nature and treatment of Gout and Angina Pectoris, being the Oration delivered before the Hunterian Society, at its thirty-sixth anniversary. By JOSEPH RIDGE, M.D., F.R.C.P. (Pamphlet, Churchill, 1855, pp. 47.)

Dr. Ridge makes the life, disease, and death of this great man the text for certain valuable comments upon gout and angina pectoris, which we are glad to recommend to the attention of our readers.

" Enough, I trust," says Dr. Ridge, at the end of his oration, " has been done in the development of clear and definite principles, to enable the youngest of my hearers subsequently to perceive, in large portions of his notes I have not read, the great importance of maintaining, for depurative and other objects, the fluid supplies (always without excess), even by the simple recourse to a tumbler of hot water at night; the quiet occupations and contemplative habits, the softer sentiments and more benign emotions that may be indulged in, whilst regular exercise on level ground to an extent that can be taken is demanded, to prevent accumulations of fat also, and further degenerations; to see the necessity of regarding angina, not as a mere assemblage of symptoms, but neglecting the name, as a manifestation of diagnostic signs, which, with attentive physical examinations, should lead us to an accurate knowledge of the state of the circulation at each part of the heart, and of the system at large; to understand its relations to gout through the effects of excessive and of surcharged blood, and of the deteriorated fluids and solids of the progenitor, and the reciprocal promotion of external and of internal podagrous affections, by its varying congestions, where the disposition or material exists; to notice the futility and mischief of an administration of antispasmodics and purgatives without a discrimination, as precise as can be obtained, of the condition of organs and of bloodvessels, of structures capable of spasm, and of nerve-cells, conducting tubes, contents, investing sheath, and membranes, at different portions of an entirely connected nervous apparatus, though diffusible stimulants, warm aperients, and carminatives may be urgently demanded;—of an exhibition of narcotics, which need additional caution in their use, from a tendency to diminish further cardiac and other movements in the degree to which sensation is controlled, and equally under the advantages of a local treatment of neuralgia at distant parts by sedatives which may get into the blood in dangerous amount; to recognize the care we should exert to prevent inflammation and its products, and promote absorption, without lessening power to degrees that lead to irremediable dilatations and a premature decease; and lastly (that I may appropriately include a rule formerly deduced from a prolonged clinical observation of more common forms of heart disease), to comprehend the mode in which we should limit to a removal of its causes all attempts to check that hypertrophy, which, when not opposed by obstructed coronaries, and other local and various constitutional conditions, is established, under permanent impediments, by a physiological law announced by Hunter, that provides for the requirements and the purposes of the capillaries and of the veins, and obviates, in great measure, the predominant evils of arterial and of cardiac delay."

Lettsomian Lectures on Insanity. By FORBES WINSLOW, M.D., D C.L., Editor of the "Psychological Journal." (8vo. Churchill, 1855.)

We have to apologize to our readers for not before bringing under their notice this volume. It has excited in the medical and literary world a considerable amount of attention, and the critics speak in the most unqualified terms of its contents. Dr. Winslow, when Lettsomian Professor of Medicine at the Medical Society of London, delivered three lectures before that learned body, viz., 1st, on the "Psychological Vocation of the Physician;" 2d, on the "Medical Treatment of Insanity;" and, 3d, on "Medico-Legal Evidence in cases of Insanity." These lectures constitute the volume before us. The first lecture is an elaborate exposition of the psychological or spiritual duties of the physician. Dr. Winslow enters fully into the consideration of this important matter, and points out, we think successfully, that the physician has higher, more noble and exalted duties than those commonly assigned to him. Dr. Winslow discusses at length the functions of the physician as a philosopher, a metaphysician, a poet, and as a cultivator of polite literature. He demonstrates the importance of all these branches of knowledge to the physician, not merely as ornaments, but as valuable practical agents in the practice of his profession. We do not think Dr. Winslow has at all over-estimated the importance of a more general acquaintance with polite literature, as a branch of medical study. The truly accomplished physician *cæteris paribus* is most likely, not only to elevate medicine as a *science*, but to practise his art successfully; and this Dr. Winslow fully demonstrates. When speaking of the cultivation of poetry, Dr. Winslow remarks—

"In forming an estimate of the value of any branch of philosophical inquiry, we must be cautious how we apply the interrogatory, *cui bono?*—neither must we adopt as our model of imitation the mathematician who, refusing to admit that any advantage could result from the study of a science not directly related to his own favorite study, exclaimed, when recommended to read Milton's 'Paradise Lost,' 'What does it prove?' Are the lofty emotions, the glorious imagery, the sublime speculations, the melodies that have charmed our ear, elevated our thoughts, improved our hearts, ennobled our nature, purified our manners, and thrown rays of sunshine over the dreary and thorny path of life, to be dismissed from our contemplation because they have no obvious and direct relationship to the practical business of life? Let us not encourage the vulgar prejudice against those exalted inquiries that have no apparent or intimate association with the science of medicine, which constitute the charm and poetry of life, and exercise a powerful influence upon the intellectual progress of nations, the civilization of the world, and the character, happiness, and destiny of man!

> —— 'Desolator! who shall say
> Of what thy rashness may have reft mankind?
> Take the sweet poetry of life away,
> And what remains behind?'"

Dr. Winslow dwells at length on the importance of a more general knowledge of the science of mind, and, after pointing out to the student the advantages that are likely to arise from the study of mental philosophy, he truly remarks—

"This science, apart altogether from its direct utility, has other great and obvious advantages, which, in the absence of more conclusive recommendations in its favor, ought to demonstrate to us the importance and value of a knowledge of our own mental constitution. The discipline—the training—the expansion—which the mind undergoes in the study of its own operations, are of themselves benefits not lightly to be appreciated. The cultivation of habits of accurate observation and reflection, of patient attention, of rigid induction, of logical ratiocination, qualifies the mind for the more ready pursuit of those branches of knowledge that are considered to be more closely connected with the practical and active business of life. The mental *gymnasium* to which I refer is admirably fitted for the development, regulation, and cultivation of those faculties of the mind upon the right exercise of which depends our intellectual advancement and happiness."

Dr. Winslow next proceeds to consider the physician as a logician. We have only room for one extract in reference to this topic:

"But, as medical philosophers, we must not be satisfied with this natural aptitude or intuitive perception of the principles of logic. The science of medicine is especially amenable to the rules of logical and inductive reasoning. Having to unravel the mysterious phenomena of life, the investigation and treatment of those deviations from its normal state, termed disease, peculiarly expose us to many sources of error and fallacy, unless we cautiously keep in view the great truths inculcated by the Baconian philosophy, and are guided by the unerring principles taught by its illustrious founder—

> 'The great deliverer, he who from the gloom
> Of cloistered monks, and jargon-teaching schools,
> Led forth the true philosophy.'

"There are but few gifted men in our profession, or in any other walk of modern science, of whom we could, in justice, say that they were able to dispense with the patient study of facts, or with the recognized *formulæ* of logical and inductive science. It was remarked of the immortal Newton, that he appeared to arrive *per saltum* at a knowledge of principles and conclusions that ordinary mathematicians only reached by a succession of steps, and after the result of much labor, long-continued, and profound meditation. It is only by strictly applying the principles of the inductive process of reasoning—by which we conclude that what is true of certain individuals of a class, is true of the whole class; or that which is true at certain times, will be true under similar circumstances at all times—that medicine will take rank with the exact sciences, and its cultivators have a right to claim a foremost position among the distinguished philosophers of the day. In the study of medicine, perhaps more than in any other science, we are peculiarly exposed to the danger of adopting false facts, of being seduced by specious and hasty generalizations, and led into error by deducing general principles from the consideration of a few particulars—the bane of all right and sound reasoning—the foundation of all bad philosophy. It is on this account that logic should form a part of the curriculum of our medical schools."

When referring to the importance of the physician engaged in the treatment of insanity having a knowledge of the constitution of the mind, Dr. Winslow justly observes:

" 'Great powers of reason are requisite,' says Vogel, 'to understand men destitute of reason.' To treat the various phases of disordered mind with any hope of a successful issue, requires on the part of the psychological physician qualities of mind rarely seen in combination—tact, presence of mind, judgment, a ready appreciation of intricate morbid mental phenomena, a delicacy of taste, a high *morale*, a steadiness of purpose, elevation of character, great command of temper, and volitional power and resolute determination not to allow any amount of provocation to interfere with that calmness and serenity so indispensably necessary on the part of those brought into immediate association with the insane. If the mind be the instrument on which we are to operate in carrying out any systematic plan of moral treatment—if it be the duty of the physician to perseveringly 'combat with delusions and hallucinations, and to substitute for them correct and healthy impressions; to strengthen these impressions by judicious and repeated repetitions; remove perverted trains of reasoning—replace them by correct induction, and give them the power and influence of habit and frequent association;' how, I ask, can he make any progress in this mode of treatment, so long as he is ignorant of the *material* with which he is to work—in fact, with the faculties of the human understanding? If the man who has the advantage of an ordinary medical education is, on account of his ignorance of the philosophy of mind, obviously unfitted for the serious duties of treating its disorders scientifically and successfully, what language can convey our impression of the folly, the barbarity, and heartlessness of intrusting the management of the insane to those who are not members of the profession at all, and who have enjoyed no more psychological or general education than that derived from their having acted as attendants in asylums, or that which they have received at a village school? Need we feel surprise at the little advancement made in the science of cerebral pathology, and the amount of public odium which has, alas! for so many years attached to those specially engaged in this anxious and important branch of practice, when we consider into whose hands this class has unhappily fallen? I trust, however, the day is not very remote when the psychological physician, engaged in the treatment of insanity, will take his proper and legitimate position in the ranks of honorable and scientific men; and the opprobrious epithet with which the vulgar and illiterate assail him will be expunged from the vocabulary. When that epoch arrives, the public and the profession will esteem, respect, and venerate those who, at great and heroic personal sacrifices (often of health, life, and reason), devote their acquirements, energies, and talents, for the benefit of this section of the afflicted family of man. 'I am at length rewarded,' says Müller,* 'since, after twenty-six years' intercourse with the insane, I have not become insane myself.' In a letter to Pinel it is observed, 'The laborer in lead-works is thankful if he escapes lameness, and the medical attendant of a mad-house if he does not there leave his reason. A more deliberate sacrifice to the mightiest good of mankind is not conceivable.' "†

The medico-theological duties of the physician are thus described:

" It is occasionally our painful duty to sit by the couch of the dying, and to witness the last fatal conflict between mind and matter. It is on such occasions that we have, either in co-operation with the recognized minister, or in his temporary absence, an opportunity of whispering words of comfort and consolation to the wounded spirit, and of directing the attention of the patient, and those immediately about him, to the only true and legitimate source of the Christian's hope. Let us not lightly esteem or neglect the solemn functions thus imposed upon us. It may be our privilege to co-operate with those whose sacred duty it is to inculcate the precepts of our holy religion, and to suggest, without subjecting ourselves to the imputation of officiousness, the *degree* and *kind* of conversation admissible under certain physical or mental states. A zealous but indiscreet clergyman may, by the character of his admonitions, fatally interfere with the successful progress of an acute case of disease, and inadvertently produce an amount of mental and physical depression, from which the patient may never rally. In the exercise of this serious, this important, and imperative duty, the

* Physician to the Julius Hospital, Wurzburg.
† " Aspects of Medical Life," by Dr. Mackness.

object should be to soothe, not to distract, the mind; to elevate, not to depress, the emotions; to inspire a holy reverence and simple reliance upon that Divine Being who is the Fountain of all Justice and the Reservoir of all Mercy. Our Saviour should be represented, not as the God of terror, but as a God of love and mercy."

Again, at the bed of death, at the last painful struggle, the physician may fully demonstrate his power and great usefulness:

"It is often the painful duty of the physician to intimate to his patient that the last gleam of hope has faded from his mind, and that he must prepare for the painful change which awaits us all. I would impress upon your minds, recognizing the powerful influence of depressing mental emotions upon the shattered physical condition, the great importance of not prematurely snatching from under the patient the only prop—frail and fragile as it may be—upon which his and our hopes of recovery rest. To inform a man that he must prepare for death; that his hours are numbered; to bring about his bed the wailing of deep distress; when reasonable expectations exist of his ultimate recovery, would, in certain temperaments, induce the prophetic result."

Dr. Winslow discusses many other points in connection with the psychological functions of the physician; but we have quoted sufficiently from this lecture to give our readers a notion of the author's views on this interesting branch of inquiry. We strongly recommend our readers to peruse this lecture. It occupies forty-five pages, and is replete with deeply important and suggestive matter.

The second lecture is on the "Medical Treatment of Insanity." Dr. Winslow maintains, in the introductory part of the lecture, that too little attention has been paid, in the present day, to the study of the science of therapeutics. He says, and we think with great truth,—"Extraordinary talents, enlarged capacities, high attainments, profound knowledge, great power of continuous and laborious scientific investigation, indomitable and unflagging industry, united to habits of close and accurate reasoning, are devotedly and zealously engaged in the study of the different branches of our noble science. I ask, whether the great, the original, the truth-loving minds among us have investigated, in a manner proportionate to its vast importance, that section of our art which specially and exclusively relates to the *modus operandi* of medicines, and their therapeutic influence in the *actual cure of disease?* I feel reluctant to breathe a word, or to utter a syllable, which could in the slightest degree be supposed to convey the impression that I undervalued and underestimated those essential and interesting departments of the science of medicine, to the investigation of which so many highly gifted men are devoting their talents and knowledge. The microscope has done much to enlarge the boundaries of science; it is an invaluable instrument in the hands of the scientific, experienced, and cautious philosopher, and the insight which it has afforded, and the light which it has reflected upon the minute anatomy of tissue, and into the nature of organic and pathological products and elements, have undoubtedly advanced considerably the science which we cultivate. The results so obtained have led to, and will ultimately be productive of, most important practical advantages. I say so much in this stage of my inquiry, to guard myself against the imputation of thinking lightly of these minute inquiries into the intimate nature of organic structure. I would not say a word to discourage the commendable zeal, industry, and patience of the microscopist, who toils

'From night to morn, from morn to dewy eve,'

in ivestigating the phenomena of matter, and who applies well-ascertained data to assist him in the elucidation of that mysterious and subtle principle which gives motion, animation, and intelligence to the grosser particles of our material organization. Admitting the great utility of the microscope, I would, placing my interrogatory in a suggestive form, ask, whether we have not, in these profound, intellectual, and necessary investigations, occasionally overlooked the great ostensible vocation of the physician? The erudite anatomist—the learned physiologist—the accurate stethoscopist—the profound analytical chemist—the zealous microscopist, capable of accurately delineating the minute anatomy of tissue, or the physical character, weight, and quality of each essential organic

element constituting its structure—will not, without the patient study of the phenomena of disease, and careful investigation of the *modus operandi* of the agents
of the materia medica in certain morbid conditions of the system, make either a
good or a successful physician. Have we not neglected the science of therapeutics? Have we endeavored to discover the most speedy mode of arresting
the disorganizing process, assuaging suffering, prolonging the duration of life,
and averting death, by the persevering administration of *physical* curative
agents?"

Dr. Winslow combats successfully with the *spiritual* theory of insanity, affirm-
ing that the mental disorder in any case is but the symptom of physical disturbance. He says—

"Among the causes which have unfortunately given force and longevity to the
idea that the administration of physical agents is of little or no avail in the
treatment of the disorders of the mind, one holding the most prominent rank is
the unphilosophical hypotheses which have been broached with the view of explaining the phenomena of insanity. To this source much of the fallacy, false
induction, bad logic, and the neglect in reference to the use of remedial measures
may be traced. Insanity has been considered to be a spiritual malady—a functional disease ; to be an affection of the immaterial essence ; to be a disorder of
the soul, and not simply the result of a derangement of the material instrument of
mind interfering with the healthy action of its manifestations. The brain has
been supposed to be intact; not a fibre disturbed, not a vesicle altered, not a
vessel overloaded ; the encephalon has been imagined, in the severest forms of
disturbed mind, to exist in all its integrity, so ridiculously absurd, so wildly unphilosophical, have been the notions entertained in reference to the proximate
cause of insanity. This spiritual doctrine has naturally led to the conclusion—
false in theory and destructive in practice—that for the alleviation and cure of
the spiritual malady, spiritual remedies were the most important and essential.
The clergyman instead of the physician was therefore summoned to the bedside
of the insane, and the Bible and Prayer Book displaced the physical remedies
prescribed for the cure of the cerebral disorder."

Again he says—

"The common phrase, 'functional disease,' is but another designation for the
spiritual hypothesis—it is but a phantom of the mind—a pathological enigma,
having no actual existence apart from the active imagination which gave it birth.
When we assert that the 'functional' or 'spiritual' theory will not bear the test
of serious examination—that it is at variance with all *à priori* and *à posteriori* reasoning—that it stands in direct opposition to positive, well-recognized, undeniable data, we are met by the interrogatory, Can you demonstrate to us the specific
character of the change induced in the nervous matter which it is alleged gives
rise to mental derangement? and do not the scalpel and microscope of the morbid anatomist in vain endeavor to ascertain, in many cases of positive, violent,
and unequivocal insanity, any appreciable structural lesion in the nervous matter,
in its investing membranes, or organs in close association with the brain, sufficient to account satisfactorily for the morbid phenomena exhibited during life?
One would really infer, from the reasoning and assertions of those who take these
spiritual views, and who repudiate the idea of insanity ever being the result of a
physical change in the condition of some portion of the brain or its appendages,
that the encephalon has no specific functions allotted to it ; that it is altogether a
useless and supernumerary organ ; that it was created for no wise purposes; and
that as far as the phenomena of mind were concerned, we could have done as
well without as with the brain ! If this organ be not the material instrument of
mind—if it be not the media through which the spiritual portion of our nature
manifests its powers—the centre of sensation—the source of volition—the seat of
the passions—

'The dome of thought—the palace of the soul'—

I ask, what *are* its functions, its specific uses and operations?—for what object
was this most exquisitely organized and complicated structure formed?—why
does it receive so large a proportion of the blood, and why is it so carefully protected from injury? These interrogatories naturally arise in the mind, when we

hear so unphilosophical and so unphysiological a theory propounded with reference to the possibility of the mind being *subject to disease apart from all derangement of the material organs with which it is so closely and indissolubly associated.* Can we conceive a more preposterous notion than that sanctioned by high authority, and which inculcates that the spiritual principle admits of being distorted, deluded, depressed, exaggerated, perverted, exalted, independently of any form of bodily disease, or modification of nervous matter?"

In discussing Dr. H. Munro's theory of insanity, Dr. Winslow observes—

"The most recent pathological doctrine propounded to explain the phenomena of insanity—I refer to the views of a recent writer*—that derangement of mind is the effect of '*loss of nervous tone,*' and that this loss of nervous tone is '*caused by a premature and abnormal exhaustibility of the vital powers of the sensorium*'—conveys to my mind, no clear, definite or precise pathological idea. It is true that we often have, in these affections of the brain and disorders of the mind, 'loss of nervous tone,' and 'exhaustion of vital power;' but, to my conception, these are but the *effects* of *a prior morbid condition of the encephalon* the *sequelæ* of specific inflammation of the hemispherical ganglia. To argue that insanity is invariably and exclusively the result of ' loss of nervous tone,' is to confound cause and effect, the *post hoc* with the *propter hoc;* and would, as regards therapeutical measures, act as an *ignis fatuus,* and allure us as pathologists from the right and legitimate path."

The subjoined observations on the classification of mental diseases cannot be too strongly impressed on the minds of those engaged in the study of this subject:

"The most simple classification of insanity, the one I think best adapted for useful and practical purposes, is its division into the *acute* and *chronic* forms; the insanity ushered in by *excitement* or by *depression,* into *mania* and *melancholia—amentia* and *dementia.* The minute divisions and subdivisions, the complicated and confused classification taught by lecturers and found detailed in books, may serve the ostentatious purpose of those desirous of making a pompous display of scholastic and scientific lore, but I think they have tended to bewilder and obscure the understanding, and lead the student in search of practical truth from the investigation of the *disease itself* to the study of its *symptoms* and to the consideration of unessential points and shades of difference. Adhering to this division of the subject, each form should be viewed in relation to its *complications,* as well as to its *associated diseases.* Among the former are epilepsy, suicide, homicide, paraplegia, hemiplegia, and general paralysis. The associated diseases implicate the lungs, heart, liver, stomach, bowels, kidney, bladder, uterus, and skin."

On the subject of diagnosis, Dr. Winslow remarks—

"I would premise that those inexperienced in the investigation of this class of cases would often arrive at false and inaccurate conclusions, if they were not cognizant of the fact, that the insane often describe sensations which they have never in reality experienced, and call attention to important symptoms which have no existence except in their own morbid imaginations. A patient will assert that he has a racking headache, or great pain and tenderness in the epigastric region, both symptoms being the fanciful creations of a diseased mind. This is particularly the case in the hysterical forms of insanity, in which there always exists a disposition to pervert the truth, and exaggerate the symptoms. Again, serious bodily disease may be present, the patient not being sufficiently conscious to comprehend the nature of the questions asked, or able to give intelligible replies to the anxious interrogatories of the physician. Insanity often masks, effectually obscures, other organic affections, the greater malady overpowering the lesser disease. When Lear, Kent, and the Fool are standing alone upon the wild heath, exposed to the merciless pelting of the pitiless tempest, Kent feelingly implores the king to seek shelter from the 'tyranny of the open night,' in an adjoining hovel. It is then that Lear gives expression to the psychological truth just enunciated—

'Thou think'st 'tis much, that this contentious storm
Invades us to the skin: so 'tis to thee;
But *where the greater malady is fixed,*
The lesser is scarce felt;
* * * * The tempest *in my mind*
Doth from my senses take *all feeling else*
Save what beats there.'

* Dr. H. Munro.

Disease of the brain may destroy all apparent consciousness of pain, and keep in abeyance the outward and appreciable manifestations of other important indications of organic mischief. Extensive disease of the stomach, lungs, kidneys, bowels, uterus, and heart, has been known, during an attack of insanity, to progress to a fearful extent, without any obvious or recognizable indication of its existence. Insanity appears also occasionally to modify the physiognomy and symptomatology of ordinary diseases, and to give them peculiar and special characteristic features."

On the much-vexed question of depletion in the treatment of insanity, Dr. Winslow remarks—

"In regard to the treatment of acute mania, the important and much-litigated question among practitioners of all countries, is that relating to the propriety of depletion. Need I refer to the conflicting and contradictory opinions entertained by eminent writers on this important and much-vexed therapeutical point? Whilst some practitioners of great repute and enlarged experience fearlessly recommend copious general depletion for the treatment of insanity, and cite cases in which this practice has been attended with the happiest results, others, equally eminent, whose opinions are as much entitled to our respect, fearlessly denounce the lancet as a most fatally dangerous weapon, and shudder at the suggestion of abstracting, even locally, the smallest quantity of blood! In avoiding Scylla, we must be cautious of being impelled into Charybdis. The error consists in a vain effort to discover a *uniform mode of treatment, and attempting to propound some specific mode of procedure adapted to all cases.* He who maintains that bloodletting is never to be adopted in the treatment of mania, without reference to its character, its origin, the peculiar constitution of the patient, and the existence of local physical morbid conditions, which may be materially modifying the disease, and giving active development to morbid impressions, is not a safe practitioner. Neither would I confide in the judgment and practice of the physician who would, in every case of violent maniacal excitement, attempt to tranquillize the patient and subdue excitement by either general or local depletion."

Dr. Winslow then proceeds to point out the kind of case in which the local abstraction of blood from the head is likely to be of service—

"In attacks of insanity, when the symptoms are acute, the patients young and plethoric, the habitual secretions suppressed, the head hot and painful, the eyes intolerant of light, the conjunctivæ injected, and pupils contracted, the pulse rapid and hard, and the paroxysm sudden in its development, *one* general bleeding will often arrest the progress of the cerebral mischief, greatly facilitate the operation of other remedies, and ultimately promote recovery. In proportion as the symptoms of ordinary insanity approach those of phrenitis, or meningitis, shall we be justified in the use of general depletion. Although it is only occasionally, in instances presenting peculiar characteristic features—cases occurring in the higher ranks of life, where the patient has been in the habit of living *above par,* and is of a sanguineous temperament—that we are justified in having recourse to the lancet, there is a large class of recent cases presenting themselves in the asylums for the insane, both public and private, in the treatment of which we should be guilty of culpable and cruel negligence, if we were to omit to relieve the cerebral symptoms by means of the *local* abstraction of blood. It is, alas! the fashion and caprice of the day to recklessly decry the application of cupping-glasses or of leeches in the treatment of insanity, in consequence, I think, of the slavish deference shown to the opinions of a few eminent French pathologists, who have, by their indiscriminate denunciation of *all depletion,* frightened us into submission, and compelled us to do violence to our own judgment. The local abstraction of blood is, in the hands of the discreet and judicious practitioner, *a powerful curative agent;* and yet it is the practice of some men, and men, too, of position, to discard altogether the remedy!"

The third lecture, on "Medico-Legal Evidence in Cases of Insanity," is perhaps the most elaborate dissertation on this subject in the English language. Dr. Winslow has, for so many years, occupied so prominent a position as a medical jurist in cases of disputed insanity, criminal and civil, that all he says on this difficult but deeply interesting branch of philosophical investigation, is entitled to our profound respect and attention. Dr. Winslow does not speak as a mere theorist. Having been professionally engaged in our English courts of law for the last ten or fourteen years, in nearly all the great law cases involving the question of criminal responsibility and mental competency to bequeath property, Dr. Winslow is in a position to convey to the profession most useful and valuable instruction on these points. His lecture on the subject occupies nearly 100 pages of closely printed matter. It is a volume in itself, and deserves to be carefully studied by all who are likely to be called upon to give an opinion on questions of this nature. How graphically does Dr. Winslow sketch the position of the medical witness in cases of insanity:

"Occasionally we have to give testimony in relation to matters of *fact;* to describe *physical* states—phenomena cognizant to sense. For example: in cases of sudden death from supposed poisoning, the toxicologist has certain well-defined scientific data to guide him to a right conclusion; he is in possession of well-recognized tests, which bring him almost unerringly to a sound and safe deduction; his evidence has reference more to an *exact*, than to a speculative—to a certain, than an uncertain science; his province (when in court) is simply to record the results at which, after careful investigation, he has arrived. The questions involved in the inquiry, whether death, under suspicious circumstances, was natural, self-inflicted, or the effect of extraneous violence, are not *necessarily* intricate, obscure, or difficult of satisfactory solution. How different, however, is the position of the witness, when his mind is brought to the consideration of questions connected with morbid mental phenomena? In these exalted inquiries he has no fixed or certain test—no infallible standard—no well defined rules—no principles of exact science, to aid him; no beacon to protect him from the rocks and quicksands which beset his course—no chart to refer to in times of difficulty—no compass to guide him in the hour of danger—no harbor of refuge into which he can run his fragile vessel when the tempest is howling and destruction impending. As medico-legal witnesses, the obstacles with which we have to contend are often of a grave and serious character. We have to deal with phenomena, of the essence or intimate nature of which we know absolutely—positively, nothing. It is our duty to elucidate principles of belief—to unravel motives of action—to explain erratic conduct the most anomalous and extraordinary; we have to trace the line which separates passion—the subtle and shifting transformations of wild, ungovernable, and impetuous passion—from the excitement of mania, and the morbid emotions incident to the minor forms of diseased mind: to sketch the varying frontier, the nice and shadowy distinctions, which separate lunacy from malignity—madness from brutality; to point out where folly merges into mental derangement—where *responsibility* terminates, and *irresponsibility* commences; to distinguish between *eccentricity* and *insanity*—*crime* and alienation of mind—*vice* and *mental derangement*—between the delusions of the lunatic and the false conclusions—the illogical deductions—the unphilosophical reasoning of men of sound intellect and of rational understanding,—to separate the normal rhapsodies of the healthy imagination, and the Arcadian illusions of the poet, from those *morbid* conceptions of the fancy—those

> ——'Daggers of the mind—false creations
> Proceeding from the heat-oppressed brain,'

those 'thick-coming fancies,' the products—the well-recognized, indisputable symptoms of a mind thrown off its healthy balance by *actual cerebral disease.*

"There is no possibility of our placing the diseased mental elements submitted to our critical examination in a psychological crucible or test-tube; we cannot avail ourselves, in these delicate investigations, of the aid of the microscope; there is no mode by which we can penetrate behind the curtain, or tear aside the veil that divides the *material* from the *immaterial*—mind from *matter*; there is no possibility of our obtaining access to that mysterious chamber where the spiritual portion of our nature is elaborated; we have no gauge, no square rule, by which we can ascertain in all cases, with any approach to chemical or mathematical accuracy, an accurate idea of the actual condition of the mind, when apparently under a cloud. In the elucidation of these points, we are in a great measure left to our unaided mental sense—to the uncertain guidance of our own deceptive experience, and alas! often, fallible judgment.

"We enter the witness-box, charged, under the solemn sanction of an oath, to decide the important questions as to the legal and moral responsibility of our fellow-men. In capital cases, we are called upon to declare whether the criminal was or was not insane when he committed the act; whether, by disordered mind, he was reduced to a state of legal irresponsibility. In other cases, equally important matters are submitted to our adjudication, involving points relative to the competency of persons to make testamentary dispositions of their property, or manage, during life, themselves and their affairs. In the former case, the life of a fellow-creature is made contingent upon the evidence of those deputed to examine him, and delegated with the responsibility of recording their medico-legal opinions as to his state of mind; in the latter instance, we are expected to depose to the competency of certain persons to exercise the otherwise inalienable privilege of disposing of property agreeably to their own notions of the law of inheritance and conceptions of what is just; and, in the third case, it is our province to decide, not upon the solemn question of life or death. but whether a fellow-citizen is in a condition of mind to justify the law in alienating from him his *civil rights*, depriving him of the control of his person and affairs, and destroying, by a legal declaration of lunacy, his free and independent agency. In the first case, it is our imperative duty to avert, if possible, *actual* death—a death of *moral* ignominy and of *physical* suffering; in the latter instance, it is left for us to pronounce whether legal dissolution is to be recorded against the party whose mind is the subject of medico-judicial inquiry. In the former case, it may, happily, be in our power to rescue a fellow-creature from the scaffold; and, in the latter instance, we may, by our evidence, have the not less pleasing gratification of shielding him from the expensive, but nevertheless, under proper circumstances, humane guardianship of the Court of Chancery."

Dr. Winslow then proceeds to discuss with great care and minuteness the following point:

"1. Cases in which the plea of insanity is urged in extenuation of crime.

"2. Cases where attempts are made to invalidate the legal operation of testamentary dispositions of property, on the ground of mental incompetency.

"3. When legal proceedings are instituted to invalidate a marriage contract on the plea of insanity and imbecility.

"4. In commissions 'de lunatico inquirendo,' issued by the Lord Chancellor, with the view of ascertaining the existence of unsoundness of mind, and competency of the party (the subject of investigation) to manage his person and property.

"5. Cases in which medical men are called upon to certify to the existence of insanity, justifying an interference with the person of the lunatic, and depriving him of his free agency, either for the purpose of placing him under treatment or protecting him from the commission of acts of violence to himself or others."

"1. An absolute dispossession, by disease, of the free and natural agency of the mind; partial insanity being no excuse for crime.

"2. The existence of a delusion, the criminal act being the immediate and direct result of the morbid idea; the proof of the presence of a delusion having no positive and clear connection with the alleged crime, not being legal insanity, and no evidence of the existence of irresponsibility.

"3. A consciousness of offending against the laws of God and man—in other words, a knowledge of good and evil.

"4. A knowledge of right and wrong—lawful or unlawful—the presence or absence of motive."*

---

* The judges will not permit the medical witness to infer the existence of insanity from the character of the *act itself*, apart from all other evidence of derangement of mind. In the case of Greensmith, tried for murder on the Midland Circuit in 1837, Mr. Justice Parke observed in his charge :— "Nothing could be more contrary to the law than to infer insanity from the very malignity and atrocity of the crime. It was true, that such crimes could never be committed by men who were in the possession and control of a right reason, and a proper mind; but it was his duty to inform the jury that the complete possession of reason was not essential to constitute the legal, any more than the moral responsibility of man, it being necessary that the party should have sufficient knowledge and reason to discriminate between right and wrong." This may be sound *law*, but it is not sound *psychology*. In many cases the "atrocity and malignity of the crime" afford to the practical physician invaluable evidence of the existence of insanity, the derangement manifesting itself in the

We cannot pretend in this brief analysis to lay before our readers even an outline of Dr. Winslow's medico-legal views. He has opened a wide field of observation for the thinking reader: and, although we consider some of the points mooted by our author as still unsettled and open to discussion, we *sub judice* nevertheless fully agree with him in the great and leading principles which he has enunciated for the guidance of the medical jurist in cases of insanity. What can be better than the advice which Dr. Winslow gives as to the conduct of the medical witness? The following extract is too important to omit:

"The witness should carefully divest himself of all appearance of partisanship. A quiet, calm, respectful demeanor—and a cautious and modest expression of opinion, even in cases which admit of no doubt—always convey a favorable impression to the court, and give additional weight and influence to medico-legal evidence. He should remember that in all probability the course of examination is carefully prepared, it being the object of the advocate to obtain from him a reply to a *consecutive series of questions*, thus gradually unfolding and eliciting the truth. Should he, in his eagerness and anxiety to make a favorable impression upon the court, anticipate the interrogatories, he might seriously interfere with the conduct of the case, and injure the cause he is most anxious to uphold.

"It occasionally occurs that a medical witness may be fully competent to give sound and satisfactory evidence in relation to the presence of insanity, without having the power of clearly stating the grounds for his opinion. A medical gentleman, upon being asked whether he considered a certain person of unsound mind, replied that such was his belief. He was then requested to state his reasons. He said he had formed his conclusions from the 'general manner' and 'deportment of the patient.' The witness was then asked to describe the 'manner' and 'deportment' to which he referred. He replied that the patient was 'odd in his manner, and had an insane and peculiar appearance about his eye and countenance;' but, upon being closely pressed by counsel to describe these symptoms more minutely to the jury, the witness was at once nonplussed, became embarrassed, and broke down. He had a lucid and a *right* opinion of the *matter of fact*, but had no power of describing the symptoms from which he had formed his conclusions. Many men are fully able to give testimony as to *results*, but are totally incompetent to explain the process of reasoning, or succession of thought, by which they have been led to the deduction. A man of practical good sense, who, upon being appointed governor of a colony, had to preside in its court of justice without previous judicial practice or legal education, received the following advice from Lord Mansfield: 'Give your decisions boldly, for they will probably be right; *but never venture on assigning reasons, for they will almost invariably be wrong.*' Lord Mansfield knew, says Mr. Mill, who relates the story, that if any reasons were assigned they would necessarily be an afterthought, the judge being *in fact* guided by impressions from past experience, without the circuitous process of framing general principles from them; and that if he attempted to frame any such, he would assuredly fail.* It would not be difficult to account, psychologically, for a defect of this kind. Are we not daily in the habit of meeting men who have, in relation to matters of art, &c., an *intuitive* perception of the true and beautiful, but who have no power of describing or analyzing their sensations and perceptions?

"A favorite manœuvre of counsel, is to ingeniously construct a number of hypothetical cases, apparently illustrative of the point at issue, and to place them *seriatim* before the witness, with the view of obtaining his opinion of each individual symptom of the alleged mental condition. The replies to such interrogatories, if unguardedly expressed, are often subsequently referred to, for the purpose of damaging his evidence. We should protect ourselves from these legal onslaughts, by carefully considering, before we commit ourselves to an answer, the precise bearing of every interrogatory; it must be rapidly viewed in all its relations, and if we are not thoroughly satisfied as to its character, it is our duty to request the counsel to repeat the question. If we do not clearly per-

character of the *act itself*. I willingly admit that we should cautiously act upon such evidence; but should we not be culpable if we were to set it altogether aside?

* "System of Logic," J. Stuart Mill, vol. 1, p. 254.

ceive its tendency we must protect ourselves, by carefully qualifying our answer. In a case where the validity of a will was contested, on the ground of the insanity of one of the subscribing witnesses, it appeared in evidence that he had at one time entertained some absurd delusions, and had attempted suicide; but that for a few months prior to the execution of the will he had repudiated the delusions, quietly pursued his studies, had written a book, and in fact was apparently well, with the exception of his being unusually shy, with a desire for solitude. To one of the witnesses, who had spoken in favor of the sanity of the party, the following question was put:—'Supposing he had committed murder about the time he had witnessed the will, would you have considered him as morally responsible for the act?' This question is said to have been artfully founded upon the imputed disposition of the witness to admit too readily the plea of insanity in criminal cases. The court would not allow the question to be answered, but the reply would not have promoted the object of the counsel."*

The distinction which Dr. Winslow draws between the mental incompetence resulting from advanced life and old age, and the mental unsoundness consequent upon, or the effect of insanity, or actual disorder of the mind, in a pathological point of view, is most important, and should never be lost sight of:

"It is important that we should remember that in all contested cases of lunacy, relating to the administration of property, it is a matter of moment for counsel, supporting the commission, if he cannot exact an admission of insanity, to induce the witness to acknowledge the existence of an incapacity (apart from the presence of actual lunacy) to manage both the person and property. If the question is, 'Do you consider the party of unsound mind?' and the answer should be either negatively, affirmatively, or of a doubtful character, the witness, in all probability, will be immediately asked, 'Do you consider the party capable of taking care of himself, and of managing his property?' Upon one occasion a question of this character was put to myself. 'Yes, *legally* competent.' 'Legally competent!' echoed Sir F. Thesiger; 'pray, sir, leave *us* (the lawyers, of course) to decide that point.' He was most anxious to force from me an admission that, in the ordinary acceptation of the term, the party was not in a condition to take care of herself, or to manage her property; but drawing what I conceived to be a psychological distinction between *natural* and *healthy incapacity*, and *the incapacity the effect of insanity*, I refused to make the admission he was anxious to obtain, and which, if procured, would, I have no doubt, have been turned adroitly against me. It was upon the same occasion, and during the same inquiry, that I was asked whether, if *I* thought the party were competent to manage herself and her affairs, the *world* would be of the same opinion? I replied 'that, upon intricate and disputed questions of science, I did not think the opinion of "the world" a safe guide.' Upon which Sir F. Thesiger rejoined, '*Then, I presume, you look down upon the opinions of the world?*† If I had been permitted, I might have quoted, in justification of my remark, the sentiments of a modern philosopher of no mean repute: 'The general voice of mankind, which may often serve as a guide, because it rarely errs widely or permanently in its estimate of those who are prominent in public life, *is of little value when it speaks of things belonging to the region of exact science.*‡ The opinion of the majority upon questions within the comprehension and grasp of men of ordinary intelligence and natural sagacity, is entitled to our profound respect. It may be, and often is, right. But does not history satisfactorily establish that what in common parlance is designated as the 'generally-received opinion' is occasionally very remote from the truth?

'Interdum vulgus rectum videt, est ubi peccat.'—Hor.

"There is a *legal* incapacity, and, according to law, it is the consequence of diseased or unsound mind. There is also ordinary and natural incapacity, which may coexist with a healthy and a sound understanding. This important and

* "American Journal of Insanity."
† I should regret if any of my readers for one moment imagined that I in the slightest degree complain of the course of examination pursued by this able, honorable, and justly distinguished advocate. The conduct of Sir F. Thesiger during the painful and protracted inquiry into the sanity of Mrs. Cummings, is beyond all praise. In his zeal for the interest of his client, he never deviated from the deportment of the gentleman.
‡ "History of the Inductive Sciences," by Dr. Whewell.

essential distinction the medical witness should never overlook when giving evidence."

The few extracts we have given from Dr. Winslow's lectures will, we hope, induce our readers to procure the volume, and master its contents. It will well repay perusal. It is replete with important facts and principles, and should find its way into the library of every member of the profession.

A clinical investigation into the diagnostic value of the Cracked Pot Sound (Bruit de Pot Fêlé de Laennec). By T. HUGHES BENNETT, M.D., Professor of the Institutes of Medicine and of Clinical Medicine in the University of Edinburgh. ("Edinburgh Medical Journal," March, 1856.)

One hundred patients in the clinical wards of the Royal Infirmary at Edinburgh were examined in this investigation, and the results of the examination, as to age, disease, and the presence or absence of the cracked pot sound, are carefully tabulated. These patients were taken indiscriminately as they presented themselves, the choice being in no way governed by a desire to obtain a preponderance of chest diseases. The chests of these patients were percussed with the hammer and pleximeter, the mouth being open, and the result was that the cracked pot sound was distinctly produced in twenty-nine out of the hundred. The general results were :

1. That the cracked pot sound was frequently absent in cases where our preconceived notions would have induced us to look for it. This was very observable in five cases of phthisis with all the signs of a cavity, in two of which, cavities, although of comparatively small extent, were found after death. 2. That the cracked pot sound was frequently present in pulmonary disease where there was no cavity, as in four cases of pleurisy, and in several cases of pneumonia. 3. That it was present in several cases where neither symptoms or signs gave any evidence of disease of the lungs. 4. That it was frequently observed to come and go in the same individual, evidently in consequence of changed physical condition in the lungs during the progress of the case.

With regard to the 29 cases in which the cracked pot sound was present, the particulars are: pleurisy, 4; pneumonia, 5; pleuro-pneumonia, 1; phthisis, 6; other diseases with pulmonary complications, 5; the pulmonary organs healthy, 8.

Pleurisy.—Of the 4 cases of pleurisy, 3 were acute, affecting only one side, and 1 chronic, affecting both sides. In all the three acute cases the sound was limited to a space immediately under the clavicle of the affected side, where it was unusually resonant on percussion. In the case of chronic pleurisy affecting both sides, there was resonance under both clavicles, and the sound was elicited on both sides. In another case of pleurisy, without resonance, there was no cracked pot sound.

It would seem, therefore, that a portion of spongy lung is necessary to the production of this peculiar sound. That this, however, is not the only condition, Dr. Bennett shows by a sixth case of pleurisy (No. 47 on the list), in which there was dulness over every part of the affected side, except in the space above the second rib. There the percussion was normal, and the cracked pot sound was absent. In a word, the sound was only produced where the percussion sound was unusually clear and tympanitic.

Pneumonia.—Of the 5 cases in which the sound was elicited, 2 were acute, and 3 already chronic. It was elicited sometimes when dulness on percussion was present, and sometimes when clearness was present. In 2 cases it was heard under both clavicles, although the disease was confined to a single lung. It was heard in every case of pneumonia.

Pleuro-pneumonia.—In the single case of this disease the cracked pot sound was present under both clavicles, although dulness on percussion was only present at the base of the right lung. The apex of the right lung was resonant.

Phthisis pulmonalis.—Out of 14 cases of phthisis the cracked pot sound could only be produced in 6. In these 6 cases there was dulness on percussion, with more or less moist râle, or hoarse inspiration with increased vocal resonance, where the sound was present. In 4 of these 6 the body was examined after death, and in 3 out of these 4 Dr. Bennett succeeded in producing the sound in question by percussing the dead chest, after making an opening in the trachea and keeping the edges of the incision apart with a pair of forceps. He did not always succeed on both sides, however, even though it had been heard on both sides during life. Where a cracked pot sound was producible a cavity was found; but in 1 case there was a large cavity and yet the sound was absent. Of the 8 cases of phthisis in which the sound could not be produced, there were 3 which presented signs of softening at the apex. In 2 of these, cavities were found after death. Dr. Bennett endeavors to explain the absence of the cracked pot sound in cases where this cracked pot sound is present by a possible diminution of elasticity in the chest, or by a temporary cutting off of the direct communication between the cavity and the bronchial tubes. In conjunction with other signs and symptoms, however, the cracked pot sound must be considered as highly diagnostic of a cavity.

Diseases with congestion, collapse, or emphysema of the lungs.—These were 5 in number; 3 of heart-disease, 1 of "chronic vomiting," and 1 of Bright's disease. In the 3 cases of heart-disease there was either dulness posteriorly and inferiorly, with resonance superiorly, or there were evidences of chronic bronchitis and emphysema. In the case of chronic vomiting there was dulness under the right clavicle, where the cracked pot sound was elicited; and, in the case of Bright's disease, percussion under both clavicles, was unusually clear, and the sound was heard on both sides.

Diseases without pulmonary complication.—In the 8 cases belonging to this class, 7 were below 21 years of age, and 4 of these below 15. In one man, however, nearly 60, with a perfectly well-formed chest, the sound could be produced.

Such, then, being the apparently opposing and puzzling facts to which Dr. Bennett is led by a careful analysis of these 100 cases, it now remains for us to inquire into the author's views respecting the theory and diagnostic value of the sound. And first with respect to the theory of the sound.

"Any true theory of the production of the cracked pot sound," says Dr. Bennett, "must embrace all the known facts. It follows that, inasmuch as it may be produced in cases of pleurisy, pneumonia, and even in the healthy chest, the existence of a cavity, as supposed by Laennec, or of a mixture of air and fluid, as stated by Piorry, is not essential. According to Skoda, when percussion is made over a cavity, it is compressed at each stroke, and a portion of air suddenly driven out of it into the bronchial tubes; the hissing murmur, caused by the escaping air, is mixed up with the ordinary percussion-sound of cavities, and this compound noise represents the cracked pot sound. That part of the theory, however, which considers a cavity necessary, is shown by the preceding facts to be incorrect.

"It has been noticed by various observers, especially by Graves, Stokes, Williams, Hudson, Walshe, and Markham in this country, and by Martinet, Andral, Piorry, Roger, Skoda, Winterich and others abroad, that a peculiar tympanitic tone, on percussion, is frequently produced in cases of pleurisy and pneumonia. An inquiry into the causes of these tympanitic and non-tympanitic sounds, or a review of the theories of Graves, Skoda, and others, is not my present object, and would lead me too far from the immediate subject of this investigation. Two excellent papers have recently been published regarding them by Markham[*] and Winterich.[†] The preceding facts, however, will show that the cracked pot sound is producible sometimes with the tympanitic and sometimes with the non-tympanitic percussion note, and it appears to me that, had attention been more carefully directed to the first sound instead of so exclusively to the latter phenomena, it would have probably been ascertained long since to have been as distinct and frequent as I have demonstrated it to be. Dr. Markham observes of a case, in which there was an amphoric percussion sound, that on one occasion both he and Dr. Sibson noticed distinctly the cracked pot sound, near the same spot. The post-mortem examination showed that the right lung was gorged with blood and serum, but everywhere still retaining some portion of air.

"On carefully considering what are the necessary conditions for the production of this peculiar sound, comparing these with the facts detailed, and referring

* "Monthly Journal," June, 1852.
† "Medizinischen Neuigkeiten," 5 Jahrgang.

to the well-known modes of producing the sound artificially, 1st, with the two hands crossed, and, 2d, by percussing with the pleximeter on a bladder containing a small quantity of air, it appears to me they are, 1st, A certain amount of confined or tense air in the tissue of the lung; 2d, The sudden compression of this air by a solid body in its neighborhood; 3d, Communication of this air with the external atmosphere.

" 1st. That a certain amount of air must be present is proved by its existence in all the twenty-nine instances in which the sound could be elicited. Thus in pleurisy encroaching on the lung from below upwards, percussion is clear under the clavicles. Where the entire thorax was dull, there was no cracked pot sound (No. 1). We have also previously alluded to the fact, that in one case (No. 21), as soon as the clearness of tone under the clavicle had disappeared, and, in another (No. 23), as soon as dulness invaded the apex of the affected side, the cracked pot sound could no longer be produced. The same observation applies to the cases of pneumonia, pleuro-pneumonia, congestion or collapse, proceeding from below upwards. On the other hand, where percussion is dull, as in pneumonia affecting the upper third of the lung, the confined air must exist below the diseased part, and be affected by the blow on percussion. In phthisis, with cavities, isolated or anfractuous, this condition is easily found. In healthy chests, especially in children, it may be easily demonstrated to occur, just when the chest is distended with air, as at the end of inspiration, thus affording the first essential condition.

" 2d. The sudden compression of the confined or tense air seems also to be a necessary condition in the production of the sound. This, however, may be effected in various ways. The blow of the hammer was in all the twenty-nine cases the immediate cause, but this could not operate in compressing the air unless the walls of the thorax were elastic, as we have shown it to be in most of those in whom the chest was healthy; or, unless in cases of diseased chest, the blow communicated vibrations to indurations over the lung, which thereby compressed the air. In the former case the blow would act directly, in the latter, indirectly. Hence why in some lungs with elastic thoracic walls, during inspiration, it may be produced without disease, and why when elastic indurations occur, as in pleurisy, pneumonia, or phthisis, it may be elicited in disease. I have frequently observed when percussing diseased chests, that the cracked pot sound diminishes in intensity after repeated percussions, I presume from the tensity of the air being diminished, by portions of it which have in this way been squeezed out of the space percussed.

" 3d. That there should be a communication between the air in the chest, and the external atmosphere, is proved by the invariable necessity of having the mouth and nostrils open before the cracked pot sound can be produced, and its immediate disappearance on shutting the mouth. After death, also, it can never be produced without previously making an opening in the trachea, or securing patency of the larynx. The necessity of this condition indeed serves, in my opinion, to explain how it happens in several cases where cavities exist in the lung—that is to say, where confined portions of air are present, with elastic chests or indurated surrounding tissue—still the sound is not elicited. For it is easy to conceive that in such cases, the bronchi leading to the external atmosphere, or the cavities themselves, may at various times be filled with purulent secretion, mucus, blood, or other fluid, and that swelling of the bronchial lining membrane, or compression of the tube, may cut off the communication so necessary for the production of a peculiar note on percussion. Hence it appears to me why in phthisical cavities the sound comes and goes—why it may be present or absent before death—but above all why this is no more an invariable sign of a morbid state than any other with which we are acquainted.

" Although these appear to me to be the conditions necessary for generating the sound, it is very difficult to determine the exact physical state at any one time necessary for its production. I believe, however, it will be found to reside in a mixture of solid and aeriform parts, the latter of which are capable of being compressed by the blow of percussion. Sometimes the former surround the latter, as in the case of a cavity. At others, the latter lie over, or upon the former, as in cases of pleurisy and dulness at the base; and occasionally the former lie upon or over the latter, as in pneumonia or infiltrated tubercle at the apex In healthy chests a similar condition is produced by a full inspiration with elastic thoracic walls—as it is in a dead stomach rendered somewhat tense by air—in which last case, by percussing with a pleximeter, and bringing the two walls of the organ near each other, the cracked pot sound may be produced—a statement originally made by Skoda, and the correctness of which has frequently been confirmed by myself."

As to the diagnostic value of the cracked pot sound, Dr. Bennett writes:

"A phenomenon which occurs in the general run of hospital cases, so frequently as twenty-nine in a hundred, and which is audible in twenty-one out of thirty-six pulmonary diseases in that hundred, must probably be considered a more common sign than any other with which we are acquainted. The character of the sound, also, is so peculiar and distinctive, is so easily produced when percussion is properly performed, and so little likely to be confounded with anything else, as to demand our careful attention. Yet it must be clear that it is in no degree pathognomonic, as it may be present in a variety of morbid states, and exists far more commonly in health, as we have shown, than is generally supposed. All these circumstances, however, are by no means opposed to its value in a diagnostic point of view. Indeed nothing, perhaps, has so much tended to throw discredit on the physical diagnosis of diseases of the chest, or been more mischievous in practice, than the attempts to connect particular diseases with particular signs, of which the notion that crepitation is diagnostic of pneumonia, and that dulness on percussion under the clavicle is diagnostic of phthisis, are striking examples. Hence, although *per se*, the cracked pot sound is of little value—of no more, indeed, than any other individual sign; it is, when conjoined with other signs *and symptoms*, capable, in no small degree, of assisting the physician in his diagnosis of thoracic diseases.

"Dr. Stokes noticed the existence of this sound in some cases of bronchitis in children, Dr. Walshe has repeatedly observed it in infancy, and Dr. Markham has observed it in the case of an engorged lung, containing a certain amount of air, but without a cavity. But we are not aware that any attempt has yet been made to indicate from the results of careful inquiry, the probable uses of this sign in practical medicine. It is very probable that it may subsequently be discovered in diseased conditions not yet observed by myself or others; but, among several which occur to me as very probable ones unnoticed for the present, I venture to give the following, as the results to which the present inquiry had led me, viz.:

' "1st. That the cracked pot sound is far more frequent than is generally believed.

"2d. That for its production, careful percussion, with the mouth open, should be practised with the hammer and pleximeter.

"3d. That it is not necessarily indicative of a cavity in the lungs, but may be present in various diseases of the chest, and even when the chest is perfectly sound.

"4th. That, notwithstanding, in percussing the chest, we should never omit to do so when the mouth of the patient is open, as well as shut, with a view of determining whether the cracked pot sound exists or not.

"5th. If present, it indicates either healthy lungs, with very elastic thoracic walls, or else increased density mingled with confined or compressed air in the thorax.

"6th. The youth of the patient, resonance on percussion, puerile or healthy respiration, and the absence of pulmonary symptoms, will serve to diagnose the healthy character of the lungs.

"7th. If the usual signs and symptoms of pleurisy, with dulness, be present with the cracked pot sound, it indicates that a portion of spongy lung is still performing its functions, and is not far from the thoracic walls.

"8th. If there be dulness under the clavicle with the mouth shut, and cracked pot sound when the mouth is open, it indicates a mixture of indurated tissue, and of air—a circumstance which may occur in partial pneumonia, or in phthisis pulmonalis—probably under other circumstances, such as aneurismal, or other tumors, compressing the lung.

"9th. Partial pneumonia can only be distinguished from limited tubercular deposition under such circumstances, by the general symptoms on the one hand, and by the absence of signs of a cavity on the other. If these fail, the diagnosis is most difficult.

"10th. But if there be symptoms and signs of a tubercular cavity, then the cracked pot sound indicates that such cavity has a direct communication with the larger bronchi, and through it with the external atmosphere.

"11th. As this is the most common condition of tubercular cavities, the occurrence of the sound in such cases, though far from infallible, is still highly diagnostic.

"The practical value of these conclusions, and the modifications in and extension of them, which may result from further clinical investigation, I shall not now dwell upon. It may be well to observe, however, that I have recently had a case in the clinical wards of the Royal Infirmary, where, with all the symptoms and signs of advanced phthisis indicating small cavities at both apices, there was a remarkably loud percussion note over the left mammary region, with distinct metallic tinkling immediately under the nipple, at the close both of inspiration and expiration. The sound resembled a double *tink tink*. It was supposed that pneumothorax existed, yet a careful post-mortem examination showed no formation of air, as supposed by Graves, no lesion of the pleura whatever, and no cavity where the noise was audible, but small nodules of tubercles scattered through emphysematous pulmonary tissue, with a small cavity at each apex. Was the metallic tinkling propagated downwards from the cavity at the apex? This interesting question must for the present remain unanswered.

"I have only, in conclusion, to express my conviction, that the remarkably characteristic cracked pot sound, must be of greater importance than it has hitherto been considered, and that, if rightly interpreted, it is calculated to assist us, in an eminent degree, in rendering our diagnosis more complete and exact."

On the organic and functional Disorders of the Stomach. By GEORGE BUDD, M.D., F.R.S., Professor of Medicine in King's College, London, &c. (8vo, Churchill, 1855, pp. 357.)

This work consists of fourteen lectures, of which the majority have already appeared from time to time in one of the weekly medical periodicals. They are not simply reprints, however, but they are republished with such additions and corrections as the author's subsequent experience has suggested.

It is not necessary to enter upon an analysis of the whole work, and it must suffice to say that the ordinary topics of stomach disorder are carefully considered, and that the whole has a decidedly practical bearing. Already, indeed, we have noticed several of the author's opinions as the lectures first made their appearance; and all that remains for us to do at the present is, to cite a few passages in illustration of the contents of the work before us. Let us take, then, the remarks upon perforating ulcer of the stomach as such a sample.

"From the account I have given of the symptoms and effects of the perforating ulcer of the stomach, it will be seen," says Dr. Budd, "that the disease becomes more easy of detection the longer it has lasted.

"Early in the disease the symptoms are few and equivocal. Pain and soreness at the epigastrium felt after meals, occasional sour eructations, and occasional vomiting—which are often the only symptoms then present—may result from various other causes, and even from mere functional disorder.

"After these symptoms have lasted some weeks or months, their very continuance becomes significant—it renders it highly probable that they depend on organic disease: while the seat of the pain, and the circumstance that it is always increased by eating and usually abates as the stomach gets empty, lead to the inference that this organic disease is in the stomach.

"After a time the symptoms I have mentioned are often succeeded by the sudden occurrence of profuse vomiting of blood. When this has happened, the detection of the disease becomes much easier.

"Vomiting of blood may, indeed, result from various other conditions; but these may generally be distinguished from ulcer by the nature of the illness and by the circumstances under which it occurs.

"1st. Vomiting of blood may result from a general tendency to hemorrhage, in consequence of a general fault of nutrition or a faulty condition of the blood, as in scurvy or purpura; but in such cases the hemorrhage is not confined to the stomach—blood issues from other mucous surfaces, and purpuric spots appear on the skin.

"2d. Again, vomiting of blood may result, as we have seen, from mechanical congestion of the stomach, in consequence of some impediment to the free passage of the blood through the liver or the chest. In such cases, the quantity of blood lost is usually small, and the cause of the hemorrhage is generally obvious enough from the coexistence of other symptoms, which reveal the primary disease and which show that the passage of the blood through the liver or the chest is greatly impeded.

"3d. Vomiting of blood sometimes occurs, without any organic disease of the stomach itself, in persons who, in consequence of repeated attacks of ague, or other causes, have great enlargement of the spleen. Here, also, the previous history of the patient, his cachectic condition, and the palpable enlargement of the spleen, readily lead us to the original cause of the hemorrhage.

"4th. Lastly, the hemorrhage may be vicarious of the catamenia; and this is especially liable to happen in young unmarried women,—the class of persons supposed to be most subject to ulcer of the stomach. But, in such cases, the hemorrhage usually occurs at the monthly period, and the natural discharge is suppressed or has previously been irregular; and, if no ulcer of the stomach exist, the vomiting of blood, although it may be attended with severe pain at the time, has not been preceded, and is not followed, by the long-continued pain and soreness produced by ulcer.

"In a large proportion, however, of cases even of this periodical vomiting of blood, an ulcer of the stomach does exist, and is the chief, if not the sole, source of the hemorrhage; but the blood, instead of issuing from a vessel of considerable size laid open by the process of ulceration, as in ordinary cases of simple ulcer, oozes from the minute vessels of the raw surface, in consequence of a congestion of the stomach, which takes the place of the appointed monthly congestion of the uterus. Symptoms of ulcer of the stomach are then present in the intervals of the vomiting of blood; and the hemorrhage is traced to a periodical congestion of the stomach only from its occurring at the appointed time, and from its taking the place of the natural monthly courses.

"5th. The vomiting of blood from the simple ulcer of the stomach may also be distinguished from that arising from other conditions by the characters of the blood vomited.

"When the hemorrhage consists in a mere oozing of blood, as it does in congestion of the stomach, and sometimes in cancer, the blood is coagulated as it escapes, and is vomited in minute clots or shreds. In simple ulcer of the stomach the blood usually issues from a vessel of considerable size laid open by the ulcer, it is poured out rapidly and abundantly, coagulates in a mass, and large clots are often thrown up.

"When vomiting of blood does not depend on any of the conditions which I have just mentioned, it results almost invariably (except in the case of malignant fevers) from organic disease of the stomach itself.

"When, therefore, profuse vomiting of blood occurs in a person who exhibits no general tendency to hemorrhage; who has no disease of the liver, or in the chest, which greatly impedes the passage of the blood; who has no great enlargement of the spleen; and in whom the hemorrhage cannot, from the time of its occurrence and other circumstances, be referred to disorder of the menstrual function; we are driven, in reasoning by the method of exclusion, to ascribe it to disease of the stomach itself. When such is the case, and when, moreover. the vomiting of blood has been preceded for some weeks or months by pain and soreness at the stomach, always brought on or increased by meals, hardly a doubt can remain that it actually depends on organic disease of this organ. But, in persons under the age of thirty, the only organic disease of the stomach that gives rise to profuse hemorrhage, with very few exceptions, is ulcer.

"It follows, therefore, that, from the peculiar train of symptoms which I have mentioned,—namely, pain and soreness of the stomach, always brought on or increased by meals, continuing for many weeks or months, with occasional sour eructations and occasional vomiting, but without much fever or constitutional disturbance, and succeeded, at the end of that time, by profuse vomiting of blood,—it follows that, from this peculiar train of symptoms, we may occasionally, in persons between eighteen and thirty, infer the existence of ulcer of the stomach with almost as much certainty as that of any inward disease.

"In persons above the age of thirty, vomiting of blood, preceded by disordered and painful digestion, may likewise occur from cancer of the stomach. For persons, therefore, who have reached this age, the question will arise,—Is the organic disease of the stomach, which we have inferred to exist, simple ulcer, or is it cancer? When the disease has lasted some months, it is usually not difficult to answer this question.

"Cancer in the stomach, in most cases, originates at the pyloric or the cardiac orifice, and in some degree narrows or obstructs it. It also gives rise to a tumor, which, at the end of some months, is generally palpable enough; and it *always* interferes greatly with nutrition, causing progressive, and, after a time, extreme wasting.

"Simple ulcer seldom produces any of these effects. When, therefore, from the train of symptoms I have mentioned, we have inferred that organic disease of the stomach exists, we may often proceed a step further, and conclude that this disease does not obstruct either the cardiac or the pyloric orifice; and from the circumstances that the power of digestion remains, and that there is no great wasting, we may conclude, also, that the disease involves only a small portion of the stomach.

"We are thus led to the conclusion that there is organic disease of the stomach of such kind as to cause hemorrhage,—that this disease involves only a small portion of the stomach,—that it does not obstruct the orifices,—and that it does not form a tumor large enough to be felt. The probability, in such a case, will be very great, that the disease is simple ulcer, and not cancer. The probability is the greater, the longer the previous duration of the disease. A simple ulcer may continue almost stationary—at any rate with little change in the symptoms —for twenty years. Cancerous disease, on the contrary, constantly and steadily progresses; the symptoms become, week after week, more marked; and, although life may be protracted, especially in colloid cancer, for four or five years, the patient generally dies, much emaciated, within twelve months.

"If, then, the disease has lasted this time, presenting the peculiar train of symptoms I have mentioned, and there is still no great wasting, and no evidence that the orifices of the stomach are obstructed, and no tumor to be felt, hardly a doubt can remain that the disease is simple ulcer of the stomach. The evidence is as complete and decisive as we can well have for any inward disease. Although, then, it may be difficult, or even impossible, soon after an ulcer of the stomach has formed, to distinguish it from some other diseases, the distinction may generally be made surely enough when the ulcer has existed many months.

"It is often possible to go a step further than this, and to form some opinion respecting the *size* and the *site* of the ulcer.

"The size of the ulcer may be judged of by the constancy of the pain and the severity of the other symptoms. If the pain be slight and of short duration, and the appetite be good, and vomiting occur seldom, and there be no wasting—the ulcer is small.

"The site of the ulcer is determined by the spot in which the pain is felt. If there be much *tenderness* at the epigastrium, *and no pain in the back*—the ulcer is most probably on the anterior face of the stomach."

On the Relation between Abscess of the Liver and Dysentery. By E. W. Eyre, Esq., Garrison-Surgeon, Bellary. ("Indian Annals," Oct. 1855.)

The following remarks upon the relation between abscess of the liver and dysentery, are taken from a paper entitled "Medical Notes on Dysentery."

They seem to be of considerable importance, and certainly they are deserving of careful attention, for they are written by a gentleman who (as our former pages will testify) has well vindicated his claim to being considered as an able and independent observer.

" 'The connection between abscess of the liver and dysentery, as a clinical fact, is indisputable.' Thus dogmatically does a writer in the 'British and Foreign Medical Review'* express himself. I believe there are few, if any, practitioners in India will agree with him. In the annual report on the 1st Madras Fusiliers for 1850-51, the subject of the connection between the two diseases was taken up; the following is an extract—' To ascertain the connection between hepatic disease and dysentery, the following table has been drawn up from the post-mortem reports (of the Regiment) for the last sixteen years, and points out the stations where the cases occurred.'

" To this table I have now added other cases that have since come under my notice; or that have been obtained from reliable sources.†

TABLE.

Stations.	No. of cases of fatal Dysentery.	Abscess of the Liver.		Various abnormal conditions of this viscus, induration, degeneration, &c.		Liver healthy.	
		No.	Per cent.	No.	Per cent.	No.	Per cent.
Kamptee . .	24	11	45·8	9	37·5	4	16·6
Secundrabad .	53	9	16·9	9	16·9	35	66·
Arnee . .	6	1	16·6	0	0	5	83·3
Arcott . .	6	0	0	3	50·	3	50·
Bangalore . .	10	1	10·	1	10·	8	80·
Bellary . .	6	2	33·3	0	0	4	66·6
Total .	105	24	22·8	22	20·9	59	55·2
Additional Table	13	3	23·	0	0	10	76·9
General Total	118	27	22·	22	0	69	58·47

" The first table has a column for other altered states of the liver besides suppuration. Whether they should all be regarded as disease I think questionable. In the post-mortems, the conditions of the organ is vaguely expressed by 'liver enlarged,' but enlargement, hypertrophy alone, is not always disease; besides if not weighed, the sight may deceive. The diseased states of the liver, apart from suppuration, that my opportunities have brought before me, have been cirrhosis in its different stages and appearances, not infrequent, and fatty degeneration, of which, however, I have seen but two well-marked instances. No one would connect these pathologically with dysentery, therefore they may fairly be excluded from a comparative table of inflammation and suppuration of the liver and dysentery, and if this be done, it will be found that of 118 cases of fatal dysentery, only 27 were complicated with hepatic abscess; or, 22·88 per cent. Mr. Waring's table, page 120, gives 149 out of 633 cases of primary dysentery, 23·54 per cent., a striking similarity. Do these results at all bear out the ingenious theory, first, I believe, proposed by Dr. Copeland, in the following words :— 'In dysentery, therefore, it may be inferred, that, in the progress of ulceration, phlebitis of the capillary veins of the bowels sometimes occurs; and that the matter or pus thus formed, in these veins, passes with the blood into the portal circulation, where it irritates or inflames the minute ramifications of the portal vessels, and the structure of the liver, giving rise to purulent infiltrations and collections in the organ, similar to those consequent upon phlebitis in other parts, but always occurring in the liver, and there only, because the morbid matter passes directly from the bowels into the portal circulation.' This theory has found an advocate in Dr. Budd. 'The consideration of these cases' (cases of deposit of pus in the lungs and liver) 'leads us naturally to a third cause—I

* No. xxvii. July, 1854.
† Other than those Mr. Waring has drawn.

believe by far the most frequent cause—of abscess of the liver: namely, ulceration of the large intestines * * * *. A connection between abscess of the liver and dysentery has long been noticed, but the two diseases are associated far more frequently than has been generally imagined.' Dr. Budd's conclusions were founded on 62 cases only; in nearly all, the abscesses in the liver are ascribed to deposit of pus due to injuries, operations on the rectum, and in 31 to ulceration of the intestines or stomach. There is not an exact parallel between these and Dr. Waring's cases, or those in the accompanying table, for in the former the hepatic disease is the paramount one, in the latter, dysentery. The number of cases is large, being a total of 751. If the theory of the formation of hepatic abscess be sound, how is it that 76·50 per cent. of dysentery had no hepatic disease? If so intimate a connection between the two exists, the absence of abscesses in the liver would be the exception, but it is found that its presence may rather be regarded as the exception.

" It was remarked in the report, ' It is probable that the two diseases are more associated in some stations than in others ; in H. M.'s 64th Regiment, while at Masulipatam, in 1833, it was found that the biliary functions were but little implicated, while in the same Regiment, at Bangalore, hepatic derangement was so blended with dysentery, that it was difficult to state which organ was the originator of the disease.'*

" On reading the remark at the head of this article, I thought that a collection of as many cases as were procurable, of primary dysentery with hepatic abscess supervening, might not be without its use, and had entered upon the subject when Mr. Waring's work appeared.† I have thus been anticipated, and a continuation of a full inquiry rendered unnecessary by the able manner in which Mr. Waring has performed his task. It may not, however, be without its interest to know in what light the connection of dysentery and hepatic abscess was regarded by the medical men, whose reports have furnished Mr. Waring with his statistics, and perhaps others may concur with myself in coming to the conclusion, that not one regarded the two diseases in the light of cause and effect, with the exception of Dr. Parkes, whose theory assimilates with Dr. Budd's, in supposing that the blood, contaminated by the ulcers or secretions in the intestines, and conveyed to the liver, is the origin of abscess there. These are the writer's own words: ' Dysentery has been the most formidable disease to contend with ; hepatitis less than what I had met with on the Tenasserim Coast ; in no instance abscess.' (Report on H. M.'s 45th Regiment, 1832.) 'The increase of these diseases (hepatitis and dysentery) was double in this month, and they were very frequently combined.' (Report on H. M.'s 45th Regiment, 1853.)‡ ' Dysentery greatly increased after June, and the cases were very severe and fatal, being combined with hepatitis.' (Report on H. M.'s 55th, 1839.) ' It is of great consequence to distinguish the complication of hepatic abscess with dysentery.' (H. M.'s 54th.) ' It (hepatitis) was rarely concomitant with dysentery.' (H. M.'s 57th, 1839.) 'Dysentery at Bangalore is a very active disease, and is connected in very many instances with hepatic disease.' (H. M.'s 89th, 1833.) ' Fifty-five were brought back (to Bangalore) with dysentery, and four sunk, in all there were hepatic abscesses. The general character of the dysenteric cases was severe, and in almost every instance there was structural disorganization of the liver.' (H. M.'s 39th, 1834.) 'In some instances the two diseases (hepatitis and dysentery) were combined.' (H. M.'s 39th, 1836.) ' I

---

* Other reports dwell on the frequency of the complication at Bangalore. At Belgaum it seems of frequent occurrence, hepatitis alone varies at the same station. In a report on H. M.'s Light Dragoons at Ajmeer, it is stated that " hepatic abscess was so common, that if a man came into hospital suffering under hepatitis, or any other acute disease, and eventually died, the probability was great in favor of one or more abscesses being found in the substance of the liver. At the same station, in the following year, it was almost as rare to meet with a case of hepatitis or hepatic abscess, as it had been common at the time referred to." In the D. Troop Horse Artillery, at Jaulnah, there was not a case of hepatitis between July 1839 and September 1840, while, in the following year, in the same months there were 15 cases;¹ there was nothing in the internal economy or cognizable atmospheric state to account for it.

† An " Inquiry into the Statistics and Pathology of some points connected with abscesses in the Liver "—1854.

‡ A large proportion of these cases (hepatitis) were complicated with dysentery, a great many instances of the latter disease showed well-marked symptoms of acute hepatitis. (H. M.'s 55th, 1839.)

---

¹ I do not vouch that all 15 were inflammation of the liver, probably not, some mere congestion. —

have examined the bodies of forty-eight who have died of true dysentery and have not found the liver disordered in one of them.' (Dr. Nicoll's Report.) ' If not complicated with hepatitis, dysentery in its worst form, &c.' (H. M.'s 41st, 1832-34.) ' Of these sixteen cases of dysentery, only a small number was discovered on dissection to have been true cases of colonitis, almost all of them have been found more or less complicated with organic lesion of the liver.' (H. M.'s 41st.) 'Hepatitis is frequently found complicated with dysentery, but whether as cause or effect, has not yet been satisfactorily determined.' (Essay on Hepatitis, by Dr. Nicoll.) ' In three of the cases of dysentery (out of 163 treated) the disease was complicated with extensive abscesses of the liver.' (H. M.'s 4th, 1840.) 'Our total (of dysentery) treated has been 108, with a mortality of twenty-six; of these, nine had the complication of hepatic abscess.' (H. M.'s 94th, 1840.)

" Now it is evident that not one of these writers regarded dysentery and hepatitis as dependent on each other in the light of cause and effect, but only as associated in some cases, and how few the proportion. Much negative testimony might be adduced, for other writers describe the two diseases apart, the thought not having apparently suggested itself that there was any pathological connection between them. It is not unreasonable to conclude that they are distinct diseases. Dysentery prevails everywhere;—it is the scourge of camps in all climates, it infests crowded transports and jails—but hepatitis has its localities; India is one of them, and why may not the two coexist in the same individual, though pathologically disconnected? When hepatic abscess is the primary disease, is the bowel-complaint, when present, true dysentery, i. e. colonitis? Dr. Nicoll, whom I have quoted, says, ' diarrhœa is a common attendant on that affection of the liver, which does not run into suppuration rapidly.' I have met with three cases within the last few months, of intractable bowel-complaint, not true dysentery, in which hepatic abscess was disclosed; in one, only the day before death, in the second fourteen days, in the third the post-mortem revealed it."

On the constitutional and local effects of Disease of the Supra-renal Capsules. By THOMAS ADDISON, M.D., Senior Physician to Guy's Hospital. (4to., London, Samuel Highley, 1855, pp. 44, with colored plates.)
Series illustrating the connection between Bronzed Skin and Disease of the Supra-renal Capsules. By JONATHAN HUTCHINSON, Esq., Surgeon to the Metropolitan Free Hospital. ("Medical Times and Gazette," Dec. 15th, 22d, and 29th, 1855, Jan. 19th, Feb. 23d, March 8th and 22d, 1856.)

In the work the title of which is placed at the head of this article, Dr. Addison relates eleven cases which seem to show very clearly that another disease must be added to the catalogue of human maladies, and this is a very important disease. The evidence is entirely and purely clinical, and the rationale is yet to be provided, but the fact appears to be indisputable.

The large supply of blood which the supra-renal capsules receive from three separate sources; their numerous nerves, derived immediately from the semilunar ganglia and solar plexus; their early development in the fœtus; their unimpaired integrity to the latest period of life; and their peculiar gland-like structure, all point to the performance of some important office; but beyond an ill-defined impression that these organs minister in some way to the elaboration of the blood, nothing whatever is known about the nature of that office. And hence it is that the facts to which we are about to call attention, have a physiological as well as a pathological interest.

It was whilst engaged in investigating a remarkable form of general anæmia that Dr. Addison was led to the discovery of the disease in question, and this is a fact of some interest and importance.

" For a long period," he says, "I had from time to time met with a very remarkable form of general anæmia, occurring without any discoverable cause whatever; cases in which there had been no previous loss of blood, no exhausting diarrhœa, no chlorosis, no purpura, no renal, splenic, miasmatic, glandular, strumous, or malignant disease. Accordingly, in speaking of this form of anæmia in a clinical lecture, I, perhaps with little propriety, applied to it the term 'idiopathic,' to distinguish it from cases in which there existed more or less evidence of some of the usual causes or concomitants of the anæmic state.

" The disease presented in every instance the same general character, pursued a similar course, and, with scarcely a single exception, was followed, after a variable period, by the same fatal result. It occurs in both sexes, generally, but not exclusively, beyond the middle period of life, and, so far as I at present know, chiefly in persons of a somewhat large and bulky frame, and with a strongly marked tendency to the formation of fat. It makes its approach in so slow and insidious a manner, that the patient can hardly fix a date to his earliest feeling of that languor, which is shortly to become so extreme. The countenance gets pale, the whites of the eyes become pearly, the general frame flabby rather than wasted ; the pulse rather large, but remarkably soft and compressible, and occasionally with a slight jerk, especially under the slightest excitement; there is an increasing indisposition to exertion, with an uncomfortable feeling of faintness or breathlessness on attempting it; the heart is readily made to palpitate ; the whole surface of the body presents a blanched, smooth, and waxy appearance ; the lips, gums, and tongue seem bloodless; the flabbiness of the solids increases ; the appetite fails ; extreme languor and faintness supervene, breathlessness and palpitation being produced by the most trifling emotion or exertion ; some slight œdema is probably perceived about the ankles ; the debility becomes extreme, the patient can no longer sit up in bed, the mind occasionally wanders, he falls into a prostrate and half-torpid state, and at length expires ; nevertheless, to the very last, and after a sickness of perhaps several months' duration, the bulkiness of the general frame and the amount of obesity often present a most striking contrast to the failure and exhaustion observable in every other respect."

This form of anæmia, in Dr. Addison's experience, with perhaps a single exception, has sooner or later terminated fatally, and as yet, the examination after death has failed to reveal the fatal mischief. In the case last examined the heart had undergone fatty degeneration, and so had the semilunar ganglion and solar plexus, but this was an isolated case. Now it was whilst seeking to throw some light upon this very obscure form of anæmia, that Dr. Addison discovered a disease, the leading and characteristic features of which are " anæmia, general languor and debility, remarkable feebleness of the heart's action, irritability of the stomach, and a peculiar change of color in the skin, occurring in connection with a diseased condition of the supra-renal capsules." He proceeds:

" As has been observed in other forms of anæmic disease, this singular disorder usually commences in such a manner, that the individual has considerable difficulty in assigning the number of weeks or even months that have elapsed since he first experienced indications of failing health and strength; the rapidity, however, with which the morbid change takes place, varies in different instances. In some cases that rapidity is very great, a few weeks proving sufficient to break up the powers of the constitution, or even to destroy life; the result, I believe, being determined by the extent and by the more or less speedy development of the organic lesion. The patient, in most of the cases I have seen, has been observed gradually to fall off in general health ; he becomes languid and weak, indisposed to either bodily or mental exertion ; the appetite is impaired or entirely lost; the whites of the eyes become pearly ; the pulse small and feeble, or perhaps large, but excessively soft and compressible ; the body wastes, without, however, presenting the dry and shrivelled skin, and extreme emaciation usually attendant on protracted malignant disease ; slight pain or uneasiness is from time to time referred to the region of the stomach, and there is occasionally actual vomiting, which in one instance was both urgent and distressing ; and it is by no means uncommon for the patient to manifest indications of disturbed cerebral circulation. Notwithstanding these unequivocal signs of feeble circulation, anæmia, and general prostration, neither the most diligent inquiry nor the most careful physical examination, tends to throw the slightest gleam of light upon the precise nature of the patient's malady ; nor do we succeed in fixing upon any special lesion as the cause of this gradual and extraordinary constitutional change. We may indeed suspect some malignant or strumous disease ; we may be led to inquire into the condition of the so-called blood-making organs ; but we discover no proof of organic change anywhere,— no enlargement of spleen, thyroid, thymus, or lymphatic glands,—no evidence of renal disease, of purpura, of previous exhausting diarrhœa, or ague, or any long-continued exposure to miasmatic influences : but with a more or less manifestation of the symptoms already enumerated, we discover a most remarkable, and, so far as I know, characteristic discoloration taking place in the skin,— sufficiently marked indeed as generally to have attracted the attention of the patient himself, or of the patient's friends. This discoloration pervades the whole surface of the body, but is commonly most strongly manifested on the face, neck, superior extremities, penis, and scrotum, and in the flexures of the axillæ and around the navel. It may be said to present a dingy or smoky appearance, or various tints or shades of deep amber or chestnut brown ; and in one instance the skin was so universally and so deeply darkened, that, but for the features, the patient might have been mistaken for a mulatto.

"In some cases this discoloration occurs in patches, or perhaps certain parts are so much darker than others, as to impart to the surface a mottled or somewhat chequered appearance ; and in one instance there were, in the midst of this dark mottling, certain insular portions of the integument presenting a blanched or morbidly white appearance, either in consequence of these portions having remained altogether unaffected by the disease, and thereby contrasting strongly with the surrounding skin, or, as I believe from an actual defect of coloring matter in these parts. Indeed, as will appear in subsequent cases, this irregular distribution of pigment-cells is by no means limited to the integument, but is occasionally also made manifest on some of the internal structures. We have seen it in the form of small black spots, beneath the peritoneum of the mesentery and omentum—a form which in one instance presented itself on the skin of the abdomen.

"This singular discoloration usually increases with the advance of the disease; the anæmia, languor, failure of appetite, and feebleness of the heart, become aggravated ; a darkish streak usually appears upon the commissure of the lips ; the body wastes, but without the extreme emaciation, and dry harsh condition of the surface, so commonly observed in ordinary malignant diseases ; the pulse becomes smaller and weaker, and, without any special complaint of pain or uneasiness, the patient at length gradually sinks and expires. In one case, which may be said to have been acute in its development as well as rapid in its course, and in which both capsules were found universally diseased after death, the mottled or chequered discoloration was very manifest, the anæmic condition strongly marked, and the sickness and vomiting urgent; but the pulse instead of being small and feeble as usual, was large, soft, and easily compressible, and jerking on the slightest exertion or emotion, and the patient speedily died.

"My experience, though necessarily limited, leads to a belief that the disease is by no means of very rare occurrence, and that, were we better acquainted with its symptoms and progress, we should probably succeed in detecting many cases, which, in the present state of our knowledge, may be entirely overlooked or misunderstood ; and, I think, I may with some confidence affirm, that although partial disease of the capsules may give rise to symptoms, and to a condition of the general system extremely equivocal and inconclusive, yet that a more extensive lesion will be found to produce a state, which may not only create a suspicion but be pronounced with some confidence to arise from the lesion in question. When the lesion is acute and rapid, I believe the anæmia, prostration, and peculiar condition of the skin will present a corresponding character, and that whether acute or chronic, provided the lesion involve the entire structure of both organs, death will inevitably be the consequence."

Dr. Addison then proceeds to speak of the difficulty attending diagnosis. The sallow anæmic conditions resulting from miasmatic poisoning or malignant visceral disease are the conditions most likely to be confounded with disease of the supra-renal capsules, and this Dr. Addison allows is not at all unlikely to happen in the early stages of the disease. Then follow the cases, of which we give the first in full and the others in abstract.

CASE 1.—James Wootten, æt. 32, admitted into Guy's Hospital, under Dr. Golding Bird, February 6th, 1850. Has been residing at Long Alley, Moorfields, and is by occupation a baker. States that he was attacked with a cough three years since, which he was unable to get rid of by ordinary remedies, and was finally cured at Saint Bartholomew's after taking pills for one week. From this time, his skin, previously white, began to assume a darker hue, which has been gradually increasing. Twelve months after leaving the above hospital, he was laid up from excessive weakness, the result of his cough, which had again appeared, and incapacitated him for his work. He now became an out-patient of Saint Thomas's, under Dr. Gooden, who cured his cough; and thinking that the color of his skin depended on jaundice, treated him for that disease, but to no purpose. He left the hospital in tolerable health, but subsequently lost flesh, and became so excessively weak, the color of his skin at the same time getting rapidly darker, that he applied for admission here, which was granted him.

Present appearances.—The whole of the skin on the body is now of a dark hue, and he has just the appearance of having descended from colored parents, which he assures me is not the case, nor have any of his family for generations, that he can answer for, manifested this peculiarity. The color of the skin does not at all resemble that produced by the absorption of the nitrate of silver, but has more the appearance of the pigment of the choroid of the eye. It seems to have affected some parts of his body more than others, the scrotum and penis being the darkest, the soles of the feet and palms of the hands the lightest; the cheeks are a little sunken, the nose is pointed, the conjunctivæ are of a pearly whiteness; the voice is puny and puerile, the patient speaking with a kind of indescribable whine, and his whole demeanor is childish. He complains of a sense of soreness in the chest about the scrobiculus cordis. The chest is well formed and perfectly resonant; the sounds of the heart are also healthy; there is some slight fulness in the region of the stomach. The urine is of a proper color, and he has passed in twelve hours one and a half pint, which has a specific gravity 1008, an acid reaction, and contains neither albumen nor sugar; there is also some pain, on pressure, in the left lumbar region.

February 8th.—Dr. Bird wished a likeness to be taken, so as to be able to watch any alterations in his color; and, considering the case one of anæmia, ordered Syr. Ferri. Iodidi, 3j, ter die; and middle diet. These he took the whole of the time that he was in the hospital, and was discharged in April, rather stronger, but the color remaining precisely the same.

Shortly after his discharge from the hospital, he was seized with acute pericarditis and pulmonic inflammation, under which he speedily sank and died.

The following is a report of the post-mortem examination:

Lungs universally adherent, the adhesions being very old. The upper lobe of the right lung contained some small defined patches of recent pneumonia, about the size of a crown-piece, surrounded by tolerably healthy structure. The lower lobe was extremely fleshy and without air. The left lung was bound down by old pleuritic adhesions, which were very tough and difficult to be torn through. The substance of this lung was fleshy, and contained but little air. There was no tubercle or cavity. The mucous membrane of the bronchial tubes was considerably injected, and, I believe, rather thickened. The pericardium was distended with fluid of a deep brown color, amounting to about half a pint; recent lymph was effused over the whole serous surface. The liver and spleen were both of weak texture, and easily broken down; the structure of the liver rather coarse. The gall-ducts pervious. The gall-bladder contained the usual quantity of bile, which was thin, watery, and clear. The thoracic duct was pervious throughout, and there was no obstruction to any of the veins or arteries, that I could discover. The color of the blood in the arteries had an unusually dark appearance. The kidneys were quite healthy, and of full size. The supra-renal capsules were diseased on both sides. The left about the size of a hen's egg, with the head of the pancreas firmly tied down to it by adhesion. Both capsules were as hard as stones. Intestines pale. Lumbar glands natural. No tubercular deposit was discovered in any organ. The head was not examined.

CASE 2.—James Jackson, a tide-waiter, æt. 35, married, admitted into Guy's Hospital, under Dr. Addison, 11th November, 1851.

With the exception of a single attack of rheumatism, his previous health had been good, until about six months ago, when he had an acute illness, with vomiting, constipation, headache, and debility. Much debility remained after this illness, and the skin soon began to be bronzed. The color now is a dark olive-brown, and there are pigmentary deposits in the lining of the lips.

The expression of countenance is pinched and anxious; the pulse is of usual frequency, but extremely feeble; the bowels are constipated; there is a disposition to vomit, with some tenderness at the epigastrium. At the beginning there was some numbness of the fingers, legs, and tip of tongue, but this symptom has passed off. After death (the manner of death is not stated), both supra-renal capsules were found to contain compact fibrinous deposits, resembling tubercle, but there was no tubercle elsewhere. The gastric mucous membrane was inflamed.

CASE 3.—Henry Patten, æt. 26, a carpenter, married, and intemperate, under the care of Dr. Rees, November 9th, 1854. Previous health had been very good until two or three months before the color of the skin began to change. The first symptoms were, pain in the back and right leg, followed by debility, wasting, and attacks of giddiness. The color is dark olive-brown, and there are in patches. He is thin, pale, and very feeble, and he is very liable to attacks of fainting. There is sickness and hiccough, pain in back, occasional partial loss of consciousness, angular curvature of spine, and leucocythæmia. He gradually sank into a torpid or typhoid state. Both the supra-renal capsules were completely converted into a mass of strumous deposit, and there were tubercles in the lungs. The lumbar vertebræ were carious, and there was psoas abscess. The spleen was rather large, and the blood leucocythæmic.

CASE 4.—John Iveson, æt. 22, a stonemason, admitted into Guy's Hospital 20th March, 1854. He died on the day following, and no history could be obtained, except that for several months he had been liable to pain in the stomach and vomiting, with tic douloureux. The face, axillæ, and hands, were of a dingy bronzed color. When admitted there was sickness, vomiting, and pain in the stomach, with great debility and some emaciation. He died from collapse, and the prostration preceding death was so peculiar, and apparently causeless, as to suggest the idea of poison having been taken. Both supra-renal capsules were wasted and destroyed (apparently from previous inflammatory disease), and the two only weighed forty-nine grains. No other disease.

CASE 5.—Ann Roots, an adult. This case, which is taken from Dr. Bright's reports, occurred in July, 1829. There is no history. The "complexion very dark." Extreme debility: bilious vomiting; emaciation considerable; abscess in the breast and swelling of the right parotid. "There was no indication," says Dr. Bright, "but to support her strength." She sank gradually, becoming drowsy and wandering occasionally before death. "The only marked disease was in the supra-renal capsules, both of which were enlarged, lobulated, and the seat of morbid deposits, apparently of a scrofulous character." They were four times the natural size, and the left had suppurated.

CASE 6.—R. H—, Esq., a barrister, of middle age. His surface generally is dark and dingy. The face, neck, and arms, are covered with patches of deep chestnut-brown, with patches of white skin interspersed. There is great anæmia and extreme languor, and some emaciation, but the emaciation is not to an extreme degree. Vomiting is frequent, urgent, and distressing, suggesting the idea of malignant disease of the stomach. The pulse is of good size, but exquisitely soft and compressible. These symptoms had continued for about a year. "The patient speedily sank." The supra-renal capsules were greatly enlarged, of irregular surface, and much indurated; the natural structure lost. No nucleated cells could be found.

CASE 7.—M. T—, æt. 60. This woman died of ulcerated cancer of the breast, and the diagnosis of diseased supra-renal capsule was only formed in the post-mortem theatre of Guy's Hospital, when the bronzing of the skin was first noticed. The color of the skin of the arms, chest, and face was of a peculiar light-brown and swarthy hue. The substance of both supra-renal capsules was invaded by a considerable amount of cancerous deposit.

CASE 8.—Elizabeth Lawrence, æt. 53, a servant, and unmarried. Always thin, but otherwise well. She had suffered for four months from dyspeptic symptoms, which symptoms began after she had been cured of a cutaneous eruption. The skin generally is very dark, particularly in the axilla and in the areola, around the umbilicus, and there are some patches of discoloration darker than the rest. She is emaciated and very feeble; she also suffers from irritability of the stomach. She died "from exhaustion" three days after admission into Dr. Babington's ward. After death the left supra-renal capsule was found to be destroyed by cancer, and there was cancer of the pylorus.

CASE 9.—Thomas Clouston, æt. 53, a sailor, married, and sober in his habits. About two months before his admission into Dr. Barlow's ward he began to lose appetite and to feel generally unwell; before this time he had been a healthy, muscular, strong-built man. The face is of a yellow bronzed tint, which became darker while he remained in the hospital. His symptoms were sensation of sickness without actual vomiting, weakness and loss of appetite, rigors every five or six hours, no pain, pulse 80, rather feeble, bowels irritable. He became weaker and weaker, and at the end of a month after his admission, he died. Tubercular deposit was found in one capsule, and also in the spleen and kidneys (the lungs were not examined); black pigment was also found in the omentum, mesentery, and cellular tissue of the abdomen.

CASE 10.—Jane Roff, æt. 28. This patient died of cancer of the uterus, and the discoloration of the skin was not noticed until she was on the table in the post-mortem theatre. The skin had "a peculiar dingy appearance." She died from exhaustion. The vein emerging from the left supra-renal capsule was obstructed by a malignant tubercle, and the organ itself occupied by a recent extravasation of blood, its structure being otherwise healthy. The right capsule was healthy.

CASE 11.—An adult who died of cancer of the lungs,&c., and in whom one supra-renal capsule was found to be entirely disorganized by cancer. The disease of the capsule was not suspected during life; but in the clinical notes of the case we find that "the patient's face presented a dingy hue." There were freckles about the face, and brown discoloration at the root of the nose and the angles of the month.

Since the publication of Dr. Addison's monograph, considerable attention has been directed to the subject, particularly by Mr. Jonathan Hutchinson, whose able report in the "Medical Times and Gazette" is deserving of all praise. This gentleman, indeed, has brought together the evidence adduced by Dr. Addison himself, and by others, and his comments upon the whole are of considerable value.

Mr. Hutchinson collects six cases in which the disease was unequivocally present, and nine cases in which the existence of the disease was not verified by post-mortem examination. We give the first six cases in abstract:

CASE 1.—An unmarried hawker, æt. 24, under the care of Dr. Burrows, in St. Bartholomew's Hospital, April 7th, 1854. In childhood he had had lumbar abscess. The first symptom of the present disorder was pain in the back. This was followed by emaciation and bronzing of the skin. This was eight months ago. The entire skin is of a dark copper-bronzed tint, with lighter patches on the chest and belly. The skin of the scrotum is almost black. The present symptoms are irritability of the stomach with vomiting, pain across the back with great debility, emaciation, partial loss of appetite. Death followed from the exhaustion occasioned by a dose of aperient medicine. Both supra-renal capsules contained pus, and some concrete bodies resembling hardened tubercle, and this was the only disease to be found.

CASE 2.—Charles Webb, æt. 24, a carpenter, admitted into Guy's Hospital, under Dr. Barlow, July 24th, 1855, and reported by Dr. Gull. Temperate. Previously robust. Five months ago he began to suffer from debility, breathlessness on exertion, nausea, "biliousness." The skin generally is of a sallow olive brown, and most so about the knees. There are patches of black pigment within the lips. The symptoms were nausea, vomiting, great malaise and exhaustion, emaciation. The blood was loaded with white corpuscles. Urine healthy. He died rather suddenly from exhaustion. Both supra-renal capsules were atrophied and destroyed, the left containing cysts, the right some solid concretions No other organs were examined.

CASE 3.—A man, aged 27 or 28, was admitted into the work-house, at Purton, Wilts, under the care of Mr. R. Hall Bakewell, and died in a few minutes after admission. The entire skin was of a deep brown or bronzed appearance, the color being darkest over the thighs. He died from the exhaustion consequent upon a short journey, and nothing was known about his previous history except that he had been for some weeks in a low and weak state. He was not materially emaciated. Both supra-renal capsules were completely atrophied, and contained calcareous concretions. The lungs were emphysematous, and there was fatty degeneration of the heart.

CASE 4.—A baker, æt. 20, a patient in the Middlesex Hospital, under Dr. Thompson. Previously of good health. Six weeks ago the skin began to be bronzed, and this was the first symptom of disorder. When first seen the entire skin was of a peculiar dark dirty-brown color. Three days before his death he became suddenly languid, and then sank gradually into fatal collapse. There were no rigors. Each supra-renal capsule was as large as half a kidney; its structure was quite destroyed, being converted into a firm tubercular-like material, and in parts softened down. No tubercle was found elsewhere.

CASE 5.—C. Burke, æt. 20, under the care of Mr. H. Curling, at the Royal Sea-bathing Infirmary at Margate (the case is reported by Dr. Rowe, March 24th, 1856) for strumous disease of the knee-joint. His health had always been delicate. Eight months ago the skin began to be bronzed, and now the skin generally is brown with some darker spots. His general health, however, seemed to improve until the 2d of August, when, after having suffered from diarrhœa for two days, he had an epileptic fit. During the next day and the day following he had several such fits, and he was greatly distressed with vomiting. On the 3d he was violently delirious, and on the 4th he died in a semi-comatose state. The discoloration of the skin had become much darker during the three or four weeks preceding his decease, and a disgusting odor was exhaled from the breath and skin. He was fat and muscular to the last. Both supra-renal capsules were destroyed, and contained cheesy, gritty, and semi-purulent deposit, and this was the only visceral disease which could be found.

CASE 6.—John D. Burrows, æt. 57, a publican, of intemperate habits, admitted into St. Bartholomew's Hospital, under Dr. Farre, April 1st, 1856. He suffered from delirium tremens when admitted. A year previously he had suffered from pains in the loins. The entire skin was of a peculiar yellowish brown, and this state had existed for three weeks or more. He died from delirium tremens after a fortnight's illness, sinking into a typhoid state, with low delirium, for some days before death. Both supra-renal capsules were converted into abscesses, but their cortical structure was not wholly destroyed. There were circumscribed abscesses in the loins.

Besides these cases Mr. Hutchinson collects ten cases (one communicated by Dr. Ranking) in which the symptoms during life were such as to warrant the belief in the existence of disease in the supra-renal capsules, but in which the diagnosis was not confirmed by examination after death. These cases are very interesting, but they cannot well be admitted as evidence.

Commenting upon the entire number of cases, Mr. Hutchinson says:

"In twelve both supra-renal capsules were proved by post-mortem examination to be destroyed by chronic disease, and in every one of these the change in color of the skin was marked and positive, and the death had been attended by peculiar symptoms of debility. In seven others no post-mortem was obtained, but the kind of cachexia and mode of death had very closely indeed resembled those in which, after death, the theory was confirmed. In one, the patient is still living, the symptoms quite corresponding with those usually met with, and appearing to be irremediable. In one, both organs were affected by recent suppuration, and in this only a yellowish brown tint was noticed, the disease having probably not existed long enough to produce the characteristic pigmentary change of hue. In four, the disease affected but one of the organs, the other remaining healthy, and in these only a slight (but yet positive) degree of the bronzing had been observed. It cannot be necessary to stop to point out that the but partial extent to which the change in tint of the skin had proceeded in the latter cases, so far from constituting any exception to Dr. Addison's opinion, strongly confirms it. Just in proportion to the extent to which the supra-renal organs are structurally disorganized, and to the length of time which they have been so, appears to be the intensity of the cutaneous discoloration. From this it seems fair to argue, that they probably stand to each other as cause and effect, and are not coincident effects of some other cause. Thus, then, of the whole number recorded (twenty-eight) we have twenty-five the evidence of which is more or less in favor of the theory under discussion."

Nor is it different with the three seemingly exceptional cases.

"In case No. 26, the patient recovered, and after lasting somewhat more than a month, the peculiar 'dirty brown tinge' of the skin disappeared. Now there is every reason for believing, that, in this instance, no pigmentary change had taken place, and that the state described was rather a diffused muddiness than a real bronzing. The reason for believing so is, that the change took place suddenly, and was complete in the course of a day or two. Possibly it was of hepatic origin; at any rate it may be presumed to have had a different cause from that of the change which in all the other cases was very slowly progressive, and requiring several months for its development. In the second exceptional case, a woman who died of cancer had shown no alteration in the color of the skin, and yet malignant deposit was found in both supra-renal bodies. Here, however, a considerable degree of functional vigor may have been retained, since neither organ was wholly involved, and in one, only a few small nodules existed. It is very possible that the portions remaining healthy may have sufficed for the wants of a body which had been reduced to extreme emaciation by a long-existing disease. Case 21 of the Table supplies us with what is more like a real exception than any other. It is, however, to be remarked, that no mottling of the skin had been observed, only a diffused muddy condition, and that some doubts had been expressed during life as to its being an example of true bronzing. The patient, moreover, had not been seen by the reporter for some months prior to death, and no note was made as to the state of the skin at the date of that event. On account of these circumstances of doubt, we may, perhaps, fairly hold this case as not proving anything, and if so, the whole of the seeming exceptions are disposed of."

Mr. Hutchinson's report also furnishes us with what is very necessary to enable us to form an opinion upon the subject of which it treats. It shows us that the signs of diseased supra-renal capsules are not present when these organs are healthy. This part of the report is from the pen of Dr. Wilks.

"In confirmation of the views held by Dr. Addison respecting the connection of disease in the supra-renal capsules, and a peculiar discoloration of the skin, I may state that the negative facts which we have now obtained in large numbers at Guy's Hospital, all tend to prove the same point. Since that physician commenced his researches on the subject, every opportunity has been taken to test his conclusions by a careful observation of the supra-renal organs in the bodies of all that have undergone a post-mortem examination, and during the last two years no case has failed to pass under the observation either of Dr. Habershon or myself. During this period, in the making of above five hundred inspections, only two cases have been met with where disease of these organs was found without having been previously diagnosed. In the first (published in Dr. Addison's book, Case 11, p. 39), a patient had died of cancer, and in one supra-renal capsule was discovered a large mass of cancerous disease which involved its entire structure. Before death, no particular notice had been taken of the browning of the skin, but, on referring to the clinical clerk's report, it was found stated that 'the patient's face presented a dingy hue.' This report was confirmed on more careful inspection of the skin, there being freckles on the face and a slight brown discoloration at the root of the nose and at the angles of the mouth. In the second case, a few malignant tubercles grew from the surface of one of these organs, but did not encroach upon its structure. In this the skin was not browned. In no other case has any appreciable disease been discovered, although it might have been supposed that the supra-renal bodies would not have escaped in those instances where the whole of the abdominal organs have been infiltrated with cancer or tubercle. Such, however, has not been the case; for, on the contrary, when they have been affected, the disease has generally been isolated or has occurred in independent growths. These facts, then, tend to strengthen the conclusions arrived at by Dr. Addison.

"When I speak of disease of those organs, I mean the palpable destruction of their substance by adventitious deposits, as cancer or tubercle, for the morbid changes in the supra-renal capsules, allied to the results of inflammation or degeneration of other viscera, have yet to be studied, nor can they be appreciated unless the observations of those peculiar bodies be much farther pursued, and their healthy anatomy better ascertained. That the healthy or normal appearance is not understood, is seen in the fact, that anatomists have taken different conditions as illustrating the standard of the healthy organ. Thus Frey, in the 'Cyclopædia of Anatomy,' says that the supra-renal capsule is divided into a cortical and medullary substance, the former being yellowish-brown and the latter reddish-brown: the delicacy of the medullary substance and its vascular nature making it very decomposable, and causing the appearance of a cavity after death. Kölliker gives a similar description of the cortical substance, but states that the medullary is of a grayish-white color, that its consistence is less than that of the cortical, and that after death the two portions of the organs become separated, and that often a cavity is thus formed in the centre. These appearances given by Frey and Kölliker are both met with, but that by the latter is no doubt the normal one; the former author's description is, therefore, very apt to mislead, for if the usual healthy appearance of the organ is red, as he states, the white substance, when found, may be mistaken for the result of disease, which has been sometimes the case. The account given by Kölliker, I believe to be the more correct, because in persons who have been killed by accident in whom I have purposely examined these organs, the central medullary portion has been of nearly a grayish-white color, and in those who have been the subjects of cardiac or pulmonary obstruction, or in those long dead, the centre has been generally red and soft. This, however, is not sufficient to account for the different appearances met with, and it still remains to be decided, whether they be due to disease, age, or post-mortem changes; I believe myself that the latter is the cause.

"If a section be made through what I believe to be the normal organ (a), the cortical portion will be seen in a narrow rim forming its periphery, and consisting of a rather soft substance of a yellow or yellowish-brown color, the inner edge generally the darker. This structure, as is well-known, is composed of radiating rows of tubes (b) or apparent tubes (at all events the fibrous envelopment sends in processes between the rows of vesicles), contained large oval vesicles, arranged end to end, and which structure is readily displayed by the addition of liquor potassæ to the microscopic section (c). The medullary portion is white and harder (not softer, as Kölliker says) than the cortical; it is composed of another tissue containing nucleated cells and nuclei (e). Within this again is a brownish substance of greater or less extent, immediately surrounding the supra-renal vein, sometimes altogether wanting, at other times existing, to the total absence of the normal white substance (d). In a good specimen, this white medullary part may reach to either end of the organ, but, if not, it is generally found in the middle portion surrounding the large venous trunk, for at this part a piece of the organ being as it were pinched up (and thence its resemblance to a cocked hat), it is of considerably greater thickness. It may, however, as before stated, be altogether absent and replaced by the brown soft medulla described by Frey. It is of primary importance to know the usual appearance of the organ as presented to the naked eye, but its minute anatomy is very interesting, as well as its vascular and nervous supply. The arteries coming from three different sources make it more

A.

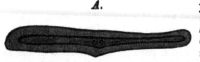

difficult to inject through them, but through the single large venous trunks it

B.

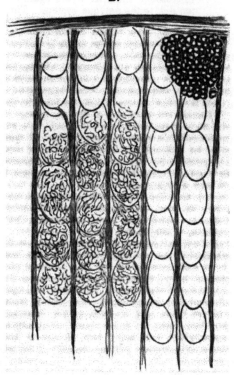

is very readily done. The distribution of nerves is remarkable from its extent.

"It will be seen that the organ requires much further study in order to ascertain if the differences in its appearance, above given, be really due to decomposition, or are in fact pathological;—other morbid changes also have yet to be observed. With reference to the amount of fat present, I may state that this varies very much in the cortical portion, both as granules in the cells, and as free globules, in the same way as in the liver and other organs. In some cases, I imagine the excess amounts to a true fatty degeneration."*

We have here, then, evidence of a new and very important disease, a disease which will, in all probability, explain the physiological uses of the supra-renal capsules. What these uses are we have yet to learn.

"Systematic physiologists," writes Dr. Gull, "have

C.

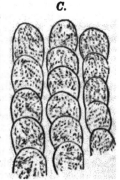

* *Explanation of the Engravings.—A.* Section-diagram of a healthy organ, showing the soft, yellow cortical portion—the inner dark border of the cortical portion—the white and firm medullary substance. In the centre of the latter are seen the cut extremities of two veins. (Not magnified.)
B. Magnified horizontal section of the cortical structure. showing the fibrous envelope sending in trabeculæ by which the columns of vesicles ⸱re separated and converted into apparent tubes. In the upper right-hand corner is seen a cluster of fat-vesicles, with pigment.
C. The cortex after treatment with acetic acid, the fibrous partitions having been rendered transparent. and the rows of vesicles alone remaining visible.
D. Section-diagram of an organ, in which the medullary portion has been converted from a whitish to a dark-brown structure. (Less than the natural size.)
E. Cells from the medullary portion.

classified the supra-renal capsules with glands, for no other reason than that they could not conceive what else they should be; but recent

D.

microscopic inquiries would again refer them, as Wharton did, to the nervous system. This celebrated anatomist, after reciting the names which had been applied to them, says, 'Many others might, probably, be given, but that which seems to me to square with them most is "glandulæ ad plexum," or, "glandulæ ad plexum nervium." After contending that these organs do not belong to the lacteal system, he en-

E.

larges on their remarkable connections with the ganglia of the solar plexus, and states an obscure hypothesis of their separating a fluid from the nervous structures into the veins.

"Though our advances in the physiology of nervous action give no support to such an hypothesis, it is yet probable that, in the remarkable nervous connections of the supra-renal capsules, he pointed out the foundation of their physiology. It is impossible for any one to survey the anatomical relations of the semilunar ganglia to these organs, without feeling how strong the probability is of such a conjecture.

"Their general and microscopical anatomy is also more or less confirmatory of such a view of their function, as well as the newly-observed clinical facts when they are diseased, namely, the great exhaustion, the feebleness of the heart's action, the nausea, vomiting, &c.

"The two structures which compose the capsules are similar in general and microscopical appearance to the two structures which compose that appendage to the brain, which we still continue to call the pituitary gland. Also the remarkable venous sinuses which bathe the one, are comparable to the numerous veins which fill the interior of the others. The most distinguished of modern anatomists have admitted that the medullary structure of the capsules is similar to the gray matter of the brain, and Kolliker, in his 'Microscopical Anatomy,' says, that he cannot but agree in those views, especially as he finds in this structure caudate cells which very much remind one of nerve-cells; and he adds, that the cortical and medullary portions entirely differ from the parenchyma of the thymus or thyroid with which the renal capsules have been associated; while the enormous supply of nerves to the medullary portion gives them a character quite peculiar, since we have no secerning organ in the body remarkable for its nervous supply."

Be this as it may, however, the pathological facts remain, and the thanks of the profession are due to Dr. Addison for the discovery of a new disease, and for the elegant and perfect manner in which he has made that discovery known.

I. *Quarterly Returns of Deaths in England and Wales during* 1855.
II. *Weekly Returns of Deaths in London during* 1855.
III. *Quarterly Returns of Deaths in Scotland during* 1855.[*]

I. Contrasted with previous seasons, 1855 proved more salubrious in England than usual, especially during its latter portion. Unlike 1854, last year was comparatively healthy, being free from any severe visitation.

Before entering into particulars, it seems interesting to state that, throughout England and Wales, the total deaths, from all causes, amounted, in 1855, to 426,242, or 11,997 fewer than in the year immediately preceding, when 438,239 fatal cases of every kind were recorded. Therefore, notwithstanding some exceptions, afterwards specified, public health appeared on the whole satisfactory, if not better than in several former seasons, when the general population was less considerable. This feature proved especially prominent during the third and last quarters of 1855, when the aggregate deaths were 185,053, instead of 241,189 in the previous six months; thus giving a diminution of 59,136, or upwards of one-fourth, if compared with the mortality recorded in the first and second quarters of last year. In reference to which result it ought, however, to

[*] As on previous occasions, we are indebted to Dr. Webster, F.R.S., for the present able Report.

be stated, the greatest increase of fatal cases occurred during the first quarter, or coldest months: when 134,605 human beings were called to their final account, thus giving 28,025 deaths beyond the number reported in the subsequent three months, or April, May, and June. This forms an instructive fact; and shows that, the public health had already become ameliorated, and so continued uninterruptedly throughout each subsequent division of the year.

Notwithstanding these general remarks, during the first three months of last year, it appears several diseases proved very fatal. Thus, in some parts of Surrey, as at Guildford and Farnham, small-pox and bronchitis prevailed extensively, owing to the severe weather and high price of provisions. Scarlatina was very rife in Kent; and at Dartford small-pox became so common that, from 40 to 50 cases occurred simultaneously: but the only deaths thereby occasioned were in persons not vaccinated. In Winchester many individuals died from pulmonary diseases, whereby the general mortality became unprecedentedly high. At Exeter catarrh seemed epidemic; and the extreme severity of the cold produced a number of deaths from diseases affecting the respiratory organs. Typhus prevailed much at Polman, a seaport in Cornwall; whilst at Truro the deaths ranged considerably above an average, in consequence of the prevalence of influenza. In some central districts the public health was by no means satisfactory. For instance, at Bedford the deaths were nearly double the average, such mortality arising from bronchitis, pneumonia, and influenza. At Dudley also, fatal cases were more numerous than in any previous quarter, particularly from pneumonia among children; 90 persons having died of that malady, 30 by bronchitis, 20 from fever, and 5 of cholera, during three months. Scarlatina proved very fatal in many districts of Lincolnshire; whilst in some parts of Lancashire the public health fell under an average. However, in Chorlton the quarter showed an excessive mortality; seeing, in the Hulme district alone, out of 564 deaths, 245 were caused by diseases of the chest and respiratory organs: occasioned mainly by intense northeast winds, which proved more than usually destructive to human life, but especially among children, and aged persons, of whom 11 were from 80 to 93 years old at death. Again, in the Regent Road district of Salford, scarlatina of a very malignant type prevailed; whilst many old people died of bronchitis. Lastly, in the Deansgate division of Manchester, the total mortality proved very high during the quarter, pulmonary diseases having carried off 164 cases, and pertussis 27, all being children. Such subjects also often became victims of other maladies, since, out of 340 deaths registered in this locality, 166 were those of young persons under 5 years of age. Some parts of Yorkshire were likewise far from healthy; Knaresborough having suffered from very malignant and fatal scarlatina. In Todmorden the deaths were also much above an average, but principally among young children and old people, by pulmonary diseases. At Scarborough, likewise, an increase in the number of deaths occurred, especially from measles and bronchitis, which proved often fatal amongst young and aged persons. Further, Penrith exhibited an excess of deaths, scarlatina having proved very fatal; the same at Cockermouth, where that disease and measles were very prevalent and fatal. In some districts of Wales, the mortality ranged likewise above an average. Thus, at Newport, scarlatina, typhus, pertussis, bronchitis, as also pneumonia, were very rife, and caused death in a great number of children. At Holywell, scarlatina and influenza were very common and fatal. Much the same may be said respecting Wrexham: where measles, scarlatina, pertussis, and pneumonia caused an increase of deaths during the early part of this quarter, when severe weather, with high-priced provisions, produced considerable effect on the health of young and old people.

During the second quarter, although the public health throughout England exhibited some improvement, compared with the previous three months, still, the mortality was greater than in the corresponding period of 1854: an actual increase being then recorded of 3918 deaths. In the Southeastern districts, several diseases were rather prevalent; for instance, at Canterbury, small-pox, scarlatina, and bronchitis seemed unusually rife. In Guilford the deaths were above an average; whilst Farnham suffered much from measles, hooping-cough, and low fever; whereby the fatal cases ranged nearly fifty per cent. more than in some former periods. Worthing also proved most insalubrious; the mortality in the district of Broadwater being sixty per cent. beyond an average; and in that of Littlehampton the ratio appeared considerably increased, owing to the prevalence of scarlatina and measles, which proved lethal amongst young children. Both at Alverstoke and in the city of Winchester the deaths exceeded the number of births; scarlatina having been fatal to many young children in the former district; whilst that disease, measles, pulmonary affections, and erysipelas were common in the latter; such sickness being referred to the protracted and unusual coldness of the season. In the towns of Bedford and Northampton an augmented rate of mortality was observed, chiefly from scarlatina and pneumonia. Again, in some parts of Cambridgeshire, as at Newmarket and Caxton, the same maladies likewise prevailed; deaths by the former disease having become unusually numerous amongst children, in the above-named celebrated horse-racing locality. Although several districts in the eastern part of England were healthier than ordinary, Norwich, Thetford, and some places besides, however, supplied a higher proportion of deaths than ordinary; small-pox, measles, and scarlatina having raged epidemically throughout certain parishes, both of Essex and Norfolk. In Wiltshire, Devon, Cornwall, and Somerset, the mortality rose higher than that reported during the previous year; although, in other parts of the southwestern division, it was about an average. The excess of deaths proved considerable in Chippenham, Stoke Damerel, and Liskeard; whilst the mining population in Cornwall by no means exhibited satisfactory sanitary conditions. Throughout Staffordshire and Warwickshire the mortality ranged lower during this quarter, than that reported in the preceding spring; but scarlatina, measles, and variola were reported as prevailing in some districts of Shropshire. In Lincolnshire the ratio of deaths was above, but in the counties of Derby, Notts and Leicester it fell below, that of the previous spring quarter. But scarlatina having proved rife in Horncastle, Caistor, Gainsborough, and the city of Lincoln, that malady caused an augmented mortality in these localities. Although at some parts of Lancashire public health was unsatisfactory, in consequence of measles and scarlatina having prevailed throughout several districts, and whilst the mortality rose higher in Manchester than during the two previous springs, Liverpool, on the contrary, seems to have been unusually salubrious. For instance, in the West Derby district of that hitherto often unhealthy commercial town, the population was reported in a very favorable state. This was said to be owing to the great extent of street and house-draining and cleansing, and to other sanitary improvements. Wigan was likewise stated as healthy; street-sewerage, drainage, and the removal of nuisances being there in active operation. At Bury, the deaths ranged also under the average; whilst the mortality of Chorlton fell below the ordinary amount; proving the healthy condition of that district. Similar remarks apply to other localities, amongst which Ashton-under-Lyne may be enumerated. Here, notwithstanding fewer deaths than usual were recorded, it appears that, amongst 179 cases of fatal disease in the Dukinfield district, actually 41 persons who died were medically attended by persons who hold no legal qualification: irrespective of those patients so treated who recovered. This is a truly lamentable condition for Ashton-under-Lyne, which ought to be investigated judicially, and, if possible, corrected by the public authorities. Throughout Yorkshire the deaths reached below an average number, the decrease being chiefly in the West Riding; particularly at Leeds and Sheffield, which were healthier than in the two previous springs. Some localities, however, of the East and North Ridings, exhibited an augmented mortality. Thus, at Beverly, Driffield, Thirsk, and Northallerton, the deaths were above an average: scarlatina in a malignant form having been very prevalent in the latter town, where three deaths took place in the same house, within two weeks, from that malady. The northern portion of England experienced an ordinary amount of sickness followed by deaths, but especially from small-pox and scarlatina, which proved fatal in some districts of Durham, as likewise in the county of Northumberland; the latter, or variola, having been very rife at East Chevington, where, however, the cases proved of a mild character in patients previously vaccinated, although severe when not so protected. In the principality of Wales nothing very remarkable was exhibited, the mortality being near an average, notwithstanding measles prevailed at Abergavenny, Crickhowell, and Swansea; in which latter place, 44 fatal cases occurred thereby in 206 deaths.

The improvement noticed in the second quarter, which, as already stated, characterized public health, continued even more remarkable during July, August, and September, than in the three months immediately preceding. The returns of deaths exhibiting, as their general result, a striking amelioration, contrasted with those reported in the summer quarter of the previous year. This feature may be further illustrated by the circumstance that, the annual rate of mortality, during these three months, was about 18½ deaths per 1000 persons living; while the average proportion of the summer quarter, in the previous ten years, reached to nearly 22 deaths per 1000 inhabitants. Viewed, however, in reference to town and rural populations, the fact is worth recording that, the annual rate of mortality in the former was rather more than 21½ deaths per 1000 residents; but in the latter the ratio scarcely exceeded 16½ per 1000; being thus upwards of 5 fatal cases more comparatively, in towns, than in the open country.

Although sanitary reports proved satisfactory from the southeastern parts of England, some districts experienced considerable sickness. Thus, fever prevailed at Bromley amongst children, and at Gillingham, on the Medway, dysentery, diarrhœa, and rubeola, were common; the deaths having been increased by fatal cases amongst invalids from the Crimea, as also of some seamen belonging to the Baltic fleet. Further, at Folkestone, the deaths far exceeded an average, caused by cholera, which had been present amongst soldiers of the British Foreign Legion. The counties of Essex, Suffolk, and Norfolk were however marked by salubrity; the mortality having fallen to nearly the same extent as in the other division. Indeed, the rate even ranged lower than that recorded during 1853, which was reported healthy. In most midland districts the deaths were also less by nearly one-fifth, than those enumerated during the summer quarter of the previous year. Scarlatina, on the other hand, prevailed in Bedford, as also diarrhœa and typhus fever; 28 persons at least having died of the above eruptive malady; amongst whom 14 were children aged 3 years and under. It should be here specially mentioned, in reference to scarlatina, notwithstanding many fatal cases of that epidemic occurred in the better classes, a great majority of deaths from this and other zymotic diseases, took place in the most drained and most densely populated localities, Bedford, in its sanitary condition, being reported as very unsatisfactory.

Throughout the southwestern counties the mortality likewise ranged below an average compared with the former parallel season; hence showing a favorable sanitary condition amongst the population: independently of any previous removal of weakly people by epidemic cholera. At Redruth, for instance, the quarter proved unusually salubrious; the healthy condition of the residents being ascribed by local authorities, to the fact that frugality in eating and drinking prevailed; whilst greater attention had been given to sanitary matters. At Bedminster, notwithstanding the deaths were under an average, it deserves notice as an instructive fact, that nearly one half of the fatal cases reported were of children under one year old. The midland parts of England, like most other districts, furnished a low rate of mortality; Wolverhampton, Dudley, and other populous localities having been salubrious. But although Birmingham lost some lives by diarrhœa, this large town, always considered healthy, proved unusually so during last summer. Cheshire and Lancashire supplied reports of a similar satisfactory character: the total deaths in these two densely peopled counties having been only 14,903, against 17,229 during the previous parallel quarter; that is 2326 fewer fatal cases. Nevertheless it should be added, diarrhœa prevailed in Chester: and one death from cholera was registered. On the other hand, Liverpool and Manchester exhibited signs of increased salubrity. In Yorkshire the sanitary improvement was equally satisfactory; especially at Leeds and Hull, which were healthier than usual. Newcastle-upon-Tyne, Sunderland, and Tynemouth, like many other localities, experienced a low rate of mortality. Whereas, Morpeth proved unhealthy, various epidemics having there been prevalent, especially scarlatina; which in one of the sub-districts, caused 19 deaths amongst a total mortality of 70; whereby the number of casualties from all diseases exceeded an average, if compared with the last six years. Lastly, in Monmouthshire, and throughout Wales, the mortuary rate, during the three months under consideration, ranged below either of the summer quarters of the two previous years; in fact, such a healthy season has seldom been experienced as the one briefly alluded to in the present paragraph.

During the last three months of 1855, the sanitary condition of both town and country districts continued to improve. Contrasted with the parallel quarter of 1854, the actual diminution amounted to 12,545 deaths. Amongst urban populations, the rate of mortality ranged 24 in 1000 residents; whereas in country parishes, it fell so low as 18 in every 1000 inhabitants; the average amount, during ten preceding corresponding seasons, being nearly 26 deaths in 1000 residents throughout large town districts; and 20 in the small town or country localities. The southeastern parts of England were comparatively healthy, the deaths being slightly below an average; Croydon and Dartford, which had formerly suffered from epidemics, being now more salubrious. Small-pox prevailed at Canterbury, and scarlatina in the Isle of Wight and at Winchester. Although the mortality was much lower in many south-midland counties, still epidemics prevailed in a few districts. Thus, variola proved fatal at Ware, in the densely populated courts and alleys of that town: where vaccination seems to be much neglected. In Royston, typhus was very prevalent: sanitary arrangements having been greatly overlooked. Scarlatina raged fatally in Welwyn, Harpenden, Chesham, Bedford, with other districts of that county; as also in Ely, Wisbeach, and Cambridge, where fever was likewise present; whilst small-pox occasioned some deaths in these counties. Mortuary reports ranged at a low figure in East Anglia; with the exception of Risbridge, King's Lynn, Saffron Walden, and several other localities. Scarlatina proved prevalent, and in a malignant type, at Downham; as also in the Ingatestone sub-district. Erysipelas, chiefly of the face, was very common in Coggeshall; whilst several fatal cases of typhus and scarlatina occurred in the parish of Ramsey, near Harwich: which is considered a most unhealthy place, being near a large marsh, and much in want of drainage. Contradistinguished to this unfavorable condition, it merits mention that, at Sudbury, not very distant, only 54 deaths out of a population comprising 8000 persons, were reported during six months: and an improvement in the health of another district, viz., Rattlesden, was ascribed to sanitary regulations; thus furnishing an instructive example for others to imitate. In the southwestern counties, the mortality was below an average, although scarlatina and fever became prevalently fatal throughout several districts.

Such was the general character of public health, in this division of England; but it should be here mentioned that, in consequence of the wreck of a large barque, near St. Keverne, in Cornwall, the burials were greatly in excess: the bodies of 93 persons having been cast ashore from the above vessel. Similar to most places of South Britain, the counties of Gloucester, Hereford, Salop, Stafford, Worcester, and Warwick, experienced a rate of mortality much below their average; the total casualties in these districts being 11,172, against 13,611 during the corresponding quarter of 1854, thus giving a diminution of 2,439 deaths, or more than one-fifth. This decrease of mortality being most striking in large towns, viz., Bristol, Clifton, Wolverhampton, Dudley, and Birmingham. In Coventry, however, there was very little decrease of deaths: many children under three years of age having died in the Holy Trinity sub-district of that city, from diarrhœa and convulsions. Lincoln, Leicester, Nottingham, and Derby proved likewise salubrious; but in Cheshire and Lancashire the improvement of public health was less extensive than in some other counties; the deaths in Liverpool and West Derby, where scarlatina prevailed epidemically, having been numerous, besides many fatal cases at Runcorn, by the same malady. Manchester and Salford, however, exhibited more salubrity. Lastly, it should be again specially noticed that, at Ashton-under-Lyne, no less than 62 persons who died, out of 248 recorded in the Dunkinfield district of that town, were actually attended by individuals *holding no medical qualification!* Surely the magistracy are sound asleep, or have abdicated their functions! Throughout Yorkshire, public health was again satisfactory, a considerable decrease of mortality having been experienced: although fever proved very fatal amongst children at Halifax. Scarlatina was rife at Knaresborough, and that eruptive malady, as also measles, raged near Northallerton. In various districts, for example, at Leeds and Hull, improved sanitary arrangements were reported as having contributed materially towards the healthy condition of residents, which facts are highly satisfactory and most creditable to all local functionaries.

The influence of various causes upon public health may be well illustrated by a reference to the township of Thornton Steward, where, in consequence of an overflow of water from the River Ure, nearly 40 cases of typhus were produced in a population of not more than 200 inhabitants. Again, although the counties of Durham, Northumberland, Cumberland, and Westmoreland manifested, speaking generally, a mortality below the average, nevertheless, scarlatina prevailed with much severity in the colliery districts of Durham, especially at two villages situated in Easington, where the epidemic was most fatal; augmented, doubtless, by the low situation of these localities, and from the soil being damp, marshy, and badly drained. At South Shields, near which many men were employed in the construction of an extensive dock, typhus and scarlatina prevailed; and in one district of Gateshead the deaths were numerous by the latter disease: hence making the aggregate mortality above an average. Lastly, in Morpeth, disease fearfully prevailed, whereby the deaths increased more than ordinary. Small-pox raged among all classes, affecting both old and young; those not vaccinated being great sufferers. Scarlatina and typhus were likewise prevalent, several cases of illness having very rapidly had a fatal termination. The Principality, on the whole, proved healthy, the aggregate mortality having been reported less than in the two previous years, although typhus and scarlatina attacked some districts, as Tremadoc, in North Wales: where, among a total of 57 deaths, 33 were children, cut off by scarlatina. Notwithstanding these exceptional facts, the public health of England and Wales exhibited unequivocal evidences of improvement.

Vaccination having recently become the subject of much discussion, even in high places, and the legislature, whilst extraordinary opinions have been enunciated, almost characteristic of the dark ages, one or two remarks on that important subject cannot seem out of place, before concluding the present outline of the sanitary condition of England.

Although cow-pox is now very much neglected in various districts, and at some places, such as Newport, Monmouthshire, there is felt a great objection on the part of the people to vaccinate their children, the operation being, as they even assert, followed by loathsome diseases, still this valuable prophylactic does not seem, according to the published reports, in so much disfavor as some years ago. It is also satisfactory to find, wherever small-pox has proved fatal, a great majority of these deaths occurred amongst children who had never been vaccinated; whilst in some places, vaccination is stated to be now more attended to than formerly. Thus, at Barnsley, in the West Riding, 440 children are reported to have been successfully vaccinated during six months. Further, it deserves being mentioned that, in St. Peter's district, Brighton, out of 1383 births registered last year, 1274 genuine cases of cow-pox were certified by qualified practitioners. These are gratifying facts, indicating improved public opinion; and if more judicious legislation were enforced, doubtless greater progress in advance would be accomplished.

When it is remembered that, prior to the introduction of vaccination, small-pox often carried off many thousand persons during a few months, even in London, which had not half its present population; whilst further, 20,000 persons are said to have died by variola in Paris during 1720; and also that it frequently ravaged many European countries, even more destructively than the plague; the recent mortality by so very loathsome a disease is by no means discouraging, notwithstanding much blind prejudice and ignorance, respecting the great benefits of cow-pox, may yet prevail amongst some classes of the community. Lastly, seeing that only 12,561 persons have died in the metropolis from variola during the last fifteen years, it is plain that vaccination must have saved thousands upon thousands.

On a former occasion, several remarks were made in reference to promoting vaccination more generally, throughout all classes, especially the ignorant and prejudiced; the chief suggestion then offered being, to compel every person, prior to accepting any public appointment, or receiving pay from Government, to prove they had first been properly vaccinated. Such regulations now work

well in other countries. Therefore, were somewhat similar rules established in
Great Britain, and carried out effectually, few outbreaks of epidemic small-pox
would be heard of, like the occurrences recently reported from ships of war on
service, or in various militia regiments. These suffered much, according to
public and authentic statements, in consequence of variola having broken out
amongst both seamen and recruits, who had never been vaccinated. Farther,
many of the metropolitan police are not protected by previous vaccination,
which deserves censure, seeing their duties often expose them to infection, even
more than most classes. The fact of small-pox having been frequently observed
amongst policemen, is shown by the number of constables belonging to that body
sent to the Small-pox Hospital during last year, when affected by this disease.
According to the registers of that public charity, which are most carefully kept
by Dr. Munk and Mr. Marson, nineteen policemen were admitted during 1855,
of whom four died. Two of the above fatal cases had never been vaccinated :
whilst the remaining seventeen were reported to have had cow-pox, chiefly in
infancy. Most of these presented cicatrices more or less perfect; but none, so
far as the able medical officers of the institution could learn, had undergone re-
vaccination. In all likelihood, had it been possible to ascertain the whole truth,
perhaps few would have been considered properly protected, when they first entered the corps. Similar reasoning applies with equal force to those regiments
of militia and ships' crews, where variola is reported to have recently broken
out amongst the recruits. Instead of idly talking so much about compulsory
vaccination, public authorities ought at once to interfere, and prevent such dire-
ful consequences in future by employing only protected persons.

To illustrate the perils that often follow small-pox, when affecting an individual,
the subjoined instructive example may be quoted from the ' Progrès d'Yvres'
newspaper, which very lately supervened in Flanders. In a cabaret called " La
Bascule," near one of the gates of Menin, four persons were playing cards at a
table in the public room, into which a child—then very ill with small-pox and
delirious—rushed from an upper apartment it had occupied. Although this
patient remained only a very short time near the guests, all four were soon afterwards attacked by variola of the most virulent kind, whereby the whole party
died successively ! Instances like these prove the value of cow-pox; and to
demonstrate the different aspect this question now exhibits, contrasted with even
not very ancient times, an observer need only look around in every large assemblage of men and women, to see how rarely any individual really bears marks
of small-pox; or to hear how very seldom an acquaintance has fallen a sacrifice
to the above, formerly so often fatal, disease. Regarding that point, the following truly graphic and most apposite account, copied from Macaulay's " History
of England," when relating the death of Queen Mary, which was caused by
small-pox, in 1694, deserves being here quoted as an apt illustration. The
great historian justly says—" That disease, over which science has since
achieved a succession of glorious and beneficent victories, was then the most
terrible of all the ministers of death. The havoc of the plague had been far
more rapid ; but the plague had visited our shores only once or twice within
living memory, and the small-pox was always present, filling the churchyards
with corpses, tormenting with constant fears all whom it had not yet stricken,
leaving on those whose lives it spared the hideous traces of its power, turning
the babe into a changeling at which the mother shuddered, and making the
eyes and cheeks of the betrothed maiden objects of horror to the lover." All
enemies of vaccination should study that picture: next ponder impartially over
the spectacle they may now almost everywhere behold : mark the great difference, and then acknowledge their erroneous opinions, in reference to the prophylactic effects of cow-pox.

II. Analogous to the country generally, London exhibited a diminished rate
of mortality during 1855, compared with the previous twelve months: although
nearly the same in amount to that of 1853, notwithstanding the recently
augmented metropolitan population. Last year, 61,506 persons died throughout
London : whereas, during 1854, the total deaths were 73,697, thus giving a decrease of 12,545, or one-sixth of the whole. Such being the aggregate mortality

of last year, it hence follows, that in the metropolis, with an estimated population of two millions and a half, the mortality ranged at the rate of 24 deaths to every 1000 persons living: or one in 41 inhabitants. This result seems, on the whole, satisfactory, considering the proportion, in some former years, occasionally rose beyond that amount; nay, even reached 30 deaths in every 1000 residents. Different metropolitan districts, however, enjoyed various degrees of salubrity. Thus, the mortuary rate ranged, in 1855, from 23 in 1000 throughout the western and northern divisions, to 25 in 1000 in the eastern districts. Again, the most unhealthy portion of the whole year was towards the end of January; whilst the periods when fewer deaths, than those reported at any other, occurred in the third week of July and the second week of October. It should, however, be remembered that, cholera prevailed like.a pestilence during the autumn of 1854; whereas last year, the same epidemic proved comparatively rare, and was very seldom fatal. But on this point, further remarks will be made subsequently.

Various diseases exhibited an augmented mortality during the past year, compared with the number of deaths by similar maladies in 1854; notwithstanding the general salubrity proved so satisfactory, as already mentioned. Amongst these complaints may be enumerated small-pox, which caused death in 1024 persons, instead of 676 during the previous year. Croup was also fatal in 535 cases, in place of 488; mortification 216 to 189; phthisis 7545 to 7107; bronchitis 5512 to 4549; disease of heart 2188 to 2062; asthma 728 to 661; gastritis 102 to 82; ascites 172 to 147; and lastly want of breast-milk was reported to have prematurely cut short the mortal existence of 358 human beings just entering into life: the number of deaths in infants, by the same cause, being 325 during the previous year. Such lamentable results—chiefly owing to the unnatural custom of employing hireling nurses by the higher classes of society—cannot be too strongly condemned, seeing its lethal effects are becoming, by every annual report, more appalling. The total fatal cases through privation of that best of food for babes—their own mother's milk—being now double in amount, compared with those recorded only five years previously.

Deaths by violence have also increased, when viewed in the aggregate. Some of the causes enumerated in this category have certainly proved less lethal, although others were oftener followed by loss of life, than in the year preceding. Thus, notwithstanding 1803 human creatures were killed by accidental causes, during 1855, throughout the metropolis, against 1767 in the previous twelve months, several serious casualties were less numerous. For instance, 100 persons died from wounds, against 108 the former year; 324 by drowning instead of 344; and 68 by other kinds of violence not specified instead of 83. Notwithstanding the results just mentioned, a very common cause of violent death proved oftener fatal last year, than the preceding, namely, burns and scalds: 341 persons having lately perished thereby, against 274 during the previous twelve months.

The precarious tenor of human life amongst the laboring population of London is well illustrated by such facts; many of whom being engaged in dangerous occupations to gain their livelihood, such deadly consequences become less remarkable and may be explained. That actually one person in every 34, of all whose mortal career was cut short, during the past year, should have died through violence, constitutes a most important fact, and ought to make some impression upon parties having the power to correct several causes by which these deaths were produced. Legislation cannot remedy every evil; nevertheless, much might be accomplished by greater care and attention on the part of those pursuing hazardous employments. Hence, such subjects merit future legislative consideration.

Contra-distinguished to previous statements, showing an augmented mortality by several diseases, others exhibited a decrease, of which the most marked seemed cholera. By this epidemic malady it appears 146 persons died, throughout the entire metropolis, during the last year, against 10,708 the preceding. In fact, this disease was rarely observed, being only partially prevalent, in the third quarter of the year, when 106 such deaths were reported. Upon which point it may be interesting to state that, in one locality, namely, the neighborhood of Golden Square, St. James's, Westminster, where.cholera severely devastated the population almost like a pestilence during the autumn of 1854, this district last year became comparatively healthy. Diarrhœa likewise proved less fatal, the deaths in 1855 being 2061, instead of 3235 during the previous year; by measles 864 died, in place of 1399; by scarlatina 2602, against 3439; by typhus 2332, against 2669; by dropsy 829, against 893; by paralysis 1180, against 1276; by convulsions 1937, against 2144; by enteritis 297, against 324; by diabetes, 38 against 62; and lastly, carbuncle, whereby 53 deaths were reported, instead of 91, as in the previous year.

Similar to what has been often previously remarked, even amongst so large a population as that congregated together in the metropolis, various diseases were characterized by a remarkable uniformity of mortuary results. For example, hooping-cough was fatal in 2415 cases, against 2471 the previous year; rheumatism and rheumatic fever 309 to 322; cancer 1055 to 1021; hydrocephalus 1531 to 1560; apoplexy 1382 to 1323: pneumonia 3992 to 3976; abscess 126 to 123; jaundice 181 to 182; nephria 200 to 195; stone 34 to 33; cystitis 37 to 37; disease of uterus 149 to 150; and finally, by affections of joints 181 fatal instances were reported, in place of 179 in the former parallel twelve months.

Reviewing the mortality of the entire year, nothing remarkable, in reference to any particular disease, seems to have occurred. It is, however, interesting to state that typhus fever, although less frequent than the two previous years, proved more prevalent in some districts of London than in others; the fewest deaths by that malady having been recorded in the central and northern divisions, the greatest number in the south and east. Thus, in central districts the mortality by typhus ranged as one to every 1264 residents; whereas, in eastern, the proportion was so high as one death by typhus fever in every 840 persons then living. Much the same remark may be made respecting small-pox: that disease having proved most fatal in the eastern and southern districts of London, but least in the western. Somewhat analogous observations apply to measles and scarlatina, the former of which was more common throughout the east, but the latter malady in south portions of the metropolis. In short, speaking generally, with reference to epidemics and zymotic diseases, all low level districts situated south of the river Thames usually prove more insalubrious, than dwellings occupying the higher positions lying north and west of that boundary.

The total deaths which were reported from the various public institutions of London next constitute a curious feature in its aggregate mortality; 11,310 residents, or 18 38 per cent., having died in these establishments, that is, nearly one-fifth of the entire number. The largest proportion, or 6552, being in workhouses, while 2956 persons died in general hospitals during 1855, almost two-thirds of whom were male patients. In workhouses the reverse prevailed : more females having ended their days within these eleemosynary institutions, than in general hospitals. On the other hand, the very few deaths recorded in prisons becomes an interesting illustration of the salubrity of such establishments. Only 71 prisoners died therein during the entire year, 14 being females. Considering the fact, that usually about 6500 inmates are confined in London gaols, whilst upwards of 43,000 individuals annually pass through those receptacles—in 1854 the actual numbers were 43,834—such a small mortality like the above indicates an unusual salubrity of London prisons, which speaks favorably of their management and sanitary disciplinary arrangements. In truth, it may be now confidently asserted—confine persons of depraved habits, defective moral principles, irregular conduct, or those who possess no control over themselves, especially when addicted to crime. If then in bad physical health they will often be restored thereby to much better condition, both mentally and bodily, than that previously manifested.

During the past year, an important addition has been made by the Registrar-General to the mortuary report of London : viz., the occupations of male persons, aged 20 years and upwards, whose deaths were recorded in the metropolis. This constitutes a very interesting feature, and is highly suggestive of much useful meditation : particularly, as it indicates the salubrity or unhealthiness of numerous employments, in which large bodies of men are usually employed. In order to convey some idea of the different questions thus mooted, the following table indicating the comparative rate of mortality, in several occupations, has now been compiled by way of specimen. Being calculated upon the number of individuals living in London, at the census of 1851, returned as belonging to the various trades and occupations then enumerated, but here divided by the actual deaths of each category during 1855; of course, the ratio thus obtained must only be considered as an approximation. Remembering always that no statistical deduction can become valuable, unless based upon a large array of facts, whilst inferences derived from very limited numbers are generally fallacious, and hence may lead to error, only those occupations in which many persons were habitually engaged have been selected, in order thereby to illustrate more conclusively the instructive questions now proposed for investigation.

Comparative Rate of Mortality in Different Occupations.

Architects and Artists	one in 64	Hatters	one in 46
Bakers	" 48	Horsekeepers, Grooms, &c.	" 64
Boat and Barge-men	" 40	Hawkers and Pedlars	" 26½
Bookbinders	" 41	Inland Revenue Servants	" 30
Booksellers and Publishers	" 54	Inn and Eatinghouse-keepers	" 39
Brewers' Servants	" 29½	Ironmongers and Manufac-	
Bricklayers and Laborers	" 34	turers	" 52½
Brush and Broom-makers	" 43¾	Laborers, General	" 42
Builders and Laborers	" 37	Legal Profession	" 55½
Butchers	" 47	Literary Men	" 58
Cabinet-makers	" 51½	Masons	" 32¾
Carmen	" 32	Medical Profession	" 77
Carpenters	" 46	Merchants and Bankers	" 58
Chairmakers	" 54	Military Men	" 28½
Cheesemongers	" 47	Musicians	" 34½
Chemical-makers	" 141	Musical-instrument-makers	" 59
Civil Service	" 49¾	Omnibus and Cab-men	" 30
Clergymen and Religious		Painters and Plumbers	" 41
Teachers	" 63	Pensioners, Chelsea	" 13½
Clerks	" 36	Pensioners, Greenwich	" 11¾
Coachmakers	" 39	Policemen	" 82
Coachmen and Postboys	" 53	Plasterers	" 35½
Coalheavers	" 29½	Printers	" 53
Coopers	" 42¾	Publicans	" 27
Cowkeepers and Milk-		Saddlers	" 37
sellers	" 41	Sawyers	" 33
Curriers and Tanners	" 67	Seamen	" 23
Drapers	" 89½	Servants, Domestic	" 66
Druggists	" 65	Servants, Inn and Hotel	" 30
Dyers	" 49	Shipbuilders and Laborers	" 27
Engine and Machine-makers	" 57¾	Shoemakers	" 46½
Engravers and Copper-plate		Shopkeepers	" 35
printers	" 53	Silkmanufacturers	" 48½
Farriers and Veterinary Sur-		Stationers	" 40
geons	" 34	Tailors	" 44½
Fishmongers	" 44	Tallow-chandlers	" 53¾
Gardeners	" 41½	Tobacco and Snuff-sellers	" 48¾
Gold and Silver-smiths	" 45¾	Travellers, Commercial	" 43¾
Green-grocers	" 38¾	Turners	" 47
Grocers	" 79	Watchmakers	" 49
Hairdressers	" 51	Wheelwrights	" 44¾

Considerable discrepancy hence becomes apparent, with reference to the varied employments in which particular persons are constantly occupied. For example, by the table, chemical-makers would seem to be a most healthy class of men, since the ratio of deaths was only one in every 141 persons so employed. Drapers come next, of whom the proportion was one in 89½; whilst policemen, being one death in every 82, occupy the third position in this mortuary scale. On the other hand, Greenwich pensioners, as might well be anticipated, exhibit a higher rate of mortality than any other class; the residents at Chelsea being, however, nearly in a parallel position. The former range about one in 12; the latter, less than one death in 14 persons living. Such results must naturally be expected; considering the often advanced ages, previous lives, and former occupations of these parties, whether soldiers or seamen. Similar remarks also apply to military or naval persons, even in the prime of life; seeing the proportion of deaths amongst the first-named class was one in nearly 28, and one in 23 of the latter category. Respecting handicrafts, it is interesting to observe that musical-instrument-makers appear to have followed the most salubrious occupation, the ratio reported being one death in every 59 persons so designated; whereas, amongst painters and plumbers, it was one in 41, and of saddlers, 37 workmen of that category. With reference to professions, medical men occupy the one in the highest position, the ratio of one death in every 77 being exhibited by that class; clergymen follow next, of whom the rate was one in 63; whilst lawyers seem placed in a much lower position, viz., one death in nearly 55 members of the legal fraternity actually alive; hence showing, that for every two medical practitioners who died last year, three men of law also succumbed to disease, if calculated according to their respective numbers residing in the metropolis.

Numerous other interesting comparisons may be made by more minutely examining the document now under review, and which will amply the repay reader's perusal. Thus, the marked diversity of mortality affecting drapers and dyers, the latter being nearly double the former. Grocers and green-grocers also occupy very dissimilar positions to each other. Cabmen likewise died in much greater proportion than coachmen and postboys. Publicans became the victims of disease in far greater numbers, or as two to one, than tallow-chandlers. Persons employed about horses appeared much more healthy than carmen, although in some respects they bear a resemblance, with reference to their occupations; nevertheless, the mortality was exactly double amongst the latter, to that furnished by the former class. Again, brewers' servants died in twice the proportion to that of curriers and tanners. Coalheavers occupied nearly a similar relative position to chairmakers; and lastly, shipbuilders, bricklayers, and housebuilders, with their various laborers, also give very different mortuary results if compared with artists and architects, or even with domestic servants; seeing nearly two deaths were reported among the first, to one in the last category; the contrast being, however, very great as to hotel and innkeepers' servants, who die in a larger ratio than persons in domestic servitude.

Another characteristic feature of this table must not be overlooked, namely, the singular uniformity which several employments therein specified furnish, as to their comparative rates of mortality. Thus, bakers and butchers, however different they may be in position, mode of existence, diet, and other physical influences—which often powerfully affect health—exhibit nearly parallel results, in reference to the calculated number of deaths. Amongst the former class, one person died to every 48, and in the latter, one to 47 then living. This analogy even appears still more interesting, when it is recollected that, bakers consume much vegetable food, are confined in a hot, close, unhealthy atmosphere for many hours consecutively, and also labor chiefly during night time; whereas, butchers seem almost constantly occupied in the open air, often eat animal food, and in order adequately to follow their particular calling, they require to be endowed with strong physical frames. Notwithstanding so great dissimilarity in many points, these two occupations appear nearly on a par with respect to mortuary results. Cheesemongers occupy the same position, whilst fishmongers, who live much in the open air like butchers, carry on business in shops which also possess free ventilation, from being without frontage towards the street, but take more fish than animal food, compared with the former—the ratio being one in 44—therefore follow even less salubrious occupations. Again, engravers of metals, printers, and persons occupied in publishing or selling books, show nearly the same results, in regard to the influence such callings produce upon the individual's health: although the mortality amongst bookbinders was considerably greater, compared with those engaged in printing and bookselling. Literary men, bankers, and merchants, likewise exhibit parallel results: whilst gardeners and persons tending cows, and milksellers also come within this category: the mortality amongst the first-named occupations being one in 58; but gardeners, cowkeepers, and milksellers, give a ratio of one death to about every 41 persons then living, and so employed. Other comparisons might be made: but it seems now superfluous to extend the list, as students may consult the table, and judge for themselves.

Before concluding these remarks on the sanitary condition of London during 1855, one or two general observations respecting the weather and atmospheric phenomena will not be inappropriate, seeing such influences often materially affect public health. Compared with ordinary seasons, last year proved drier than usual, excepting 1854, the amount of rain being 21 inches and a fraction; whereas in 1853, the quantity reached 29·6 inches, and in 1852 it rose so high as 34·4 inches, or nearly two-fifths beyond the gauge of the period now under review, which hence was the reverse of humid. The mean temperature of the air ranged less than that recorded in any previous year, ever since the Registrar-General's Reports were first published, the highest daily average being greatest during spring, and least in autumnal months, but especially towards the latter portion of the year: it having then seldom varied beyond eleven degrees in one day during the last ten weeks, and generally about nine; which constitutes a very slight change in the variable climate of England. Such a limited diurnal alternation of the thermometer, as that now mentioned, contributed greatly to the good physical condition of the people, which characterized that portion of the year. Indeed, physicians may confidently expect, whenever much difference of temperature is observed betwixt day and night time, particularly should dryness of the air alternate with humidity, if diminished electrical tension prevails, or the barometric pressure ranges low, with a still, hazy atmosphere, then sickness more frequently supervenes, and mortality appears augmented in consequence. When opposite atmospheric phenomena obtain, assuredly public health will be promoted, and the season prove *pro tanto* salubrious.

III. Scotland having established, after much discussion and some delay, through adversely interested parties, an official registration of births, marriages, and deaths, resembling the plan now pursued in England, the adopted measure promises great and beneficial results, supplies a desideratum long felt, and removes the opprobrium that North Britain was almost the only country in Europe, where such a system was unknown. Nevertheless, although in various respects excellent, respecting one special point, it is defective and highly objectionable, viz.:—that any medical man who shall have been in attendance during the last illness until the patient's decease, must transmit, within fourteen days after death, under a penalty of forty shillings, a certificate of such event to the district registrar. This proceeding seems most arbitrary, and has justly given great umbrage to professional men. If legislators consider penalties advisable, in cases of that description, they should place the responsibilities on the deceased's relatives—certainly not on the attendant, who perhaps may only casually have seen the patient in question. What renders this compulsory clause more unjustifiable is, that no remuneration is provided for the party thus forced to supply important information. When recently visiting Scotland, the writer met various medical friends, who complained seriously of this grievance, and stated that, some had even been called upon, under penalty, to certify respecting the death of individuals, to whom they had only given casual advice, and of whose disease, and its subsequent fatal termination, they retained scarcely any distinct recollection. This summary mode appears, indeed, over-legislation, and should be altered forthwith. No similar tyrannical treatment towards medical practitioners prevails in England; whilst there the existing system acts satisfactorily, notwithstanding the certifiers are also not remunerated. Therefore, any penalty is wholly superfluous, besides being unjust; and instead of proving useful when dealing with gentlemen, it will more likely even produce an opposite effect; and hence may tend to prevent accuracy in returns thus obtained gratuitously.

The registration of deaths, now under review, having only come into operation on the 1st of January, 1855, no comparison can consequently be instituted with previous mortuary details; so that any remark which is subsequently made, upon the sanitary condition of North Britain, must be wholly confined to the past year. During the above period, the total deaths registered amounted to 62,154; being in the proportion of about one death to every 48 persons living. This indicates a rather favorable state of public health: although it must be recollected, at the same time, as the system of registration was new, and the people not yet fully accustomed to its working, every fatal termination of disease may not have been communicated. Nevertheless, last year's rate of mortality seems to have ranged lower than in England. As might be expected, however, the proportion of deaths, taken in the aggregate, is more or less exceeded by all those counties where a large number of the population reside in towns. Thus, in Lanarkshire —the Lancashire of Scotland—the ratio of mortality was so high as nearly one in 37; whereas, in Orkney, it was one in 67; in Peebleshire, also, one in 67; but in the county of Clackmannan the proportion of deaths was reported as one in 68 persons then living; being almost half that of Lanarkshire.

On the other hand, the difference as to mortuary details among town inhabitants, compared with residents in rural districts, was strikingly manifested during the past year.

Throughout the former localities, which had a population of nearly one and a half millions, and contained every large town, the percentage of mortality reached one in 38; whereas, in country parishes, with an equal population, the amount of deaths was only one in 58 residents; thus showing a greater loss of human life, from influences connected with urban residences, than elsewhere. In other words, ordinary dwellers in towns, even during the recent healthy ages, died at the rate of 261 out of every 10,000: while the rural population only furnished 169 deaths among the same number of persons. According to these authentic data, Scotland may be stated to have manifested considerable salubrity, and remained free from any general epidemic; that satisfactory condition being, doubtless, in part, owing to atmospheric influences and weather, which often affect physical health. The proportion of deaths, however, ranged higher during the first part of the year, or cold months, than in the mild seasons of summer and early autumn; but they again augmented towards winter; whereby, the most healthy period was August and September; the least salubrious, March and February. The total deaths, amounting to 7227 in February, contradistinguished to 4047, in September; thus showing 3180 less during the latter month, or actually 44 per cent. diminution.

Viewed in reference to particular seasons, the first three months of 1855 were characterized by great mortality—reported as mainly owing to the cold, and other atmospheric phenomena. During this quarter, 19,685 deaths were registered; which gives the large proportion of one in 38 persons living, the majority being females. Although the average mortality over Scotland was thus high, that of some districts, viz., the counties of Berwick, Peebles, Selkirk, and Clackmannan, ranged remarkably low: the rate being only one death in every 53 residents. On the other hand, mortuary reports attained their highest figure in Lanark and Renfrewshire. The ratio giving one death to every 38 persons living, throughout the former, and one in 29 residents of the latter county. Such increased mortality having been produced by an excessive number of deaths, among the over-crowded populations resident in Glasgow, Paisley, and Greenock. One remarkable feature deserves also special notice: namely, the mild and sheltered island of Bute, which, although hitherto generally considered salubrious, proved quite the reverse. Here, the ratio gave one death for every 34 persons living, and thereby exceeding the average of all Scotland, taken in the aggregate.

During the second quarter of last year, a great improvement became evident in the general health, 15,312 deaths being then reported amongst the entire population. Consequently, instead of the ratio of mortality ranging one death in every 37 persons, the proportion fell to about one in every 49 residents. This result, however, varied considerably in some divisions and counties. Thus, in the northwestern districts, whose population is almost entirely rural, the mortality was only one death in every 61 persons living; whereas, in the southwestern parts of Scotland, where most of the large manufacturing towns are situated, the proportion of diseases terminating fatally, reached so high as one case for every 36 residents. This difference may be made more intelligible by stating that, the districts embracing all the most populous towns, and which comprise half the entire population of North Britain yielded 9173 deaths, during the quarter now under consideration; while, the remaining rural districts, embracing an equal population, furnished only 6139 deaths, viz., 3034, or one-third decrease.

If an improvement in the public health was great during the second quarter, the amelioration proved not less marked throughout the three months ending the 30th of September. In that period, the total deaths only amounted to 12,988, being 2324 fewer than those recorded during the previous quarter: and actually 6697 below the numbers reported for January, February, and March. These figures consequently give an estimated proportion of one death to every 57 persons then living. This ratio, however, varied in different localities: the mortality being scarcely without exception highest in those counties where the amount of town inhabitants is greatest; but lowest in districts having an almost entirely rural population. Nearly two thirds of the total deaths, viz., 8093, being reported from the former, and about a third, 4895, from the latter, or rural portion.

Although rather under the first two quarters of last year, the aggregate deaths during the fourth exceeded, but not materially, the number registered in the three months immediately preceding. During the quarter, 1416 deaths were reported throughout Scotland. That gives the low proportion of one case of disease having a fatal termination, in every 53 persons then living. This result, however, varied considerably in different counties: having been noted in Nairn and Sutherland as one death in every 108 persons, whilst throughout the whole northern districts, the ratio ranged at one in every 82 residents. On the other hand, in the southwestern or manufacturing counties, the proportion reached to one death in 44 inhabitants. But restricting such estimates to Lanarkshire alone, the mortality rose so high as one death in every 23 persons residing in that county. Respecting the different rates noticed in town and rural populations, a discrepancy was strikingly manifested during this quarter. Thus, in the divisions which include all the populous towns, 8934 deaths were recorded; while the remaining, or rural districts, having the same amount of inhabitants—or half the entire population of Scotland—only furnishes 5228 deaths; thereby showing that a loss of 3706 lives probably originated from influences mainly connected with residence in towns. At all events, the marked distinction now mentioned amply merits special consideration.

Notwithstanding the generally healthy condition of the public throughout North Britain, particularly during the latter half of last year, virulent epidemic attacks of small-pox and scarlet fever prevailed in different localities. Still, in every place where variola broke out, it deserves to be mentioned that, nearly all the fatal cases from this malady occurred among those who had not been vaccinated. Indeed, by many persons, that invaluable safeguard appeared wofully neglected—hence throwing much discredit upon public authorities, as also the people generally. This conduct doubtless originated either in gross ignorance, wilful neglect, or obstinate prejudice against the protective influence of vaccination; and even that occurred in a country much famed for its often intellectually cultivated population. These remarks respecting variola apply, in a special manner, to such places as Dundee and Greenock, where the above loathsome disease has, for some years past, caused nearly double the average mortality thereby recorded in English towns: which hence makes this fatality truly excessive.

Various questions of exceeding interest might be mooted in reference to the sanitary condition of residents, in that part of the British Empire now under review. But only one point will be in conclusion noticed, namely,—the very large proportion of young children who were cut off, either by disease or otherwise, below five years of age, and often much younger. This peculiarly striking feature portrayed by mortuary details, was especially observed in town populations. The amount being generally greatest in Glasgow, Dundee and Greenock. In these localities, the death-rate of such children often exceed 50 per cent. of the total mortality. Nay, during the month of last September, it was 61 per cent.; and in August immediately preceding, the returns show that 64 deaths in every 100 actually took place amongst young persons under five years of age. Such lamentable results are much to be deplored, and show some social evils must prevail, causing an infantile mortality so high as that recently observed in urban districts. Farther, the number of still-born infants ascertained to have come into the world, but who died at, or previous to their birth, seems likewise to have been considerable. For instance, in Dundee, during most years, the ratio of such casualties was seven and nearly one-fifth per cent.: while in Glasgow, although the proportion was less, it still ranged upwards of seven still-born cases in every one hundred births.

Compared with other large towns, or even capitals, both in England and on the continent, the amount of still-born infants does not often attain so high a figure, as that recorded in several districts of Scotland. Thus, in London, the ratio is about three and three quarters per cent. of the total deaths registered. At Stockholm, the proportion is less than four per hundred. In Berlin it fell under five per cent. In various large towns of France the number of still-born infants is below either Glasgow or Dundee, besides various other Scottish districts. For example, in Bordeaux the rate ranges under 2½ per cent.; in Rouen it is less than 5¾; in Lyons 6¾; in Paris 7¾, or nearly the same amount as in Dundee; but at Marseilles the rate rose higher, being 7¾ in that populous commercial community. These varied statements are both curious and instructive, whilst they illustrate the very grave question now brought under discussion. Indeed, with reference to that portion of the British dominions, which has been but briefly noticed in the present report, all vital statistics of the above description, based upon official documents, seem so remarkable, and assume such an important feature, that they demand serious attention by the legislature and philanthropists, with a view to mitigate or prevent, if possible, similar calamitous consequences in future. Few investigations could be of greater importance, or fraught with more benefits to the poor and laboring classes of the community.

The data upon which useful deductions could be fairly inferred being yet only of a rather limited character, it appears somewhat premature to compare, with any precision, the salubrity of particular localities; especially in reference to the special diseases which have proved most fatal in various districts. Nevertheless, one or two general remarks may very legitimately be made respecting three of the most populous towns of North Britain, in order to show how far the mortality occasioned by several diseases—not epidemics—differed during the past season. Take, for example, Aberdeen, situated on the east part of Scotland, which has about half the population of Edinburgh, likewise lying on the eastern coast, and compare these cities with Glasgow, located on the western portion of the island, but containing double the number of inhabitants to Edinburgh. Some very interesting results may then be obtained; seeing diseases of the respiratory organs, such as pneumonia, bronchitis, and croup, proved much more fatal in Glasgow, than either in Edinburgh or at Aberdeen. Thus pneumonia caused twice as many deaths in Glasgow as in Edinburgh, and near four times as many as in Aberdeen. Bronchitis exhibited analogous results also amongst the residents of each of these towns; whilst croup was five times more deadly in Glasgow than in Aberdeen.

Again, enteritis prevailed with greater severity at Glasgow than in either Edinburgh or Aberdeen. Indeed, that disease proved three times more fatal in the first named city, compared with the latter: whilst apoplexy oftener caused death in the capital, than elsewhere. On the other hand, phthisis seemed nearly uniformly destructive throughout all populous towns: whereas, typhus became much oftener a fatal disease in Aberdeen and Glasgow than in Edinburgh. This appeared to have been likewise the case with dropsy; that malady having occasioned upwards of twice the number of deaths, at Aberdeen, in reference to their aggregate populations, if compared with the Scottish metropolis. Reviewing the whole subject, it may then be very confidently asserted that Glasgow, comparatively speaking, is much more insalubrious than any other city, not only in Scotland, but also in Great Britain. This may be confidently asserted, but, at the same time, it is only justice to state (and it gives us much pleasure to be able to make this statement) that this sad stigma will soon be removed by the sanitary improvements which are now being carried out on all hands, by the energetic and intelligent municipality of this city.

II.

REPORT ON THE PROGRESS OF SURGERY.

On Aneurismal Sacs. By W. Colles, Surgeon to Steevens' Hospital, Dublin.
("Dublin Quarterly Journal of Medicine," Feb. 1856.)

In this paper Mr. Colles advances a doctrine originally propounded by his late father in 1810—that *the striated substance contained in the sac is an effusion of lymph poured out by the sac itself,* and not (as is usually held) a deposit, in some unaccountable way, from the blood coagulated within the sac. He says—

"If we examine blood extravasated within the body, we find it coagulates; that it becomes enveloped by a layer of lymph effused by the surrounding parts; that this sac encloses and finally absorbs the clot, or, if it be too large to be absorbed, or if any cause excite inflammation, this sac pours out pus, and the cure is effected by suppuration, as in abscess: but we never find the coagulum as if endowed with any action of its own, to be separated into layers.

"We know that if we make an artificial cavity without exposure to the air, as in subcutaneous sections, lymph is effused, which forms a sac if there be any foreign body or blood extravasated; if not, it is poured into this space; this lymph becomes organized, fills up the cavity, and approximates the divided parts, and is either itself absorbed or goes to form new tissues; hence we would expect the sac of an aneurism to be subject to the same laws, and to pour out lymph with the same object. If an increased action be excited in many of the cavities of the body, we find lymph will be effused, and this lymph will often assume the appearance of layers; it is observed in the peritoneum, pleura, pericardium, trachea, bladder, but I think most frequently in the subcutaneous bursæ, especially in that of the patella. Why this lymph at times is effused in layers, and at others not, is not very satisfactorily understood, though the fact has been frequently observed, and attributed to renewed attacks of inflammation. In aneurismal sacs the constantly dilating force of the blood may renew the irritation, and cause a separation of the outer layers, whose tendency is to contract, from the sac which is forced to enlarge, and thus give rise to a fresh deposit."

Now this view enables us to account for certain peculiarities of aneurism, and it also involves certain important modifications in treatment.

If the laminæ of fibrin within the sac of an aneurism are deposited from the blood we should expect to find the outer layers more degenerate than the inner layers, and quite independent of the sac. But the reverse is the case, for the outer layer is firm and of the yellow color of lymph, it is better organized and its attachment to the sac is such that it cannot be separated without some difficulty and much pain, and, on the other hand, the inner layers are softer, more or less tinged by the coloring matter of the blood, and often detached and shreddy as if broken up and acted upon by the current of the blood. If the layers are deposited from the blood we should expect to find them in all aneurisms, but in reality they are seldom found when the lining membrane is perfect. (They are seldom found under these circumstances because it rarely happens that the lining membrane of the other parts takes on a tendency to pour out lymph, or to adhere to a coagulum if a coagulum forms in contact with it.) If the layers are deposited from the blood we should expect that the great majority of cases of aneurism would eventually tend to a natural cure. On the other hand, the history of aneurism is more intelligible on the supposition that the layers within the sac are formed by secretion from the sac, and this is pointed out by Mr. Colles at considerable length, and with much clearness and cogency of argument.

This view, moreover, is shown to lead to a more accurate plan of treatment.

" We should have," writes Mr. Colles, " two objects in view,—to oppose, to lessen, or entirely stop the current of blood which distends the sac at each pulsation, and by its constant action forces it to work 'its way through the most firm resistance ; at the same time to support the sac in its efforts to resist this distending force by throwing out layer after layer of organized lymph, to strengthen its walls, and fill up its cavity. Thus we find many cases recorded where attention to only one of these objects has resulted in a cure, but the combination of both is, in general, requisite. The first is the principal one, and that which has chiefly occupied the attention of the surgeon ; and I should consider nothing would more effectually promote this object than a closer observance of the practice of the older surgeons : keeping the patient quiet, on low diet, and subjecting him to small bleedings at short intervals ; this may be also assisted by the exhibition of such remedies as control the formation of blood, or the force or frequency of the heart's action. Of the local remedies to effect the same object, recourse is frequently had to the ligature of the vessel, a practice latterly supplanted by the temporary compression on the artery, which retards or obstructs the flow of blood into the sac or breaks the force with which it acted in distending the sac ; so that now the sac goes on contracting, and filling up the cavity with layers of lymph, and is not disturbed in this operation.

· " The latter object, to support the sac, seems to have escaped the consideration of the surgeon, because the idea formerly was that, unless he could make pressure enough to obliterate the sac, or so as to allow the blood in it to coagulate, pressure was useless. But the records of surgery give us innumerable examples of cases in which this moderate pressure was alone sufficient, and often materially assisted in promoting the cure of the disease, especially when combined with frequent small bleedings, though the authors did not endeavor to explain the manner in which this pressure acted. This pressure should be moderate, its only object being to give support ; if more, it would excite inflammation or absorption of the sac, and it would be more effectual when it could be applied so as to control the lateral dilating force of the circulation, as well as the perpendicular pulsation, that is, in cases where the sac is superficial, and the fingers can be passed on all sides of it.

" There is another inference to be drawn from the preceding observations, that is, we should not consider the patient perfectly cured, nor allow him to return to his previous mode of life, or his former exertions—not only till all pulsation within the tumor shall have ceased, but until we consider that there has been time for all blood to have been absorbed from the cavity, and its place supplied by these protruded layers of lymph, which are then in their turn to be removed ; and if, unfortunately, it should so happen that the pulsation does reappear, we are not to despair of effecting a cure, but again have recourse to the pressure, or whatever other means we had been before employing, and which had made such progress in the treatment.

" We perceive that the ligature of the artery below the sac can offer very small chance of success, as it does not moderate, but rather increases the force of the circulation in distending the sac. We see also, that a coagulum in the sac, if large, is a great impediment to the cure adopted by nature, and may even give rise to suppuration within the sac, or may cause only temporary cessation of the pulsation, the disease returning if by any means any fluid blood passes from the artery into the sac. And, therefore, these artificial and chemical means proposed and tried, of causing this coagulation, are, at best, uncertain and too often dangerous, by exciting an inflammation generally of an unhealthy character, and so destroying the patient ; or if he escapes this danger, he must be subject to all the inconvenience of a tedious treatment ; for his cure cannot be perfect,—he will be liable to a relapse any moment, before the complete absorption of the coagulum, and the deposition of firm, solid, adhering lymph in its place.

"From the foregoing considerations we should also be led to infer, that we would have a more rapid cure in those cases in which the sac is soft, not containing many of these layers of lymph; because in old sacs the layers are more firm and unyielding, being acted on by pressure of the blood, and this pressure being removed, the subsequent filling up will be more slow than in a case where there are few laminæ : for, the current being interrupted, the sac itself will close in and contract to a considerable extent, and the subsequent effusion of lymph, being formed free from the action of the pressure of the circulation, will be more considerable, in thick layers, and with a greater tendency in itself to contract.

Asphyxia, its rationale and remedy. By MARSHALL HALL, M.D., F.R.S.

(*Lancet*, March 1, and April 12, 1856.)

The following remarks are deserving of very serious attention, and we give them without any comment, for they are as plain and intelligible as they are important and useful.

" The term asphyxia, which ought to be exchanged for apnœa, designates that condition of the animal system which results from the suspension of respiration.

" Respiration involves two processes—the inhalation of oxygen and the exhalation of carbonic acid.

" *The remedy* for the suspension of respiration is, on every principle of common sense, the restoration of respiration. This view might be considered, irrespective of physiological inquiry and proof, as self-evident ; but that proof is amply supplied by physiology.

" Of the two functions suspended, it is certain, from physiological inquiry, that the retention of the carbonic acid is by far the more fatal, and that, in a word, asphyxia is the result of carbonic acid retained in the blood, which becomes, in its excess, a blood-poison.

" If this view be correct, it is evident that restored respiration is to the blood-poison in asphyxia what the stomach-pump is to poison in the stomach ; and that it is *the* special remedy, the *sine quá non* in asphyxia.

" But this blood-poison is formed with a rapidity proportionate to the circulation, which is, in its turn, proportionate to the temperature. To elevate the temperature or to acclerate the circulation *without* having *first* secured the return of respiration, is therefore *not to save*, but in reality *to destroy life !*

" Now, let me draw my reader's attention to the *Rules* for treating asphyxia, proposed and practised by the Royal Humane Society. They are as follow :

" ' 1. Convey the body carefully, with the head and shoulders supported in a raised position, to the nearest house.

" ' 2. Strip the body, and rub it dry; then wrap it in hot blankets, and then place it in a warm bed in a warm chamber free from smoke.

" ' 3. Wipe and cleanse the mouth and nostrils.

" ' 4. In order to restore the natural warmth of the body,—

Move a heated covered warming-pan over the back and spine.

Put bladders or bottles of hot water, or heated bricks, to the pit of the stomach, the arm-pits, between the thighs, and to the soles of the feet.

Foment the body with hot flannels.

Rub the body briskly with the hand ; do not, however, suspend the use of the other means at the same time ; but, if possible, immerse the body in a warm bath at blood heat, or 100 deg. of the thermometer, as this is preferable to the other means for restoring warmth.

" ' 5. Volatile salts or hartshorn to be passed occasionally to and fro under the nostrils.

" ' 6. No more persons to be admitted into the room than is absolutely necessary.'

" My first remark on these rules for treating asphyxia is, that 'to convey the body to the nearest house,' is doubly wrong. In the first place, *the loss of time* necessary for this purpose is—*loss of life !* on the contrary, not a moment should be lost; the patient should be treated instantly, on the spot, therefore. In the second place, except in very inclement weather, the exposure of the face and thorax to the breeze is an important auxiliary to the special treatment of asphyxia.

"But most of all, the various modes of restoring the temperature of the patient, the warm-bath especially, are objectionable, or more than objectionable; they are at once inappropriate, unphysiological, and deleterious.

"If there be a fact well established in physiology, it is that an animal bears the suspension of respiration in proportion, not to the warmth, but, within physiological limits, to the lowness of the temperature, the lower limit being about 60° Fahr. A warm-bath of 100° Fahr. must be injurious.

"All other modes of inducing warmth are also injurious, if they divert the attention from *the one remedy* in asphyxia—artificial respiration,—or otherwise interfere with the measures to be adopted with the object of restoring this lost function.

"Such, then, are the views which the scientific physician *must* take in regard to the late rules for treating asphyxia promulgated by the Royal Humane Society.

"I now proceed to state the measures by which those rules must be replaced.

"I revert to a proposition already made: as asphyxia is the result of suspended respiration, the one remedy for the condition so induced is, self-evidently and experimentally, the restoration of respiration.

"But there is an impediment to artificial respiration never before pointed out. It is the obstruction of the glottis or the entrance into the windpipe, in the supine position, by the tongue falling backwards, and carrying with it the epiglottis—an event which can only be effectually remedied by adopting *the prone position.*

"In this position the tongue falls forward, drawing with it the epiglottis, and leaving the ingress into the windpipe *free.*

"But even when the *way* is patent, there remains the question, how is respiration to be effected? The syringe or the bellows may not be at hand, and if they were, the violence used by them is apt to *tear* the delicate tissue of the lungs. The mode proposed by Leroy, of compressing the thorax by means of a bandage, and allowing its expansion by the resilience of the costal cartilages, is proved by experiment to be futile, chiefly, no doubt, from its being attempted in the supine position, with the glottis obstructed.

"The one effectual mode of proceeding is this: let the patient be placed in the prone position, the head and neck being preserved in their proper place. The tongue will fall forward, and leave the entrance into the windpipe free. But this is not all, the thorax and abdomen will be *compressed* with a force equal to the weight of the body, and expiration will take place. Let the body be now *turned* gently on the side (through rather more than the quarter of a circle), and the pressure on the thorax and abdomen will be removed, and inspiration— effectual *inspiration*—will take place! The expiration and inspiration are augmented by timeously applying and removing alternately pressure on the spine and ribs.

"Nothing can be more beautiful than this life-giving—(if life *can* be given)— this breathing process.

"In one series of experiments, twenty cubic inches of air were expelled on placing a corpse in the prone position, and ten cubic inches more by making pressure on the thorax and ribs, the *same* quantities being *inhaled* on removing that pressure, and on rotating the body on its side. But I must give the experiments in detail:

"A subject was laid on the table, and pressure made on the thorax and ribs, so as to imitate the procedure of Leroy. There was no result; a little gurgling was heard in the throat, but *no inspiration* followed. The tongue had fallen backwards, and closed the glottis or aperture into the windpipe! All inspiration was prevented.

"Another subject was placed in the *prone* position. The tongue having fallen *forwards*, and the glottis being free, there was the *expiration* of twenty cubic inches of air, a quantity increased by ten cubic inches more on making pressure along the posterior part of the thorax and on the ribs. On removing this pressure, and turning the body through a quarter of a circle or rather more, on the *side, the whole* of the thirty cubic inches of air were *inspired!*

"These manœuvres being repeated, ample respiration was performed·!

"Nay, there may be a question whether such considerable acts of respiration may not be too much.

"It is to be observed, however, that, in this mode of artificial respiration, *no force* is used ; the lung therefore is not injured ; and that, as the air in the trachea and bronchial tubes undergoes little or no change in quantity, the whole inspired air passes into the air-cells, where the function of respiration is alone performed.

"It deserves to be noticed, that in the beginning of this experiment in the prone position, the head had been allowed to hang over the edge of the table : all respiration was frustrated ! *Such is the importance of position.*

"Reserving the full exposition of this method of *postural respiration*, this these-opnœa (from θεσις, position), for another occasion, I will conclude by reducing these views into the simplest *Rules* for the treatment of asphyxia.

"*New Rules for the Treatment of Asphyxia.*

"I. Send with all speed for medical aid, for articles of clothing, blankets, &c.

"II. Treat the patient on the spot, in the open air, exposing the face and chest freely to the breeze, except in too cold weather.

"I. *To excite Respiration,*

"III. Place the patient gently on the face, (to allow any fluids to flow from the mouth).

"IV. Then raise the patient into the sitting posture, and endeavor to *excite* respiration.

"1. By snuff, hartshorn, &c., applied to the nostrils ;

"2. By irritating the throat by a feather or the finger ;

"By dashing hot and cold water *alternately* on the face and chest.

"If there be no success, lose no time, but—

"II. *To imitate Respiration,*

"V. Replace the patient on his face, his arms under his head, that the tongue may fall *forward*, and leave the entrance into the windpipe free, and that any fluids may flow out of the mouth ; then

"1. Turn the body gradually but completely on the *side, and a little more*, and then again on the face, alternately (to induce *inspiration* and *expiration*) ;

"2. When replaced, apply pressure along the back and ribs, and then remove it (to induce further *expiration* and *inspiration*), and proceed as before ;

"3. Let these measures be repeated gently, deliberately, but efficiently and perseveringly, *sixteen times* in the minute, *only;*

"III. *To induce Circulation and Warmth,*

"1. *Continuing* these measures, rub all the limbs and the trunk *upwards* with the warm hands, making *firm pressure* energetically ;

"2. Replace the wet clothes by such other covering, &c., as can be procured.

"VI. *Omit the warm-bath until respiration be re-established.*

"To recapitulate, I observe that—

"1. If there be one fact more self-evident than another, it is that artificial respiration is the *sine quâ non* in the treatment of asphyxia, apnœa, or suspended respiration.

"2. If there be one fact more established in physiology than another, it is that within just limits, a *low* temperature conduces to the protraction of life, in cases of suspended respiration, and that a more elevated temperature destroys life. This is the result of the admirable, the incomparable, work of Edwards.

"3. Now, the *only* mode of inducing efficient *respiration* artificially, at all times and under all circumstances, by the hands alone, is that of the postural manœuvres described in this paper.

"This measure *must* be adopted.

"4. The *next* measure is, I have stated, to restore the *circulation* and *warmth* by means of pressure firmly and simultaneously applied *in the course of the veins*, therefore *upwards*.

"5. And the measure *not to be adopted*, because it tends to extinguish life, is *the warm bath, without* artificial respiration.

"This measure *must* be relinquished.

"These conclusions are at once the conclusions of common sense and of physiological experiment. On these views human life may, nay, must sometimes depend."

On the Average Duration of Life in patients with Scirrhous Cancer of the Breast. By JAMES PAGET, F.R.S., Assistant-Surgeon to St.-Bartholomew's Hospital. ("Lancet," Jan. 19, 1856.)

In a lecture delivered at the Royal College of Surgeons, about four years ago, Mr. Paget stated that the average duration of life in cancer of the breast, when the disease is left to itself, is thirteen months greater than in cases where the diseased breast is removed by operation. Mr. Paget, however, finds that this is an erroneous estimate.

"Records which I have made or collected of 139 cases of scirrhous cancer of the breast, watched to their conclusion, or to their survivals beyond the average duration, give," he says, "the following result:—

"In 75 not submitted to operation, the average duration of life, after the patient's first observation of the disease, has been 48 months. In 64 submitted to operation, and surviving its immediate consequences, the corresponding average has been a little more than 52 months. The longest duration of life, in the former class, has been 216 months; in the latter class, 146; the shortest in the former, was 7 months; in the latter 7½.

"The proportionate numbers of the deaths[*] in each year, after the first observations of the disease, may be represented by the following table:—

			With Operation. Per Cent.		Without Operation. Per Cent.
"In the first year, there died	.		4·7	. .	8·
" second "	.		6·25	. .	22·6
" third "	.		21·8	. .	24·
" fourth "	.		14·	. .	9·37
" fifth "	.		20·	. .	7·3
" sixth "	.		11·	. .	5·3
" seventh "	.		9·37	. .	9·37
" eighth "	.		3·12	. .	2·66
" years after the eighth	.		9·37	. .	12·

"When the extremes of duration are so widely different as they are here shown to be, a perfectly reliable average cannot be obtained, unless the numbers of cases are, on both sides, larger than those supplied by my records.[†] I believe, therefore, that the results here stated are only near the truth, and that the collection of more cases will in some measure alter them.

"Thus, it is nearly certain that the averages stated above are, on both sides, rather too low, for twenty of the patients (i. e., one-seventh of the whole number) are, or were, still living, after having survived the average time of duration with the disease. Moreover, as cases of the longest duration are the most likely to be lost sight of before their record is completed, it will generally happen that a collection of cases will include a disproportionately large number of those of short duration. Allowing, however, for these causes of reduction in the calculated average durations of life, there appears no reason to expect that any number of completed and unselected cases will prove an average duration of more than five years from the first observation of the disease.

"The sources of error above referred to would, I think, especially reduce the estimate of the average duration of the cases in which no operation is performed; for unless cases are kept with an express intention of recording all that occur, without any selection whatever, there will be a tendency to omit a disproportionate number of those which are not made interesting, either by operations, or

---

[*] With the deaths, I have included in this table the numbers of those who are still living beyond the average period. The omission of them would have made no difference in relation to the question concerning the influence of the removal of the cancerous breast.

[†] I could have easily made the numbers larger by including doubtful, or only probable cases of cancer of the breast, but tables so made up seem worse than useless.

by some of those striking events which are most common in acute cases. Hence, the records will generally contain too few of the most chronic cases in which no operation has been performed. I have expressly avoided this error in my own note-books, by avoiding everything like a selection of cases for record; but I cannot be quite sure that the same rule has been observed in some of the records from which I have derived cases observed by others. I can find, however, no reason to believe that any full and accurate tables of cases will bring out, as a result, that patients, in whom cancer of the breast is left to pursue its course, live longer, on an average, than those from whom it is removed. Rather, I believe that, if care be taken in the discrimination of the cases appropriated for the operation, and in the rejection of those that are unfit, there will appear a gradually increasing, though it may be always a small, advantage in favor of the cases in which the breast is removed. Probably it may be ascribed, in some measure, to such care, that the additional and continued cases, which I have tabulated in the last two years and a half, make the average duration in those operated on rather longer, and that in those not operated on, rather shorter than it appeared in 1853.

"With regard to the rules that may be observed in the selection of the cases most fit for operation, I may refer to the published lecture; continued observations having only confirmed the statements made therein. I will only refer to one fact, which the table printed above shows—namely, that the proportion of deaths, in the first two years of the disease, is much less in those who are operated upon, than in those who are left, amounting in the former to less than 11 per cent., in the latter to more than 30 per cent. Such a result, while it justifies the operation in cases of acute cancer, which are not attended with evident cachexia, may be fairly set against the mortality from the operation itself, which I still believe to be not less than 10 per cent."

Three cases of Stricture of the Rectum treated by Incision. By George Murray Humphrey, Esq., Surgeon to Addenbrooke's Hospital, Cambridge. ("Assoc. Medical Journal," Jan. 12, 1856.)

Mr. Humphrey tells us that he was induced to resort to the knife in the following cases, in consequence of the very indifferent success which had attended the treatment of stricture of the rectum by bougies; and most certainly the result is well calculated to satisfy his expectations, and to furnish much matter for profitable reflection to all surgeons.

We leave the cases to tell their own tale, merely adding that they suggest to Mr. Humphrey the three following hints for the future: 1, to prevent the bowels from acting for several days by means of opium, after having first secured (if possible) their complete evacuation; 2, to divide the sphincter ani as well as the stricture; and 3, to endeavor to insert a tube into the bowel after the division of the stricture. The cases are as follows:

CASE 1.—W. H., æt. 30, a healthy-looking man, was admitted, Dec. 17th, 1852, with the usual symptoms of stricture of the rectum. Of these the chief was great difficulty in passing motions, which were never larger than a tobacco-pipe. Sometimes they were loose; at others, nothing passed without the aid of medicine. The stricture was situated about two inches from the anus, with a sharply defined edge encircling a narrow orifice that would not admit the tip of the finger. Several warty excrescences surrounded the verge. There was a fistulous opening in the perinæum, discharging feculent matter; and the presence of the same matter in the urine, with dirty, purulent discharge from the urethra, and pain in making water, proved that a communication existed between that canal and the rectum.

He said, that about seven years ago, when serving as a soldier in India, he had an attack of dysentery. Shortly after his recovery, he was troubled with "piles." A difficulty in passing the motions soon followed, and increased till a twelvemonth ago, since which it had continued about the same. The piles were cut in 1848, which, he thought, aggravated his symptoms. He stated that he never had syphilis.

For some weeks I persevered with the cautious use of the bougie; but making little or no progress, I determined to divide the stricture with the knife. Accordingly, having passed my left forefinger through the narrow orifice, I introduced a blunt-ended bistoury upon it, and freely divided the stricture and adjacent wall of the rectum on one side, including the sphincter ani. This was followed by very great relief. He was soon able to pass the motions with ease, and continued so much better, that, in the latter part of February, he was discharged for a time, at his request. In April he returned, stating that he was still able to pass motions without difficulty, or pain; but the fistula in the perinæum remained, and there was still a brownish discharge from the urethra. Accordingly, I laid open the fistula into the bowel. In June he had nearly reacquired the complete control over the sphincter, though, when the motions were loose, they sometimes escaped. He had no difficulty in passing the evacuations, and the discharge from the urethra had ceased. Still there was some contraction of the bowel in the situation of the stricture.

I have not been able to hear any more of this patient.

CASE 2.—A stout woman, æt. 35, admitted in January, 1855. She had syphilis ten or twelve years ago, and suffered from pain and difficulty in defecation; with discharge from the anus, for eight or nine years. About three years ago a gathering formed, burst beside the bowel, and left a fistula. Others had subsequently formed and burst. There were several integumental excrescences about the anus. The finger found the lower part of the bowel uneven and indurated, and encountered a tight stricture about two inches and a half above the anus. The left side of the buttock was indurated, and there were three fistulous orifices; one, four inches behind the anus, through which the probe entered the bowel a little above the external sphincter; a second, three inches to the side of the anus; and a third more in front. The probe introduced into these did not enter the bowel.

Jan. 27th.—When the patient was under the influence of chloroform, I laid open all the fistulæ, tracing their course with the probe as I cut along, to be sure of following them out. Two entered the bowel below the stricture; the third was continued up alongside the stricture. As I could trace it no further, I pressed my finger through the stricture, and pushing the bistoury alongside it in the ischio-rectal fossa, from the termination of the fistulous track, completely divided the stricture, and laid open the bowel in its lower three or four inches. The incisions requisite to effect all this were very extensive. One vessel bled freely, and was secured by a ligature. A slight attack of erysipelas followed. It did not last long, nor extend far. When it had nearly subsided, I introduced my finger, and finding the passage quite clear, inserted a small speculum vaginæ, securing it there for twenty-four hours by a bandage. Two days afterwards I passed a large rectum bougie into the colon. No other treatment was adopted, except the occasional introduction of the bougie by herself. Gradually the wounds healed; she acquired the power of retaining the motions, and has not, from the time of the operation, experienced any difficulty in passing them. She reported herself quite well when I saw her about a month ago.

CASE 3.—S. H. æt. 35, a delicate woman, admitted in July, 1855, had suffered six or seven years from stricture of the rectum, which had gradually become worse, in spite of the ordinary treatment resorted to on several occasions. Each introduction of the bougie was followed by so great an increase of irritation, that its use was discontinued, and she derived more benefit from cold water clysters than from any other means. Her distress from discharge, frequent worrying action of the bowels, and straining to void the motions, was so great, that she was quite incapacitated for work, and obliged to live by herself. The aperture of the anus was granulated, the lower part of the bowel rather indurated; and the stricture, about two inches above the anus, was so tight, that I could scarcely find the orifice. Encouraged by the case last narrated, I passed my finger through the stricture when she was under the influence of chloroform, and guiding a bistoury upon it, cut through the stricture. I endeavored to insert a tube into the bowel, but relinquished the attempt on finding that it had a tendency to pass into the exposed cellular tissue, where the stricture had been divided, instead of continuing its course in the bowel. Unfortunately the bowels continued in a highly irritable state, and the frequent passage of the motions caused much pain and purulent discharge. These symptoms were combated, to a certain extent, with opium; but the case did not go on so satisfactorily as I could wish. I made no attempts to pass bougies after the operation, because the introduction of my finger, on one occasion, increased her pain for some days. She gradually recovered; and though she still suffers a good deal from slimy discharge and irritation, consequent on a diseased state of the lower bowels, she is able to pass the motions with much less difficulty.

On Mr. Liston's Method of Holding the Knife in Lithotomy. By WILLIAM FERGUS-SON, Esq., F.R.S., Professor of Surgery in King's College, &c. ("Medical Times and Gazette," April 12, 1856.)

The object of the author in this paper (which was read before the Royal Medical and Chirurgical Society, on the 25th of March), is to draw attention to a remarkable error, (as he conceives,) in the illustration of this operation, as portrayed in the works of Miller, Pirrie, Erichsen, and even Liston himself. Mr. Fergusson maintains that it was Mr. Liston's practice to cut with the knife underhand, and not overhand, as is represented in all the works just named; and he accounts for the mistake in the engravings by supposing that Mr. Liston's artist, while intent upon the anatomy of the parts, and the position of the point of the knife, had considered the attitude of the hand as of minor importance. He maintains that Mr. Liston has actually misrepresented his own operation; and that his pupils, while professing to describe it, have taken his representation as the model, and so perpetuated an error which in time might possibly lead to much misapprehension, if not to evil consequences. The paper is accompanied by excellent diagrams, representing, on a large scale, the illustrations from the works alluded to, as well as from the author's own work; and it contains many passages illustrative of the great manual dexterity of the late Mr. Liston, and highly complimentary to that surgeon.

A practical treatise on Diseases of the Testis and of the Spermatic Cord and Scrotum. With numerous wood-engravings. By T. B. CURLING, F.R.S., Surgeon to the London Hospital, &c. Second edition, revised and enlarged. (8vo., Churchill, 1856, pp. 519.)

In this edition some new chapters have been added, many chapters have been rewritten or altered, and all the chapters contain additional facts of practical importance and interest. The work, indeed, is more than ever entitled to be considered as the standard authority on the subject of which it treats.

The author divides his subject into three heads,—diseases of the testis, diseases of the spermatic cord, and diseases of the scrotum. Under diseases of the testis the subjects treated of (a chapter is devoted to each subject) are congenital imperfections and malformations, atrophy, injuries, hydrocele, hæmatocele, orchitis, tubercular disease, carcinoma, cystic disease, fibrous tumor, cartilaginous tumor, calcareous deposits, loose bodies in the tunica vaginalis, fœtal remains in the testicle and scrotum, entozoa, spermatocele, nervous affections, sympathetic and functional disorders, and castration; under diseases of the spermatic cord, the subjects are varicocele, adipose tumors, and spasm of the cremaster, producing retraction of the testis; under diseases of the scrotum the subjects are injuries, prurigo, varicose veins, pneumatocele, œdema, diffuse inflammation, mortification, elephantiasis, adipose tumors, fibrous tumors, cystic tumors, and carcinoma. In each of these chapters we might find abundant matter for quotation, but it must suffice to say that everywhere we have evidence of a well-informed and practical writer. The remarks upon cystic disease may serve as a favorable example of the rest, and with these we will content ourselves. After some preliminary remarks, chiefly upon the anatomical characters of the disease, Mr. Curling proceeds:

"Considerable doubt has long existed in respect to the nature and mode of origin of this disease of the testicle. Sir A. Cooper, who described it under the

name of 'hydatid disease,' evidently supposed that the cysts might be formed
of enlarged and obstructed tubuli; for he remarks, 'although at first sight they appear to be cysts, when traced they are not distinct bags, but send out solid
processes by which they are connected with other bags.'* In this opinion I
was disposed to concur, the disease appearing to me to be analogous to the cystic
tumors of the breast which originate in a morbid dilatation of the lactiferous
tubes. But having subsequently observed in several specimens of cystic testicle
healthy tubuli seminiferi forming a layer spread over the morbid mass, generally
at its upper part, I was at a loss to reconcile the tubular origin of the disease
with this condition of the organ, until the difficulty was solved by careful inquiries which I made in a case favorable for investigation, owing to the early stage
of the cystic development.

"In December, 1852, a man, aged thirty-seven, consulted me on account of
an enlargement of the testicle, which was first observed about seven months
previously. Having no doubt that the disease was either carcinomatous or
cystic, I recommended its removal, and performed the operation. The patient
recovered favorably, and has since remained quite well. On making a section
of the tumor, I found the tubular structure spread over a part of its surface just
beneath the thinned tunica albuginea. The morbid mass was a marked specimen of cystic disease. Some of the larger cysts measured half an inch in
diameter, but the majority were much smaller; and many were no larger than
millet seeds. A great many of the cysts contained a transparent limpid fluid,
others a bloody fluid, a few coagulated blood, and several a solid whitish opaque
matter. The cysts were embedded in fibrous tissue, which was particularly
dense towards the centre of the growth. On examination of thin slices of the
tumor in the microscope, the origin of the cysts in a dilatation of tubes was
clearly made out. Thus, in some specimens, a tube could be traced to a termination in a dilated pouch. In others a cyst appeared to arise from a lateral
dilatation of a columnar tube, or at the extremity of a loop; whilst in others the
dilatation appeared to be uniform. These dilated tubes and cysts were lined by
a tessellated epithelium, and many of them contained a dark granular matter.
The opaque whitish substance found in several of the larger cysts consisted
chiefly of a mass of modified tessellated epithelial scales, and corresponded to
what is called cholesteatoma. No spermatozoa was detected in any of the cysts
or morbid tubes.†

"The minute examination of this specimen fully establishes the origin of the
cysts in a morbid condition of the ducts. The circumstance of the healthy
tubular structure being found external to the morbid growth, shows that the ducts
affected are not the tubuli seminiferi. If the latter were the seat of the disease,
we should expect to find the tubes which remained sound, pushed to one side,
or at any rate near, or mixed up with, the diseased ducts, and not spread over
the surface and distinctly separated from the morbid growth. Nor can the diseased ducts be those of the epididymis, for I have invariably found this part
unaffected or wasted and lost in the morbid mass. If the disease sprang from
the tubes of the epididymis, the tubular structure of the gland, unless destroyed
by pressure, would certainly be found in a mass enclosed in its own tunica, distinct from the morbid growth, and not extended over its surface.

"It being clear, then, that neither the tubuli seminiferi nor the ducts of the
epididymis are the tubes which undergo the changes constituting the cystic
disease, its seat may be considered as conclusively traced to the ducts of the rete
testis. Why they alone are subject to the morbid change, I admit my inability
to explain.

"I have remarked that small masses of enchondroma are frequently mixed
up with the cystic growth. It is clear from recent observations that the enchondroma is originally formed within the tubes and their cystic dilatations. I have
examined with Professor Quekett several specimens of cystic testicle in which
the intratubular development of the cartilage was quite manifest. The cartilage occurs in elongated portions, which are easily detached from the cysts en-

* "Observations on the Diseases of the Testis." p. 83.
† A fuller account of these investigations, illustrated by plates, will be found in a paper communicated to the "Medico-Chirurgical Transactions," vol. xxxvi. p. 449. These observations have since
been confirmed by examination of another specimen of the disease.

closing them. Enchondroma may be developed so abundantly as to encroach upon and obliterate the cysts, and to form the chief bulk of the tumor. This appears to have been the case in a testicle excised by Mr. Hancock, which I have had an opportunity in examining. It weighed four pounds six ounces, and is the largest cystic testicle I have met with. The development of the cartilage within dilated tubes in this specimen is described and figured by Mr. Hogg in the 'Transactions of the Pathological Society.'*

"The minute examination of these cystic tumors shows the non-malignant character of the disease, which, moreover, is fully confirmed by the accounts of those cases in which the history has been preserved, patients having lived many years after the excision of the organ, and died of a different disease. Yet cases occasionally occur, which strongly tend to shake our confidence in this conclusion. Some years ago, a medical friend, aged thirty-two, was attacked with disease of the testicle. It continued to increase in size, and at the end of eighteen months was excised. On a cursory examination of the tumor, I found it to exhibit the ordinary appearances of cystic disease, blood being, however, extravasated in two or three places, which was attributed to some exploratory punctures made previous to the operation. The patient never regained his health, but remained cachectic. In about six months he suffered from hæmoptysis, which was followed by attacks of severe lumbar pain, and subsequently the liver enlarged to a great size. He died eighteen months after the operation. On examination of the body, masses of medullary cancer were found in the lumbar glands, lungs, and liver.

"In a visit which I paid several years ago to the Museum of St. George's Hospital, Mr. Cæsar Hawkins showed me two specimens of well-marked cystic testicle which had been removed by operation, the patients having died within two years afterwards by internal tumors, and he expressed to me his opinion that this disease was a malignant affection. I have recently made a careful examination of these preparations. The soft matter from the cysts of both tumors, when placed under the microscope, was found to consist of a mass of nucleated cancer-cells. Some of them contained numerous dark granules; and where the diseased mass was the softest, the granules were more abundant than the cells, the cell-walls in these instances having been most probably destroyed. In some of the masses portions of ducts filled with cells might be observed. No epithelial scales could be detected in either of the specimens. In one of them there were some small portions of enchondroma.†

"It seems clear from these facts that cystic disease occurs in the testicle in two forms, a malignant and non-malignant, the former being far the more rare. And if the histological observations be fully confirmed, the presence in the cysts of tessellated epithelium will indicate the character of the non-malignant, and the presence of nucleated cancer-cells the nature of the malignant. We shall thus be furnished with the means of determining a most important distinction in practice.

"In describing a malignant form of the disease, I do not comprise cases of encephaloid cancer in which two or three cysts may be found mixed up with the cancerous matter, but tumors the great bulk of which is composed of cysts of various sizes. Indeed, in a specimen of this form of the cystic disease which I have recently examined, the appearances so closely resembled those of the non-malignant form of this affection, that it was impossible to distinguish the difference without the aid of the microscope. It seems probable, however, that although in the early stage of the malignant form the cystic structure prevails, that at a later period the cysts become destroyed by the rapid growth of carcinomatous tissue. This had probably occurred in a specimen in the Hunterian Collection (No. 2416). It is a section of a large tumor of the testicle, the upper part of which is composed of a multitude of small cysts, whilst the remainder exhibits the usual appearances of medullary cancer. The patient died of internal cancer a few weeks after the removal of the diseased organ.

"In the preceding account of a cystic testicle I have noticed the occurrence,

* Vol. iv. p. 180.
† Cruveilhier has described and figured a diseased testicle, which appears to have been a well-marked specimen of malignant cystic disease with enchondroma. This case has already been referred to at p. 303.

in a few well-developed cysts, of a solid whitish matter, exhibiting the characters of cholesteatoma. I have observed isolated formations of the same kind in other cystic testicles, both malignant and non-malignant. In a diseased testicle removed by Mr. Henry Thompson last April, and kindly sent to me for examination, I found a combination of cholesteatoma, enchondroma, and encephaloma, with cysts within the dilated and thinned tunica albuginea. The cholesteatomatous matter existed in great abundance, forming with numerous small deposits of enchondroma a portion of the tumor, the upper, distinct from the larger mass below, which consisted principally of encephaloid growths and cysts. The two portions were separated by loose seminal tubes. The tubes between the cysts were in some parts unaltered, and in others dilated and filled with changed cells.* The patient, a man aged 25, died about five months after the operation of medullary cancer of the lumbar glands, lungs, and other internal parts. In this case, also, it seems probable, that the cystic structure was more perfect in the early period of the disease than at the time of the operation.

"*Symptoms.*—The swelling to which the cystic disease gives rise takes place imperceptibly, very slowly, and without producing pain. After existing for several months, it occasions a chronic indolent tumor of an oval shape and elastic feel, which is scarcely at all tender or painful. The surface of the tumor is generally smooth and even, but is occasionally irregular. There is sometimes fluctuation consequent on the presence of a thin layer of fluid in the vaginal sac surrounding the cystic growth. When the tumor attains a large size it is inconvenient from its bulk, and unless well supported, it occasions a dragging sensation and uneasiness in the loins. The disease usually commences at the middle period of life: I have not myself met with it later than between the ages of forty and fifty. Its origin is often ascribed to some accidental injury of the part.

"*Diagnosis.*—Cystic disease of the testicle may be mistaken for hydrocele, hæmatocele, and encephaloid cancer. The diagnosis from vaginal hydrocele is extremely easy. The tumor is of an oval shape, not pyriform, as in hydrocele; it feels heavier, and fluctuates less distinctly; and there is an absence of the pain experienced in compressing the part usually occupied by the testicle in hydrocele. The swelling also is not transparent. Notwithstanding these distinctive marks, Sir A. Cooper considered that the surgeon was very liable to err, and he admitted that he had been two or three times mistaken, and had put a lancet into the part expecting to find water issue, and a few drops of blood only have followed. The distinction from hæmatocele is much less marked, as the latter has a somewhat solid feel, weighs heavy in the hand, is not transparent, and fluctuates less distinctly than a hydrocele. The absence of pain in compressing the back of the tumor will be the best guide to distinguish the cystic disease from a hæmatocele. As I have remarked in the previous chapter, the characters of the cystic disease are in general so similar to those of encephaloid cancer, that I can give no satisfactory directions for distinguishing them. The surgeon must be guided in his opinion by inquiries into the history of the case, and by noticing the condition of the cord and of the lumbar glands, and the state of the patient's health, which are unaffected in the cystic disease, but are liable to suffer in malignant enlargements of the gland. The tumor produced by the latter affection is also less even and regular, and makes more rapid progress than that occasioned by the cystic disease.

"In cases of difficult diagnosis the doubt may, in general, be safely removed by introducing a trocar into the front of the tumor. A hydrocele or a hæmatocele will be at once made evident by the free escape of serum or blood, and a great reduction in the size of the swelling. If the case be cystic disease, only a small quantity of serum tinged with blood will flow; and if it be a soft cancer, blood of a bright color will probably escape somewhat copiously without producing any diminution in the size of the tumor. In some instances, the existence of the latter disease may be rendered yet more certain by the detection of cancer-cells in the soft matter or fluid found in the canula after its withdrawal. In performing this exploring operation the surgeon should use a common-sized

* For fuller particulars of the minute examination of this tumor by Dr. A. Clark and myself, vide " Transactions of Pathological Society," vol. vi, p. 241.

hydrocele trocar. The bore of the exploring trocar, and the groove of the exploring needle, the instruments commonly used, are not of sufficient size to allow of the ready escape of the grumous blood of an old hæmatocele, or of the matter of soft cancer. The wound of the trocar is quite unimportant. In cases in which an operation is likely to be required, it will often be convenient to defer this exploratory examination until arrangements have been made for further proceedings, if necessary.

" *Treatment.*—No kind of treatment, either local or general, is of any service in this disease, the morbid changes being quite beyond the influence of remedies. The only means that can be adopted is the removal of the tumor, which should be performed as soon as the surgeon is satisfied that the disease will not yield to treatment. The morbid growth should afterwards be submitted to a minute examination, and if no cancer-cells be found, or if the cysts contain tessellated epithelium, he will be able, with some confidence, to assure his patient of his permanent recovery, and immunity from all risk of a relapse."

Amputation of the Knee-joint, illustrated by cases which have occurred in American practice, and mainly by those which have been treated in the New York Hospital. By THOMAS MARKOE, M.D., Surgeon to the New York Hospital. (New York Journal of Medicine, January, 1856.)

In a former volume ("Abstract," XX) we directed attention to the subject of amputation at the knee-joint, and related four cases in which the operation had been recently performed in this country and in France. In our opinion, indeed, the operation is one of great importance, and we are, therefore, very glad to meet with the very able paper of Dr. Markoe now before us.

In this paper Dr. Markoe relates the particulars of eighteen cases in which the leg has been amputated at the knee-joint during the last four or five years. All these cases occurred in America, ten were in the New York Hospital and three were under the care of the author himself. In addition to the cases also Dr. Markoe furnishes us with some valuable comments, and it is upon these that we propose to dwell.

The results of the operation in these eighteen cases agree with the results of European experience in showing that amputation at the knee joint is a less fatal operation than amputation through the thigh. Comparing the joint experience of Europe and America in this respect, there is a difference of 6½ per cent. in favor of amputation at the knee-joint.

Knee-joint.	Whole number.	Death.	Percentage.
European practice	28	12	43
American practice	18	5	28
Total	46	17	37
Thigh.			
Phillips' cases	987	435	44
American cases	68	29	43
Total	1055	464	43½

In studying the history and watching the progress of the ten cases which have fallen under our own immediate consideration, the following appear to Dr. Markoe as favorable points of comparison between amputation at the knee-joint and amputation through the thigh:

" 1. The crowning advantage of an amputation through the knee joint, over an amputation through the femur, and the consideration to which all the others are subordinate, and from which they derive their main importance, is, that the stump left, by the former operation, is a useful one, while that left by the latter is a useless one for any purposes of progression. Those who have not been in the habit of observing the adaptation and working of artificial limbs may not be aware that, in the stump left after amputation through the thigh, no pressure can ever be borne upon its extremity, be the bone ever so well covered by soft parts.

The extremity of the bone is so small, that any pressure upon it, sufficient to assist in sustaining the weight of the body, would soon be followed by ulceration, and protrusion through the cicatrix. In these cases the artificial limb is so arranged, that the support of the body takes place at the hip, by bands passing round under the tuberosity of the ischium, and round the trochanter; so that, in fact, the patient sits in a sort of cushioned ring, carefully adapted to fit these two bony prominences, while the stump of the femur is received into a conical opening of the artificial thigh, and is only used to direct the forward movements of the limb, and to steady the apparatus, which is bound to it laterally, as firmly as it will bear. It is evident, therefore, that in this apparatus, the patient walks, as Velpeau remarks, as if he had an anchylosis of the hip-joint, all his motions being made by the pelvis, and not at the coxo-femoral articulation. This mode of progression, as may be conceived, is not only exceedingly awkward and ungainly, but so laborious that very few persons have strength enough to walk, under these circumstances, with any freedom, or to any great distance. These remarks apply to those who have the means of commanding an artificial limb of the best construction; but, to the laboring man, amputation through the thigh is an absolute and inevitable condemnation to the crutch for life. On the other hand, the stump left after amputation at the knee, if it be a good one, is perfectly capable of sustaining the pressure of the body on a simple cushion. This fact is fully demonstrated by the cases published both here and abroad. To the poor man this single circumstance makes all the difference, between his being able to earn his living by active employment and his being laid by for life a hopeless cripple. To the rich man, who is able to secure the aid of an artificial limb, it makes the difference between a point of support at the knee and a point of support at the ischium; in fact, it is practically the difference between amputation below, and amputation above, the knee.

" 2. The operation at the knee is farther from the trunk than that through the thigh, and is, therefore, probably attended with less constitutional shock or depression. I say probably, because this is not a fact which is positively proved by statistical deduction; but, at the same time, it is so entirely in accordance with analogy, and so consonant with the opinion and practice of surgeons in other cases, that it may safely be taken for granted till disproved. I would, myself, be disposed to go further, and say that, from the nature of the parts cut in the two cases, the thigh operation, where enormous surfaces of muscular tissue are divided by the knife, would be much more depressing to the powers of life than the knee operation, where almost nothing but integument is involved in the incisions,—a consideration which might be of moment in a case where, from shock or injury or from hemorrhage, the reactive forces were so reduced, that a single ounce of blood or a single degree of further depression might fearfully compromise the favorable issue.

" 3. The section at the knee-joint is, in reality, less extensive than in amputation higher up. No parts are cut but the integuments, and though a large surface is exposed when the flaps are complete, it must be remembered that a great portion of that surface consists of the cartilaginous covering of the femur, a natural, not a wounded surface, and whatever inflammatory changes we might a priori fear would take place in it, yet experience thus far clearly shows that this surface plays almost a perfectly passive part in the earlier processes, finally accommodating itself to the adhesive reparative actions in a manner which is not entirely interrupted under the most unfavorable circumstances of exposure and suppuration.

" 4. In the operation under consideration no muscular interspaces are exposed by the knife, excepting those of the heads of the gastrocnemius, which muscle being divided near its origin, is of small extent and depth. There is, therefore, less chance of suppurative inflammation travelling upwards, in case such inflammation attacks the surface of the stump: for it is a well-known fact that it is along these interspaces, and among their soft areolar tissue, that abscess is most apt to burrow up the thigh, when the operation is done by section through the bellies of these muscles. The muscles moving the leg upon the thigh are, it is true, divided; but it will be observed that the quadriceps extensor is divided through the ligamentum patellæ, and the flexors, as well as the gracilis and sartorius, are cut at their tendinous portions and immediately retract in their sheaths, so as to be entirely out of the way; and it is well known that a clean cut of healthy tendon is almost never followed by any but the simplest and most healthy reparative action.

" 5. The operation at the knee-joint requires fewer ligatures than amputation of the thigh, and these few consisting usually of the popliteal, the two sural, and the two inferior articular arteries, are cut in such a manner that their orifices are all close together in the centre of the popliteal space. By making, therefore, a small opening through the integument, of which alone the posterior flap consists, we are enabled to bring all the threads of the stump, by a short and direct route, in the most depending position, and thus the space between the flaps and the condyles, where we are most anxious to procure adhesive inflammation, is not fretted into suppuration by the presence of the ligatures crossing it, to be brought out between the lips of the wound.* This procedure was adopted in several of the cases. In several instances no vessel in the anterior flap required ligature, thus leaving the posterior leash of ligatures the only ones in the stump.

" 6. In the knee-joint operation, the muscular attachments, which are concerned in the movements of the limb, are not divided. Those which are severed are merely for the movements of the leg, all the muscles proper of the thigh being left untouched. A singular circumstance results from this, viz., that the patient is able to move the stump with a freedom and facility which is astonishing. This is well seen in the case of a little child on whom Dr. Markoe operated, and the same thing is strikingly noticeable in his second patient,—case No. 3,—so much so that, within a week after the operation, even before the first inflammation had subsided, he was able with ease to lift up, and hold up, his stump, without assistance, to be dressed. From this also it happened that the twitching and jerking so common and so painful in all newly-made stumps, gave him but little pain, and the little he did suffer seemed to be mainly from the stump being drawn up against the bedclothes, and was entirely prevented by a band passing over the middle of the thigh, and fastened loosely to the bed, so as to prevent the stump from rising high enough to strike the coverings above.

" 7. An advantage belonging to the knee-joint section, which may be considered as directly resulting from the last-mentioned, is found in the fact that no retraction of the cut muscles can take place after the healing of the wound; by which gradual retraction, it is well known that the muscular covering is generally withdrawn from the end of the bone, and what is called a conical stump is left, in which nothing covers the bone but integument or cicatrix tissue. Dr. Markoe's experience would lead him to think that, in all cases where divided muscles are united over the end of a bone, as in flap amputation through the thigh, the ultimate result is a complete disappearance, by combined absorption and retraction, of the muscular tissue, which, on the first healing of the wound, gave a thick and promising covering to the end of the bone. It will be found, if the limbs be examined a year after they are healed, that the conical stump above described is the rule and not the exception, and that, in four cases out of five, nothing but cicatrix tissue covers and protects the end of the bone. In the stump left by the exarticulation at the knee we have, it is true, nothing but integument on the face of the stump, but that integument is applied over a large, smooth, natural surface, well adapted to receive and sustain pressure, while the cicatrix, if the operation be properly performed, is thrown backwards in such a manner as to be entirely protected from pressure, in the deep fossa between the projection of the condyles.

" 8. Last, and not least, of the advantages which the knee-joint section promises over the thigh amputation, is, I think, to be found in the fact, that in one the bone is unwounded, and that in the other it is severed with a degree of violence, the effects of which, perhaps, are not fully appreciated. The effects of this violence, both upon the bone and its envelopes, and of the exposure of the cavity of the medullary membrane, to the action of air and pus, are seen in several of the accidents which occur after amputation, some of which are merely of sufficient gravity to annoy the patient, and prolong the period of his cure; while others are of so great severity and danger as materially to influence the safety of the opera-

* This method of bringing out the ligatures through the posterior flap was first suggested and adopted by M. Blandin.

tion with regard to life. Thus, for example, among the slighter mischiefs of which the injured bone is the source, we have the exfoliation of a narrow ring of dead bone, which has been killed by the direct violence of the saw. The separation of this ring, with its attendant suppuration, keeps the wound unhealed; and the parts around tender and painful, until the process is complete and the dead bone comes away, perhaps during twice or thrice the period which would be necessary to heal the wound without this complication. Another and much more serious trouble is found in the formation of those long tubular sequestra, which are sometimes found in stumps two or three, or even four months after amputation. The existence of these peculiar sequestra has attracted the notice of most of the systematic writers on surgery; but I have not met with any explanation of the mode in which they are produced, except that Mr. Syme alludes to them, as produced by injury done to the medullary membrane, by which the bone, nourished by that membrane, dies and exfoliates in a tubular form. This is unquestionably correct, as far as it goes; but it leaves unexplained the nature of the injury to the membrane in question, which has such important consequences. This injury may be the result of suppurative action extending along the membrane, and separating it from the bone; but, if this is a possible explanation, the absence of all symptoms of undue inflammation in the cases which have occurred in our hospital forbids its being received as the usual cause of the mischief. I regard it as produced by the severing of the nutritious arteries of the bone, either by the saw, while it is passing through its bony canal, or by the catlin before it has reached the nutritious foramen.* The supply of blood thus cut off from the medullary membrane can only be restored by the anastomosis which it has with the vessels of the spongy portion above. These vessels, however, are supplied with blood from small twigs, which enter the bone at various points around the extremity, and, of course, are contained in unyielding canals. The necessary increase in their calibre, therefore, to supply the wants of the medullary membrane can take place but slowly, and, in the meantime, the small vessels which the medullary membrane sends into the bone are not properly filled, and the death of the bone is produced up to the point where the anastomotic supply is sufficient to save it. The medullary membrane itself, probably, never dies from this cause; but is gradually restored by the supply from above, and goes on secreting new bone on the inside of the sequestrum, while the periosteum is converting the old bone into a thick involucrum outside, so that when it is ready to come away, the sequestrum is found inclosed in a double cylinder, formed by the periosteal involucrum outside, and a smaller medullary involucrum within. These sequestra vary in size from three to seven, or even in one instance on record, to nine inches in length. They are, most commonly, complete cylinders with here and there an opening through them. Through these openings bony granulations may sometimes shoot, if the sequestrum be left too long, by which it may be locked fast in its bed, and may require a serious and troublesome operation to extricate it. While thus remaining in the stump, these pieces of dead bone produce all the annoyance to which necrosis of the shaft of the long bones always give rise. The wound does not heal; the end of the stump enlarges by the new bony deposit which forms the involucrum; and extensive suppuration continues from the various sinuses which lead down to the bone, while new abscesses are constantly forming. The suffering and discharge thus continuing are sufficient to keep the patient in a constant state of constitutional irritation, which, in a feeble person, might have the most serious, or even fatal, consequences; and his only relief is to be found in a removal of the cause of offence. When this is taken away (and it can usually be done by seizing the exposed end with a strong pair of forceps, and drawing the sequestrum carefully from its bed), the relief is immediate: the suppuration dries up, the abscesses heal, fever ceases, and the stump rapidly heals. I have dwelt more particularly on this accident, because there is but little said of it in our surgical treatises, and I think it must occur more frequently than is commonly supposed; indeed, Mr.

* In order to satisfy myself as to the usual point of entrance of the nutritious artery into the bone, I examined forty-five femora, contained in two of the museums of this city, and found that in twenty-three the nutritious foramen was about the junction of the middle and upper third, and in twenty-two it was at or near the centre of the bone. In several instances it was double. The direction of the canal is always from below upwards.

Syme makes this one of the considerations which induced him at one time to proscribe, altogether, amputation through the middle, compact portion of the shaft of the femur; he insisted that, to avoid this, as well as other accidents liable to occur in amputation through the middle of the thigh, it was better to make the section of the bone sufficiently high up to pass through the spongy tissue, which has sufficient vitality to enable it to resist the dangers liable to happen when the compact structure is sawed through.

"The effects of this violence to the bone, and of its exposure in a suppurating wound, are also more seriously and more fatally exhibited in those cases where from some previous vitiation of the system, phlebitis attacks the bone with its destructive and often rapidly fatal consequences. Happily, in our well-ventilated and healthy hospitals, we very rarely see instances of this disease; but, if we may credit the report of some of the surgeons of Europe, suppurative phlebitis of the bones is, with them, a common cause of mortality after amputation of the limbs in their continuity."

Dr. Markoe also enters into several other points, which are of interest to the practical surgeon. He shows that the dangers apprehended from opening so large an articulation as the knee have been greatly exaggerated, and that they are practically of rare occurrence. He also advances reasons for concluding that the best mode of operation, when we have a choice, is by the large anterior and short posterior flap. But for these points, and the rest, we must be content to refer to the paper itself—a paper which will well repay careful perusal.

III.

REPORT ON THE PROGRESS OF MIDWIFERY AND THE DISEASES OF WOMEN AND CHILDREN.

On the action of Digitalis upon the Uterus. By W. Howship Dickinson, Esq., late Obstetric Assistant at St. George's Hospital. ("Medical Times and Gazette," Dec. 15, 1855.)

In October, 1854, a patient in St. George's Hospital, who was suffering under most severe menorrhagia, was cured (Mr. Dickinson informs us in a paper recently communicated to the Royal Medical and Chirurgical Society) by the infusion of 'digitalis, exhibited for the relief of a cardiac affection, from which she also suffered. In consequence of this, the author was induced to try, by the permission of Dr. Lee, the same treatment in a series of cases of uterine hemorrhage which had occurred in the hospital. These cases, of which a table is given, are seventeen in number, and the general results of the treatment is as follows:—In every case of uterine hemorrhage unconnected with organic disease requiring the employment of active remedies, admitted into the Hospital after October, 1854, the administration of digitalis was had recourse to as the sole treatment, and the discharge was invariably arrested by it. The time which elapsed before the hemorrhage subsided varied with the dose in which the digitalis was exhibited. When large doses were given, as an ounce to an ounce and a half of the infusion, the discharge never appeared after the second day; when smaller doses, it never continued beyond the fourth day. In uterine hemorrhage connected with organic disease, the remedy acted with less certainty; its exhibition was required for a longer time, and the effect was sometimes transient. The author then speaks of the mode in which the digitalis operated in controlling uterine hemorrhage; and, after concluding that its effect could not depend on the sedative influence of the drug in the heart and arteries, he shows, by various experiments and observations, that the arrest of the hemorrhage is due to the action of the digitalis on the ganglia of the uterus, by which the organ is stimulated, and muscular substance powerfully contracted.

Since the reading of this paper we have had repeated opportunities of putting this treatment in practice at the Westminster Hospital, and in this way we are able to confirm what is here stated respecting it. We have no doubt indeed as to the very marked and special influence of digitalis in arresting hemorrhage from the uterus; but we have some difficulty in agreeing with Mr. Dickinson about the *modus operandi* of the medicine. Digitalis is unquestionably a sedative in its action, and we cannot see why it should not cause the muscular fibres of the uterus to contract by virtue of this sedative action (*v.* "Abstract," XXII). Be this as it may, however, the clinical fact remains, and this is one of no small practical importance.

On Flooding before delivery, and especially on a new principle and method of treatment of Placenta Prævia. By Dr. Barnes. ("Medical Times and Gazette," December 29, 1855.)

The paper, of which the abstract is subjoined, was read before the Medical Society of London on the 22d of December, 1855. In this paper the author

passes in review the actual state of obstetric science and practice in relation to
the pathology and treatment of placenta prævia, and shows that the prevailing
belief is, that so long as the delivery of the child is not effected there is no security against hemorrhage, and that hence the rule in practice of proceeding to
forced delivery as early as practicable was almost universally inculcated, the only
exception consisting in the more or less general substitution of the plan of totally
detaching the placenta. The author thus shows that, while the practitioner was
anxiously waiting for the moment when the dilatability of the cervix uteri would
permit the passage of the hand, for the purpose of turning, the patient might
perish of flooding; and that, therefore, in the most severe class of cases, those
of central placenta, some other resource, some means of placing the patient in
security against renewed flooding, before the full dilatation of the os, is eminently
desirable. Dr. Barnes then explains the physiological course of a labor with placenta prævia, and the mode in which Nature sometimes arrests the hemorrhage
before the expulsion of the child. He shows, by the help of an ingenious and
interesting diagram, that a stage of labor arrives when the recurrent contractions
of the womb do not entail any further flooding; that the pains return in their
usual course, with the usual effect of further dilating the os uteri, and forwarding
the labor, but without causing any further flooding; that the labor was in fact
resolved into a natural one, and would be safely concluded by the natural powers.
Reflection upon these cases has led Dr. Barnes to doubt the truth of
the obstetric dogma, which declares that there is no security against hemorrhage, so long as he presence of the liquor amnii or the child in the womb
prevents full contraction. Dr. Barnes then unfolds the anatomical, physiological, and clinical facts which lead him to the conclusion that, under proper restrictions, Nature might in many cases be trusted to with more confidence than was generally believed. The clinical facts, he says. had come to
him first, and led him to examine into the anatomical and physiological bearings
of the case. He relates cases in illustration, and quotes a commentary upon one
of these cases from a memoir he had published ("Lancet," 1847), in order to
establish his priority in the enunciation of the views he now laid before the
Society; and adverted to the fact that he had, since the publication of that memoir, constantly taught in his lectures on midwifery. the same doctrine; and
stated that, even the original of the diagram now exhibited, rudely sketched, was
also figured in the memoir referred to. He has, therefore, believed his views to
be original, and was surprised to find, in several numbers of the "Berlin
Monatschrift für Geburtskunde" for the present year, a controversy between Dr.
Cohen, Dr. Credé, and Professor Hohl, in which Dr. Cohen for the first time
expounded similar views to his own, whilst Dr. Credé referring to writings of
1853-54, also claimed them; and Professor Hohl assigned them to Dr. Zeitfuchs,
so far back as 1843. Dr. Barnes acknowledged, with pleasure, that Dr. Cohen's
views of 1855 fully confirmed those put forth by himself in 1847; but he found
in the writings of Credé and Zeitfuchs, nothing whatever to show that either had,
in the remotest degree, possessed himself of the points in question. But Cohen
had gone beyond the author in proposing a new operation based upon the physiological and clinical facts expounded. This operation consists in—1. Determining the side of the uterus to which the smaller flap of the placenta is attached;
2. In rupturing the membranes and detaching the placenta from this half of its
circumference; 3. Exciting uterine contraction; 4. Hooking finger over edge
of placenta, tearing membranes from the freed border of the placenta; and 5.
In separating the placenta in a circumference of 190° to 200°. The greater half
of the placenta, now freed from the dragging of the lesser half and membranes,
is now drawn back, just as in placenta lateralis, with the uterus. From this
moment there is no further danger. Cohen insists, like the author, on the impropriety of hastening labor unless urgent complications arise. Dr. Cohen refers
to his experience to prove the efficacy of this method, but does not recite any
cases in illustration. Dr. Barnes pointed out that the difference between his memoir and that of Dr. Cohen consisted simply in this:—Cohen had, in 1855, carried forward the principle Dr. Barnes had enunciated in 1847, by proposing the
artificial partial detachment of the placenta, instead of trusting, as Dr. Barnes
had recommended in certain cases, the execution of this operation to the powers

of nature. The author then quotes from Sir Charles Hill, passages showing that the anatomical distribution and physiological action of the muscles of the uterus accorded with and explained the clinical facts observed in the course of intermissions and cessations of hemorrhage from placenta prævia as set forth by Dr. Barnes. The author then explains the mode and mechanism by which the hemorrhage in placenta prævia is arrested. The opening of the mouth of the wound, and the detachment of the placenta adhering to this part, are effected by the active contraction of the longitudinal muscles of the uterus; this active contraction shortens the cervix, when it intermits, a passive contraction goes on, which maintains or even increases the shortening of the cervix. This shortening necessarily compresses the torn mouths of the vessels and checks the flooding caused by each successive detachment of fresh placenta, until the detachment has gone to the boundary line, beyond which point the further expansion of the cervix has no effect, and when all fear of flooding is at an end. It was not therefore necessary that the uterus should be empty in order to arrest the flooding. This arrest depended upon the contraction of the cervix, which went on, although the fundus and walls were prevented from contracting. Dr. Barnes submitted the following as some of the conclusions deducible from his researches:—

1. In cases of placenta prævia the hemorrhage is sometimes arrested spontaneously before the complete detachment of the placenta, before the discharge of the liquor amnii, and consequently before the expulsion of the child, or the pressure of its head against the cervix.

2. That this spontaneous arrest of the flooding is owing to the sealing up of the vessels torn by successive detachments of placenta, and the attainment of a stage of labor when no further detachment can take place until after delivery.

3. That dangerous and even fatal flooding sometimes occurs while the os uteri is still closed, and so undilatable as to render it impossible or inexpedient to have recourse to forced delivery.

4. That in such cases it is eminently desirable to possess some means of diminishing the hemorrhage until the hand can be passed through the os uteri.

5. The spontaneous or artificial detachment of the cervical portion of the placenta competes with two most formidable operations, dangerous to mother and child—forced delivery, and the total separation of the placenta. The new principle of treatment may, in many cases, supersede forced delivery altogether; since the patient being secured against further flooding, to resort to turning when the flooding has ceased is an unnecessary proceeding, although the os uteri may admit of it. In many more cases this principle will be the means of gaining the necessary time to admit of turning or other modes of forced delivery being performed with safety. In almost every case it may supersede the practice of wholly detaching the placenta, since the end in view being the arrest of the flooding, it is better to detach only just so much of the placenta as will effect this end, than by detaching all, to destroy the child.

Dr. Barnes concluded by a particular exposition of the application of his views to the varieties of placenta prævia occurring in practice.

Tabulated account of sixty-nine cases of Labor in which the Ergot of Rye was administered. By R. U. WEST, M.D., of Alford, Lincolnshire. ("Medical Times and Gazette," Dec. 22, 1856, and Feb. 9th, 1856.)

The object of this tabulated account is to obtain an answer to the question whether or not the use of ergot of rye in obsteric practice is so injurious as some late writers would have us to believe. The question is one of some difficulty, but there is no reason to doubt that blame has been ascribed to the ergot where no blame was due. This is well seen in a case of twins which occurred to Dr. R. U. West in 1853.

"When I first arrived at the house of my patient, finding the os uteri in a thick, rigid, and undilatable state, I waited," says Dr. West, "a few hours without doing anything. I then, when the os was in a more favorable condition, gave a full dose of ergot, because the pains were very inefficient. In an hour, the child was born—dead. Now, the pains had been anything but continuous; on the contrary, the intervals were unusually long and complete; that between the two last pains which attended the expulsion of the head having been at least five minutes in duration. The child had every appearance of having been alive up to the time of birth, and though there was no pulsation in the funis, yet the umbilical vessels felt full. This, then, thought I, must be an example of the specific bad effect of the ergot. But, when the child was removed, I placed my hand on the abdomen of the mother, and found there was another child. And in a quarter of an hour a second child was born *footling*, very lively and vigorous. Now, surely any specific poisonous influence of the ergot must have been experienced by both children, and more by the second than by the first, in proportion to the greater length of time during which it was exposed to it."

This being the case, Dr. West thought it desirable to endeavor to arrive at something like a conclusive opinion upon the subject, and in order to this he decided on tabulating the essential particulars of a number of *consecutive* cases in which he might from any reason think it expedient or useful to administer the ergot. These cases, which are sixty-nine in number, are related with great care, the state of the os uteri when the ergot was given, the interval between the dose and the birth of the child, the condition of the fœtus, the character of the pain produced, the previous condition of uterine action, the manner in which the mother recovered, and several other points of interest, all being carefully noted. Our space will not allow us to give the table, and we must therefore content ourselves with referring to it, and with giving Dr. West's conclusions:

"With reference to the probability of the ergot causing the death of the fœtus, I may observe that, in the whole number of 69 cases, there were 9 still-births, viz., in cases 2, 5, 16, 19, 23, 33, 39, 56, 67. All the other children were born more or less lively and vigorous. Of case 25, where the fœtus survived its birth only half-an-hour, I ought to observe that the mother usually gave birth to still-born or similarly feeble children. Certainly, her three previous children were in this condition, no ergot having been given. From this list of 9 still-births we may at once exclude cases 19 and 33, the putridity of the fœtuses in these two cases having proved that they had died some days before the commencement of labor. Cases 5 and 39 were attended with considerable hemorrhage during or immediately preceding the labor, a circumstance of itself quite sufficient to account for the death of the children. In case 67 the death of the child was undoubtedly caused by pressure on the funis during the difficult delivery of a hydrocephalic head in a case of feet presentation. Four still-births remain to be explained, viz., in cases 2, 16, 23, and 56. Let us examine these cases. In case 2, although the pains were improved, yet they could scarcely be said to be *ergotic*, the intervals of ease between them being unusually long and perfect. The child was born fifty minutes after the administration of ergot. The case resembles that reported in the *Association Journal*, as far as regards the first-born of the twins, with this exception, that the funis was not round the neck. I cannot explain the death of the fœtus in case 2, when I compare it with the other cases in this report. In case 16 we had the same long intervals between the pains, and the woman was much longer under the influence of the medicine. The head lay for an hour on the perinæum, and the funis was prolapsed over the shoulder. Now, this shoulder had a very congested appearance; and I am inclined to think that, during the lengthened period of the head lying on the perinæum, the funis was compressed in that situation, so as to stop its circulation, so that the child's death need not be attributed to the poisonous influence of the ergot. Nay, further, I would maintain that the ergot, by hastening the birth, would be more likely to prevent the death of the child, in such a case, than to cause it. I think that, if the vectis had been used much sooner than it was, the child might have been saved. In case 23 the woman had excessive œdema of the lower extremities, extending to the vulva, and was in a bad state of health generally. The labor was unusually severe, and the child's head was much pressed during the dilatation of the very rigid cervix uteri. There were surely here other causes of danger to the fœtus than the ergot. In case 56 the child died manifestly from congestion of the head, caused by pressure in a severe instrumental primiparous labor. So much for the danger to the fœtus. Do the cases just referred to, when compared with the large number in which, under all sorts of unfavorable circumstances, and with a duration of the labor process, under the influence of the ergot, varying from a quarter of an hour to three and four hours, the fœtus was born lively and vigorous, prove anything whatever against the ergot of rye? I certainly think not.

"Neither do I think that the ergot does the mother any harm. In all the cases tabulated, the mothers recovered; in the great majority of them without any bad symptoms whatever. No. 5 had an alarming attack of tympanitis, simulating puerperal fever, but she had been much weakened by hemorrhage in the commencement of the labor. Case 22 does not need any observations. No. 55 had precisely the same symptoms after her first confinement as in this, her third; and that first confinement was so quick, that her child was born before my arrival, no ergot having been given, of course.

"All the women recovered. But this was not the case with all that I attended during the period included in what I may call these experiments, viz., from January 1, 1854, to November 25, 1855. Nos. 2235, 2300, and 2349, in my register, died within the month, and none of these had had the ergot during their labors. No. 2235 died of mania on the 20th day. No. 2300 had had dysenteric diarrhœa for more than a month before her confinement, which was premature, and was followed by adherent placenta. She had had no medical advice until her labor commenced, and her child was born before my arrival. She died of exhaustion on the 11th day. No. 2349 died of uterine phlebitis, of which she felt the first symptoms during the second week, her death taking place on the 20th day of lying-in; a young primipara confined of twins; easy labor, both footling; no ergot given.

"Has the ergot any effect in producing or preventing retention of the placenta? Neither the one nor the other. During the period of these experiments I had six cases of retained or adherent placenta, requiring the introduction of the hand, viz., in cases 2169, 2237, 2298, 2300, 2400, 2435. The ergot was given in case 2169, but in none of the others.

"It will have been observed, that in many of the cases the ergot was given while the os uteri was nearly closed, rigid, and undilatable. As this practice is contrary to the rules, for such a condition made and provided, I must make a few observations on the subject. In such cases as Nos. 5 and 39, in both of which the labor had commenced with profuse gushes of hemorrhage, the placenta having been, probably, implanted somewhere near the os uteri, the practice is, I believe, sanctioned and enjoined by the best authorities. But what of other cases, where there is no risk to the patient in waiting for Nature to play her proper part in the business, which she is certain to do———in time! Why, surely something may be urged on the side of the accoucheur. It is no joke to be carried off seven or eight miles away from home, and to find, on your arrival, that your patient has taken the alarm at the first little twinge, and despatched her husband, 'bloody with spurring, fiery hot with haste,' for the doctor. John Chamomile arrives; there is a prospect before him of having to wait perhaps twenty-four hours. He has a large practice, and no assistant, and all his patients must be neglected: perhaps the Squire's, or the Rector's lady may be hourly expecting her little affair to come off, and, with her double or triple fee—that bright oasis in the desert of poor Chamomile's experience, may fall into the hands of his gaping rival—him of the 'opposition brass plate!'* If he hint at the propriety of his leaving the patient, and returning home for a few hours, the husband, anxious to behold the face of his first-born, and all the old wives, who have been summoned to assist at the interesting event, protest vehemently against such a proceeding; besides, John Chamomile, being no judge of horse-flesh, is generally cheated by his kind neighbors in that article, and, consequently, cannot afford to make two long journeys where one will do, let alone his own bodily fatigue,—pretty sure, as he may be, that the hot-headed husband will, reason or none, fetch him again in a few short hours. What is poor Chamomile to do in all this perplexity? Having a resource within his

"Chamomile has a great deal at stake in this matter besides his fee:—there is his social position! —It is really *ȟϊν ἤ θαρϊϊν* with him; for is he not "well with the squire, and on dining terms with the rector?" Vide Sketch of John Chamomile, in the "Times" leader, January 23, 1851.

reach, which will, in all probability, send him on his way rejoicing, back to the delights of Opodeldoc Lodge, in three or four hours at the furthest, it is small blame to him, if—

> ' He gently prevails on his patient to try
> The magic effects of the ergot of rye.'—TENNYSON.

"Does he do any harm either to mother or child? Let my Table answer that question. I need only refer to Case 35, in which the efficacy of the medicine was strikingly apparent in rendering the os uteri dilatable, when it had been very rigid during many hours of useless suffering. In many cases of rigid os uteri, it is uterine action that is wanted. The patient may have pains, but they are not of the right sort, until after the grand specific has been taken. It is best, however, to wait a few hours, say three or four, before giving the medicine, and if you can then manage to get the tips of two fingers into the os uteri, it may be safely given, and with certain advantage.

"I think I may conclude this paper in the words with which I concluded my report of the case of twins above referred.to :—' I am quite sure that the ergot of rye, when given with the ordinary precautions, does no harm to the mother, and I am very doubtful about its hurting the child.' "

Case of Spontaneous Delivery after the death of the mother. By M. DECHAMBRE. ("Gaz. Hebd. de Méd. et. Chir.," Feb. 22d, 1856.)

The following case is taken from the Parisian journal "La Presse," by M. Dechambre, the learned and accomplished editor of the "Gazette Hebdomadaire de Médecine et de Chirurgie." It made a great sensation in the Fauborg du Temple in Paris, where it occurred, as it appears, in February last, but it is not given with any circumstantiality. There need be no doubt, however, as to its authenticity.

Commenting upon this case, M. Dechambre is disposed to ascribe the expulsion of the foetus to the pressure exercised upon the uterus by the development of putrid gas in the abdomen after death. To us, however, the case has a different signification, as may be gathered from the views we hold in connection with muscular contraction (v. "Abstract," XXII). But be this as it may, the fact is of extreme interest both in a physiological and clinical point of view, and we must not neglect to preserve it in our pages.

CASE.—The patient was a lady, Madame X—, æt. 24, who had died of typhoid fever after an illness of three or four days. All the arrangements for the funeral were complete, and the coffin containing the corpse was exposed at the entrance of the house. The mourners were also assembled, and the time for placing the corpse upon the hearse was drawing nigh, when all present were horrified by seeing blood dripping from the badly made coffin upon the pavement. The report spread to the neighborhood like wildfire, and an immediate examination of the corpse was demanded. An examination was made, and this led to the discovery that Madame X— had been in the fourth month of pregnancy, and that she had been delivered in her coffin about seventy hours after death. There are no further particulars, except that the examination was made by two physicians, under the inspection of M. d'Agnèse, Commissary of Police.

INDEX TO NO. XXIII.

THE

HALF-YEARLY ABSTRACT

OF THE

MEDICAL SCIENCES:

BEING

A PRACTICAL AND ANALYTICAL DIGEST OF THE CONTENTS OF THE PRIN-
CIPAL BRITISH AND CONTINENTAL MEDICAL WORKS PUBLISHED
IN THE PRECEDING SIX MONTHS.

TOGETHER WITH

A SERIES OF CRITICAL REPORTS ON THE PROGRESS OF MEDICINE AND
THE COLLATERAL SCIENCES DURING THE SAME PERIOD.

EDITED BY

W. H. RANKING, M.D., CANTAB.,

PHYSICIAN TO THE NORFOLK AND NORWICH HOSPITAL,

AND

C. B. RADCLIFFE, M.D., LOND., L.R.C.P.,

ASSISTANT PHYSICIAN TO, AND LECTURER ON MATERIA MEDICA AT, THE WESTMINSTER HOSPITAL.

Apparatu nobis opus est, et rebus exquisitis undique et collectis, arcessitis, comportatis.
CICERO.

NO. XXIV.

JULY—DECEMBER, 1856.

———

PHILADELPHIA:

LINDSAY AND BLAKISTON,

NO. 25 SOUTH SIXTH STREET.

1857.

TERMS.

Two Dollars per annum, free of postage, *if paid for in advance.*

LINDSAY & BLAKISTON,

Publishers.

NOTICE TO CORRESPONDENTS.

The Editors request that all communications be forwarded (free) to Mr. Churchill, *New Burlington Street, London.*

The Editors are compelled to remind their American correspondents, that no parcels are taken in, unless the entire charge be paid upon them.

C. SHERMAN & SON, PRINTERS,

19 St. James Street.

CONTENTS OF NO. XXIV.

PART I.—MEDICINE.

I.—*General Questions in Medicine.*

II.—*Special Questions in Medicine.*

(a) *Concerning the Nervous System.*

(b) *Concerning the Respiratory System.*

(c) *Concerning the Circulatory System.*

(d) *Concerning the Alimentary System.*

(e) *Concerning the Genito-Urinary System.*

PART II.—SURGERY.

I.—General Questions in Surgery.

(a) Concerning Tumors.

(b) Concerning Wounds and Ulcers.

(c) Concerning Diseases of the Bones and Joints.

(d) Concerning Operations.

II.—Special Questions in Surgery.

(a) Concerning the Head and Neck.

(b) *Concerning the Chest, Abdomen, and Pelvis.*

(c) *Concerning the Upper Extremity.*

(d) *Concerning the Inferior Extremity.*

PART III.

MIDWIFERY, AND DISEASES OF WOMEN AND CHILDREN.

(a) *Concerning Pregnancy and Parturition.*

(b) Concerning the Diseases of Women.

(c) Concerning Diseases of Children.

REPORTS ON THE PROGRESS OF THE MÉDICAL SCIENCES.

I.—Report in Medicine.

II.—*Report in Surgery.*

III.—*Report in Midwifery and Diseases of Women and Children.*

IV.—*Report on Pyschological Medicine. By Dr. Robertson,* . 245

ABSTRACT OF THE MEDICAL SCIENCES,

&c. &c.

PART I.

PRACTICAL MEDICINE, PATHOLOGY, AND THERAPEUTICS.

SECT. I.—GENERAL QUESTIONS IN MEDICINE.

(A) HYGIENE.

ART. 1.—*Effects of Color upon Health.* By "A Correspondent of the Builder."
(Edinburgh Medical Journal, June, 1856.)

"From several years' observations in rooms of various sizes, used as manufacturing rooms, and occupied by females for twelve hours per day, I found that the workers who occupied those rooms which had large windows with large panes of glass, in the four sides of the room, so that the sun's rays penetrated through the room during the whole day, were much more healthy than the workers who occupied rooms lighted from one side only, or rooms lighted through very small panes of glass. I observed another very singular fact—viz., that the workers who occupied one room were very cheerful and healthy, while the occupiers of another similar room, who were employed on the same kind of work, were all inclined to melancholy, and complained of pains in the forehead and eyes, and were often ill and unable to work. Upon examining the rooms in question, I found they were both equally well ventilated and lighted. I could not discover anything about the drainage of the premises that could affect the one room more than the other; but I observed that the room occupied by the cheerful workers was wholly whitewashed, and the room occupied by the melancholy workers was colored with yellow ochre. I had the yellow ochre all washed off, and the walls and ceilings whitewashed. The workers ever after felt more cheerful and healthy."

ART. 2.—*The relation of Teetotalism to the diseases of Europeans in India.*
By Mr. WARING.

(Indian Annals of Medical Science, April, 1856.)

In some admirable notes on the diseases of India, Mr. Waring gives a table which tends to point out that in India a teetotaller is more liable to fever than a person who drinks moderately, or even immoderately. Thus:

Showing the Sickness and Mortality amongst three classes of Men with Fever, in six European Regiments, serving in the Madras Presidency, in 1849.

Class.	Strength of each Class.	Fever Admissions.	Fever Deaths.	Per cent. of Admissions to Strength.	Per cent. of Deaths to Strength.	Per cent. of Deaths to Admissions.
Teetotallers,	450	141	1	31·33	0·22	0·70
Temperate,	4318	768	1	17·78	0·02	0·13
Intemperate,	942	190	2	20·16	0·21	1·05

Though teetotallers are more liable to fever in India, they are, however, more exempt from some other diseases, and the balance of chances after all inclines considerably in their favor. This appears in another table which Mr. Waring gives in an appendix to his paper, and which represents the experience of the European troops in the Madras Presidency in 1849:

Classes.	Teetotallers.				Temperate.				Intemperate.			
Strength.	450.				4318.				940.			
Diseases.	Admissions.	Deaths.	Per cent of Admissions to Strength.	Per cent of Deaths to Strength.	Admissions.	Deaths.	Per cent of Admissions to Strength.	Per cent of Deaths to Strength.	Admissions.	Deaths.	Per cent of Admissions to Strength.	Per cent of Deaths to Strength.
Fevers,	141	1	31·33	0·22	768	1	17·78	0·02	190	2	20·16	0·21
Cholera,	...	...	...	...	17	13	0·39	0·30	7	6	0·74	0·63
Dysentery,	52	3	11·55	0·66	344	31	7·96	0·71	112	15	11·88	1·59
Diarrhœa,	50	1	11·11	0·22	348	4	8·05	0·09	108	...	11·46	...
Other diseases of stomach and bowels,	23	...	5·11	...	337	6	7·80	0·13	112	2	11·88	0·21
Hepatitis,	26	...	5·77	...	249	16	5·76	0·37	96	2	10·19	0·21
Disease of lungs,	43	...	9·55	...	478	17	11·06	0·39	113	4	11·99	0·42
Disease of brain,	14	...	3·11	...	108	1	2·50	0·02	82	5	8·70	0·53
Rheumatic affections,	27	...	6·00	...	487	...	11·27	...	143	1	15·18	0·10
Venereal affections,	94	...	20·88	...	1414	1	35·06	0·02	447	...	50·63	...
Other diseases,	119	...	26·44	...	1464	10	33·89	0·23	584	5	61·98	0·53
	589	5	130·88	1·11	6114	100	141·59	2·315	2024	42	214·86	4·45

The following short table will place the above figures in a stronger light:

Class.	Strength.	Total Admissions.	Total Deaths.	Per cent. of Admissions to Strength.	Per cent. of Deaths to Strength.	Per cent of Deaths to Admissions.
Teetotallers,	450	589	5	130·88	1·11	0·84
Temperate,	4318	6114	100	141·59	2·31	1·63
Intemperate,	940	2024	42	214·86	4·45	2·07

The influence of intemperance on sickness and mortality is shown here in a forcible manner.

ART. 3.—*The influence of Occupation upon Mortality.*
By (1) the Registrar-General, and (2) Dr. LETHEBY.

1. (*Fourteenth Annual Report of the Registrar-General.*)
2. (*Association Journal,* Oct. 25, 1856.)

(1) The different mortality in the twelve occupations mentioned below, in the decennial period, ranging from the age of 45 to 55, is very remarkable. It is thus stated :

1. *Farmers.*—Of the twelve classes under consideration, farmers are the longest livers, their rate of mortality being not quite 12 in a 1000 (11·99). The number of English farmers of all ages in 1851, including 2429 graziers, was 225,747, of whom there were 53,608 between the age of 45 and 55. In that year the total number of deaths among farmers of all ages was 6426, very much below the numbers which would have been registered had these individuals been engaged in other pursuits. These facts prove that the pure air, the daily exercise, the substantial fare, and the other aids to health enjoyed by this substantial class, considerably modify the influence of unfavorable weather, bad seasons, open ports, peculiar burdens on land, and all the other ruinous things which farmers' friends have been accustomed to depict in such gloomy colors.

2. *Shoemakers* hold the next place to farmers, their rate of mortality between 45 and 55 being 15·03 in 1000. They are followed by—

3. Weavers, ...	15·37 in 1000.
4. Grocers, ...	15·79 "
5. Blacksmiths, ...	16·51 "
6. Carpenters, ...	16·67 "
7. Tailors, ...	16·74 "
8. Laborers, ...	17·30 "

As will be seen on inspection, there is among these seven occupations a gradual increase in the rate of mortality, which, considering their great diversity, is quite remarkable. The near approach of these occupations to each other in the scale of mortality arises from the circumstance that they have peculiar dangers which tend to counterbalance each other. Thus it is to be noticed, that "the tailor is not exposed to the explosions which are fatal to the miner, and the laborer has exercise which is denied to the tailor."

Ascending this scale of danger, we pass to—

9. Miners, ...	20·15 in 1000.
10. Bakers, ...	21·21 "
11. Butchers, ...	23·10 "
12. Innkeepers, ...	28·34 "

A great disparity is observable in passing from laborers into the class of miners, telling a tale of dangers, many of which result from criminal neglect. Between laborers and the last four classes in this table, there is a most remarkable hiatus. In the classes previously noticed, the difference in no case is more than one in a thousand, and in some instances less. Here the difference begins with three, and mounts up to nine, in a thousand.

The returns show that the highest rates of mortality are found among the butcher (23·10 in 1000), and the class of innkeepers and licensed victuallers (28·34 in 1000).

The extraordinary mortality of butchers is a fact for which we are indebted wholly to the last census. The "red-injected face" of the butcher has produced a wrong idea as to the healthy nature of his occupation. This idea is now corrected by scientific induction, and proper sanitary means will overcome the evil thus brought to light. To quote the significant remarks in the report conveying this fact, here is an important problem for solution: "On what does the great mortality of the butcher depend? On his diet, into which too much animal food, and too little fruit and vegetables enter? On his drinking to excess? On his exposure to heat and cold; or, which is probably the most powerful cause, on the elements of decaying matter by which he is surrounded in his slaughter-house and its vicinity?"

If the rate of mortality among innkeepers, licensed victuallers, and beershop-keepers, should be seized with avidity by the advocates of teetotalism, they must not be forbidden its use; at the same time they must be reminded, that "many highly respectable men of this class lead regular lives, and are of steady habits; but others, exposed by their business to unusual temptations, live intemperately and enjoy less quiet at night than the rest of the community. They are exposed also to zymotic diseases, by intercourse with large numbers of people."

(2.) The influence of trade and occupation upon mortality, as exemplified in the City of London, is further seen in the following extract from Dr. Letheby's first report of the sanitary condition of the City of London:

The results of this investigation must be looked upon only as approximations to the general truth, and as evidence of what is yet to be done in this department of State medicine.

The expectancy of life among young men, generally, at twenty years is up to sixty. That is nearly the expectancy in London with shopkeepers and domestic servants; for the mean age at which they die is 58·8 and 58·6. Butchers, poulterers, and fishmongers, live to the age of 53·8. Clerks, accountants and messengers reach to the age of from 52 to 52·3. The same is about the mean age of blacksmiths, gasfitters, and the workers in the coarse metals generally, while publicans, wine-merchants, waiters, tailors, laborers, and shoemakers, live to the age of from 49·9 to 50·3. Cabmen, and ostlers, and draymen, live only to 49·4, and soldiers, sailors, and policemen, reach only to 48 years. A like difference exists in the longevity of women, for, while the wife of the shopkeeper will live to be about fifty-seven years of age, and the domestic servant to 51·5, the wife of the publican and beershop-keeper, and the wife of the cabman and ostler will only reach to 44·2 and 48 years of age; and the needlewoman sinks into the grave at 42·6 years of age.

These facts show that the influences which are at work in shortening the duration of life are not merely general, but that they are affected by the habits of the people. Where there are bad food, close confinement, filthy dwellings, and improvident, or vicious habits, there the lifetime is short; but where the conditions are of an opposite character, as in the case of servants and shopkeepers, it is nearly as long as it is in England generally. This is further borne out by the percentage causes of death, for consumption and fever are most fatal with shoemakers, cabmen, laborers, and needlewomen; and, though a large mortality from fever occurs amongst domestic servants and nurses, yet this is easily explained by considering the infectious character of the disease, and the circumstances under which the subjects of it are placed.

That home influences alone have much to do with the shortening of life is evident from the fact, that the wives of the several classes are correspondingly short-lived. In the case of the laborer there is an apparent exception, for the longevity of the wife is greater than that of the shopkeeper; but this is explained by the fact that the laborer's wife is generally unprovided for at the death of her husband, and she seeks an asylum in the workhouse, where she reaches to a good old age; in fact, about thirty per cent. of the deaths among the wives of laborers occurred in the workhouse.

During the past year, the total number of deaths in the workhouses was 456, of which 231 were males, and 225 females. Of these, 52 belonged to the laboring class, 41 to the porter, 10 to the clerk, 23 to the tailor, 17 to the metal-worker, 13 to the publican, 34 to the shoemaker, 15 to the soldier, 23 to the carpenter, 15 to the cabman, 29 to the shopkeeper, 6 to the butcher, 39 to the domestic, and the rest are not specified. In all about 15 per cent. of the deaths occur in the workhouse.

ART. 4.—*Fœcal Fermentation as a cause of disease.* By Dr. ROUTH.

(*Lancet*, June, 1856.)

In this paper, which was read before the Medical Society of London, on the 17th of March, 1856, the author first referred to the conditions insisted upon in a former paper as favorable to emanation—*i. e.*, evaporation of morbid miasmata: 1st. A certain amount of temperature, and a light state of atmosphere. 2d. Moisture in the air. 3d. The existence of ammonia always present in contagious diseases, and in the decomposition of organic matter. Whereas the opposite state, a low temperature, and heavy state of atmosphere, and dryness favor the deposition of such miasmata to the surface of the earth, and their solution in water. From such data, when known, we could almost always argue *a posteriori*, as to whether the poison were imbibed in water, or respired in air. At very low temperatures, 0° Fah., and even some degrees above that, he believed emanation was impossible. Vapor at 0° Fah., contained only 0·856 of moisture; at 95° Fah., 17·009. Even at 11° Fah., it was nearly 0; at 50° Fah., 2·5. In reference to this point, Dr. Routh alluded to the views of Dr. Barton, of America, on yellow fever, as confirmed by Dr. Hunt, of Buffalo, who had shown that yellow fever never occurred except when heat and moisture concurred with what they called terrene causes—*i. e.*, upheaval of soil and decomposing organic matters. Dr. Routh then spoke of the nature of some of these miasmata, some which were like perfumes, detectible by their effects on the body, but not chemically; others, like carburetted hydrogen, sulphuretted hydrogen, and phosphuretted hydrogen, were discoverable as such, and no doubt concurred in the production of symptoms. These emanations required a certain amount of heat for their development—according to Chisholm, from 60° to 90° Fah., above or below which they were destroyed. But in many cases something more was needed, and it was a favorable electrical state of the atmosphere. It was known that the electric effects varied with the degree of moisture in the air; and, sometimes, as in typhus, the mucous membranes give positive electricity, and the skin negative, which was the reverse of what was observed in health. Dr. Routh then proceeded to consider the injurious influences of fæcal emanations, in proof of which he quoted the evidence of Drs. Sutherland, Grainger, and Lewis. In the case of the Christchurch Workhouse, Spitalfields, where the emanations of a manure-manufactory, especially when the wind blew from the manufactory towards the workhouse, gave rise to typhus and typhoid fever, and gave a malignant character to measles, smallpox, &c. The same thing was observed in St. George's, Southwark, in the summer of 1847, where, from a similar cause, intractable diarrhœa resulted. The mortality in places exposed to the effluvia of night-soil, as in the potteries of Kensington, the Witham suburb of Hull, was always very much greater than in other ordinary localities. The author then alluded to the objection which had been raised about the healthiness of Montfaucon, near Paris, and its neighborhood. Statistics in reference to the relative sanitary condition of this locality, as compared with others in Paris, were, however, wanting; but it was a known fact that, when the wind blew from that quarter towards the Hôpital St. Louis, puerperal fever was generated in the lying-in wards. If the workmen of Montfaucon themselves escaped typhus, it was due rather to the strong animal food they indulged in, as compared to other workmen of Paris, than to their occupation. Debility and bad food had been shown, both by Drs. Alison and Corrigan, to make persons very obnoxious to typhus.

If the views above enunciated were correct, the remedies called for were such as would check fermentation. These were, alkalies, mineral acids, concentrated vegetable acids, volatile oils, alcohol, sea-salt, the metallic salts, especially mercury, sulphurous acid, arsenious acid, chlorine, creosote, &c., and charcoal. A lesson might, moreover, be learnt in regard to treatment in these cases, from the processes employed for deodorizing manure. One way was, by collecting the slime and mud of large rivers, which being burnt, owing to the organic matter contained in it, yielded charcoal in very minute divisions. Peat cinders (the refuse of carbonized peat), the bran of sawed wood, and some kinds of mould, had a similar effect. Hydrochloric acid, the tribasic phosphate of soda, and the mother-liquor of salt-works, were equally good disinfectants. Amongst this list one could not fail to be struck in recognizing those remedies which have been found most efficacious in the treatment of many of the diseases before referred to. Thus, in cholera, sulphuric acid, charcoal, saline injections, common salt, and mercury; in diarrhœa, creosote; in dysentery, sulphate of copper, alum, and charcoal; intermittent fever, charcoal and arsenic; typhus, mercury, effervescents, &c. There could be no doubt that for every disease generated by fermentation there was a peculiar antiseptic most fitted for selection; thus arsenic might be the best for skin diseases, because it acted chiefly on the gelatinous tissues; so there was probably one most applicable to diseases of the mucous membrane, glands, &c., but few of these were known certainly. These remedies, however, only applied to the individual; something more was required for the sanitary condition of communities. Two of these general remedies have been lately much spoken about—viz., charcoal and sea-water. *Charcoal* had been alluded to before as an antiseptic. From Dr. Stenhouse's inquiries, however, it appeared to be also a destroyer of ferments, as well as a deodorizer, the first property being due to the large quantity of oxygen contained in its pores, which burnt, as it were, the decaying matter. Dr. Routh then alluded to the series of papers on this subject, published in the "London Journal of Health," by Dr. Richardson. Charcoal filters applied over our gully-holes and water-closets might, in great measure, destroy the bad odors; still all the gully-holes could not be closed, as mud and rain must descend into the sewers; hence it was imperative to deodorize the sewers themselves. The price of hydrochloric acid, chloride of lime, and ordinary charcoal, rendered the chance of their general employment quite improbable; but charcoal prepared according to Mr. Salmon's method, by the combustion of the Thames soil, would suffice for all purposes. All that would be necessary would be, its admixture with the water by which the sewers were ordinarily flushed, which could be done by forcible agitation of the water and charcoal prior to its diffusion. —*Sea-water:* As a supply of water had been of late recommended by Mr. Fuller, Dr. Routh was fearful, from what he had observed at the sea-side, and in marine as compared with fresh-water vivaria, as also from some experiments made, that organic matters would putrefy much more readily in sea-water than in fresh. If sea-water therefore were used, it must also be mixed with charcoal; and this might readily be done with the foul Serpentine or Thames water, which would be thereby completely deodorized and purified, and this would be effected at much less expense. If the matter of sewers were in this manner collected at some distant point, we should obtain, moreover, an excellent deodorized manure, and our London streets and river would be comparatively sweet and pure, and as a result disease would be less frequent and fatal.

ART. 5.—*Revival of Urn-burial.* By the Editor of the "Edinburgh Medical Journal."

(*Edinburgh Medical Journal,* Nov. 1856.)

"A curious discussion has been raised by the Académie de Medecine of Paris, on the mode of disposing of the dead. Several of the leading Paris journals, particularly the 'Presse' and the 'Siècle,' defend with great boldness the assertion of the Academie, that the vicinity of Père-la-Chaise and the cemetery of Montmartre is gradually introducing new diseases amongst the working classes; and that in summer time the hospitals are crowded with the victims of pestilence engendered by the foul air of the graveyards in the neighborhoods of Paris. The discussion is likely to lead to some result and to become a party question; for a new journal, to be devoted entirely to this one subject, has just appeared. This journal, called 'La Cremation,' is edited by two of the first writers of the 'Presse,' and is supposed to be quite in accordance with the sentimets of the Government. M. Alexandre Bonneau proposes to replace all cemeteries adjoining to all great cities by an edifice to be denominated a 'sarcophagus.' This edifice to occupy the highest spot of ground in the city, 'where the corpses of both rich and poor should be conveyed, there to be laid out on a metallic tablet, which, sliding by an instantaneous movement into a concealed furnace, would cause the whole body to be consumed in the space of a few minutes.' With true French instinct, M. Bonneau proceeds to urge not only the utility to the public, but also the interests of art in this new method of disposing of the dead, for he points out with great complacency the new element of prosperity to the artists existing in the furnishing of funeral urns, which he declares would soon open a new source of expense and luxury to the rich. 'For who would not love to preserve the ashes of his ancestor? The funeral urn would soon be found to replace on our consoles and mantel-pieces, the present ornaments of bronze clock and china vases now found there.' All this may seem a misplaced pleasantry to English minds; but in Paris these things find serious men to write and fight in their defence; and we cannot help feeling rather startled on reading the sanitary report which first led to their discussion. 'The vicinity of the cemeteries is a constant source of mortality. No matter from what quarter the wind blows, it must bring over Paris the putrid emanations of Père-la-Chaise, of Montmartre, or Montparnasse; and the very water which we drink, being impregnated with the same poisonous matter, we become the prey of new and frightful diseases of the throat and lungs, to which thousands of both sexes fall victims in the spring and autumn of every year. Thus the *angine couenneuse*, which baffles the skill of all our most experienced medical men, and which carries off its victims in a few hours, is traced to the absorption of the vitiated air into the windpipe, and has been observed to rage with the greatest violence in those quarters situate on the outskirts of the town, and, consequently, the nearest to the cemeteries.'

"The latter argument has created many converts to the opinions of M. Alexander Bonneau; and the first number of 'La Cremation' has excited much interest. After a long interval of desuetude, Sir Thomas Browne's 'Urn-burial' may come to be consulted as a work for practical details—and the urns in our museums, instead of representing obsolete utensils, may become models for those vases which present such charms for M. Bonneau. Perhaps, however, the vase theory is a step too far in advance, and the Parisians, if they see their way to consumption by fire, may prefer burying the ashes of their friends in the earth, as was done with the remains of Shelley's burned body, rather than that the dust of humanity, however rich the enclosing caskets, should be chimney ornaments in drawing-rooms.

"The utilitarian character of the English, as distinguished from the more fanciful temperament of the French, is exemplified in the mode of interment adopted in the case of the late Sir William Temple, as detailed in the 'Times' some days ago. The body was interred in a bed of charcoal, whilst the gases from the coffin are conducted by a pipe to the outside of the church. The leading journal speaks in high terms of the conserving influence thus exercised on the lungs of worshippers; but we are not so sanguine as to the benefits of the system. It may do in rare instances of intra-mural burial, but if universally adopted, congregations would be saved at the expense of the general public. Cremation is a process to which the British mind will not soon be reconciled, and the only graveyard reform presently within reach is distant cemeteries and deep sepulture amongst charcoal or other deodorizing substances."

ART. 6.—*On the defects of Hospitals in respect of Ventilation, &c.* By Mr. ROBERTON.

(Reprinted from the *Transactions of the Manchester Statistical Society*.)

The principal object of this paper is to draw attention to the necessity of constructing hospitals in such a way that the air of one ward will not mix with and pollute the air of another ward. The hospital at Bordeaux (of which a plan is given), in which the wards are in reality detached buildings arranged around a large quadrangle, and separated by gardens, and into which the air can freely enter and pass out again through oppositely-placed windows, which reach from the floor to the top of the ceiling, is pointed out, and very properly pointed out, as a model of what a hospital should be. Indeed the paper contains many excellent remarks which deserve to be studied by those who are concerned in the formation of buildings for the reception of the sick and wounded.

ART. 7.—*Poisonous effects of the Vapor of Sulphuret of Carbon in Caoutchouc manufactories.* By M. DELPECH.

(*L'Union Médicale*, May 31, 1856; and *Assoc. d.*, Sept. 20, 1856.)

The symptoms produced by this vapor upon the workmen exposed to it are developed in different degrees. They are thus arranged by M. Delpech.

"1. *Disturbance of the intellectual functions.*—Impairment of memory is the most common and most marked of the symptoms of this class. The workmen forget what they have to do, and make great mistakes, to the injury of the manufacture. Every moment they search for the tools which they have just laid aside; they are vague in their ideas, and cannot keep their attention fixed on any one subject. Two patients, observed by M. Delpech, could not find words to express their ideas. Some became violent and irritable, being angered at the least cause, striking all who came in their way, and breaking objects near them. Want of sleep, restlessness, fatiguing dreams, and awakening with starts, were observed in almost all M. Delpech's cases: during the day, these patients were depressed, and without energy; and, whether from want of sleep, or more probably, from the influence of the sulphurous vapors, they felt a strong propensity to sleep.

"2. *General sensation* is not very severely affected; however, there is almost always some heaviness of the head, more or less severe headache, sometimes very intense, and extreme vertigo. The pain, it has been observed by M. Bouchardat, occupies the top of the head, and is sometimes transient, lasting only two or three hours, sometimes obstinately persistent. In several cases, there have been observed pains in the limbs like chronic rheumatism, and general creeping and pricking sensations. M. Delpech has never observed well-marked anæsthesia; but M. Bouchardat has noticed slight loss of sensibility in the arms and hands. In one of M. Delpech's cases there was complete insensibility to pain—common tactile sensibility remaining; in another, there was marked hyperæsthesia.

"3. *Special senses.*—Though no structural lesion could be discovered in the eye, the sight was, in M. Delpech's cases, greatly weakened. The pupils were mobile, but generally dilated; a thick cloud seemed spread between the patients and the objects at which they looked. Hearing was temporarily affected in several. The food of the patients, their tobacco, and all odorous subjects, appeared to them impregnated with the fumes of sulphuret of carbon.

"4. *Generative functions.*—In nearly all the cases, the sexual appetite was lost. Coition was almost impossible. As the patients were young healthy men, this fact is more remarkable: and perhaps this impairment of the sexual function is one of the most marked symptoms of poisoning by sulphuret of carbon. The same effect has been observed in females.

"5. *Motion.*—One patient had frequent painful cramps of the limbs; another had involuntary contractions of the upper eyelid; and another had a kind of transient contraction of the flexor muscles of the fingers. M. Bouchardat and M. Delpech have observed a stiffness of the fingers, and of the upper limbs in general. In all the patients, muscular weakness was strongly marked, both in the lower and the upper limbs. There was in all the patients a degree of hesitation in their movements approaching to general tremor; but it appears to have reached a high degree in one case only. The muscular debility was accompanied by marked atrophy. In one case, the arms were so reduced that there was a depression in the interosseous space of the forearm; and the muscles of the thenar eminence were greatly reduced. The power of contraction, under electricity, remained in the muscles of all the patients who were submitted to this test.

"6. *Digestive organs.*—The symptoms have generally begun by slight disturbances of the digestive functions. Loss of appetite has been constant, and has reached so high a degree as to amount to disgust for all food, from the idea that it tasted of sulphur. The appetite reappeared in several when they had passed some hours in the air. Another symptom has been constant nausea, not always, but generally, amounting to vomiting. The vomiting returned at various times; sometimes during work, when the ejected matters were greenish and bilious; sometimes after breakfast, when the food was rejected. The vomiting was generally accompanied by extreme *malaise* and cold sweats, and left the patients much exhausted. Salivation, properly so called, was not observed; but several had their mouths frequently full of saliva. Colic was an habitual symptom, occasionally very severe: it was not regularly accompanied by either diarrhœa or constipation. The fæcal matters very often smelt strongly of sulphuret of carbon: some of the patients complained much of flatulence.

"7. *Respiration.*—The breath generally smells of sulphur. There is generally some breathlessness after walking; the respiration is short; but M. Delpech has only twice discovered any abnormal physical signs.

"8. *Circulation.*—The heart seemed healthy in all the patients. Several felt palpitation at various periods. In the cachectic patients, *bruits de souffle* were heard in the vessels of the neck. No constant febrile phenomena have been observed. In some there have been sudden rigors, with acceleration of the pulse, especially during the night.

"9. *Secretions.*—The urine in these cases has not been sufficiently examined; but in some it has been at times colored brown by alkalies, and at other times has contained a large amount of sulphates and carbonates. Several of the patients have felt pain during micturition—due, if their observation of the odor of the urine be correct, to the presence of sulphur. M. Delpech has observed an odor of sulphuret of carbon in the urine kept for his examination. The slight irritation of the urethral mucous membrane may be also explained by the presence of salts in abundance.

"10. *Cachexia.*—The patients fall into a more or less marked state of cachexia; they are pale, their skin is pasty, their mucous membranes lose color, and anæmic murmurs can be heard. Most frequently, this cachexia is complicated by the complete or partial persistence of the symptoms of which it is the sequel. General weakness, loss of sexual power, and a sensation of vagueness in the mind, are the most usual concomitant phenomena."

ART. 8.—*On Arsenic-eating.* By Mr. W. B. KESTEVEN.

(*Assoc. Journal*, Sept. 20,·1856.)

The following is a summary of the information respecting arsenic-eating, which is elicited in these very interesting papers:

1. The evidence upon which the statements have been made, is simply the loosest kind of second-hand hearsay evidence. Neither Dr. Von Tschudi, Mr. Boner, Dr. Johnston, Dr. Kaltenbrenner, nor Dr. Vitzhum, have personally observed or watched the arsenic-eater, although the two latter are resident in parts of Styria where it is alleged that arsenic-eating prevails. All these gentlemen have received their information from other persons.

2. No chemical examinations of the excretions of those alleged to be taking arsenic have been made; neither has any necroscopic examination or chemical analysis been made of the bodies or organs of those who have died after having indulged in arsenic-eating.

3. No analysis of the substance said to be eaten as arsenic has been attempted, in order to ascertain that primary essential point.

4. The alleged tonic and stimulant effects of arsenic taken in the manner reported, are totally at variance with all other experience of the action of this poison; while the consequences which, it is pretended, follow on the discontinuance of the habit of arsenic-eating, are consistent only with those witnessed in all other parts of the world as the result of the long-continued and persistent administration of this substance, and these disappearing on the withdrawal of the drug, in all other instances except those of the pretended Styrian arsenic-eater.

5. No mention has been made of the effects of arsenic upon the systems of those unaccustomed to its action—the beginners in the practice; and surely no one would be so bold as to assert that the Styrian peasant can do what no other human being can do; that is, swallow a grain or two of arsenic, for the first time, without experiencing consequences of any kind. There is, moreover, a total want of any statistical information as to how many are killed off in the process of becoming accustomed to the effects of the poison—a fact which of itself throws the gravest doubts upon the story, since even a very slight inquiry inevitably must have revealed a certain mortality from this cause, more surely than from the alleged occasional excess, or want of the poison.

6. No information has been tendered as to how long this alleged practice may have existed. It is quite certain that it could not have suddenly sprung up without having attracted the attention of resident medical practitioners: since some of those who have been reported as indulging so depraved an appetite, are said to have so done for periods of twenty or thirty years. Dr. Von Tschudi reports. that one man had followed the practice for forty years, and had derived it from his father. As these persons must have learnt the practice from others, when did the indulgence

originate? and how is it that it has only lately come to light, and that merely through the passing curiosity of a traveller? Strange, if true.

7. In the districts of Cornwall where arsenic is largely prepared, no such practice as arsenic-eating has ever been known. Supposing the truth of the statements respecting the Styrian peasantry, the same might fairly have been expected of the Cornish peasantry; the absence of the practice, therefore, in the latter case, augments the incredibility of the former. On the other hand, it must be noticed that the destruction to the lower animals and to vegetation, together with the symptoms of chronic poison by its inhalation, and of chronic skin-disease by its external irritation, observed in the mining districts of Cornwall, has been altogether overlooked by the searchers for marvellous stories among the arsenic-works in Styria, where this deadly poison is said to bestow health, vigor, and beauty.

How different is the gloomy picture of these cases of chronic poisoning from the glowing colors in which this fearful agent is dressed up to charm the innocent and the ignorant, in the pages of Dr. Johnston's romance. How great a discrepancy is here seen—a discrepancy fatal to the credibility of the entire tale, with those who will take the pains to reflect thereon. So dominant, however, in most minds, is the love of the marvellous, that, no matter how improbable, the tale is taken up and repeated until, by frequent repetition, it gains so firm a hold upon public credence, that to doubt is to be guilty of heretical scepticism.

So indisposed, or so incapable, to investigate any scientific matter are too many, that they will readily save themselves that trouble by indulging their credulity.

It has been stated in the outset, that the medico-legal importance of this question induced the writer to investigate its grounds. It has been shown, now that the story wants verification, that so far as information has been procurable, up to the present time, the assertion of the practice of arsenic-eating is totally destitute of all the elements of proof which are invariably demanded, and have always been produced, before statements assuming a scientific character can be received as trustworthy, or regarded as facts.

To urge, therefore, as probable, such a fabulous explanation of the presence of arsenic in a human body, is mere idle talk, and an affront to the common sense of a jury—a mere trick unworthy a highminded advocate. If, however, the plea should be put forth, it will, as in the late Burdon slow poisoning case, be blown to the winds, as utterly untenable and irrelevant to the question before the court. It is hoped, moreover, that medical witnesses will not again admit inferences from such unsupported statements, as having the same weight and value as those drawn from indisputable fact.

Not only was it desirable on medico-legal grounds to show the fabulous character of this story, but it is also of the last importance thereby to warn those who are not competent to detect the fallacious and superficial nature of its evidence, that they must not dare to tamper with so virulent a poison, under the belief that it may be taken with impunity. Notwithstanding all that has been written about its power to bestow a healthy hue, and to heighten the charms of beauty, it still remains a potent poison;—as they may too late discover, if they suffer themselves to be led away by the specious misrepresentations of the lovers of the marvellous.

The conclusion drawn is, that the story of the Styrian arsenic-eaters is not only unsupported by adequate testimony, but is inconsistent, improbable, and utterly incredible.

ART. 9.—*On the influence of Artificial Heat upon the Atmosphere of London.*
By Dr. Chowne

(*Medical Times and Gazette*, Oct. 18, 1856.)

The following particulars are extracted from a paper which was read by Dr. Chowne, on the opening of the present session of the Medical Society of London:

" The well-known effect of clouds, in reflecting back the heat radiated to them from the earth and terrestrial objects, induced me to make some experiments on the subject. These experiments were made in the winter months, when the agents for producing artificial heat are in general operation. It might be easily imagined, that the vast amount of heat generated in the metropolis, and in all large manufacturing towns, by the use of furnaces, by domestic fires, by gas-lights, &c., must exercise considerable effect on the temperature of the atmosphere of these localities. During the year 1850, in order to ascertain the temperature of the London atmosphere on fine clear nights, when compared with that of moderately cloudy nights, as well as on intensely dark and cloudy nights, when radiation would be most obstructed, a cylinder of three inches in diameter, and twelve inches long, was inserted vertically in the earth, and a thermometer was placed within it. The upper orifice of the cylinder, being just level with the ground, was covered by a piece of zinc plate, merely laid upon it; the lower extremity of the cylinder was closed by a disc of the same metal, and soldered. At the same time another thermometer was suspended, nearly over the cylinder, at the height of about ten inches from the ground, and in the free air. The state of the sky was carefully examined during all the experiments. The same general fluctuations of temperature occurred, as have been observed within certain limits, by Mr. Wilson, Mr. Six, Dr. Wells, Melloni, and others; but on intensely cloudy nights, the quantity of heat reflected back by the clouds was sufficient to raise the temperature of the exposed thermometer to a higher degree than that indicated by the thermometer in the cylinder, and partaking directly of the earth's warmth. The experiments were made in one of the gardens at the back of Connaught Place West, Hyde Park. Thus it is satisfactorily proved that on the moderately cloudy nights, when compared with those of the three fine nights (namely, the 27th, 28th, and 29th of November), the thermometers indicated the presence of reflected heat in a degree not differing from what might have occurred in the open country; but that on the densely clouded nights, they indicated a degree of heat sensibly above what they could have derived from the earth's surface. Other thermometers were suspended at the same time in pairs; one of each pair was placed in a situation where it was more or less sheltered from the sky; the other was placed about two feet from it, and at the same height from the ground, but fully exposed to the sky. The result was that, on the intensely dark and cloudy nights, the temperature of the exposed thermometers attained a higher degree than that attained by those that were sheltered. This occurred on the nights when it was found that the exposed thermometer already spoken of as being suspended near the ground, attained a higher temperature than that in the cylinder within the ground. Hence, although in ordinary circumstances the air under a shed is, during the night, warmer than the unsheltered air, yet on extremely overcast nights, the relative temperatures are reversed, and are rendered analogous to those which exist on sunny days, when thermometers exposed to the sun's rays indicate a higher temperature than those sheltered from them. Dr. Wells, when he had changed the place of his experiments on dew from the open country to Lincoln's Inn Fields, considered that the surrounding houses had an influence on his thermometers. He says, 'In situations where large masses of bare solid matter exist, . . . a greater heat will be received by the exposed body than what is radiated by itself. For example, it seemed certain to me that the houses surrounding Lincoln's Inn Fields had an influence upon my thermometers during my experiments there at night, beyond what arose from their merely returning a quantity of heat, equivalent to that which they received from the surface of the garden.' It does not appear that Dr. Wells attributed the various effects produced on his thermometers to any influence of artificial heat translated by processes of combustion from the earth to the clouds, and reflected by them back again; indeed, at the time when his experiments were made, two great sources of heat now in operation, the making and the burning of gas, had but a very limited existence. It may likewise be remarked that the consumption of gas for lights had added almost incalculably to the quantity of heat communicated to the open air. The experiments were repeated on nights more or less foggy, and the results were in accordance with what had been observed by the authorities already mentioned, namely, that fog does not exercise the same power as clouds in reflecting back the heat emitted by radiation or otherwise from the earth." Dr. Chowne then dwelt on the important inference which appeared to be deducible from the fact that so large a body of artificial heat can be thrown back upon terrestrial objects, a probable consequence being to augment the atmospheric capacity for holding aqueous vapors; and this circumstance renders the subject one of interest in regard to the atmosphere, not only in its physical relations generally, but also in its relations to our sewers, and the openings from them at the gratings in the streets. Although in a room where gas is burning, the hygrometer (Mason's indicates a decrease of the difference of temperature between the dry bulb and the wet one, owing to the quantity of vapor generated by the process of combustion, yet the fact of such formation in the open air would but slightly interfere with the aggregate results of combustion going on by other means at the same time.

The quantity of aqueous vapor supplied by the surface evaporation from the streets of London, except when they are wet with rain, or from other causes, is extremely small; and the same might be said of that from the surface of the Thames, when compared with the vast extent of the metropolis. The Thames, moreover, is remote from the great mass of the populous districts. On calm, still nights, when there is scarcely wind enough to move our atmosphere along; and when, moreover, there is the absence of rain, any increase of temperature, such as the experiments described show to take place, must have a powerful influence, not only on all the pneumatic relations existing between the open atmosphere and the atmospheres of dwelling-houses and of sewers, but also on the chemical relations affecting all dead and decomposing organized matters. This led the author to a consideration of the emanations from sewers under the atmospheric conditions just noticed, and which lead us to the general question of means and ends connected with sanitary improvements. Meteorological and physical phenomena in the grand operations of nature we cannot control, whether they affect us for good or for ill; but what belongs to the class of artificial operations might hereafter find a remedy; there is, however, very much to be changed before that can be brought about. The author then referred successively to openings in the streets as not fit places of escape for subterranean exhalations; the transmission of the atmosphere of the sewers by means of the house-drains into our houses. With regard to the temperature of the sewers, the author had no opportunity of ascertaining the state of the case. On the intensely cloudy nights to which the experiments detailed in this paper refer, the inference, however, would be, that a strong analogy would be found in the results to the fact already recorded. The circumstances under which currents of air take place, and the direction of their movements, next came under consideration, and the author proceeded to detail investigations carried on in respect to the direction of currents from gulley-holes; but in respect to the data obtained, remarked that the results could not be fully explained without a better knowledge as to the pneumatic influence which particular parts of the sewers are under at the time of making the trial. With regard to dwelling-houses, the author had ascertained, in very many instances, that great quantities of foul air passed from the sewers to their interiors, steadily and constantly contaminating the atmosphere of the house, although generally the admitted effluvia, owing to its being diluted by the atmosphere of the house, does not betray its presence by a strong odor. Dr. Chowne concluded by remarking that the bearing of these experiments was to show that the condition of the atmosphere, produced by the various sources of artificial heat referred to, could not fail to have a powerful influence, not only on the sanitary state of the metropolis, but also of all large manufacturing towns.

(B) ACUTE DISEASES.

ART. 10.—*On the treatment of Typhus and Typhoid Fever.*
By Professor DIETL, of Cracow.

(*Wien. Wochenschrift*, 44, 50, 1856.)

In this paper Dr. Dietl advocates a nourishing and tonic plan of treatment in fevers. Pure air and good nourishment (not mere slops) are, in his opinion, of far greater importance than pharmaceutical remedies; but at the same time a free use of acids, especially the phosphoric, and of quinine in large doses, is believed to be of the greatest utility. Dr. Dietl even objects to cold applications to the head, on the ground that the head symptoms in fever are the result, not of simple cerebral congestion, but of a dyscrasia, which does not require and will not bear any depressing agencies whatever. The sentiments and practice of Dr. Dietl are indeed, very similar to the sentiments and practice of Dr. Stokes, and others of the same school.

ART. 11.—*On Typhus in the Crimea.*
By M. BAUDENS, Surgeon-in-Chief of the French Army.
(*American Quarterly Journal of Med. Science*, Oct. 1856.)

M. Baudens has lately addressed a letter from Constantinople to the President of the Parisian Academy of Medicine, in which he states that the typhus which reigned amongst the French troops is not identical with typhoid fever, notwithstanding a certain amount of analogy as to cause, periods, and sequelæ.

Typhus, as lately observed in the Crimea, is engendered by want, and crowding, either in prisons, hospitals, or on board vessels; the disease may, indeed, be called forth and removed at will. This is not the case with typhoid fever and other epidemics, as cholera, which, in spite of all precautions, break out suddenly and disappear without any appreciable cause. Typhus is propagated both by infection and contagion; the latter mode of transmission, which is doubted by some as to typhoid fever, is quite evident as to the Crimean typhus.

The difference between typhus and the generality of epidemics is, that the latter reign only temporarily, according to the duration of certain atmospheric influences, whilst typhus continues until the causes of infection have been removed. The Crimean typhus has presented less regularity and uniformity in the accession of symptoms than the ordinary typhus described by Hildenbrand. This irregularity may be ascribed to various causes, amongst which should especially be noted scurvy, dysentery, and the intermittents, which were excited by the marshes of the valley of the Tchernaya. There were mostly no premonitory symptoms, as lassitude, sleeplessness, lumbar pains, horripilatio, tension in the head, and vertigo, so common in typhoid fever. The Crimean typhus began at once by shivering, frontal cephalalgia, stupor, muttering or violent delirium, total prostration, more or less discharge from the eyes, the nares, or bronchi, intense thirst, and a foul state of the alimentary canal. The burning skin was covered in two or three days with an exanthematous eruption, different from that which is seen in typhoid fever, and presenting irregular groups of round spots of a dull red, smaller than a split pea, and not disappearing upon pressure with the finger. There were generally neither petechia nor sudamina. The fever proved continuous, with from 100 to 130 beats in a minute, but was interrupted by one, or sometimes two, regular paroxysms in the twenty-four hours, somewhat similar to fits of ague, which circumstance has given the Crimean fever a peculiar character. The abdomen was generally soft, painless, and without either tympanitis or that gurgling in the iliac fossa peculiar to typhoid fever. Instead of the diarrhœa which generally accompanies the latter affection, constipation was present in the Crimean fever, except in those cases where dysentery existed before the attack. The inflammatory period lasted five or six days, and was followed by cerebral symptoms of the ataxic and adynamic character. The latter lasted only four or five days, and were slight in the cases which recovered.

The short duration of this fever contrasts strikingly with the length of time during which typhoid fever generally lasts. Death has often occurred on the third day, sometimes on the second, and even on the first. The latter were fearful cases. The fever continued rarely beyond the twelfth or fifteenth day, save when complications occurred, such as congestion of the viscera of any of the three splanchnic cavities. Convalescence almost always took place within the first ten days, the patient passing at once, as it were, from death to life. Coma and delirium left him as by magic, but sleep continued heavy, and there remained deafness, weakness of sight, and some loss of memory. No falling of hair, as happens after typhoid fever, was noticed. The favorable changes were often preceded by epistaxis, diaphoresis, critical urine, and sometimes mumps. Convalescence, which advances so slowly in typhoid fever, is rapid in typhus, and errors of diet have no unpleasant results. This is owing to the absence of inflammation of the intestinal follicles, and the non-congestive state of the mesenteric glands, the reverse being one of the principal characteristics of typhoid fever.

The liver and the spleen, in the Crimean typhus, were often found gorged with blood, and softened; the lungs, when congested, were either clogged or hepatized; the meninges injected; opaline effusion in the arachnoid, sometimes with pseudomembranous patches; cerebral surface dotted, softened, or presenting on its surface a layer of pus.

ART. 12.—*Influence of Season upon Cholera in India.*
By MR. WARING.

(*Indian Annals of Med. Sci.*, April, 1856.)

The connection between cholera and *drought* has been commented upon on a former occasion. The present facts are very striking:

"During the years 1851, '52, and '53, the deaths, in Bombay, from cholera amounted to 6494; the proportion which died in each month or season is exhibited in the following table:

Months.	1851.	1852.	1853.	Total.	
February, ...	905	91	3	999	
March, ...	1013	160	13	1186	} 3062, or 61·8 per cent.
April, ...	601	271	5	877	
May, ...	373	149	16	538	
June, ...	339	151	9	499	} 1281, or 19·7 per cent.
July, ...	73	165	6	244	
August, ...	37	66	6	109	
September, ...	25	19	6	50	} 438, or 6·7 per cent.
October, ...	19	10	250	279	
November, ...	20	6	571	597	
December, ...	207	24	240	471	} 1713, or 26·3 per cent.
January, ...	408	23	214	645	
	4020	1135	1339	6494	

"On turning to the meteorological abstracts in the appendix for an explanation of the great mortality of the first and fourth quarters, as shown above, and the comparative exemption of the second and third quarters, we were at once struck by the fact of the two latter quarters (the second and the third) constituting the regular monsoon, or rainy season, of Bombay. If, instead of taking quarters, we divide the above cases into half-years, we find the figures stand thus:

Rainy season (May to October, inclusive), ... 1719 deaths,
or, 26·4 per cent.
Dry season (November to April, inclusive), ... 4775 deaths,
or, 73·5 per cent.

"A careful comparison of the above figures with the meteorological abstracts, leads naturally to the conclusion that (in Bombay at least) the humidity of the air, in the wet season, is unfavorable to the generation and development, or operation, of the choleraic poison, be that what it may; and that, on the other hand, the dry season is, in some mode, yet unexplained, favorable to its generation and operation. We notice that, in the six dry months in each year, the pressure of the air, as shown by the barometer, attained its maximum, and likewise, that the mean range of the pressure was greatest in these months; also the thermometer showed the widest ranges, and the humidity of the air was comparatively small. One other circumstance marks the dry from the wet season, which deserves notice, namely, *the prevalence of the land winds*, so much dreaded by most natives of Southern India, especially on the western coast. I am unable to trace the connection between them, by comparing the mean number of hours the land wind prevailed and the deaths from cholera; but it is certain, that the mean number of hours the land wind blew during the dry season, when cholera was most rife, is above three times greater than in the wet season, when, as we have seen, cholera is comparatively rare."

ART. 13.—*On the Cholera which visited Her Majesty's Black Sea Fleet in the autumn of* 1854. By Dr. BABINGTON.

(*Lancet*, Aug. 23, 1856.)

This report is compiled from the returns of the medical officers of the fleet to queries drawn up by the Cholera Committee of the Epidemiological Society. It was read on the 4th of August, 1856, at a meeting of this Society.

Dr. Babington commenced by observing that the medical officers of the navy were, from the double examination which they had all passed through, first under the general professional authorities of the empire, and then under the authorities connected with the service, well qualified to answer inquiries, and the more so from their isolated positions and probable freedom from preconceived theories. The superior opportunities of observing disease at its onset, and of knowing the habits, occupations, diet, &c., of the ship's crew, were pointed out, as also the advantage of being able to trace all particulars regarding first cases. The great facility which a ship possessed of being able to move from place to place was particularly dwelt on; after which the writer proceeded to enumerate the ships in the Black Sea fleet—twenty-five in number—in which cholera occurred; also those—three in number—in which diarrhœa occurred; and, finally, those in which there was neither cholera nor diarrhœa. He then read the queries which the Cholera Committee had circulated to the fleet, and explained an elaborate table which he had drawn up of all those circumstances in the answers to those queries which admitted of tabulation. He next took into consideration those subjects in the queries which did not admit of tabulation, the first being the question as to whether the crews of boats communicating with the shore suffered more, and at an earlier period, than the men who were confined to the ship. A summary of the answers showed that in seven ships those persons having communication with the shore *were* first affected with the disease; and that in fourteen ships the disease did not appear first in those who were in communication with the shore: while in the remaining ships there was no evidence either one way or the other. To the question regarding the number, if any, of cases without premonitory symptoms, a summary of the answers showed that out of 711 attacked of cholera, reported in the Black Sea fleet, there were, without premonitory symptoms, 134 cases, or more than one in six. The following is a summary of the opinions of the medical officers: first, on the chief predisposing and exciting cause of the outbreak; second, on the comparative immunity of certain of the ships; third, on the treatment of the disease; and fourth, on the best preventive measures. The question regarding predisposing causes is answered by the medical men of fifteen ships only, and their opinions are all comprised under one or other of the following heads: exposure to sudden changes of heat, cold, and moisture, and to night air; bad food and clothing; intemperance; the immoderate use of fruit and vegetables, or the use of unripe fruit or decayed vegetables; the drinking cold water when hot; over-fatigue; crowding; bad ventilation; the use of impure water; finally, diarrhœa, as a consequence of the foregoing causes, whether singly or in combination. With respect to the exciting cause, the question is answered by the medical men of sixteen ships only. Of these, ten consider it to have been atmospheric influence; one considers the poison to have been atmospheric, but that it was rendered contagious by evacuations from the sick, and by foul air; while the remaining five, without mentioning the term, evidently lean to the side of contagion. The question regarding the cause of comparative immunity received answers from the medical men of sixteen ships, who attribute it to the shifting of locality; to cleanliness, dryness, and thorough ventilation; to keeping the men out of the sun, and fully occupying them; to their excellent health and regular habits, and their non-communication with the shore; to the free use of chloride of zinc; to the use of quinine wine as a preventive; to the avoidance of unripe fruit, and the early treatment of diarrhœa. On the subject of treatment, there are answers from all those ships which were visited by either cholera or diarrhœa, but there were twelve which escaped altogether. It seems to have been a very frequent practice to commence with a large dose of calomel and opium, and to proceed with small doses at frequent intervals. In at least eighteen of the ships, calomel seems to have been the leading medicine. Stimulants, both internal and external, were much used. Dr. Billing's plan, by oft-repeated small doses of tartar emetic, is extolled by one gentleman, and Dr. Stevens's saline plan by another; but no such amount of success seems to have followed any mode of treatment as to recommend it emphatically beyond the rest. The only novelty noticed is the application of numerous cupping-glasses over the limbs and body, which in one ship is said to have had a good effect in restoring warmth and preventing cramp. The suggestions offered with regard to prophylaxis admit of division into those which respect the ship and those which respect the men. As to the former, the chief recommendations are cleanliness, ventilation, fumigation, and whitewashing, dryness, the free use of chloride of zinc, and a shifting of locality. In one instance it is suggested that in steamships the bilges should be lined with metal, to prevent the absorption of grease, and that they should be flushed with alkaline hot water previously to purification by chloride of zinc. The preventive measures as applicable to the men are a generous diet with fresh provisions when procurable, recreation, amusement, comforts, warm clothing, including the use of flannel, especially round the abdomen, the use of quinine wine, a strict surveillance and immediate attention to diarrhœa, the serving out of tea and coffee before going on deck in the early morning, a supply of clean bedding well aired, the prevention of intercourse with any ship or locality where cholera exists, abstinence from unripe fruits, from excesses of all kinds, from exposure to night air, wet, hot sun, or the early morning air without food, the avoidance of fatigue, especially in the sun, and exposure to sudden chills or to long fasting. Returns were received from seven Baltic ships, which, having subsequently joined the Black Sea fleet, received the queries there. Some opportunity of forming a comparison, though an imperfect one, was thus afforded. Dr. Babington, in concluding his report, made a few remarks on it, of which the following is a short abstract. The most encouraging fact it contained, he considered to be the great disproportion between the number of attacks of cholera amongst the officers and those amongst the men. Out of 884 officers in the Black Sea fleet, there were but 5 who had the disease, and of these one was a gunner, and one a boatswain, whose habits probably assimilated more to those of foremast men than of quarter-deck officers. There were in the Black Sea, 11,488 seamen, amongst whom there occurred 705 attacks. These numbers give a proportion of 1 to 177 in the former case, and 1 to 16·3 in the latter. In the Baltic, where, in the ships which sent reports, there were 183 officers and 1841 seamen; there was a perfect immunity from cholera amongst the former, and 49 attacks, or 1 in 37 57 amongst the latter. Dr. Babington thought the difference chiefly owing to a difference in the predisposing, and in a great measure preventible causes. Amongst the men in the Black Sea fleet, the proportion of deaths to attacks was 1 to 18, and in the Baltic as 1 to 2·88. Comparing the seamen with the marines, it was found that in the Black Sea the attacks of the marines, who in number bore a proportion of 1 marine to 38 sailors, was 1 to 12; and the proportion of deaths to attacks, as 1 to 1·16, the disease being therefore somewhat more fatal amongst them, and notably more frequent than amongst the seamen. In the Baltic, on the contrary, where the proportion of marines to seamen was nearly the same, the number of attacks amongst the former was only 1 in 42·6, and there was only 1 death, or 1 in 384. Of all the suggestions as to preventive treatment, Dr. Babington thought that which recommends a shifting of locality the most valuable, as it proved successful in several instances. The report concluded with an apology for its length, which was unavoidable if justice were to be done to the subject and to those meritorious medical officers who had with so much courtesy furnished the materials.

ART. 14.—*On concurrent Scarlet Fever and Measles.*
By Mr. W. B. KESTEVEN.

(*Journal of Health, Oct.* 1856.)

"Difficulties of diagnosis have, within a period of the last three or four years, frequently happened to the author in regard to scarlatina and measles. His number of cases, however, not having been sufficiently great to serve the purpose of any useful statistical comparison, the writer has contented himself with stating the general features of the cases to which he refers, as illustrated by the subjoined (as they may be termed) representative cases.

"In the month of September of this year the writer attended five children in a house in Albany Street, Regent's Park. In each case there was indisposition for four or five days, consisting of simple febrile or catarrhal symptoms, with cough, coryza, watering and redness of the eyes. On the fourth or fifth day the severity of the symptoms abated coincidently with the appearance of an eruption of a dull reddish color, not, to the sense of touch, elevated above the surrounding cuticle; when viewed through a lens about a quarter of an inch distance, many of its apices appeared to be desquamating on the second day. At first it looked very like the early eruption of confluent smallpox, but wanting the raised hard and granular feeling to the finger of that disease. The eruption was scattered over the body and limbs. On the face, neck, chest, and arms, it presented the irregular shaped clusters seen in measles. The tongue was furred, and its apex was as red as a boiled lobster. The throat, in three instances, was slightly sore, and was of a scarlet color. The pulse was rapid, but soft. The bowels rather costive. Urine scanty, but not high colored, and free from albumen.

"These were the most prominent features observed. The variations were, that in two of the children the eruption was more distinct, the spaces of clear skin between the spots being of greater extent. Head symptoms were seen in one child, subsiding with the fever and eruption. The eruption continued apparent for from three to five days, and then rapidly disappeared; the cuticle subsequently desquamating as in scarlatina. An interval of a fortnight occurred between the subsidence of the disease in three of these children, and the first appearance of the symptoms in the two youngest. A period of two days only intervened between each case of the three eldest. Some of the children in this family had been to a school where several of their schoolfellows were absent on account of illness—said to be measles. The author had himself attended the elder children in measles two or three years previously.

"Irregularity, very similar to that described in the preceding cases, as already stated, has been met with on many occasions during the last three or four years. In some cases the first symptoms have corresponded less to those of measles than above related.

"The cases here recorded are regarded by the writer as furnishing instances of the concurrence of measles and scarlatina, the symptoms respectively of each of these fevers masking those of the other, and causing embarrassment to the diagnosis. They have, in most instances, presenented a striking resemblance to the description of measles given in his 'Practice of Medicine' by Cullen as that met with in his day; while they possessed also the undoubted characteristics of scarlatina.

"This conjunction of eruptive fevers, if admitted as the correct view of these cases, presents an exception to the principle so emphatically laid down by John Hunter, and to a very great extent adopted by his successors, that two different fevers cannot exist in the same constitution at the same time. There is little doubt, however, that this principle cannot be accepted rigidly and without modification. Many parallel instances have been cited by Mr. Marson from his own experience at the Smallpox Hospital, and communicated to the Royal Medical and Chirurgical Society in a paper read May 26th, 1847. 'Thus,' concludes Mr. Marson, 'either from personal observation, or from the writings of others, I present examples of the simultaneous occurrence of variola and scarlatina, variola and rubeola, variola and pertussis, variola and vaccinia, rubeola and scarlatina, rubeola and vaccinia, rubeola and pertussis, varicella and vaccinia, pertussis and vaccinia.'"

ART. 15.—*Treatment of Scarlatina Anginosa.* By Mr. P. H. CHAVASSE.

(*Assoc. Journal*, March 15, 1856.)

The paper, of which the substance is as follows, was read before the Medical and Chirurgical Society of Birmingham, on the 4th of March, 1856. After referring to the fortunate result of his practice, Mr. Chavasse proceeds:

"My plan, of late years, has been so uniformly successful (not having lost a case of scarlet fever for upwards of seven years), that I have not deemed it necessary to keep a record of cases. The system I adopt, in a case of scarlet fever, is to keep the bedroom cool—I may say cold—and to have a thorough ventilation through it : I, therefore, throw open the windows, be it winter or summer, and have the curtains and valances of the bed removed. If it be winter time, I allow the patient to have one blanket and a sheet ; if it be summer time, a sheet only to cover him. If the throat be not seriously affected, I merely order a narrow strip of flannel once round the throat. If the tonsils be much enlarged, I apply a barm and oatmeal poultice to the throat, changing it night and morning. I prescribe an acidulated infusion of roses mixture, that is to say, infusion of roses, with an excess of acid, made palatable with an additional quantity of syrup, to be taken every three or four hours. This is the only medicine I give. When the child is old enough, I find roasted apples, mixed with raw sugar, very grateful to the patient.

 " Here let me pause, to advise my medical brethren always to make medicines for children pleasant. The administration of nauseous medicine to children oftentimes causes sickness, disgust, and irritation, which frequently do more harm than the medicine does good.

 " But to return to our subject: I avoid purgatives in scarlet fever. I never, on any account, give a particle of opening medicine for the first ten days at least. It is my firm conviction, that the administration of purgatives in scarlet fever is a fruitful source of dropsy, disease, and death. When we take into consideration the sympathy that there is between the skin and mucous membranes, I think that we should pause before giving irritating medicines. The irritation of purgatives on the mucous membrane may cause the poison of the skin disease to be driven internally, to the kidneys, throat, pericardium, or brain. You may say, Do you not purge if the bowels be not open for a week? I say, emphatically, No !

 " Now with regard to food. If the infant be at the breast, keep him entirely to it. If he be weaned, and under two years old, give him milk and water, and cold water to drink. If he be older, give him toast and water, and plain water from the pump, as much as he chooses ; let it be quite cold—the colder the better. Weak black tea, or thin gruel, may be given, but caring nothing if he take nothing but cold water, unless he be an infant at the breast. Avoid broths and stimulants of every kind.

 " Now, you must warily watch for a change of temperature of the skin. As long as the skin is hot, the above plan I steadily follow ; but the moment the skin of the patient becomes cool, which it will do, probably, in five or seven days, instantly close the window, and immediately put more clothes on the bed. But still do not purge.

 " You will find the acidulated infusion of roses most grateful to the little-patient ; it will abate the fever, it will cleanse his tongue, it will clear his throat of mucus, it will, as soon as the fever is abated, give him an appetite. I believe, too, the acid treatment has some peculiar properties of neutralizing the scarlatina poison. I do not pretend to explain how, or why, or wherefore.

 " When the appetite returns, you may consider the patient to be safe. The diet must now be gradually improved. Bread and butter, milk and water, and arrow-root, made with equal parts of milk and water, may be given for the first two or three days. Then a light batter or rice pudding may be added ; and, in a few days afterwards, a little chicken, or a mutton chop.

 " Within the last few years I have had some fearful cases of scarlet fever ; but, relying on this plan of treatment, I have given, even in very bad cases, a very favorable diagnosis. I have had cases where there have been violent headache and delirium ; where there have been immense swellings of the parotid and submaxillary glands ; where there have been enormous enlargement and ulceration of the tonsils ; where a great portion of the fluid that has been taken by the mouth has escaped down the nostrils ; where there has been a purulent discharge down the nose, which discharge has in many instances quite excoriated the skin over which it has travelled ;—and yet in such cases the patients have invariably recovered.

 " There is another important regulation I lay great stress upon. I never allow a scarlet-fever patient, even if the attack be mild, to leave the house under the month in the summer, and then not if the wind be in the east or northeast ; nor under six weeks in the winter. During the last seven years, I have never had anasarca from the scarlatina ; and I attribute it entirely to the plan I have just recommended, and in not allowing my patients to leave the house under the month—until, in fact, the skin that has peeled off has been renewed. Dr. Watson, in his valuable lectures, gives some advice on this subject. From the sixteenth to the thirtieth day I watch the case assiduously, to assure myself that there be no dropsical approach, carefully examining the urine, ascertaining that there be plenty of it, and that it be not albuminous.

" Let me now sum up the plan I adopt:

" 1. Thorough ventilation, a cool room, and scant clothes on bed, for the first five or seven days.

" 2. A change of temperature of skin to be carefully regarded. As soon as the skin is cool, closing the windows, and putting additional clothing on bed.

" 3. Infusion of roses with an excess of acid, sweetened, the only medicine to be given.

" 4. Purgatives to be religiously avoided for the first ten days at least, and even afterwards, unless there be absolute necessity.

" 5. Leeches, blisters, emetics, and cold and tepid spongings, inadmissible in scarlet fever.

" 6. A strict antiphlogistic diet for the first week, during which time cold water to be given *ad libitum*.

" 7. The patient *not* to leave the house in the summer under the month; in the winter, under six weeks.

" My firm conviction is, that purgatives, emetics, and blisters, by depressing the patient, sometimes cause scarlatina anginosa to degenerate into scarlatina maligna; for although I have had numerous cases of scarlatina anginosa (my practice being much among children), and some of the cases very severe ones, I have never had, since I have adopted my present plan of treatment, one single case of scarlatina maligna. I have such faith in my present plan of treatment, that, if it be duly followed out, I should seldom despair of even the worst of cases recovering.

" I am aware that some of our first authorities advocate a different plan to mine. They recommend purgatives, which I may say, in scarlet fever, are my dread and abhorrence. They advise cold and tepid spongings—a plan which I think dangerous, by driving the disease internally. Blisters, too, have been prescribed: these I consider weakening, injurious, and barbarous, and likely to irritate the already inflamed skin. They recommend leeches to the throat, which I am convinced, by depressing the patient, lessen the chance of battling against the disease, and increase the ulceration of the tonsils. Again, the patient has not too much blood: the blood only is poisoned. I look upon scarlet fever as a specific poison of the blood, and which will be eliminated from the system, not by bleeding, not by purgatives, not by emetics, but by a constant supply of fresh and cool air, by the acid treatment, by cold water as a beverage, and for the first few days by a strict antiphlogistic diet.

" Sydenham says, that scarlet fever is oftentimes ' fatal through the officiousness of the doctor.' I conscientiously believe that a truer remark was never made; and that, under a different system to the usual one adopted, scarlet fever would not be so much dreaded."

(C) CHRONIC DISEASES.

ART. 16.—*On Leukhemia.* By Professor VIRCHOW.

(*Dublin Hospital Gazette,* Aug. 15, 1856.)

Professor Virchow, in a paper which appeared in the "Gesammelte Abhandl. zur Wissenschaft. Med.," early in this year, adds some important facts to those which have hitherto been collected regarding this malady. Professor Virchow published his first case of this disease (which he met with and had an opportunity of examining after death, in the Charité Hospital at Berlin, on the 1st of August, 1845), in the 780th number of Froriep's "Notizen." He then gave it the name of "Leukhemia," or white blood; but Professor Bennett, of Edinburgh, in his elaborate work on this subject, has preferred the name leucocythemia, as expressing more literally the leading pathological features of the disease. In the paper, however, from which the following is extracted, Professor Virchow states, that he sees no sufficient reason to set aside the name which he originally adopted; he is of opinion, also, that the study of leukhemia is at the present day more advanced than that of many of the diseases described by the physicians of old; and among diseases of the blood, one can hardly name any better known in its development, its progress, and the details of its symptoms.

The blood normally contains a certain proportion of white corpuscles; these corpuscles increase in number under the influence of certain physiological conditions, as during digestion, pregnancy, and some pathological states, as inflammatory and typhoid affections; but these transitory states are no more the expression of a true dyscrasia, than heat and acceleration of the pulse after a meal are analogous to fever.

Up to the present time, continues Professor Virchow, almost without exception, this disease is permanent, surely running its slow and fatal course; and towards the close of life the white corpuscles are in immense excess. In one case, the proportion of the white to the red corpuscles was as 2 to 3; in another, observed by Vogel, as 1 to 2; in a third, by Schreiber, as 2 to 3. The numbers given by Pury 1 to 7, 12, 19, and 21, do not correspond with extreme degrees of the complaint; nevertheless, they express a very marked and singular alteration in the blood, when one thinks that the normal proportion is as 1 to 357 or 355.

Blood which flows spontaneously, or is obtained artificially during life, is not so modified that one can judge from its color and with the naked eye of its alteration; but when it has been defibrinated and let stand for a time, the red corpuscles fall to the bottom, and the white form a layer over them of a yellowish-white purulent appearance. This separation takes place in the dead subject in a manner no less distinct, for in the right side of the heart and pulmonary artery are found soft, unresisting clots of a yellow color, apparently formed of pus.

The quantity of white corpuscles is not the same in all parts of the body of a patient suffering from leukhemia; and the physiologists Lhéritier, Beclard, Lehmann, Kölliker, have pointed out this unequal distribution, independent of any specific disease.

If certain organs have the property normally, or under certain pathological conditions, of actively contributing to the destruction of the red globules, the venous blood quitting such an organ should contain a large proportion of white; and such is the case of the spleen, for analysis has shown that in leukhemia the blood of the splenic vein is twice as rich in colorless globules as that of the jugular.

According to Professor Virchow, two forms of leukhemia exist (*splenic and lymphatic*), the one introducing into the blood the element constituting the pulp of the spleen; the other, elements analogous to the parenchyma of the lymphatic glands. As the disease of the glands is found more marked, so are the lymphatic elements found more abundant in the blood, and the coincidence of an affection of the spleen does not cause the blood to lose the characters which it gets from the admixture of the histological principles of the lymphatic glands; and *vice versa*, when the alteration of the spleen is predominant, and the neighboring glands are secondarily affected, the modification of the blood retains its splenic character.

The chemical analysis of the blood in leukhemia has furnished interesting results: the researches of Vogel, Parkes, Robertson, and Drummond have shown that the albumen, the fibrin, and the salts of the serum, are in their normal proportions, that water is in excess, and that the solid elements, especially the red globules, are diminished; in fact, that there is no change in the composition of the blood plasma, but merely a substitution of the white globules for the red.

The swelling of the lymphatic glands is ordinarily slow in its progress, but not invariably so; thus in the case given by Rinecker, the disease made its appearance after a cold bath, and commenced by swelling of the cervical glands, which rapidly acquired a considerable size; later the axillary and inguinal glands became affected, there was fever, and the glandular enlargements were hot and painful. And in two other cases reported by Mohr and Vogel, the symptoms followed the same course. Sometimes, on the other hand, the tumors grow very slowly; in one case, the patient, aged 42 years, had been for two years the subject of indolent glandular hypertrophy; in another the glandular swelling dated twenty years back, occupied different regions of the body, and it was during his residence in hospital that any disposition to inflammation of the lymphatic vessels first appeared.

The glands do not in general show any morbid material in their structure, merely a simple increase of their normal elements; externally they seem soft and elastic, having a sort of false fluctuation, their surface is smooth, sometimes shining, and of a color varying from white to yellow or gray. On section, the cortical portion is found thickened, and the cavernous tissue of the hilum also hypertrophied. The cortical portion is more homogeneous, gray, or of a reddish white. The normal division of the follicles is hardly to be distinguished, the parenchyma is soft and friable, and there exudes a milky fluid. The mass, under the microscope, resembles the infiltration of the intestinal follicles in typhus.

The lesions of the spleen are more complex. As to the development of the tumor, we find its progress and symptoms sometimes chronic and insidious, spreading over many years, yet sometimes proceeding with rapidity, accompanied with fever and pain. Uhle has observed, as Virchow has also pointed out, the excretion of a great quantity of uric acid and urates in the urine during febrile attacks; and this condition of the urine may be the more surely regarded as connected with the affection of the spleen, as Scherer has found uric acid and hypoxanthine in that organ.

The spleen is almost always very much increased in volume, attaining occasionally twelve or fifteen times its normal weight; there are generally found very manifest traces of perisplenitis, the capsule is almost always thickened, opaque, milky, having spots and thickenings scattered more or less widely over its surface, the latter sometimes half cartilaginous. There also exist adhesions to the surrounding parts, particularly the diaphragm and retro-peritoneal tissue. The specific gravity of the organ seems increased, it is more resisting than natural, and its tissues often seem bloodless; it is of a pale or yellowish red, sometimes brown.

The large vessels only seem to be of large calibre and to remain open; the follicles are small, often badly defined, and indistinct. However, they are to be found on a close examination, since, by their whitish color, they can be distinguished from the red pulp. The spleen pulp is exceedingly abundant, very resistant, almost elastic, and hard to tear; the thickened trabeculæ are easily seen. The examination with the microscope shows everywhere the normal elements, but more abundant and more condensed than natural; the substance intermediate between the cells and the pulp is more considerable and more solid than it should be; it is not unusual to find some pigment passing from yellow to red, or from gray to black. Very often points are met with, more or less scattered on the surface, of a red color, so intense as to mark them out from the rest of the tissue; later this redness assumes a hemorrhagic appearance, and the spots, at first slightly raised, dip in at a more advanced period, become compact and dry. The color alters from red to yellow or a dirty gray; the little mass becomes caseous or tuberculous, and at length ends by being transformed into a sort of yellow, greenish, or red cicatrix. Examined microscopically, the normal elements of the spleen are discovered in a state of dissolution.

Another organ, besides the lymphatics and the spleen, is attacked in the course of this disease—the liver, which becomes the seat of an hypertrophy, so that its weight increases from eight to fifteen pounds; usually as it increases in weight it does so also in density, and sometimes resembles the cirrhosed liver. Uhle has discovered many little granules of a dirty white color, presenting the appearance of semolina. In one case Professor Virchow saw in the liver small white points scattered through its parenchyma, of the size of an hepatic lobule, and, indeed, they seem to have taken the place of the lobule; one of these white points was developed to the size of a pea, and there was extracted from it a fluid which contained the elements of the lymphatic glands.

Much still remains to be learned as to the commencement and early stages of this disease, of which there is not, at the present time, one single case whose cure can be positively stated. With regard to it in its more advanced degree, the following facts seem to be distinctly ascertained :—The disease is always febrile, and the fever assumes the hectic form; the patient dies in a state of marasmus; the digestive and respiratory derangements take place early; the disposition to diarrhœa is interrupted by occasional attacks of constipation; the dyspnœa is carried sometimes to such a pitch, that it cannot be accounted for by muscular or pulmonary disorder, but seems to depend directly on the intimate constitution of the blood.

ART. 17.—*Case of Idiopathic Gangrene of the Four Extremities, resembling Gangrenous Ergotism.* By Dr. BERNARD HENRY, Surgeon to the P. E. Hospital, Philadelphia.

(*The Phil. Examiner*, March, 1856.)

This case presents many points of interest. It resembles very closely the gangrenous form of ergotism, of which a case was recently related in the "British and Foreign Medico-Chirurgical Review," by Dr. T. Camps (*v.* "Abstract," xxii); but, at the same time, it differs from this affection in the absence of spasmodic symptoms, and in the fact that the intellect remained comparatively clear up to a very short period before death. The patient, it appears, had eaten rye-bread shortly before her illness began, but there was no evidence that this was of bad quality. On the contrary, it was ascertained that she had always had abundance of good food. Dr. Henry remarks, that there were many points of resemblance between this case and the cases of "dry gangrenous leprosy" which had fallen under his notice in the Hospital of St. Lazarus, at Bahia. The case itself occurred in the P. E. Hospital, Philadelphia.

CASE.—J. C—, widow, æt. 42, sempstress, dark hair and eyes, was admitted November 22d, 1855. She was a native of Maryland, but for some time past had resided in this city. By her own account she had led a very irregular, dissipated life, and had been very intemperate. She had been treated for syphilis in the Blockley Hospital; had given birth to nine children, besides having had frequent abortions intentionally produced.

On admission, she stated that she had been laboring under a persistent diarrhœa during the past summer, which did not yield to remedies, and by which her health and constitution were much impaired.

The symptoms of the present disease made their appearance about two weeks previously. November 9th, on returning from the yard, where she had been washing some articles, she felt a stinging sensation in the hands and feet. They were rendered more painful by scratching, and assumed a dusky red color, which became more livid and intense up to the date of her admission into the hospital.

Dr. West, who had previously seen her, considered that she was laboring under purpura, to which disease her symptoms then bore a strong resemblance.

When she first came under my care, her condition was as follows: the countenance icterode, with an anxious expression, the conjunctivæ yellow, eyelids puffy, the intellect remarkably clear, the hands and forearms, for about a third of their length, of a leaden hue, deepening off to the fingers; these were flexed on the hand, black in color, and dry and shrivelled in appearance. The feet and lower third of the legs were in a similar state. The tip of the nose and the skin over both patellæ were of a dusky color, as though brushed over with bronze paint. The tongue was not much coated, but was marked with two longitudinal reddish-brown stains. The pulse was 80, quick and small.

The affected extremities were icy cold to the touch, and sensibility was so destroyed that the prick of a pin inserted in them was not felt. Sensibility above the line of discoloration was acute.

Movement gave much pain; the weight and warmth of the bed-clothes could not be borne; the cold air was more agreeable. The cartilages of the ears showed a commencing similar condition. The bowels at this time were constipated, and the urinary secretion small in quantity.

She was ordered milk punch, opium, and nutritious diet. Dr. West had previously prescribed a draught containing a drop of creosote, every four hours. The legs were enveloped in cotton wadding; this was afterwards removed at her own request.

November 24th.—The discoloration of the extremities has extended up an inch higher, no line of demarcation is perceptible, the livid hue shading off into the normal color. The pulse remains small, and the urine scanty. Ol. Terebinth., gtts. x, every fourth hour, were added to the treatment.

26th.—Vesications, filled with a dark red serous fluid, made their appearance at the edges of the discolored parts. A specimen of urine was obtained passed before breakfast. It was high colored, of a reddish tinge, sp. grav. 1010, reaction alkaline, and exhibits mucus and purpurine.

The case progressed without much alteration in the general symptoms. The lines of demarcation between the sound and affected parts by degrees became more distinct. There was a copious discharge of serous fluid from the vesications. Morphia was given at night to procure sleep, and laxatives to regulate the bowels.

30th.—Ordered Sulph. Quin., gr. j; Tinct. Cinchon., 3ij, every two hours; milk punch, opium, &c., to be continued.

December 3d.—The parts are now quite black and dry. The lines of demarcation are distinct, and a slight odor is for the first time perceptible; she sleeps well, and expresses herself as feeling better generally.

Sp. grav. of urine 1010, with an acid reaction. Directed light warm water dressings.

7th.—Pulse in right carotid and brachial artery 92, small and soft. Tongue reddish brown and dry. Temperature under the tongue 102° Fah., in right axilla 96°, in left axilla 100°, right foot and leg 62°, left do. 61°. Temperature of ward, 62°.

During the following five or six days her condition underwent very little change. The suppuration increased, with a most offensive, peculiar odor, unlike that of ordinary gangrene. The limbs were dressed with solution of chloride of soda. It was necessary to increase the doses of the opiates to produce sleep; the urine was secreted in very small quantities, insufficient for examination, and she was ordered to take acetate of potassa, the creosote to be discontinued.

11th.—Her symptoms more unfavorable, appetite bad; urine still deficient; pulse 80, small. Directed as a diuretic, Potass. Bitart., grs. iij; Potass. Iodid., grs. ij, to be substituted for the acetate of potassa. Beef tea to be added to the diet.

12th.—Complains of burning pain in her stomach; great desire for cold drinks. Vomiting. Tongue dry and brown, passed very little urine, pulse 100°, small. The process of separation more advanced upon the arms than upon the legs, it having extended nearly down to the bone. Upper part of left leg somewhat swollen and infiltrated; changing and removing the dressings causes great pain. From this date to the 15th, no change.

The spirits terebinth. discontinued, owing to the irritability of the stomach.

20th.—Rather better. Urine still scanty, tongue moist. Takes 2 grs. sulphate morphia at night, ½ gr. every three hours during the day. Complains much of gagging and disposition to vomit, caused apparently by fetor. Her appetite continues very bad, with great irritability of the stomach. The line of separation on the arms is complete. The gangrenous portions are dark, dry, shrivelled, resembling an Egyptian mummy, united only by bone and tendon to the sound parts, which show a disposition to granulate.

26th.—As she appeared rather better than usual to-day, the tongue moist, pulse soft, bowels naturally opened, and urine more abundant, the right hand was removed by sawing through the exposed bones. The granulations were dissected up, to make as fair a stump as possible under the circumstances. No vessels were taken up, but the cut extremities of the bone bled freely. She experienced very little pain, and no inconvenience from the operation. I wished to remove the left hand also, but postponed it at her own request. Directed comp. spts. of lavender, with syrup of ginger and mineral water, to allay thirst and vomiting, with an opiate injection at bedtime.

28th.—Removed the left arm. No disturbance to the patient, the bone, as in the first instance, perfectly sound, and bled freely. Arrested hemorrhage by cold water. No vessels secured.

30th.—The patient seemed better this morning, having slept soundly for a couple of hours. Tongue pale and clean, pulse small and soft; temperature under the tongue 100°; appetite bad, disposition to vomit.

Very little change took place during the following week; the stumps showed a disposition to heal well, and the line of separation between the sound and gangrenous parts of the lower extremities was so marked as to justify their removal by amputation, did her strength permit.

Her appetite, however, continued bad, she rejected nearly all food, and sleep was procured only by means of large doses of opium.

Tonics and stimulants were administered whenever they could be retained.

On referring to the notes, I find, January 13th, that for the last two days she has been sinking; her mind, which, up to the present, has been remarkably clear begins to fail, she has become irritable, and her sensibilities appear blunted. She partially recognized those around her, but could not speak.

January 14th.—She remained in a comatose state during the day, and died at half-past five in the evening.

Autopsy, thirty hours after death.—Emaciation not very great. On opening the thorax and abdomen the viscera were found remarkably dry, scarcely any moisture; very little blood in cutting across the large arterial trunks. The whole venous system appeared engorged with black, thick blood. The lungs were perfectly healthy. Adhesions of the right pleuræ. On opening the pericardium, no fluid was found. The heart was rather small, the coronary veins engorged, as was the whole venous system. The tissue, also, of this organ was more soft than natural, with a tendency to fatty degeneration, and slight fatty deposits in the valves. The pulmonary artery and valves were natural in their structure, but contained a venous clot. The auriculo-ventricular opening was contracted, so as with difficulty to admit the finger. The valves of the aorta were normal; a coagulum was found in the descending aorta. The brachial and femoral arteries were dissected up and examined; they presented no unnatural appearance, but were found adherent to the bone, and closed at the line of demarcation.

On opening the abdomen, the liver presented itself fatty and very much enlarged. There appeared to be commencing cirrhosis; there was resistance to the knife on cutting through the lobuli of that viscus.

The other organs presented nothing remarkable.

ART. 18.—*On the transmission of Syphilis from the Fœtus to the Mother.* By Mr. HUTCHINSON, Surgeon to the Metropolitan Free Hospital.

(*Medical Times and Gazette*, Oct. 11, 1856.)

The following are the general conclusions, arising out of a table of fifty cases, in which a syphilitic taint was believed to be communicated from the fœtus in utero to the mother:

1. That women pregnant by fathers suffering from constitutional taint are very liable to receive the disease from the fœtus.

2. That, when this occurs, the form of disease manifested by the mother will resemble closely that of the father.

3. That syphilitic cachexia, and symptoms of the late tertiary class (palmar psoriasis, fissures of the tongue, leucorrhœa, serpiginous cicatrizing ulcers, and nodes) are the most frequent manifestations of taint thus derived.

4. That the reason why, under these circumstances, severe outbreaks of symptoms of the secondary class so very rarely occur is, that the father has, in almost all cases, long passed that stage, and possesses only a taint of the blood or late tertiary manifestations.

5. That the disease thus derived is not zymotic, *i. e.* that its severity will depend directly on the amount of the contagious material received, and on the constitutional vigor of the recipient, and that increase of symptoms and relapses may be produced by repetition of exposure to contagion.

6. That proneness to abort is not nearly so frequently observed in this class of cases as in that in which the mothers have themselves had primary syphilis.

7. That contamination by pregnancy offers a satisfactory explanation of most of the cases of so-called contagion of secondary syphilis.

8. That it is extremely doubtful if "contagion by the seminal fluid" be possible, cases being extremely rare in which married women, who have never conceived, become the subjects of constitutional taint, without having had primary symptoms, and are, in all probability, to be explained as errors of observation. (The author had met with but one case of this class.)

ART. 19.—*On Mercurial Fumigation in the treatment of Syphilis.* By Mr. HENRY LEE, Surgeon to King's College and the Lock Hospitals.

(*Medical Times and Gazette*, Aug. 2, 1856.)

The paper, of which this is an abstract, was read before the Royal Medical and Chirurgical Society on the 24th of June, 1856.

After giving a sketch of the early history of fumigation in syphilitic complaints, its use, abuse, and abandonment, chiefly on account of the cumbrous and inconvenient apparatus employed, the author proceeds to notice the more modern procedure recommended by Mr. Langston Parker. He then points out the practical objection to the use of the gray oxide of mercury, arising from its very uncertain composition as procured from the shops, and finding, from experience, that it was the light-colored oxide alone which volatilized and produced its effects upon the constitution, and having reason to believe that the light color was due to the presence of calomel, the author performed a series of experiments with calomel alone, or mixed in a certain proportion with the gray oxide, the general result of which went to satisfy him, that for the purposes of mercurial fumigation, 5 or 10 grains of calomel alone, are, in ordinary cases, quite sufficient; and that when the gray oxide is used, the admixture of a few grains of calomel will facilitate its sublimation, and insure its medicinal action. Upon making comparative trials with the calomel alone, and combined with steam (as in Mr. Parker's apparatus), it was found to act more certainly and with greater regularity in the latter case. The following simple plan was suggested by the author: Two small spirit-lamps are used; over one of them is a thin metallic plate, upon which the metallic is placed; over the other a cup of hot water. The patient sits upon a caned-bottom chair, placed over the lamps, enveloped in a blanket; or, if greater economy be necessary, the patient may heat a thick tile in the fire, place it in a night-stool, with a gallipot of hot water upon one corner of it, sprinkle the calomel over the surface of the tile, and sit over it enveloped, as before, in a blanket. The advantages of this simple mode of administering mercury to the system are, rapidity of action, while at the same time but little constitutional disturbance is produced, and all the severe train of symptoms of irritation and debility attendant upon the prolonged internal administration of the mineral are avoided. The small amount of heat used for the purpose of volatilizing the calomel in this apparatus, constitutes the essential difference between Mr. Lee's mode of using the vapor of calomel, and any former trials with that form of mercury; for if the temperature be very high, the calomel is at once converted into vapor and dissipated. The paper is accompanied with a tabular view of twenty cases in which the gray oxide was used, either alone, or in combination with calomel, and calomel was used alone, and shows the age, sex, form of disease, preparation of mercury used, and the time at which the mouth became affected by the fumigation; the result being, to prove that the patient's system can be as readily influenced by a small quantity of calomel in vapor as by a large quantity of the gray oxide or bisulphuret of mercury.

SECT. II.—SPECIAL QUESTIONS IN MEDICINE.

(A) CONCERNING THE NERVOUS SYSTEM.

ART. 20.—*A case of Softening of the Brain in a child.* By Dr. F. CHURCHILL.

(*Dublin Quarterly Journal of Medical Science*, Aug. 1856.)

This case, which is related in the Transactions of the College of Physicians in Ireland, is preceded by a slight sketch of what is laid down in books upon such cases—a sketch which leads to the inference: 1. That inflammation and softening of the cerebral substance is somewhat rare in children. 2. That it is generally said to be accompanied with pain, obscuration of the intellect, disorder of the senses, convulsions, or paralysis, or all of these symptoms, according to the severity and duration of the attack. 3. That, however rare, cases have been recorded in which few or none of these symptoms were present, and yet the patient died of ramollissement—whether inflammatory or not, may be disputed, but in which the disease appeared as a primary affection. 4. That such cases, from their rarity and difficulty of diagnosis, possess great practical interest; and that it is only by the collection of individual cases that we can hope to arrive at any positive conclusions.

CASE.—"On Tuesday, the 21st of March, I first saw A. B., æt. 9½, a little girl, of a slight, delicate appearance, with very fair skin and red hair, and of unusual intellectual activity—a member of a family rather obnoxious to head affections: first complained of severe headache on Monday, March 17th, 1856. We have since found reason to believe, however, that she had been unwell for more than a week, but, as she was anxious to compete in some school examination, she concealed her illness from her mother. On the Monday, however, the pain was too violent to be longer hidden, and it continued without intermission, though with aggravated paroxysms, until I saw her. During this time she slept well, and had some appetite, but no fever. She insisted upon going to school on Wednesday, and was sent home, much the worse for the exertion and the excitement.

"I found her in bed, complaining of severe pain and throbbing in the head (especially at the top), which increased occasionally to an almost intolerable degree. There was neither intolerance of light nor sound at that time. Her intellect was as active and clear as usual; she spoke freely, nor did she dream when asleep. There were neither startings, convulsions, nor stupor. The pulse was 74; neither full nor feeble, but slightly irregular. She had vomited once or twice, but, upon inquiry, I found that it was always after taking food or medicine; however, she took many things without vomiting; she complained of no nausea; the tongue was loaded, but furred and moist; the bowels were quite regular. The sensitive and motive powers were perfectly natural.

*   *   *   *   *

"I found it impossible to come to any positive conclusion, and, if I have clearly described the case, it will be probably conceded to me, that the wisest thing I could do was, to suspend my judgment until the course of the disease should elucidate its nature. Meantime I treated the case very cautiously, so as to meet the possibility of its being inflammation of the brain or its membranes. Leeches were applied, and the legs were fomented; a brisk purgative was given, followed by Hydrargyrum cum Creta and James's powder at short intervals.

"Whether the course of the disorder did elucidate its nature, remains to be determined; but, omitting *daily* reports, I shall state merely the changes in the symptoms throughout, in a more connected though cursory manner, premising, that the patient died on Wednesday, April 2d—the sixteenth day of her illness.

"The headache continued as bad as ever throughout the entire illness, unless, perhaps, the last two days, increasing in paroxysms, and accompanied by moaning. Still she slept very well at night, from which I infer, that the pain must have remitted; but she almost always awoke with it. The sleep for the most part was sound and natural, but one or two nights it was so deep, as to resemble stupor while it lasted. Her intellect was clear throughout; there never was anything like delirium. At first she spoke freely; but as the disease advanced, she either could not or would not make the effort to speak—I rather think the latter, as she occasionally spoke a few words, quite intelligibly, up to the last day; up to within an hour of her death, she evidently recognized those around her. She never had either startings, squinting, the least convulsion, or loss of power. Occasionally, but not frequently, she yawned. The vomiting ceased entirely the day after I first saw her, and never returned. There was no thirst up to the twelfth day, and no appetite; the bowels required, at first, a little medicine, but afterwards she was troubled with mercurial diarrhœa. The urine was secreted in the usual quantity, and of the usual appearance; but towards the end she had twice some delay or difficulty in passing it, which speedily disappeared.

"The senses at first seemed more acute, both light and noise annoyed her, but, after a few days, this diminished; a strong light seemed disagreeable, and throughout, although the pupils answered to the light, I should say that, considering the position of her bed, facing the window, they were ordinarily more dilated than one would have expected.

"The pulse, I have mentioned, was at first about 72, and slightly irregular; but this irregularity disappeared after two days, and never returned; when asleep it was below 70. This continued up to the twelfth day, when suddenly, in the afternoon, a smart outburst of fever occurred; the skin became hot (having been quite natural previously), the pulse rose to 120, and there was great thirst. I do not think the headache was worse, and no nervous symptoms were developed. This attack lasted five or six hours, and then subsided, without perspiration. She fell asleep, and in the morning I found a complete remission. The same attack was repeated on the thirteenth, fourteenth, and fifteenth days, but rather less severely each day; so that on the day she died, the prospect seemed rather less dark than previously; although the exact nature of the disease seemed, if anything, rather more obscure.

"Thus, on April 2d, at 9 o'clock, of the sixteenth day, she took beef tea, swallowed well, recognized those around her, and seemed unusually free from headache and fever. At 10 o'clock she suddenly became insensible, but not convulsed; the breathing became laborious and rattling; the pulse quick and weak; lips blue; countenance livid; and at 11 o'clock she died quite calmly.

"However puzzled I might be to explain satisfactorily the nature of the attack, it was quite clear that there were grounds for very serious apprehension, and that the wiser plan would be to treat the case as disease of the brain, with such modifications as the symptoms called for; and in this view I was fortunate to have the concurrence of Sir H. Marsh, who saw the patient with me soon after the commencement of my attendance, and up to the day but one before she died. We applied leeches to the head and feet, blisters constantly renewed to the neck and head; ice to the head; mustard cataplasms to the legs; gave Hydrargyrum cum Creta, subsequently calomel and James's powder, until diarrhœa had set in, and afterwards James's powder alone, and mercurial frictions; but I cannot say that even temporary relief appeared to result from any of these measures.

"Having obtained permission to examine the head, Dr. M. Collis was good enough to make the post-mortem dissection, about twenty-four hours after death. There was no congestion of the scalp, but on raising the skull, we found the superficial vessels of the brain were somewhat fuller than usual; there was no opacity of the arachnoid, no tubercular deposition, and no effusion. The substance of the brain was natural to a considerable depth, but we found the posterior portion of the great commissure of the brain, the fornix, and septum lucidum, so much softened as to be semifluid. It was of much the usual color, neither yellowish nor reddish. A superficial layer of the corpus striatum was also softened. The ventricles contained a considerable quantity of opaline serum; and there was more beneath the arachnoid of the cerebellum, and at the base of the brain, but nowhere did the membrane exhibit marks of inflammation.

"Thus we see that we may have fatal softening and effusion, with an absence of almost all the symptoms which are usually attendant on these affections; for the only permanent symptom in this case, and, I may add, aspect of serious disease, was the headache. Neither fever (at first) nor disorder of the senses or intellect, no starting, convulsion, nor paralysis, no continued vomiting nor obstinate constipation, marked the disease. Towards the end, indeed, a change took place, and then the aspect of the complaint rather resembled remittent fever than anything else.

"There is, however, a very important question remaining for consideration, viz., the relation, in point of time at least, of the softening and the effusion. Was the case one of inflammation of the brain running on into softening, followed by effusion; or was it a case of arachnitis, in which the softening was a secondary consequence, as noticed by Rilliet and Barthez? So far as we may venture to draw an inference from the history of the case, I think it is in favor of the softening being the primary disease, for we know, as in the case to which I alluded in the commencement of this notice, that ramollissement of the central nervous structure may exist with but few symptoms; whereas I believe it to be extremely rare, if it ever occurs, that meningitis should run a course of sixteen days at least, with such an utter absence of the ordinary characteristic symptoms.

"My own impression is, that the primary affection was inflammation of the central portions of the brain, and that the membranes participated in the morbid action, about the time when the febrile action set in; but that the effusion did not occur until the morning of the day on which she died, and that it was the immediate cause of death.

ART. 21.—*Delirium Tremens in a young child.* By Dr. WEISS.

(*Pr. Ver-Ztg.*, viii, 1856; and *Schmidt's Jahrb.*, v, 1856.)

This case is briefly related as follows:

CASE.—Pat. —, æt. 4½, the son of a publican, had for some time had such a love of alcoholic stimulants that he would employ all manner of tricks to get them. On ordinary occasions he would sleep off the attacks of drunkenness which were caused when these tricks succeeded, but on the present occasion, having been severely punished by his father, he fell into a spasmodic condition, and fancied that mice were running over him—he fell, in short, into a condition in which all the symptoms of delirium tremens were present. It was necessary to give full doses of morphia before the symptoms yielded. The author states, that the love of stimulants had arisen out of the doses which had been given by the parents when the child was quite an infant, with a view either to strengthening or else to quieting him; and he also refers to an analogous case in a child, æt. 5½, which is recorded in Constatt's "Handb.," iii, p. 156.

ART. 22.—*Case of incipient Mania, cured by large doses of Opium.* By Mr. PYE H. CHAVASSE, of Birmingham.

(*Assoc. Med. Journ.*, Sept. 6, 1856.)

The value of full doses of opium in many cases of insanity, a fact sufficiently known to many, though not yet properly appreciated by all, is well illustrated in the following case:

"CASE.—Miss T—, housekeeper, æt. 41, of melancholic temperament, had amenorrhœa in the summer of 1854, which lasted three or four months; but, in the September of the same year, she became 'regular,' and continued so until I commenced attending her—that is to say, until and during the beginning of her attack of mania.

" My attendance upon her commenced on the 13th of August, 1855. The following particulars of her previous history are all that I was able to glean. She had been a little nervous and eccentric, and had complained of occasional pains in her head, principally at the top and back of the head, and could not sleep well at night; otherwise, she was able to attend to her duties. Not feeling quite well, she returned to her father's house.

" A few days before I was called to see her, decided symptoms of mania showed themselves. She became morose and taciturn, sitting for hours without speaking a word, and staring upon vacancy. When spoken to, she would answer only in monosyllables, and even then not always to the purpose. Her natural disposition was gentle, obliging, and affectionate. She could not sleep at night; she had not slept for many days. Although usually taciturn, she occasionally sang a few words, repeating the same over and over again, to a low and monotonous tune. It was necessary to watch her night and day; as, from her manner and gestures, there were indications that she meditated self-destruction. She occasionally became very violent, requiring two or three persons to hold her down. At these times, her father and friends urgently requested me to send her to a lunatic asylum. I begged them to have a little patience, and to let me try for a short time longer the plan of treatment I was then adopting, before sending her from home.

" *Treatment.*—I first gave two grains of solid opium and one grain of Castile soap, made into a pill, every night and morning, for two or three days. These doses had no effect in producing sleep; I therefore increased the dose of opium to three grains every night and morning. She continued these increased doses for several days. Still no sleep. I then enlarged the dose to four grains every night and morning. She now had snatches of sleep: but did not sleep more than half an hour or an hour in the day and night. I now gave her five grains of opium every night and morning; and with the happiest results. She now slept six or seven hours in the night without waking, and all symptoms of insanity left her. As soon as she could sleep, I gradually reduced the quantity of opium; so that in a short time she only took two grains of opium every night: and, after a few weeks, I was able to discontinue it altogether. She is now, I am happy to say, quite well.

" I may state, that as long as she was taking *moderate* doses of opium, the bowels were constipated, requiring aperients; as soon as I resorted to *large* doses the bowels acted without the necessity of administering a particle of opening medicine.

"August 25th, 1856.—A year has now elapsed, and I have the satisfaction of recording the fact, that she has not had the slightest return of maniacal symptoms. Since her illness she has not been again 'regular;' although, for two or three months after her recovery, I endeavored to make her so, by giving her preparations of iron. She considers herself to be quite well."

ART. 23.—*Hydrochlorate of Morphia and Coffee in Cephalalgia.* By M. BOILEAU.

(*Rév. Méd.-Chir.*, Feb. 1855.)

M. Boileau informs us in this paper that he has often found hydrochlorate of morphia, dissolved in a strong solution of coffee, of the greatest service in severe headache; and he relates a case in illustration, in which a headache of the most intense character, and brought on by the most trivial causes, as exposure to a slight draught, was relieved in this way. In this case, moreover, the pain had resisted the morphia and the coffee given separately. M. Boileau's practice is, to give a dose—about half a grain of morphia in a small cup of hot, strong coffee—as often as the pain recurred, and to do this as often as was necessary; and his experience goes to show that the attacks will rapidly become less and less frequent, until at last they cease altogether.

ART. 24.—*On Neurosis of the Vagus.* By Dr. C. J. SHEARMAN.

(*Medical Times and Gazette*, Sept. 20, 1856.)

"Since 1849, my attention has been engaged by a class of cases which have presented symptoms of peculiar characters, and deranging both mental and bodily functions. The essential mental symptoms have been—depression of spirits, leading to a gloomy view of the position of the patient, everything in the world being against his comfort and happiness; his judgment so impaired as to be incapable of drawing, by any means, a correct conclusion from premises; so great vacillation of the mental faculties as to effectually prevent any plan devised from being pursued to a satisfactory result; impairment of memory; exaltation of imagination, and excessive deficiency in the acts of volition; a kind of dreamy *laissez faire* taking the place of the command which a healthy man feels he has over the circumstances of life.

"The symptoms of bodily affection are those of lassitude and malaise, most marked in the morning, always less in the evening, and almost completely removed by indulgence in society; a feeling of exhaustion located at the epigastrium, relieved by outward pressure, the ingestion of food and exhibition of stimulants; frequently a sensation of gnawing, tearing, or indescribable uneasiness, is added to this feeling of exhaustion; cough, without expectoration; yawning, sighing, and nausea, occurring between the meals, but never following them; palpitation on the least exertion or annoyance; vertigo, tinnitus aurium, and incomplete direction of muscular effort, with deficient muscular sense; constipation, and free urinary secretion, with dry skin. The whole of these symptoms observe a periodicity, sometimes tertian, at others quotidian; and, under both forms, the period of exacerbation is antemeridional, almost a perfect immunity existing each evening.

"The symptoms being those of derangements of the gastric, pulmonary, and cerebral system, and from not being able to ascertain the existence, in most of the cases, of any cerebral, cardiac, pulmonary, pleural, or gastric structural disease, I was limited to one of two affections to account for them,—viz., disordered gastric secretion, or some neurosis of the gastro-pulmonary nervous group. I could never ascertain the existence of the former, and I attributed, therefore, the affection to some disorder of the latter.

"During the course of the cases, I found that the small quantity of food frequently indulged in, which was borne in such small quantities at first, was succeeded by a power of full repletion afterwards; the appetite became in many cases almost ravenous, and this led me to look for sugar in the urine. I found it, and subsequently found sugar in the cases of only recent origin. From palsy frequently succeeding hyperæsthesia of the nerves of sensation, and the vagus nerve being known to be chiefly an afferent nerve, I formed the conclusion that this disease, in its early stage, was one of the vagus nerve in some course of its tract, either centric, peripheral, or intermediate; of irritation in its early stages, of palsy succeeding that irritation, and designated it, in my note-book, 'sinking dyspepsia,' and treated it as

I would have done neurosis of any other centripetal nerve, and with satisfactory results.

"Bernard's discovery of the formation of sugar in the liver, and its passage into the urine, on irritation of the origins of the vagus nerve, also of the influence of irritation of the centric portion of the divided vagus in the production of saccharine urine, as corroborated by Pavy, have, I consider, decided the accuracy of the diagnosis, and enable me to raise hyperæsthesia of the vagus from the position of merely an attendant symptom of disease to that of an idiopathic affection.

"The experiments of Magendie, Reid, Flourens, Legallois, and others—the cases recorded by Brodie, Romberg, James, Johnson, Goolden, Gibb,—the observations of Bernard, Barreswill, Lehmann, Schmidt, and Pavy,—enable me to draw from sixty cases of this disease (of which twenty-two were unassociated with any other affection, and thirty-eight with various neuroses, cachæmic affections, &c.,) the following conclusions, and which I can (I think safely) substantiate by cases to be detailed in this and subsequent papers.

"1. One of the functions of the vagus nerve is the communication to the sensorium of the condition of the stomach.

"2. That two forms of neurosis of this nerve exist; one of hyperæsthesia, the other of anæsthesia.

"3. Hyperæsthesia is attended by irritability of the stomach, increased feeling of necessity of respiration, altered reflex action of muscles of respiration, and of laryngeal function.

"4. Anæsthesia is attended by boulimia, and diminished necessity of respiration.

"5. Both forms obey the ordinary laws of diseased action of centripetal nerves, and are amenable to the rational treatment of the same.

"6. Both are attended by altered blood-formation, with its ordinary effects on the various organs of the body, and many by irradiated or reflex sensations (in the form of vertigo, tinnitus, deafness, neuralgia, dyspnœa, &c.), and reflected muscular actions, as epilepsy, catalepsy, various forms of spasm of bronchial tubes, intercostal muscles, hiccough (spasm of diaphragm), clonic spasm of voluntary muscles, &c.

"7. Both forms by saccharine urine.

"8. That hyperæsthesia of the vagus induces disturbance chiefly of judgment; secondarily, of memory, imagination, and the power of association of ideas.

"The urine, in all the cases of neurosis of the vagi, is passed frequently and in small quantities; its amount in the twenty-four hours is rarely two quarts, but is increased by indulgence in malt liquors — is alkaline when voided, of a clear pale, gooseberry-wine color; no marked odor, excepting that of sugar; sp. gr. 1016 to 1030; acid fermentation not commencing under four or five days, when it becomes ropy and filled with vegetable growths; after this passes off the usual alkaline fermentation ensues. The urea is not increased in amount relatively to the other solid contents, but diminished in proportion to the water; uric acid is diminished, also the alcoholic extracts relatively to the whole contents of the urine; its chief characters are alkalinity and saccharine condition.

"In testing for sugar, I have always removed the ammonia and rendered acid by hydrochloric acid, and used Trommer's test, or Barreswill's, and from time to time obtained an alcoholic extract, from which I have obtained the characteristic indication of sugar."

Then follow several illustrative cases, of which we give three:

In March, 1854, a woman, æt. 42, was struck over the left ear. Two days afterwards she felt extreme sinking sensation at the epigastrium; constant desire for food, the digestion of which produced flushing and swelling of the features, vertigo, tinnitus, great heat of the palms of the hands and the soles of the feet, and a sensation of formication over the whole of the body. These were followed in three days by severe tic of the same side, engaging the frontal, orbital, malar, inferior maxillar and cervical regions. Four days after the accession of the tic I saw her, and ordered quinine and aconite internally. These seemed to be of no use; and from swelling occurring under the lobe of the ear, I suspended that treatment, ordered leeches to the swelling, and, on its subsidence, gave quinine and arsenic. The epigastric symptoms first, the facial and cervical subsequently, yielded, and she rapidly recovered. Has had tic neither before nor since the blow.

A woman, in 1853, applied to me for relief for shingles. Some months before I saw her she fell with the right side of the head against a chest, and received the blow somewhere behind the ear. She thought nothing of it; but in a few weeks found herself suffering from all the symptoms I have described attending hyperæsthesia of vagus, and to this succeeded the shingles of the same side. She had the periodicity of symptoms and the mental affection well marked. She was relieved rapidly, and subsequently cured by Argenti Nitratis, gr. ½; Opii, gr. ½; Ext. Anthemidis, gr. iv, ter die; Quinæ Disulphatis, gr. ij; Acid. Nitrici Diluti, ℥xx; Aquæ Fontanæ, ℥iss, ter die. In both cases the urine was saccharine, and possessed the other qualities described, all of which disappeared under the treatment. In July, 1856, a young man, æt. 18, applied to me for relief from epilepsy. Two years ago he was struck by a stone opposite the superior posterior angle of the parietal bone of the right side; lost some blood, but no other immediate injurious result seemed to follow; but he noticed that soon after the blow he passed much more urine than he had been accustomed, and passed it unconsciously in the bed; also he had all the symptoms of hyperæthesia of the vagus, which have gradually passed into those of anæsthesia. During the last eighteen months he has had epileptic fits at intervals of seven or fourteen days, generally on the Saturday. He has now an enlarged thyroid body encroaching on the carotid region; saccharine alkaline urine, and still the vagus affection with diurnal exacerbation. Under nitrate of silver, gr. ½; Indian hemp extract, gr. ½; Extract. Anthemidis, gr. iv; and quinine, his epigastric sensations are relieved, and the fits diminished in frequency, and the urine lessened in amount and in its saccharine character. He is still under treatment.

The treatment adopted by Dr. Shearman is intended—

1. To diminish the sensibility of the extremities of the afferent nerves engaged in the disease, the nitrate of silver, or the chloride (held in solution by ammonia), with opium, I have found the most expeditious; it rarely purges, and is far more useful than bismuth, prussic acid, and alkalies.

2. The exhibition of nervine tonics, quinine, iron, arsenic, zinc, salts, when there has appeared to be only functional derangement; but, where any head affection has been suspected, it has been removed previously.

3. The exhibition of alkalies is of great value. There is no doubt now that sugar is an agent of great value in the metamorphosis of the system, independently of its being food for respiration; it is found in large quantity in the egg, and increases (not diminishes) during incubation; it bears an intimate connection with the formation of bile; also, it has some influence on the solution of carbonate and phosphate of lime in the blood; but, inasmuch as it is rapidly transformed before it reaches the lung, and transformed, too, almost immediately after its production in the liver, where one of the great blood-forming functions is carried out; we see the necessity of not only restoring to the liver the function of forming a fermentable (in connection with albuminous matter) sugar, which is arrested during disease of the vagi, but of rendering the blood such as will allow of this fermentation. An acid state of the blood will not allow it, an alkaline facilitates it; and with this view an alkaline treatment should be conjoined with the special treatment of the neurotic affection. Liq. potassæ, in one-drachm doses, reduces the sugar in the urine, and renders the latter acid in this disease; it restores the blood, in all probability, to such a state as to transform the sugar so soon as the liver has regained its functions from alleviation of the affection of the vagi.

4. Nutrition of the body must be regained during convalescence; the value of fatty matter in this function is too well known to allow of its inutility after emaciation; besides, there is reason to consider that sugar is formed from two sources in the liver; partly from albuminous matter, partly from olein. The portal blood normally contains more olein than the hepatic, and fat in the solid residue of portal blood is as 3·225§ to 1·885§ in the hepatic; by the oxidation of glycerine and oleic acid we obtain the elements of grape sugar and cholic acid. Schmidt, Bernard, and Lehmann are strongly disposed to believe that the olein is one of the sources of both sugar and cholic acid. These are sufficient reasons for the exhibition of cod-oil; and I can speak very strongly in favor of its use in the treatment of neurosis of the vagus, and in cases of neuralgia depending on that disease.

ART. 25.—*Favorable cases of Hydrophobia.*
By Dr. J. LEWIS SMITH, Physician to the Northwestern Dispensary.

(*New York Journal of Medicine*, March, 1856.)

" It is a matter of interest, and of practical importance," says Dr. J. L. Smith, in one of a series of admirable papers on hydrophobia to which we had occasion to refer in our last volume, "whether hydrophobia is necessarily fatal. That its occurrence may be prevented by a little treatment, when unequivocal prodromic symptoms have appeared, is clearly ascertained. In the records already examined by us, instances of this are mentioned, and occasionally the threatened attack was more than once averted.

" Hear, also, the remarks of that eminent physician, and profound medical philosopher, Dr. Elliotson, on this point ('Lond. Lanc.' May, 1829): 'Usually, I believe (he speaks of the premonitory stage) there are symptoms of weariness, general indisposition, dizziness, chills, and flushes ; sometimes a pain has been felt in the bitten part. I think it very possible, from an occurrence which happened in my own practice, that these symptoms may go no further ; that the disease, if I may so speak, may go off. Two little girls, standing at their father's door, were bitten by the same dog ; a dog passing, snapped at both of them, and bit them in the face. She who was bitten the second, became hydrophobic, and died. The other, at exactly the same time, experienced the same premonitory symptoms as her sister—heaviness and general indisposition,—but they all went off.

" ' If then, an attack of hydrophobia may be prevented after its premonitory stage has commenced, may not the disease itself, though fully established in some instances, be thrown off, and the patient be saved ?

" ' The observations of Mr. Youatt, upon the dog, have shown that, in this animal, hydrophobia may occasionally have a favorable termination. In commenting on the second case in table (No. III) he says, speaking of one of his canine patients : " The dog was suspected to have been bitten. It was in a manner certain that it had been bitten, but the wounded part could not be detected, and he was not operated upon. The disease approached ; it established itself. There was the perversion of temper ; the suspicious scowl ; the eager watching of imaginary objects ; the darting at some phantom of the imagination ; the depraved appetite ; and the characteristic howl. The malady pursued its regular course during more than twenty-four hours, and then came a gradual calm—the dog quieted down to his usual appearance and habits—he became well. * * * Another and another case succeeded. Once in a hundred times, or more, the constitutional affection admitted not of a doubt * * and the patient got well.' "

" The fact that hydrophobia may terminate favorably in the dog, does not furnish certain proof that it may likewise in the human species ; but certainly it is an argument of great weight, in support of such a doctrine. The belief is pretty general, that canine madness is uniformly fatal in man. Instances of recovery are reported in the journals, but they have attracted little attention, from the fact, that other diseases possessing a strongly marked nervous element may be mistaken for true rabies. No doubt there has frequently been an entire misapprehension of the nature of the affection, and several records in my collection confirm this opinion ; but the most cautious statistician, it seems to me, must admit that in a part, at least, of the following cases, genuine hydrophobia was present."

Favorable Cases.

No.	Sex.	Age.	Part Bitten.	Incuba-tion.	Duration of Prod.	Duration of Disease	Treatment.	Authority.
1	M.	Ad.	Hand.	3 m.	6 d.	...	Purgatives, stimulants, &c.	Wm. Grant, G. Doane, *Med. Gaz.*, July 10, 1830.
2	F.	35	Finger.	8 d.	5 d.	...	Purgatives, arsenic, incision.	T. Tomkin, E. G. Varenue, *Lon. Lan.*, Aug., 1835.
3	M.	Ad.	Arm.	12 to 14 m.	2 w.	...	Purgatives, leeches, opiates.	Dr. Du Heaume, *Med. Gaz.*, Dec., 1837.
4	"	17	"	3 w.	Several d.	...	Purgatives, Hyd. Chlor. Lib. opiates.	Dr. Hooper, *Medical Times*, May 17, 1847.
5	"	...	Thumb	12 d.	2 d.	...	Hyd. Chlor. Lib., in-cision.	W. F. Haines, *Lond. Lan.*, 1847.
6	F.	30	Wrist.	About 3 m.	About 3 w.	...	Opiates, anæsthetics, &c.	Prof. Jackson, *Amer. Journ.*, 1849.

"An abstract of the histories and symptoms of these six cases will enable us to judge whether the disease was really hydrophobia."

CASE 1.—The wound which was inflicted by a dog, whose condition is not given, healed after the lapse of several weeks.

November 14th.—About three months subsequently to the reception of the bite, the patient was seized with headache and rigors, which were relieved by a purgative. On the 20th of the same month, the presence of water distressed him, and attempts to drink caused the characteristic spasms of the neck. The cicatrix had an inflammatory appearance, and he was seen to rub it. He was timid and distrustful, and a viscid secretion began to form in his mouth and throat.

This condition continued till the 21st, when he was placed in a warm bath, and all these untoward symptoms vanished.

The amendment lasted till the evening of the 22d, when he again became restless, and, on the 23d, relapse was complete. The dread of water was so great, that the bath was not repeated; but 280 drops of laudanum were administered. He slept six hours, and awoke refreshed and free from spasms. On the evening of the 25th another relapse occurred, attended by a flatulent condition of the bowels.

The records do not state how long the spasms continued; but the patient grew progressively weaker, so as "to require brandy and broths plentifully." On December 14th he was nearly insensible; pulse 130; extremities cold, and hiccough constant. He was fed with chicken broth, jellies, and stimulants; and, contrary to all expectation, a gradual improvement followed, and on the 8th of January he was able to leave the place.

CASE 2.—Bitten by a favorite dog, which was killed in a week, with the salivary glands enlarged. The wound was trifling, and healed in three days.

June 30th, eight days after the injury was received, she was suddenly seized with cephalalgia and dimness of vision. These symptoms were momentary; but they recurred at intervals for several days, accompanied by an uneasy sensation in the neighborhood of the bitten finger.

July 4th.—When drawing beer from a cask, she became giddy; but recovered, on stopping the cock. The following day her eyes were bright, prominent, and intolerant of light, and she complained of pain in the left side.

6th.—Constipation; aversion to food and drinks, and each attempt to take them followed by a convulsive fit.

7th.—Intolerance of light, and aversion to liquids increased; complains of pain extending up the arm from the bitten finger; pulse weak and fluttering, and neck tumid; the paroxysms last about five minutes.

8th.—One of the cicatrices slightly inflamed, and the symptoms of yesterday continue. She has been treated with aperients and the liquor arsenicalis. Treatment to-day,—excision of the cicatrices, and the application of veratrine ointment over the neck and arms.

9th.—Has improved since the excision; feels less pain in the throat, and none in the arm, and has had only one paroxysm.

15th.—Continues improving, but deglutition difficult; gums swelling, probably from the arsenic which she has continued taking.

August 10th.—Has had no return of the complaint. Mr. Youatt commented at length in the "Lancet,"on the above case, entertaining, apparently, no doubt of its genuineness.

CASE 3.—Was bitten by his own Newfoundland dog, which two years subsequently, when the records were published, was alive and well. It inflicted the bite from provocation, and did not show, before or afterwards, any suspicious symptoms.

The cicatrix, before the occurrence of hydrophobia, had occasionally been painful, and at the inception of the disease it presented a reddish appearance.

After two weeks of anxiety and melancholy, he was taken, February 11th, 1837, with attacks of convulsive respiration.

12th.—Respiration as yesterday; face flushed; pulse quick; bowels flatulent; pupils dilated but contractile; rational; quantity of saliva, increased. Twenty-four leeches were applied to his temples; blisters to the calves of his legs, and purgative enemata administered.

9 P.M.—Much excited by the vesication; countenance anxious, and eyes brilliant. Has spasms when water is offered.

13th.—Symptoms as before. The noise of a carriage in the street, the touch of an orange to his lips, and pressure upon the cicatrix, occasion paroxysms.

14th.—Pulseless, insensible, and extremities cold. Had no spasms during the night, but at twelve o'clock to-day a paroxysm occurred, lasting two hours. After this he gradually convalesced. During the latter part of his sickness he took opiates, stimulants, and mercurials.

CASE 4.—The wound was severe, and inflicted by a dog known to be rabid.

The disease was ushered in by restlessness and melancholy, lasting several days, and when fully developed, the paroxysms were severe. The sound of water, the least noise in the room, opening a door, increase or diminution of light, and the sight of a glass vessel, caused either convulsions or great distress. He complained of thirst, of a constriction across his chest, and of itching in the cicatrix. He was ordered—Tr. Camph., and Tr. Opii, aa, ʒij, to be repeated in half an hour, and a mercurial.

On the following day he was better. The cicatrix had given way and was discharging. There was no delirium; the paroxysms were less frequent and severe; and he slept four hours in the morning.

After this he gradually convalesced. He was salivated, but not till the improvement had commenced. A year subsequently he was seen by Dr. H. in his usual health.

CASE 5.—Bitten slightly in September, 1846, by a dog which had been four or five weeks in a singular state, and at the time the bite was inflicted, showed symptoms of rabies, viz., spasms, dread of water, and increase of saliva.

On the twelfth day after the injury, the wounded part became hot and prickly. The day following it was better, but the third day it became worse again, and headache, thirst, and restlessness commenced. He now complained of pain in his throat; his deglutition was difficult; and five or six times hourly, the characteristic spasms took place.

On the nineteenth day after the infliction of the bite, convalescence was established   The treatment consisted in scarifying and poulticing the bitten part, and in mercurialization.

CASE 6 —The wounds received by this patient were slight, and inflicted by a strange dog, running in the street.

After three months the cicatrices became red, slightly tumefied, and painful.

One festered and discharged a few drops of greenish matter, and then healed, giving no further trouble. The other remained hard and painful, and pain extended from it up the arm to the shoulder.

This condition continued a few days, when one morning, as she was drinking, she experienced a sudden shuddering sensation. The following evening the same sensation occurred from putting her hand in water, and violent spasms of the throat, with a sense of suffocation on attempting to drink; currents of air produced no unpleasant effects; the fauces were dry, and she retained her senses perfectly. Counter-irritation and antispasmodics were prescribed.

On the following day (October 29th) there was an apparent amendment. She had had no spasms since the previous day, and had passed a quiet night. She took water readily, and her pulse was natural; but the affected arm had lost its sensibility and there was deep-seated pain in the course of its nerves.

She was ordered antispasmodics with rhubarb and mercury, but the first dose brought on violent spasms threatening suffocation. The paroxysms now recurred frequently, produced by trifling causes, as the waving of the hand, and sometimes occurring spontaneously. Chloroform was administered, and the red and tumid cicatrix excised; but the spasms continued, and the sight of a silver spoon and the brushing away of flies, were sufficient to induce them.

The record for October 31st states that she had passed a comfortable night, and that the wound was discharging freely.

From this time she gradually convalesced. Cicatrization had taken place, and the pain had ceased in the arm by the second week in December, but the shoulder and axilla remained tender, and occasionally painful till the 1st of January, when her health was permanently restored.

Dr. Smith adds, in another place—

"The striking similarity, we may say identity, of symptoms in the above cases, with those which we have seen to be characteristic of hydrophobia, leave little doubt, that these patients suffered that appalling disease. This opinion receives confirmation from the fact that, at least four of the dogs which inflicted the bites were at the time, or soon after, either rabid, or in such a condition as to excite the strongest suspicion of rabies.

"But the most convincing proof that the above were genuine cases lies, perhaps, in the fact, that in all six, the bitten part was the seat and source of some unusual sensation, or that it presented some unusual appearance, at or before the commencement of the disease. We may then consider it settled, that hydrophobia, though so commonly fatal that one affected with it can indulge no reasonable hope of recovering, does, in rare instances, have a favorable termination."

ART. 26.—*Inhalations of Chloroform in the treatment of Chorea.*—By Dr. GERY.

(*Bull. Gén. de Thérap.*, March, 1855.)

On several occasions lately, chloroform inhalations have been used at the Hôpital des Enfans, in Paris, in obstinate and unmanageable cases of chorea, and the effect has always been to quiet the movements, and procure sleep for a time varying from 10 to 30 minutes; and this without producing any injurious consequences. In this way time was gained for the administration of food and appropriate remedies. The quantity inhaled varied from $2\frac{1}{2}$ to 5 drachms by weight. Of course, the usual precautions were taken in conducting the inhalation.

ART. 27.—*On "Intermittent Rheumatic Contractions."* By M. TROUSSEAU.

(*Gaz. des Hôpitaux*, No. 72, 1856.)

Under this name M. Trousseau describes certain nervous symptoms of more or less gravity, and resembling more or less intimately, as the case may be, hysteria, epilepsy, eclampsia, or catalepsy; unaccompanied by any obvious disease of the brain or cord; and occurring most frequently in nursing women. In some of these cases, the blood presented a buffy coat, as in rheumatism, or symptoms of rheumatism alternated with the nervous symptoms. But there appears to be no very good reason why M. Trousseau should have applied the term "rheumatic" to the nervous symptoms. Indeed, there appears to be no good reason for discarding the good old friendly term *hysteric*.

ART. 28.—*On the treatment of Epilepsy.* By DR. JOHN OSBORNE, Physician to Mercer's Hospital.

(Dublin Quarterly Journal of Medicine, Nov. 1856.)

In this paper, Dr. Osborne records the result of his hospital experience in the treatment of epilepsy, an experience embracing twenty-six cases, and extending over twenty-seven years. Dr. Osborne's theory is, that sleep and epilepsy are very closely allied, and that the cure for the treatment of epilepsy is to be taken from the right knowledge of the cause of sleep. Now sleep, in his opinion—

"Is produced by turgescence of the choroid bodies, they being essentially erectile structures, in the lateral and third and fourth ventricles of the brain, compressing the origin of the spinal marrow and from the nerves proceeding from that region; whilst at the same time, by the occupation of so much of the cavity of the cranium, the quantity of blood circulating at the surface of the hemispheres is proportionately diminished, and thus a double impediment is offered to the perception of external objects, and communication with the external world is cut off during the portions of time required for nutrition and repair of the nervous centres."

The object of treatment is to lessen this erectile turgor, and in order to do this, the tumultuous action of the heart is to be quieted by digitalis, and the distended capillaries stimulated to contraction by cantharides. One formula is the following:

"Infusion of digitalis, and water of acetate of ammonia, of each two ounces; pennyroyal water, four ounces; mix. One ounce to be taken mid-day, evening, and night; and the tincture of cantharides to be added, commencing with five drops, and increasing by one drop each dose. When it appeared desirable to give digitalis in a lesser, and cantharides in a greater proportion, then the following was used:—Infusion of digitalis, three ounces and a half; tincture of cantharides, half an ounce; mix. Forty minims to be given in milk thrice daily, and progressively increased."

The results of this treatment, in Dr. Osborne's opinion, were very successful.

ART. 29.—*On Lactate of Zinc in Epilepsy.* By M. HERPIN.

(Bull. Gén. de Thérap., Nov., 1855; and *Méd. Chir. Rév.* July, 1856.)

M. Herpin points out the fallacy of deductions from cases treated *en masse* by any remedy, without classifying the cases, and taking the prognosis into consideration. He divides cases of epilepsy into three groups. 1. Where the prognosis is *favorable.* This embraces cases in which there have been less than 100 attacks. 2. *Little favorable* cases, where there have been from 100 to 500 attacks. 3. *Unfavorable* cases, where there have been above 500 attacks. The duration of the affection, together with the age and sex of the subject, also influence the prognosis. All things being equal in respect to the number of fits, the most recent cases are the most favorable. Under five months' duration, the chances of recovery are twice as great as from five months to a year. After ten years, success is rare. Of all ages, old age is the most favorable; then youth and infancy; and least of all, adult age. In M. Herpin's hands there have been twice as many failures with males as with females. Adult men are most unfavorable subjects. To apply this sort of division to the cases treated by lactate of zinc:—of 41 epileptics, the treatment was only sufficiently advanced in 35 for any decision as to its effect being arrived at. Of these 35, 15 were favorable cases, 12 little favorable, and 8 unfavorable. Of the 8 unfavorables, 2 have improved to an extent which militates strongly in favor of the remedy. Of the 12 little favorable cases, in 2 children, aged respectively eight years and twenty-one months, the fits were suppressed: and a remarkable amelioration took place in one man. Of the fifteen favorable cases, 4, in which various other remedies had failed, were uninfluenced by the lactate; one of these had suffered ninety attacks in fifteen years and a half; a second, aged forty-four years, had symptoms of commencing general paralysis; a third, aged four or five years, had a hydrocephalic head; and a fourth, which had lasted three years and a half, was otherwise favorable. In 6 of the remaining 11, the attacks were suppressed; and of the 5 others, 3 have had the intervals so much prolonged as to afford hope of complete cure on continuance of the remedy; the remaining 2 were amended. The remedy was given for a period of from five or six to twelve months.

ART. 30.—*On the rational treatment of Epilepsy.* By Dr. RUSSELL REYNOLDS.

(*Lancet*, July 5, 1856.)

In this paper, which was read before the Medical Society of London, May 24, 1856, the rational treatment of epilepsy is distinguished from two other kinds—viz., the empirical, or non-rational, and the *a priori*, or falsely rational. It consists of the application deductively to particular cases, of inductively acquired knowledge of the disease in general, and of remedies in general. The measure of success attending treatment is, in the long run, the measure of its rationality; for such application to particular cases is the experiment by which we may test the correctness or incorrectness of our interpretation of phenomena, both of disease and medication. This is, however, true only when we have attained to an accurate measure of success. The so-called accidental cures are not accidental, but are dependent upon undiscovered laws; neither are they exceptional, for there are no exceptions to natural laws; but there are few laws so accurately comprehended in the sciences of pathology and therapeutics, that we can announce them without the aid of percentages, averages, and means. The latter are, then, numerical expressions, not of the whole truth, but of such fractions of the truth as we are for the time being able to perceive. These numerical expressions are means which we may employ in the search after truth; they are not the end of scientific investigation. It is not the object of this paper to present numerical results, but to indicate certain broad, general truths, ascertained with regard to epilepsy and epileptics, which may serve as the guides towards a rational employment of those agencies which lie within our reach. There are three steps in the process by which we arrive at a rational treatment of a disease. They are—1st, the appreciation, so far as possible, of the real nature of that disease; 2dly, the recognition of the general effects of different courses or modes of treatment; and 3dly, the application of particular remedies to particular cases. Upon each of these steps it is proposed to offer comments.

I. The appreciation of the real nature of the disease in question. It is not intended to assert that we have arrived at a knowledge of the ultimate essence of the malady: but we may recognize its phenomena; and not leaving these as an unsifted heap of pathological facts, we may, by their partial interpretation, reduce them to their "lowest terms." In epilepsy, the three modes or phases of life present some more or less notable modifications. Thus, there are symptoms referable to the mind, to the motor apparatus, and to organic life, and we may therefore class them into mental, animal, and vegetal. Regarding the epileptic not merely during the accession of a fit, but in the inter-paroxysmal period, we may state the prominent features of his disease to be the following:—1st, deficiency of will; 2dly, excessive susceptibility to the induction of involuntary movements; 3dly, an altered condition of the organic processes.

1. Deficiency of will, exhibiting itself in the absence of due control over thought, emotion, and simple sensation, and reflective movement. As it has been argued at another time,[*] this diminution of will produces, phenomenally, loss of both apprehension and memory, alternating or coexisting with a vague, wandering condition of mind, which, under accidental circumstances of excitement, may display itself in delirium. The emotions are easily disturbed; they exert an undue influence upon the inner and outer life; their expression is uncontrolled; delusive ideas are not unfrequently entertained; sudden impressions upon the senses startle the patient, unnerve him, and make him tremble; he is not master of himself; and all these morbid conditions are but illustrations of a deficiency of will which reaches its maximum—viz, the complete extinction of volition, in the unconsciousness of the attack.

2. Excessive susceptibility to the induction of involuntary movement is evident

[*] On the Inter-paroxysmal Condition of Epileptics (*vide* "Abstract" XXII.)

during the attacks from the spasms which are then present; but during the intervals of seizure there are feebler but not less characteristic indications of the same
tendency. Muscular agitation, in the form of tremor, choreic spasm, or choreiform
movements, occurs in 73 per cent.; and this exaggeration of motor activity we
may confidently refer, as Dr. Marshall Hall long since pointed out, to the spinal
centre. I say "confidently," for there is no evidence of increased muscular irritability, on the one hand; nor, on the other, can we affirm, in the greater number of
cases, the existence of any undue irritation. As examined by percussion and the
galvanic current, the muscular irritability of epileptics is constantly below the
average of health; and although we may often refer the commencement of attacks
and their recurrence to indigestion, loaded intestines, disturbed emotions, and so
forth, these irritations ought not to be considered the efficient causes of epilepsy or
epileptic attacks, since they neither exceed in degree nor differ in kind from the
irritations to which hundreds and thousands are daily exposed without suffering
any such catastrophe as an epileptic fit. Failing, then, to find the source of this
excessive motility in either the muscles themselves or in the nature of the irritation
to which afferent nerves may be exposed, we must, *pro tempore* at all events, refer
it to that which lies *between* the stimulus and the contraction—viz. the spinal centre;
and in this centre we recognize an undue readiness or susceptibility of reflective
action.

3. Altered or morbid conditions of the organic processes are found in many epileptics; but it may be most confidently asserted, that there has not yet been pointed
out any one condition which necessarily exists. Frequently there is organic debility; but this, so far as my experience extends, is by no means invariably present.
Amongst seventy-one cases which were analyzed for the paper already referred to,
there were no discoverable signs of debility in twenty-nine; it was notably marked
in eleven only. The organic conditions vary indefinitely; but there is this, however, which is common to them all—viz., the existence of a *change* from the previous condition of the patient, or from that of health. The existence of such changes
as those attendant upon dentition, the commencement of puberty, or pregnancy, or
of such as may belong to the condition of general anæmia and the like, cannot but
exert a perturbing influence upon the nervous centres, which are placed in such
intimate relation with the entire organism. The nature of such perturbation we
may not understand, but we cannot question its existence, or doubt the importance
of its treatment. But when there are structural lesions in the nervous centres
themselves, or in their appendages, such as tumors of the brain, or chronic meningitis,—and when there are positively morbid blood conditions, such as that of
urinæmia induced by Bright's disease, &c., &c.,—we do not, in my opinion, have
to deal with epilepsy, but with epileptiform or allied convulsions, dependent upon
other and recognizable diseases.

II. The second step in arriving at a rational treatment of epileptics, is taken by a
recognition of the effects of different therapeutic agents, considered in their general application to the disease in question. If the interpretation already given of the
prominent features of epilepsy be correct, there are three classes of objects to be
attained. These are—1, the education or increase of volitional control; 2, the
diminution of excessive susceptibility in the spinal centre; and 3, the correction or
counteraction of what may be morbid in the organic system.

1. The education or increase of volitional control is to be attempted by two classes
of means, having relation to the circumstances which have either caused, or served
to maintain, the deficiency of will. The former class includes all those means which
should educe that self-control which, through hereditary, constitutional, hygienic,
or social conditions, has undergone but an imperfect development; the latter embraces those agencies or modes of treatment which should screen the patient from
such excitement or perturbation as may have succeeded in overmastering the will.
If the mind and will are not duly exercised, they will waste; if they are overtaxed
or overstrained, they will wear. We have to avoid these two extremes, enjoining
judicious discipline and healthy educational exercise for the child who has been too
fondly tended, and allowed to pass its time in indulged idleness at home; and enforcing absolute rest, or even entire seclusion from the worry of the stock exchange
or the anxiety of professional life, when these have injuriously absorbed the thought
and sapped the mental strength of the individual.

2. The diminution of excessive susceptibility in the spinal centre requires for its attainment two kinds of treatment: viz., the scrupulous avoidance of all sources of undue irritation, and the exhibition of such agents as shall diminish the amount of irritability already existing, such as hyoscyamus, and allied medicines.

3. The removal or correction of those morbid conditions which exist in the organic system cannot be too carefully or perseveringly attempted. For the attainment of this object, the guides are those which we have in regard of all other diseases, and they need no further notice here.

III. The application of particular remedies to particular cases forms the third step in the process of arriving at a rational treatment of epilepsy. In order to gain this end, we may divide epileptics into three classes, and the recognition of a particular case as belonging to one or another of these groups will mainly guide us in the direction of treatment. The three classes may be separated from each other by the predominance, in those individuals who compose them, of one or another of the three main features of the disease, as it exists during the inter-paroxysmal period. Thus, in the first, the mind is predominantly at fault; in the second, the most characteristic symptoms are those of exalted muscular activity; and in the third, there are the signs of an abnormal organic condition. Cases of epilepsy require treatment for each of the three groups of symptoms, but some require especial attention in one direction, and others necessitate a different kind of management.

In illustration of these principles, the author read the records of nine cases of epilepsy, three belonging to each of these groups.

ART. 31.—*On Tetanus in India.* By Mr. WARING.

(*Indian Annals of Medical Science*, April, 1856.)

We take the following facts and remarks from the same "Notes on the Diseases of India," to which we have already referred on more than one occasion in the present volume:—

"Frequent as this disease (tetanus) is represented to be in Demerara, Trinidad, St. Domingo, and in some other localities in the West Indies, no comparison, I think, can be instituted between its frequency in these places and in some of the towns of India, Bombay especially, as will be seen by a perusal of the following statement:

Showing the Deaths from Tetanus in the Town of Bombay, for a period of three years, 1851-52-53.

Year.	Total Deaths.	Deaths from Tetanus.	Proportion.				
1851	14,724	332	1 death from tetanus to 44 from all causes.				
1852	13,763	341	1	"	"	40	"	"
1853	14,164	239	1	"	"	39	"	"
	42,651	912	1	"	"	46	"	"

"Large as this number is, both absolutely and comparatively, it is still below the mark, as under the heading of 'Total Deaths' are included 'still births,' whilst under that of tetanus is excluded that puerperal form of the disease, which, we shall subsequently see, is both frequent and fatal. We have no means of comparing the proportion of tetanic deaths in Calcutta and Madras with those of Bombay, but if an opinion may be formed from hospital returns, we are justified in saying that the disease is not of so frequent occurrence in Calcutta as it is in Bombay. Thus in the Calcutta General Hospital,[*] during five years (1847–51), only 56 were admissions with tetanus, whilst at the Jamsetjee Jejeebhoy Hospital[†] in Bombay, during a period of seven years (1845–51), the admissions under this heading amounted to 195.

* Dr. Jackson, "Indian Annals of Med. Science," No. 1, 1853, p. 58.
† Mr. Peet, "Bombay Med. Trans.," No. 1, N. S., 1853, p. 1.

"Compared with more temperate climates, the ratio of deaths from tetanus appear still more striking ; thus we find the following proportions to exist:

Place.	Period.	Total Deaths.	Deaths from Tetanus.	Proportion.
London, ...	1850-3-4	224,515	73	1 in 3075
Ireland, ...	1831-51	1,187,374	238	1 in 4987
New York, ...	1819-34	83,783	112	1 in 748
Bombay, ...	1851-3	42,651	912	1 in 46

"The proportion existing in Bombay, taken in this light, cannot but be regarded as very formidable.

"*Influence of Seasons.*—In seeking to ascertain the cause of so prevalent a disease, one of the first questions which presents itself to the mind is, what were the atmospherical and meteorological conditions of the locality during the period of its prevalence. Fortunately we have here good data to judge, from which we here subjoin :

Month.	1851.	1852.	1853.	Total.	
February, ...	28	32	14	74	
March, ...	26	35	24	85	} 242 or 26·5 per cent.
April, ...	26	36	21	83	
May, ...	28	22	25	75	
June, ...	21	34	21	76	} 220 or 24·1 per cent.
July, ...	27	21	21	69	
August, ...	29	24	17	70	
September, ...	31	28	18	77	} 226 or 24·9 per cent.
October, ...	30	24	25	79	
November, ...	29	35	22	86	
December, ...	39	29	14	82	} 224 or 24·8 per cent.
January, ...	18	21	17	50	
	332	341	239	912	

"This table, I think, satisfactorily shows that seasons *per se*, exercise no influence on the mortality of this disease, each quarter presenting us with very nearly the same proportions of deaths from this cause. A slight increase is observable in the month preceding the rains (May), but nothing sufficiently marked to allow us to place any stress upon it. For some other cause, therefore, must we look ;—it cannot well be lowness of site, as both Madras and Calcutta are, equally with Bombay, very slightly elevated above sea-level. So likewise it cannot be poverty, wretchedness, or want of drainage, otherwise Calcutta and Madras would produce quite as many cases as Bombay. Its cause yet remains to be discovered."

ART. 32.—*On the Characteristics of Strychnia Tetanus.* By Dr. R. ADAMS, Surgeon to the Richmond Hospital.

(*Medical Times and Gazette*, Aug. 16, 1856.)

In a paper containing an account of a case of suicidal poisoning by strychnia, Dr. Adams draws the following comparison between ordinary tetanus and strychnia tetanus :

1. Strychnia tetanus resembles ordinary tetanus in its spasms, particularly when they assume, as they frequently do, the form of opisthotonos.

2. A rigid condition of the muscles exists in both cases, not only during the actual paroxysms, but also during the intervals between them

3. Strychnia tetanus, in its progress to a fatal result, is much more rapid in its course than ordinary tetanus.

4. The commencement of this last is silent, and the expression of the counte-nance is peculiar and characteristic.

5. The beginning of the former is announced by loud and repeated screams and moanings.

6. The hands in strychnia tetanus are early and severely affected ; in ordinary tetanus the hands are the parts of all others the last and least affected.

ART. 33.—*A case of Writer's Cramp, cured by Electricity.* By M. SECCAMINI.

(*Gaz. Med. de Italiana (Lombardia)*; and *Gaz. Med. de Paris*, March 15, 1856.)

The patient in this case was a lawyer's clerk, æt. 40, well in other respects, who had suffered for some time from a paralysed condition of the right hand. When he attempted to write, the fingers grasped the pen convulsively, and writing was out of his power. The case is not given circumstantially, and we are not told how long these symptoms had continued, but enough is said to show that they were those of ordinary writer's cramp, which had been brought on by an excessively pro-longed use of the pen, and that there was no disease in the great nervous centres or elsewhere. Examining the arm by means of the electrical apparatus of Duchenne, the sensibility was found to be in a perfectly natural state, but not the motility. The flexors of the fingers and the adductors of the arm contracted normally ; the pronator teres contracted imperfectly ; and the extensors of the arm contracted very slightly. The electricity was applied by means of two moistened sponges, and the paralysed muscles were excited by acting powerfully upon their antagonists, after the plan laid down by M. Duchenne; and the result was that the use of the hand was perfectly restored, after fifteen sittings of about half an hour each.

ART. 34.—*Case of Spinal Apoplexy.* By Dr. ISAAC F. PORTER, of New London, Connecticut.

(*American Journal of Medical Science,* July, 1856.)

Cases of this nature, or even of spinal congestion, terminating fatally, are met with so rarely, that any new case is necessarily possessed of considerable interest. Dr. Porter's diagnosis, it is true, is not confirmed by a post-mortem examination, but there can be no reasonable doubt as to its correctness.

CASE.—A talented and opulent merchant, largely employed in commerce, was busily engaged from early dawn until afternoon of an intensely hot day in Septem-ber last, in getting to sea one of his ships. He was 40 years of age, and his general health good, although there is in the family a proclivity to plethoric, congestive, and paralytic diseases. He had drank freely, though prudently, of cold liquids, and, after the ship had sailed, went into a barber's shop, about 5 o'clock P.M., and had his head "shampooed," as he had occasionally done before. Heated and exhausted as he was, the irrigation of the water, as it flowed over the back of his head and neck, was, for a time, very grateful, though it had been standing, as was said, the most of the day in the room. He soon, however, became chilly, and was seized with a violent pain in the lower part of his back, and, on attempting to leave the shop, became partially paralysed ; and he was obliged, soon after, to stand motionless in the street for some minutes. The powerlessness then seemed gradually to leave him, and he was able to walk, though with difficulty, his gait being noticeably changed, as observed by his friends. About half an hour after, he was again seized with pain in the back and numbness, and loss of power in the lower limbs, attended with a very severe chill ; yet the palsy was not severe enough to prevent his walk-ing home at 6 P.M., when he went immediately to bed. By advice of friends, he took hot stimulant drinks and teas, hot pediluvia, and had bottles of hot water placed around him. He soon emerged from the chill, and moderate reaction came on, but complained greatly of pain in the back, and numbness of his extremities. A little before 10 o'clock P.M., I saw him—intellect perfect; countenance anxious, though disposed to think lightly of his disease, saying he should be at his store in the morning ; shaking with the cold at the slightest motion of the bedclothes ; gentle perspiration, but the hands cold and clammy when exposed to the air. The pain in the back, and numbness, still continued, and new distress, like colic, had lately manifested itself in the abdomen, with a most urgent desire for a passage from the bowels. A free motion had occurred just before the attack, and, previous to my arrival, he had endeavored to use the close-stool, but immediately on rising, with help, into the upright position, he had fainted. Insisting on making a second attempt, he arose with help, but rather *fell* than *sat* in the chair. Immediately his head dropped on his chest, his breathing became stertorous, and the muscles began to show convulsive action. Contrary to my express command, he afterwards made another attempt, with the same result, and on coming to himself he said: " I am truly in a critical situation, and will make no further effort." There was desire to pass water, but it was by no means so urgent, and none passed him during life. From 11 o'clock P.M. of Tuesday night until 4 P.M. of the following day, when he expired, he maintained the horizontal position, except as he vomited twice in the night, and slightly turned from side to side, with restlessness and jactitation from pain in the bowels and back. His pulse, as I entered the room, was a mere thread, contrasting strongly with his flushed and congested countenance. The slightest pressure annihilated it, and after effort on his part it was entirely gone.

The aspect of the case, at the outset, was almost hopeless, and the symptoms progressed with rapid strides towards a fatal termination. About 4 o'clock in the morning his acute distress left him ; the pulse slightly rose in volume and power under the use of stimulants and nourishment, and by crowding them it was for a short time maintained, but soon either the stomach rejected them, or they ceased to have anything more than a momentary influence. He soon after became somnolent, though he was aroused without difficulty until within an hour or two of his death, and always showed a good share of intelligence, and answered questions promptly and properly. While apparently asleep, he occasionally uttered incoherent expressions, but on being aroused, was perfectly conscious. Showing how naturally and spontaneously our thoughts flow in their accustomed channels, shortly before he expired he said, in a firm voice, " I believe that everything is aboard," which were his last words. " Even in our ashes, live their wonted fires."

Soon after dissolution, remarkable evidence of venous engorgement presented itself.   The entire surface of the body appeared as if deeply ecchymosed or cyanosed. The color was uniform and permanent.

There were unusual reasons for preserving the body as long as possible, and the weather was very hot and oppressive. Much as a post-mortem examination was desired, yet these reasons, and the mechanical difficulties to be overcome being so great in exposing the vertebral canal, and the want of suitable instruments, all conspired to render it impracticable.

The treatment in this case was directed, at the outset, to obviating the alarming prostration. Ignorant, at that time, of the cold douche, the chills in the barber's shop, and the subsequent loss of muscular power, the debility was referred to some unknown *functional* derangement, and alcoholic drinks, sulph. ether, and aromat, spts. ammo. were freely used, with animal broths; and externally, fomentations were applied to the abdomen, and Granville's lotion, sinapisms, and a blister to the back. Leeches were proposed to the medical gentlemen in consultation, but declined on account of the adynamia. The influence of medication was momentary and trifling.

(B) CONCERNING THE RESPIRATORY SYSTEM.

ART. 35.—*The influence of Sea Voyages and Warm Climates on the progress of Pulmonary Consumption.* BY M. JULES ROCHARD.

(*Edinburgh Medical Journal*, Oct., 1856.)

The following conclusions are arrived at on this subject by Mr. Rochard, after a most elaborate investigation of the subject. His paper is published in the " Memoirs of the Academy of Medicine of Paris," for 1856, and is an " ouvrage couronné dans la séance publique du 11 Décembre, 1855."

1. Sea voyages accelerate the progress of pulmonary tuberculization, much more frequently than they retard it.

2. This disease, far from being rare among marines, is, on the contrary, much more common among them than in the land army. It prevails with equal intensity in the hospitals of our ports, in our stations, in our fleets. The "officiers de marine,"

the physicians, the commissaries, all who are afloat, in a word, are subjected to this general law.

3. With rare exceptions, which must be admitted, considering some facts recorded by men of credit, phthisis advances on board ship with more rapidity than ashore.

4. The naval profession should be interdicted, in the most decided manner, to all youths who appear to be menaced with phthisis.

5. The consumptive can get no advantage from sea voyages, except they be on board under certain special hygienic conditions, and change climate and locality according to the seasons and atmospheric vicissitudes; things which cannot be realized on board of ships with a mission to fulfil. Journeys by land, and prolonged stay in a well-selected country, allow of all the same objects being attained, with much less expense and danger.

6. Warm countries, taken as a whole, exercise an injurious influence on the progress of pulmonary tuberculization, and accelerate its course.

7. Those situated in the torrid zone are especially injurious, and stay there should be formally interdicted to the phthisical. - The opinions of the physicians-in-chief of our colonies, and of the English colonies, comparative statistics of colonial and of European regiments in the two sets of countries, the frequency of phthisis in our tropical stations, and in those of England in the same latitudes, and a multitude of special observations, demonstrate this completely, and the examination of each particular locality confirms it.

8. Most hot climates, situated outside of the torrid zone, are equally injurious to the tuberculous. Some points on the confines of this region, and concentrated in a narrow space, are exceptions. This is owing to local conditions. To sojourn in them protects the phthisical from acute affections of the respiratory passages which accelerate the progress of tuberculization, permits a mode of life better adapted to keeping up the general strength, prolongs existence sometimes, and contributes always to a more easy termination of the same.

9. It is in the first stage of phthisis that there is any hope from emigration, and any reason to expect good results from it.

The localities to be recommended to the consumptive M. Rochard divides into four series, according to their respective advantages:

1. Madeira. 2. Hyères, Venice, and Pisa. 3. Rome, Nice, of which the reputation is constantly decreasing. 4. Menton, Villa Franche, Bay of Spezzia, Lake of Como, the Balearic Isles, the Shores of Greece, the North of Egypt, Algeria.

ART. 36.—*A Mode of Restoration in Pulmonary Consumption.*
BY DR. THEOPHILUS THOMPSON, F.R.S.

(Lancet, May 17, 1856.)

" When we speak of the cure of phthisis, the idea usually suggested to the mind is that of a closed vomica; the accidental tissue which encloses the cavity being contracted, and drawing with it the pulmonary substance, so as to produce external puckering; whilst within, there is presented an imperfect cicatrix of fibrous material. This change, however, I suspect is not so frequent as that to which I propose to invite the attention of the profession, occurring in certain cases where the tubercular deposits is in small masses surrounded by healthy portions of lung. The exudations poured out around a tubercular deposit may prove nutritive, and conduce to its maintenance; but, on the other hand, if incapable of development, they may rapidly degenerate, and softening may ensue; and the pulmonary tissue may become infiltrated with tubercular pus, abounding in solitary molecules, masses of fat globules, nuclei, and incomplete cell formations. The process of disintegration thus set up, unfavorably affecting the surrounding texture, the process of destruction extends: but under more favorable circumstances, the tubercular substance may undergo a different kind of metamorphosis, and, its development ceasing, it may waste, in consequence of the withdrawal of nutritive material; the organic elements may be absorbed, leaving only calcareous salts, combined with aggregate fat globules, pigment masses, and plates of cholesterine. This change is not uncommon. It may, I think, often be traced in a certain class of delicate dyspeptic individuals whose vital powers have been husbanded. One of the most remarkable signs which I have found accompanying this form of tubercular disease, is the modification of the respiratory sound, which I have ventured to designate 'wavy inspiration,' because it conveys to the ear the impression that the air enters by a succession of waves instead of a continuous stream. There are several varieties of wavy inspiration, more or less extensive, variable, and transient: one, dependent on bronchial affection, usually accompanied with rhonchus; a second, of high key, associated with rheumatism of the muscles of the chest; a third, combined with pleuritic friction sound, and increased by pressure; but the variety which has special reference to the affection under consideration, is a delicate, somewhat distinct sound, limited in extent, and usually persistent until superseded by signs of more advanced disease. Several of these varieties of wavy inspiration may, indeed, be associated in the same individual, but may still be distinguished and interpreted, as in the patient whose case I proceed to describe."

CASE.—Mr. C—, a gentleman, æt. 32, residing in one of the suburbs of London, applied to me, on the 16th of March, 1854, complaining of weakness and of slight cough. He was five feet ten inches in height, and weighed nine stone eleven pounds. At the General Exhibition, in 1851, he weighed nine stone twelve pounds, but soon afterwards lost flesh; subsequently he increased in weight, but recently had again declined. One of his sisters died of phthisis, another had threatenings of the disease, but recovered. Two years since he had slight hæmoptysis in streaks, and had lately occasionally awoke with blood in his mouth. There was slight dulness on percussion near the acromial end of the right subclavicular region, but the principal physical signs were on the left side, consisting of wavy inspiration over the whole apex before and behind, at some parts accompanied with friction sound, and increased by pressure, and attended with superficial pain. The pulse was 88 in the sitting, 116 in the standing, posture; the gums presenting the festoon common in consumptive subjects; tongue rather white; bowels regular; urine depositing lithates. I prescribed a turpentine liniment, a grain of extract of colchicum every night, and saline draughts, with hydrocyanic acid.

March 20th.—Wavy inspiration of lower key, and less extensively heard; a little above the left nipple sounding distant, and not increased by pressure; expectoration dotted with blood, and, under the microscope, found to contain pus globules, granules, and *elastic tissue of the lungs*, teased out as though long imprisoned; also much large angular epithelium from the fauces. In correspondence with this last observation, the fauces were flushed and granular. I prescribed lemon-juice, prussic acid, and tincture of hop, with infusion of cascarilla.

26th.—Weight, nine stone ten pounds; wavy inspiration still marked; fauces very granular. I directed a continuance of the mixture, two drachms of cod-liver oil twice daily, and an application to the fauces, composed of equal parts of trisnitrate of bismuth, mucilaginous mixture, almond oil, and rose water.

On the 3d of April, the throat appeared better; the pulse was 84; other symptoms as before, excepting that there was much night perspiration, for the relief of which I prescribed four grains of oxide of zinc, and four of extract of henbane, to be taken every night.

On the 18th of April there was some click ("humid crepitation") above the left nipple; pulse 88; weight, nine stone nine pounds. The dose of cod-liver oil was increased.

May 1st.—He was somewhat improved in feeling and appearance, but there was "dry glass-rubbing sound" at some points of the left apex. A blister was therefore applied over this region.

17th.—Weight, nine stone twelve pounds; pulse reported to be 66 when he awakes in the morning. To have of iodide of potassium two grains, ten minims of solution of potash, with infusion of cascarilla, three times a day, and to continue the oil.

June 10th.—Weight, nine stone thirteen pounds; throat decidedly better, but the click continuing.

18th.—Weight advanced to ten stone one and a half pounds, although for some days rather free hæmoptysis had occurred. After a few doses of sulphate of magnesia, with infusion of roses, the spitting of blood ceased; but the bowels being confined, diluted aloetic pills were administered.

After this date the click near the left nipple extended. On August 15th the patient's weight had fallen to nine stone eleven pounds, and the pulse risen to 92.

The throat was relaxed, and the tongue white. The dose of cod-liver oil was increased, and he was directed to have a tannic acid gargle, and a mixture of nitro-hydrochloric and hydrocyanic acid. During the two following months there was little change, excepting slight increase of weight. There was slight hæmoptysis and some night perspirations, but the latter symptom yielded to oxide of zinc. On the 16th of October his general feelings were improved, but the pulse was 92, and there was wavy inspiration of high key in the left subscapular, and crackle ("dry crepitation") in the middle subclavicular region. In addition to his other medicine, a grain of quinine was prescribed, to be taken thrice daily. On the 31st of October his weight was ten stone four pounds, being an increase of six pounds in a fortnight; pulse 88.

November 21.—There was slight hæmoptysis, and extensive wavy inspiration before and behind. Half a drachm of iodine, a drachm of iodide of potassium, to be dissolved in half an ounce of spirit, for an application to the left subclavicular region.

28th.—Weight, ten stone seven pounds; pulse 76; some pain on the left side of the chest. Chloroform and laudanum, with soap liniment, to be applied; other medicines continued.

During the first three months of 1855, the click extended a little downwards, and there was pain near the left nipple, but these symptoms disappeared. The expectoration, which had varied much in quantity, gradually diminished, and at one period in the month of May was accompanied with a little *calcareous matter tinged with blood*. The treatment during this period was not altered materially, excepting by the addition of free inunction of coco-olein, having a grain of iodine dissolved in each ounce. In June this patient weighed ten stone ten pounds, and his pulse varied from 60 to 70; there was slight bronchophony in the middle subclavicular region on the left side, but no click, and near this point a little delicate wavy inspiration, but the high-keyed wave was no longer to be detected. From the time of the calcareous expectoration the marked fluctuations of condition were no longer observed, he steadily improved in condition, and is now able to walk six miles, and attend with comfort to his ordinary professional avocations.

It may be difficult to determine the relative influence of the different remedies employed in promoting the satisfactory result; but there can be little doubt that, irrespective of general hygienic measures, the cod-liver oil was of essential service, and that its good effect was increased by the contemporaneous administration of quinine. The endermic introduction of coco-olein and iodine has also appeared to me in the present and some other instances to be useful.

"In the case next to be described, a similar process appears in the first instance to have occurred, followed, however, under less favorable circumstances, by a renewal of disease."

CASE —A medical practitioner, æt. 27, in the year 1852, had dull percussion over a small portion of the lung, corresponding to the second intercostal space on the left side. In January, 1853, he had a little calcareous expectoration, the size of a split pea, mixed with a little blood. The dulness disappeared, and he remained tolerably well until about the autumn of 1854, when he contracted influenza and cough, which he thinks were rendered severe by bad diet and exposure to the weather in the Caffre war. He was a seven-months' child, and could never eat butter or fat. Hair abundant on head and arms, but remarkably deficient on the chest. He had suffered severely from shingles.

On the 14th of April, 1855, he applied to me in consequence of slight morning cough, accompanied with expectoration of a little thick, yellow mucus, sometimes resembling milk when falling through water. I found dull percussion at the acromial end of the right subclavicular region, and wavy inspiration at the summits of both lungs, but chiefly of the right, where there was also prolonged expiratory murmur. Pulse 88, sitting; 108, standing. I prescribed sarsaparilla with solution of potash and taraxacum, and an appropriate place of recreation in the country. This plan, however, he was prevented from carrying out, but went to the north of England, where, after much professional exertion and responsibility, he had an attack of hæmoptysis.

June 13th.—I found marked increase of dulness, and bronchial respiration, where

·formerly wavy inspiration was the principal sign. He felt weaker; his eyes were pearly-looking; his general aspect unpromising; *the expectoration submitted to the microscope was found to contain much pulmonary tissue.*

This case must be regarded as a second attack of phthisis, which in the first instance had pursued (like the case first described) a progress towards recovery. I know of several instances in which, after a repeated recurrence of such conditions, ·the disease has remained in abeyance, and the patient become able to discharge a full share of the duties of life.

"Such cases occur chiefly amongst patients in constitutional conditions rather delicate than unsound, and of active habits, easily fatigued, subject to neuralgia, often hypochondriacal (and not unfrequently having jugular murmur), but remarkably varying in efficiency for the discharge of active duty, according to the extent to which hygienic rules can be observed. Wavy inspiration is a principal local manifestation. This sound indicating, as I believe, a free expansion of the neighboring portion of lung, the result of a condition favorable to the happy termination of the disease, with calcareous metamorphosis of the tubercular deposit."

ART. 37.—*On the treatment of Pneumonia and Pleurisy.* By Dr. NIEMEYER, Professor of Clinical Medicine in Greifswalde.

(*Prager Vierteljahrssch.*, Bd. iv, p. 121; and *Med.-Chir. Review*, July, 1856.)

Professor Niemeyer is much opposed to the employment of general venesection in pneumonia and pleurisy, and only uses it exceptionally with a view to prevent impending suffocation, and to facilitate the reflux of the blood from the brain, but not for the purpose of arresting the inflammation. He agrees with the observation of Dieck, that the convalescence is more rapid in those cases that have been treated without than in those which have been treated with venesection; and he explains the fact by the increase of fibrin, and diminution in the amount of the red corpuscles, induced by the venesection.

The treatment adopted by Professor Niemeyer consists in the application of compresses wrung out in cold water over the affected part of the thorax, and their renewal as often as they become warm. The great relief experienced by the patient is a sufficient guarantee that the repetition of the application will be carefully attended to. The only internal remedy employed was nitre, in doses of two drachms in the course of twenty-four hours. Although employed at different ages, and in various forms of the disease, no metastasis or other evil consequences have ever been noticed by the author. He has seen persons attacked with very tumultuous symptoms, enabled by this treatment to return to their occupation on the seventh day after seizure. Professor Niemeyer recommends an early exhibition of steel in the convalescence from the diseases under consideration.

ART. 38.—*Pneumonia originating in the Pulmonary Capillaries.* By Dr. GORDON.

(*Dublin Quarterly Journal of Medical Science*, Aug. 1856.)

This form of pneumonia appears to be essentially a blood-disease, and sometimes comes on very suddenly, at other times more slowly; like all diseases of this type, it is often epidemic; it sometimes supervenes on other diseases, but often attacks persons who were previously in apparently good health. The great chemical alteration which the blood would appear to undergo, consists in the augmentation of the fibrin, but this augmentation taking place, amongst other modes, by the conversion into it of a more or less considerable quantity of the albumen: we thus have two distinct morbid actions taking place within the sanguiniferous system, one consisting in the removal of the great nutrient or formative power in the blood, and the other in the sudden engorgement of the capillaries with a great mass of, most probably, crude fibrin, which, partly from depressed vital action, and partly from mechanical over-distension, they are unable to transmit.

The symptoms and physical signs with which this form of disease is attended are such as are not merely easily reconcilable with this improved condition of the blood, and engorgement of the pulmonary vessels, but such as we might naturally expect to be produced by such amount of morbid action. It rarely happens that we have an opportunity of examining the lungs of a patient who has died in the very early stage of this affection. I have said above that the disease is frequently epidemic; it would seem to have been so in the year 1841, at which time I was resident clinical clerk in the Hardwicke Hospital; it then attacked several patients who were recovering from fever, and their strength being already greatly reduced, some died within a few hours from the commencement of the attack; these cases were carefully noted by me at the time, and the post-mortem appearances were exhibited at different meetings of the Pathological Society, by Dr. Corrigan, physician to the hospital. Cases apparently similar were also noticed about the same time by Dr. Stokes and Dr. O'Ferrall. One of Dr. Corrigan's communications on the subject terminates as follows:—" The circumstances I have mentioned, if confirmed by future observations, would go to establish an idiopathic form of disease, characterized chiefly by an atonic state of the vessels, *and in which the symptoms were not amenable to any of the usual modes of treatment.*"

The appearance of a lung when seen in the *very early* stage of this form of pneumonia is very unlike that produced by acute inflammation of the air-vesicles of the lung. When first seen after the opening of the thorax, it presents a dark blue color. This appearance, however, is very evanescent, and is almost completely lost in the course of three or four hours after the lung has been removed. When grasped in the hand, it feels like muscle; but, unlike what is usually termed carnified lung, it is increased rather than diminished in size, but is not so much increased as in the more ordinary form of pneumonia: it is firm and heavy, and sinks in water, but does not appear to have any tendency to pass into any form of hepatization, nor does it afford any feeling of crepitation, or anything allied thereto. This description, which I have borrowed from my reports of the cases above alluded to, and from Dr. Corrigan's demonstration of the appearances before the Pathological Society, as well as from subsequent examination of other similar cases, appears to me to indicate a modification of pulmonary disease altogether different from ordinary vesicular pneumonia, nor yet to be confounded with pulmonary apoplexy, or " the collapse of the lung as connected with bronchial obstruction," described by Gairdner and others.

The symptoms which existed in those who died in this very early stage, were great and sudden collapse, sudden lividity, and coldness of the surface; the lips beame purple, and a dark flush arose on the face; they complained of excessive weakness; there was great depression of strength—in fact, "in no case could the asthenic character be better marked." In some cases the patient complained of difficulty of breathing; but even when there was no complaint uttered, the increased rapidity of the respiratory acts—in one case they amounted to sixty in the minute —indicated great pulmonary obstruction. The respiration was usually diaphragmatic; the tongue was moist and dark-colored; the pulse small, feeble, and very rapid; the surface of the body almost cold; there was seldom any complaint of cough, but there was frequently pain in the side, which was not always referred to the part where the physical signs showed the existence of disease. These physical signs were, great dulness on percussion over a certain portion of the chest, according to the extent of lung engaged, which did not seem to follow any precise rule; in some instances the upper part of the lung was affected, sometimes the lower, sometimes portions of both lungs; and, corresponding to the amount of dulness, there was either absence or great feebleness of the respiratory murmur.

Patients dying in this stage of the disease, died generally of collapse. I have never seen those extreme symptoms to attend this disease, except in individuals who were greatly reduced by previous illness, or some other cause; they generally, but not always, prove fatal. Several recovered during the epidemic in 1841, and within the last two months I saw a very well-marked case of it, which recovered, under Dr. Corrigan's care, in the Hardwicke Hospital.

The symptoms which attend the disease, as it generally comes under our notice, and which seem to distinguish it from ordinary pneumonia, are, that 1. The peculiar heat of the skin, so forcibly dwelt upon by Addison, as almost pathognomonic of pneumonia, does not exist; the skin is never very hot, sometimes dry, often cool, and even perspiring; but it very early acquires a peculiar *jaunâtre* aspect, which it retains throughout, and often does not lose for some time after all physical evidence of disease has vanished. This symptom was very strongly marked in several cases lately in hospital. some of whom are still under observation. 2. The cough is altogether different in character from that of ordinary pneumonia: it is very short, frequent, and performed without any apparent muscular effort whatsoever—very unlike the painful and distressing cough so often witnessed in vesicular pneumonia. 3. There is seldom any expectoration; when it does occur, it is not viscid, nor homogeneous, nor tenacious. 4. There is seldom much pain in the side; never the acute, stabbing pain, which occurs in vesicular pneumonia from the pleura being implicated, because we rarely find pleurisy existing in this form of disease, and, as we remarked before, we often find the patient refer the pain which he does complain of to a part of the chest where we have no other evidence of disease existing. 5. The high fever which attends vesicular pneumonia is absent; the pulse is seldom remarkably frequent; it is always feeble, and soon acquires a peculiar jerking feel, which it owes to the tenuity of the blood. The patient has frequently a listless and careless manner, and appears unwilling to speak even about his illness. Such was the case in a boy, about nine years of age, who was admitted into the Hardwicke Hospital, on June 5th, with solidification of almost the entire of one lung; yet neither he, nor his parents, who came with him, mentioned any one symptom from which such disease might be inferred. The prominent symptom for which they requested relief was constant vomiting. In some cases the pulmonary affection is accompanied by an attack of herpes labialis. There is always complete loss of appetite for solid food, but often great thirst; considerable modification of the voice often exists, amounting in some instances very nearly to aphonia; there is sometimes restlessness, and often insomnia. The physical signs are very constant: there is a dull sound on percussion over the affected portion of the lung or lungs, and at first very feeble respiratory murmur, which, however, maintains somewhat its vesicular character, but soon becomes very decidedly bronchial. The peculiar crepitus of vesicular pneumonia is never audible. If the patient recovers, the progress of the physical signs is very remarkable; sometimes within twenty-four hours the extreme bronchial respiration and bronchophony are replaced by a feeble or even ordinary vesicular murmur, proving that the air-cells merely suffered obliteration from pressure, which, being removed, they again expanded.

The patient seldom dies in this stage; when he does, it is generally found that a very great portion of the lungs is engaged in the disease; they are very tough and heavy, and a section of them exhibits a uniform light gray color. But the progress of this affection is very rapid (it seldom extends over a period of weeks, like some cases of vesicular pneumonia, which has passed through all its stages), and the lung seems readily to pass into a condition somewhat allied to gangrenous degeneration. Effusion now takes place into the bronchial tubes, and the patient dies asphyxiated. Post-mortem examination usually shows the lung to be of a dirty gray color; there is no well-marked suppuration, but a species of general softening, and commencing decomposition.   *   *   *   *   *

I would infer that the amount of albumen which may appear in the urine of a patient affected with this form of pneumonia, is not indicative of the amount of pulmonary disease, nor does its accumulation prove the extension of the pneumonia; but that, on the contrary, from the appearance of albumen in the urine in such cases, we may anticipate an amendment in the original disease; and that, from a sudden disappearance of albumen from the urine, we may dread a relapse of the pulmonary affection.   *   *   *   *   *

Perhaps one of the best-marked features of this disease is, " its not being amenable to any of the usual modes of treatment." I need not here allude to the more than inefficacy of abstraction of blood in any form to meet its requirements. The treatment by tartar emetic is equally inapplicable; and the mercurial plan of treatment, as it is termed, is also powerless to control this formidable affection. The treatment by the internal use of oil of turpentine, so advantageous in the suppurative stage of vesicular pneumonia, does not appear to have any influence on this form of disease. Wine and the usual diffusible stimulants support the patient's strength, and add to his vital energy, and so are of use; but they seem to have no specific power over the disease, such as is evidently exercised by the sulphate of quina. During the last eight months I have treated with quina all the cases of this form of pneumonia which I have witnessed, and I had the opportunity of observing several cases similarly treated by Dr. Corrigan in the Hardwicke Hospital. On the

19th of April last, Dr. Corrigan presented to the Pathological Society a specimen of this form of pulmonary disease, when he took occasion to allude to the efficacy of quina in its treatment. The result of this treatment has been that, of the cases which came under observation before effusion had taken place into the bronchial tubes, none proved fatal; while some few recovered, even after the lips had become blue, the face congested, and mucous rales were audible in the bronchial tubes.

ART. 39.— *On the connection between certain forms of Pneumonia and Renal Disease.* By DR. B. Z. M'DOWELL, Physician to the Whitworth and Hardwicke Hospital, &c.

(*Dublin Quarterly Journal of Medicine*, May, 1856.)

Dr. M'Dowell's object in this paper is to direct attention to a combination of morbid conditions, which does not appear to have been *specially* noticed,—the frequent coexistence, namely, of certain suppurative inflammations with chronic renal disease, but more especially to the combination of the latter with the suppurative and gangrenous forms of pneumonia, of which several cases have recently come under his notice.

At a recent meeting of the Pathological Society of Dublin (19th January, 1856), Dr. M'Dowell exhibited a specimen of gangrenous pneumonia, in which a diseased condition of the kidneys likewise existed (this case is the second of the two cases here selected); and his remarks at the time were thus reported:

" Dr. M'Dowell particularly directed the attention of the Society to this combination of disease, and stated his belief, that chronic renal disease had a great influence on the development of suppurative inflammations. This he had especially observed in pneumonia, as, for the last eighteen months, during which period he had paid particular attention to this subject, *he had not met with a fatal case of suppurative pneumonia in which renal disease was not also found to exist.* His opinion was, that pneumonia, in the great majority of instances, passes through certain regular phases, which naturally tend to a restoration of the healthy condition of the lung; but that when pneumonia occurred in a person in whom renal disease had pre-existed, the tendency of the disease then was to assume the suppurative, or the gangrenous form."

Dr. M'Dowell gives twelve cases in illustration, of which we copy two.

CASE 1.— *Double pneumonia. Purulent infiltration of the lungs. Bright's disease of the kidney. Death on the sixth day.*—Thomas Wood, a carman, æt. 32, was admitted into the Hardwicke Hospital, under Dr. M'Dowell's care, August 5th, 1853. Patient was a man of very intemperate habits. Three days before admission (Sunday) he got drunk, and was exposed all night to wind and rain. He returned home early on Monday, feeling chilled and ill; violent rigors followed, with cough and oppression of the breathing.

On admission (fourth day, Wednesday), the face was darkly flushed, the dyspnœa intense, and there was total prostration of strength. Respiration, 44; pulse, 130 in the minute; skin, extremely hot; there was frequent cough, with thin, scanty, colorless expectoration; and pain on inspiration in the left side.

Double pneumonia was found to exist, the right lung being principally engaged; more than half of this lung gave the signs of solidification; over the lower portion of the left lung friction likewise existed, denoting the coexistence of pleuritis.

Fifth day. Right lung wholly solidified.

Respiration, 52; pulse, 140; raved incessantly all night; dyspnœa more urgent; vomiting; died on Thursday evening, sixth day of the disease.

Autopsy.—Thoracic viscera.—Double pneumonia, with pleuritis on the left side. The right lung was solidified throughout, and infiltrated with dark-colored pus; the tissue of the lung was very friable and non-crepitant. The left lung was solidified in patches, in all of which pus was diffused. The uninflamed portion of the lung was emphysematous. The pericardium was extremely adherent to the heart; in some places the adhesions consisted of bands half an inch long. The heart was enlarged and hypertrophied, weighing 16 oz. when separated from the pericardium. Its tissue was slightly softer than natural, but its valvular apparatus was perfectly healthy.

Abdominal viscera.—The liver was large and pale. The spleen softened, but of natural size.

The kidneys were extensively diseased; externally both were pale, smooth, and mottled. The tubular structure had nearly altogether disappeared, and white, soft, fatty-looking material occupied the greater bulk of the organ. _ The left was much diminished in size. The right weighed 5½ oz., and the left 2½ oz. only; in the latter a fibrinous clot of a brown color lay in a small cavity, with the walls of which it had but a very slight connection. ("Pathological Register of the Whitworth and Hardwicke Hospitals.")

CASE 9.—*Pneumonia of the left lung, terminating in gangrene. Fatal in seventeen days. Both kidneys extensively diseased.*—Eliza Champion, æt. 28, was admitted into the Hardwicke Hospital, under Dr. M'Dowell's care, December 31st, 1855. On Saturday, the 22d, had a severe rigor, followed, after three days, by cough and fetid expectoration. Two days after her admission she miscarried of a fœtus at the seventh month. On the day following, January 2d, she was much prostrated, weak, and sunk. Pulse rapid and small; expectoration copious, dark-colored, thin, and fetid; bright circumscribed flush on each cheek; pupils contracted; cough very troublesome. Respiration 56; pulse 136; the breath was fetid. On examination amphoric blowing was found to exist over the greater portion of the back of the left lung; metallic resonance of the voice, and gurgling, were likewise evident; but there was no splash heard on succussion; whilst abnormal tympany, and the signs of excentric displacement, were absent. The diagnosis of a large gangrenous cavity in the left lung was not therefore difficult.

She was ordered eight ounces of wine daily, and an ounce of a mixture containing six drachms of syrup of bark, three drachms of solution of chloride of soda, one drachm of tincture of opium, and six ounces and a half of water, to be taken every fourth hour. Treatment did not seem to influence the progress of the disease; the expectoration became greater in quantity, and more and more offensive; soon it gurgled up from the throat with little effort on the part of the patient; presently, shreds of a stringy substance, like fragments of lung, were coughed up, and from this time the fetor became almost insufferable; yet the strength did not seem to give way much until the eighth, when diffused inflammation of the left parotid region appeared; then came rapid sinking, and death ensued on the following morning.

Autopsy.—The left lung was found in a state of absolute putrefaction; what remained of it hung in loose shreds, revealing a dissection of the tubes and vessels; recent lymph, contrasting by its white color with the black mass beneath, lay in thick patches on the pleural surface. The *right lung*, which was nowhere solidified, was found studded with several gangrenous vesicles, from which, when they were cut into, fetid gas and grayish-colored pus escaped, whilst the substance of the lung beneath was found deeply disorganized. The *kidneys* were symmetrically and extensively diseased; a section showed a great increase in the depth of the cortex, an adventitious deposit, absorption of the central cones, and an excessive deposition of fat towards the pelvis.

The order of the morbid changes in this case was, probably, the following: first, pleuro-pneumonia of the left lung, which rapidly passed into gangrene (owing, as I believe, to the existence of extensive renal disease); secondly, the gases thus generated were absorbed, giving rise to a putrescent condition of the blood; as the result of which we had, thirdly, cellulitis of the parotid region, and gangrene in isolated patches (not preceded by inflammatory consolidation) of the right lung.

"These cases, twelve in number," Dr. M'Dowell proceeds, "constitutes the evidence in support of the opinion, already several times expressed, that between pneumonia in its worst and most fatal forms, and structural disease of the kidneys, some definite relationship exists. If this opinion be adopted, and if we regard the combination of diseases illustrated by these cases, as representing parts in one great chain of pathological sequences, then the order of these sequences is easily traced out. It is no new doctrine that a diseased condition of the kidneys cannot long exist without an impairment, more or less serious, of the great function of excretion. A morbid condition of the blood is established as the result of imperfect depuration; hence arise certain secondary affections, of which (in connection with diseased kidneys) serious inflammations and affections of the brain and heart have attracted the most attention. But it is probable that the secondary affections which depend on organic renal disease, will vary according to the stage of the disease, or according to the peculiar form under which it is manifested.

"'Bright's disease,' we now know, is a generic term which includes several dissimilar diseased conditions of the kidney; and whilst inflammation of the serous membranes may be more frequently associated with one particular form of disease —viz., the small, contracted, 'granular' kidney—pneumonia in its worst forms (gangrenous or suppurative) may be more particularly the secondary result of the large, smooth, pale kidney, which was so uniformly found to coexist in the cases already detailed.

" In these observations my object has been to avoid theorizing, and to furnish a simple statement of clinical facts; and I am perfectly ready to adopt or reject the opinions here advanced, as more extended observations may either confirm or refute them.

" At another time I hope to be able to furnish some evidence of the influence which renal disease exercises on the development of pyemia in general; and, in fine, will very briefly state the conclusions which I think may naturally be deduced from the cases given in the preceding pages:

" 1. That in fatal cases of pneumonia renal disease is very frequently found to exist.

" 2. That where such a combination of disease exists, suppuration of the lung will be very constantly met with.

" 3. That a similar morbid condition of the kidney is often found in gangrene of the ung.

" 4. Or, it may be conversely stated, that where pneumonia supervenes in a person, in whom renal disease has previously existed, it is very apt to assume the suppurative or the gangrenous form.

" 5. That pneumonia, when it occurs in such fatal forms, and under such circumstances, is probably one of the 'secondary affections' of 'Bright's disease.'

" It has not been my intention to convey the idea that pneumonia has never been enumerated by authors as one of the complications of ' Bright's disease;' though some writers are silent on the subject, others have distinctly noticed it, especially Rayer. But it will be found that the pneumonia described in this paper is of a different nature from that noticed by Rayer. The pneumonia which he describes as secondary to 'albuminous nephritis' comes on at a late period, and after the dropsy and other symptoms of the renal disease have been fully pronounced; and hence he observes:—'The symptoms of such pneumonias are more or less marked by those of dropsy, or by the symptoms of cardiac disease, or other concomitant pulmonary lesions.' In none of the cases above described was renal disease suspected to exist; all were apparently in the enjoyment of good health up to the moment of the sudden development of the pulmonary affection. Neither do the cases of pneumonia, alluded to by Rayer and other authors (Bright, Gregory, Christison), resemble, in their anatomical characters, those detailed in the preceding paper. Suppuration and gangrene, either of which was found in all these instances, were not observed by any of these authors. One of Rayer's cases, however, is an exception to this statement—Case 38—in which external suppuration of the lung was found to exist. In the other two (for only three cases are given by Rayer in illustration) red hepatization and œdema, with engorgement of the lungs, were the principal morbid changes."

ART. 40.—*On the pathology of Hooping-cough.* By Dr. HYDE SALTER, Assistant-Physician to Charing-Cross Hospital, &c.

(*Lancet,* July 5, 1856.)

The paper of which the abstract is here subjoined, was read before the Medical Society of London, May 24th, 1856:

After enumerating some of the many discrepant and imaginative theories of the nature of hooping-cough that writers on the subject had indulged in, the author stated, in answer to the question—To what category of derangements do the most constant and characteristic features of the disease the most intimately unite it?—

that, in his opinion, it was to the contagious fevers—to those diseases which consist of the assumption into the body of some specific *materies morbi* introduced from without, and undergoing a certain process of self-multiplication within the system—to the zymotic diseases; in fact, in favor of this view, he said, there was this three-fold evidence :—1st. That hooping cough was contagious. 2d. That it runs a definite course, having certain premonitory signs: certain phenomena when the disease has attained its height, and certain sequelæ. 3d. That it is self-prophylactic; a person having had it once does not have it again.

Now the three circumstances—contagion, definite course, and self-prophylaxis, are, he maintained, *par excellence*, the three characteristic circumstances of the contagious fevers, and the possession by any disease of these three features would always be, to him, a sufficient warrant for its admission into that family of disorders. The author then thus stated, in more exact terms, his views:—That the catching of hooping-cough depends upon the inoculation of the system with a specific poison; that this poison chooses for itself a certain eliminatory surface as its emunctory; that the surface that it so chooses is the respiratory tract of the mucous membrane, from the conjunctiva to the ultimate bronchial tubes, although the whole of the tract need not be involved in every case; that its material presence gives rise to an exalted sensibility and inflammation of the part; and that the exalted sensibility and inflammation constitute the proximate cause of the specific symptoms. The author's conviction of the correctness of the above theory was based on the following considerations:—*a*. The premonitory symptoms of catarrh, injection of the eyes, coryza, &c. *b*. The symptoms of vascular disturbance of the trachea, bronchial tubes, large and small, down even, in many cases, to the ultimate lung-structure, that generally accompany or follow the cough. *c*. The intermediate position with regard to time, of the laryngeal, between the nasal and the bronchial symptoms, implying a creeping down of the condition of the mucous membrane, in a regular course. *d*. The power which one child will have who does not hoop, of communicating the disease to another who will; showing that the spasmodic part of the affection is non-essential. *e*. The eliminatory power of the surface, which is consistent with the supposed final cause of its being affected. *f*. The support derived from the whole weight of the argument of analogy. Dr. Salter concluded by considering, in succession, certain objections to his theory, which he could conceive others to make, but which, from want of space, we are unable to enumerate.

ART. 41.—*On obstruction of the Pulmonary Artery.* By Dr. G. H. KIDD, Assistant-Physician to the Coombe Lying-in Hospital.

(*Dublin Quarterly Journal of Medicine*, Nov. 1856.)

A case of obstruction of the pulmonary artery occurring in the Coombe Lying-in-Hospital, and recorded in this paper, together with the cases related by Cruveilhier and others, affords, in Dr. Kidd's opinion, a series of symptoms sufficiently general, at least, to direct attention to the condition of the pulmonary artery. First, there is a degree of fever, with impaired appetite, scanty or suppressed secretions, and vomiting, as usually occurs at the onset of phlebitis elsewhere; a sense of pain at the precordium, and tightness of the chest may be complained of; the countenance gradually assumes the well-known and remarkable phlebitic aspect; great debility is evident, attended, it may be, with a tendency to syncope; along with this there is great quickness of the pulse, which is at the same time small, weak, soft, and compressible. The debility is greater than there is anything in the other symptoms to account for, and evidently depends on the diminished current in the arteries, and deficient supply to the nervous centres and to the muscles. The languid circulation and congested state of the venous system are still further shown by the violet patches, the œdema, and tendency to sloughing of the integuments. The over-burdened right ventricle relieves itself by regurgitation: hence the swollen, and, perhaps, pulsating jugulars. The respiratory movements are rapid, attempting to compensate by increased action for the limited portion of the lung that is taking part in the aëration of the blood, and vesicular emphysema may now occur, as observed in Dr. Gordon's case.

The constitutional symptoms of phlebitis may now increase in gravity, miliary or red eruptions appear, and the patients gradually fall into the typhoid state, and die.

All this time, the uterus, if it be a puerperal case, may manifest no sign of its veins being affected; or, if they had been affected, as in Cruveilhier's case, the disease may have yielded at an early stage to treatment. Instead of terminating thus, the patient may be cut off suddenly, at an earlier stage, after some unusual muscular exertion whereby the systemic circulation has been hurried, and the great centres deprived of blood more quickly than the diminished stream from the lungs could renew their supplies; or the progress of the case may even yield hopes of a recovery, the graver symptoms subsiding, but the same sad fate ensuing on any sudden exertion.

Of 32 cases of obstruction of the pulmonary artery, from various causes, that have been published, including this, that came under Dr. Kidd's notice, death occurred suddenly—that is, either in apparent health or in apparently favorable convalescence—in 10 instances. In 6 it occurred during serious illness, but without any symptoms to cause it to be foreseen. In 12 cases its approach seems to have been gradual; and in 4 the mode of its occurrence is not stated. Of the prognosis or treatment of a disease which has hitherto been recognized only by dissection after death, it is almost idle to speak, yet the appearances found in one of the cases already quoted from Mr. Paget afford reason to believe that nature has effected a partial cure. Three of the cases recorded by Dr. Cheevers presented very similar traces of a disease that was in process of cure; and certainly, reasoning from analogy, there is no ground for regarding the case as utterly hopeless. How far Art may be able to assist Nature in her attempts at a cure may be questionable. Certain salts, it is believed, as the nitrate of potash, have the power of hastening the solution of fibrinous deposits, and are perhaps, deserving of a trial. One thing, however, is certain, that in all cases where the existence of an obstruction may be suspected, the most absolute quiet, in the horizontal position, and freedom from emotion or muscular exertion, should be maintained till the pulse regain its fulness and lose its frequency, and the ease of the respiratory movements indicate the perfect performance of the function of the lungs.

ART. 42.—*On Chloroform in affections of the Chest.* By Dr. BREITHAUPT.

(*Méd. Zeitung*, No. 39, 1856; and *Medical Times and Gazette*, May 24, 1856.)

Dr. Breithaupt states that he has found chloroform useful not only in pneumonia, but in the form of bronchitis that nearest approaches to this, the bronchitis cruposa capillaris, in which the small bronchial tubes become filled with fibrous exudations. It is, in fact, just at the most dangerous periods of these diseases it becomes most useful, viz., when the accumulation of exudation takes place in the cells of the lungs or in the finer bronchi, inducing great dyspnœa, and impeding the de-oxygenation of the blood. The author, after frequently employing chloroform in catarrh, and in the first stage of pneumonia or bronchitis, has come to the conclusion, that it exerts no special action, nor is attended with any mischievous effect, although it cannot always be given with impunity in large and frequent doses. It at once diminishes the dyspnœa and irritating cough, but does no more, and should not be trusted, to the neglect of venesection, except in those slight cases in which a mere antiphlogistic regimen suffices for a cure. But while in the early stages it is a mere adjuvant, it is at a later period a means of great value, when from the obstruction of the cells and smaller bronchi a severe degree of dyspnœa is produced and paralysis of the lung threatened. While the means usually employed, as arnica, benzoin, or camphor, are useless or only aggravate the condition, the chloroform proves of great utility. Dr. Breithaupt believes it acts on the one hand by expanding the obstructed part, and aiding by this, as well as by its locally stimulating influence, the expectoration; and, on the other hand, by the calming influence it exerts upon the irritated nervous system of the respiratory organs. In the cases related, the patients seemed as if suffocated, and the sensorium had begun to be disturbed; freer and deeper respiration followed when the sense of pain and anguish had been removed. Such freer expansion of the lung necessarily gave rise to a freer pulmonary circulation and a better oxidation of the blood. The best proof of this influence is seen in its employment for the paroxysms of dyspnœa in phthisis. Here, where blisters, analeptics, opiates, &c., not unfrequently add new inconveniences to those in existence, chloroform, in its tranquillizing and reviving effects can scarcely be surpassed by any other agent.

ART. 43.—*"The ready method in Asphyxia."* By Dr. MARSHALL HALL.
(*Lancet*, Oct. 25, 1856.)

Several important additions and improvements having been made in this mode
of treatment, Dr. Hall thinks it right to lay the last and best form which it has
assumed before us.   Dr. Hall proceeds:

"It will be obvious to us all, that our main objects are—to renew respiration
and improve the circulation.   Our *means* are physiological and physical; our Rules
as follow:

"All obstruction of the glottis being removed by placing the patient in a *prone*
position, in which any fluids and the tongue itself fall forward (Rule I), our *first*
effort is to *excite* respiration physiologically (Rule II); our *second*, if this fail, is to
imitate the acts of respiration mechanically (Rule III); our next object is to
endeavor to improve the circulation, which is done by promoting the flow of the
venous blood, and to restore warmth in the limbs (Rule IV); we again, as we proceed, revert to the physiological principle of *exciting* respiration from time to time
(Rule V).

"RULES.

"1. Treat the patient, *instantly*, *on the spot*, in the *open air*, freely exposing the
face, neck, and chest, to the breeze, except in severe weather.
"2. Send with all speed for medical aid, and for articles of clothing, blankets, &c.

"I. *To clear the throat—*

"3. Place the patient gently on the face, with one *wrist* under the forehead; [all
fluids and the tongue itself then fall forwards, and leave the entrance into the windpipe *free.*]

"II. *To excite respiration—*

"4. Turn the patient slightly on his side, and
   "(i) Apply snuff or other irritant to the nostrils, and
   "(ii) Dash cold water on the face previously rubbed briskly until it is
       warm.

"If there be no success, lose no time, but,

"III. *To imitate respiration—*

"5. Replace the patient on his face.
"6. Turn the body gently, but completely, *on the side and a little beyond*, and
then on the face, alternately; repeating these measures deliberately, efficiently, and
perseveringly, fifteen times in a minute, *only;* [when the patient reposes on the
thorax, this cavity is *compressed* by the weight of the body, and *expiration* takes
place; when he is turned on the side, this pressure is removed and *inspiration*
occurs.]
"7. When the *prone* position is resumed, make equable but efficient *pressure
along* the spine; removing it immediately before rotation on the side; [the first
measure augments the *expiration*, the second commences *inspiration.*]

"IV. *To induce circulation and warmth—*
continuing these measures.
"8. Rub the limbs *upwards*, with *firm pressure* and with *energy*, using hand-
kerchiefs, &c.
"Replace the patient's wet clothing by such other covering as can be instantly
procured, each bystander supplying a coat or a waistcoat.
"Meantime, and from time to time—

"V. *Again, to excite inspiration.*

"10. Let the surface of the body be *slapped* briskly with the hand; or—
"11. Let cold water be *dashed* briskly on the surface, previously rubbed dry
and warm.
"The measures formerly recommended and now rejected by me, are—removal

of the patient, as involving dangerous loss of time; the bellows, or any *forcing* instrument, and the warm bath, as positively injurious; and galvanism and the inhalation of oxygen as useless.

"The inhalation of dilute pure ammonia has in it more of promise."

ART. 44.—*On Jugular Venesection in Asphyxia.* By Dr. STRUTHERS.

(*Edinburgh Medical Journal, May,* 1856.)

A paper on this subject was read before the Medical and Chirurgical Society of Edinburgh, March 19th, 1856, by Dr. Struthers. The object of the paper, which was illustrated by preparations and drawings of the valves in the cervical veins of the human subject, was to ascertain whether distension of the right side of the heart could be relieved by opening the external jugular vein in the human subject. The experiments of Drs. John Reid, Cormack, and Lonsdale, had satisfactorily shown that, in the lower animals (dogs, cats, and rabbits), the right side of the heart could be thus disgorged so as to restore its action, which had been arrested by a simple mechanical cause, over-distension. He considered that the indication of restoring the heart's action by jugular regurgitation, had not received that attention which Dr. Reid's suggestive paper demanded for it. Dr. Struthers described the anatomy of valves which he had found in the cervical veins, as well as those usually alluded to as present in the external jugular. A pair of valves at or within the mouth of the internal jugular vein; a pair in the subclavian vein immediately external to the point of union with the external jugular; a pair at or within the mouth of the external jugular; a second pair in the course of the external jugular, at the upper end of its sinus, or large portion, about an inch and a half above the clavicle, and various lesser valves at the mouths or within the tributaries of the external jugular. The varieties, and relative position of the two portions of each pair of valves was described, as he had found them in numerous careful examinations. With the view of ascertaining whether regurgitation could take place notwithstanding these valves, Dr. Struthers performed a series of experiments on the dead subject. A pipe was fixed in the femoral vein, and tepid water thrown freely upwards. The general result was, that the external and other jugular veins very soon became distended, and that when the lancet opening was made, at about an inch above the clavicle, the fluid regurgitated freely. At first a jet came, emptying the distended sinus, and then it continued to flow, never in a jet, but in an active stream across the neck, escaping by the wound with a wriggling motion, evidently due to the obstruction offered by the valve which it had overcome. Care was taken to ascertain that the fluid came by regurgitation, not from above; but, if allowed, it also came freely from above, having ascended by the internal jugular. The introduction of a probe so as to hold aside the guardian valve of the external jugular did not much accelerate the regurgitative flow. When the catheter was introduced, however, the fluid came very freely by it—as freely as from a distended bladder.

It is easy to introduce a common male catheter to the vena cava or right auricle, by directing it backwards and inwards, as well as downwards, from the point of venesection. But as soon as the catheter has entered the subclavian vein, the fluid comes as freely as when it is pushed farther. As soon as the point of the catheter is withdrawn into the external jugular, the fluid ceases to come by it. In one subject the fluid could not be made to regurgitate. This was at the time attributed to the circumstance that the cranium had been opened for the removal of the brain, the fluid pouring out by the cranial sinuses; but, on dissection, two pairs of valves were found in the external jugular below the lancet opening, besides the pair above it, as usual. Regurgitation seems to be prevented by two pairs of valves, though one pair may be overcome. In these experiments the veins of the arm did not become distended, and no regurgitation took place from a lancet opening in the axillary vein, although afterwards it was seen that only two pair of valves had stood in the way, between the heart and the opening. By "pair," Dr. Struthers meant the two separate portions which act together as one valve. He (Dr. Struthers) drew the following conclusions: 1. No venesection can be of any use in asphyxia, except in the neck, on the principle of regurgitation; which, however, may also relieve congestion of the head. 2. That, besides warmth and friction, and (the most simple and effectual of all means) continued artificial respiration by alternate compression and relaxation of the sides of the chest, jugular venesection should be tried. 3. With reference to Dr. M. Hall's recent recommendation of the prone position, to prevent the tongue falling back and closing the glottis, the question occurred—Does the tongue fall back, under passive circumstances, in the supine position? Is not the closing of the superior glottis, under all circumstances, a muscular act—both the carrying down and back of the tongue and epiglottis, and the lifting upwards and forwards of the larynx? The mouth, however, should be cleared of frothy mucus. 4. That to obviate the evident risk of entrance of air into the veins, the wound should be closed as soon as regurgitation is about to cease, and artificial respiration be then commenced; the jugular venesection having been performed as early as possible.

(C) CONCERNING THE CIRCULATORY SYSTEM.

ART. 45.—*The Physical Signs of Adherent Pericardium.* By Dr. ROBERT LAW, Professor of the Institutes of Medicine in the School of Physic, Ireland.

(*Dublin Quarterly Journal of Medicine*, Aug., 1856.)

This sign is " *the persistence of the same extent of dulness to percussion in the præcordial region, no matter what position the individual may assume.* The area of dulness on percussion in the præcordial region will be the same under every varying position of the body. The heart becomes so braced up that it cannot move as it does in its normal state, when, if examination be made, the patient either lying, or sitting, or standing, the results of percussion will vary accordingly, the dulness being greater in the first position, and less in the two latter. The individual himself, also, is quite conscious of the existence of some solid resisting body within his chest, which does not move in the changes of posture of his body, but impedes its motion.

" I have proved this sign in cases where I have seen the patients all through their attack of pericarditis, and also in cases where the adhesion had been already formed, and have never found is to disappoint me. I, therefore, claim for it that it is *the physical sign* that may be relied on in proof of an adherent pericardium."

This quotation is taken from a paper upon pericarditis.

ART. 46.—*On the origin of " Bruits Vasculaires."* By Dr. TH. WEBER.

(*Archiv für Physiolog. Heilkunde*, t. 14, p. 40, 1855.)

Dr. Th. Weber has published a memoir of considerable length on " Bruits vasculaires," in which he shows experimentally—

1. That the bruits which are perceived in tubes traversed by a fluid, depend upon the vibrations of the walls of these tubes, and not upon the friction of the fluid particles upon those walls.

2. That these bruits are more readily produced in tubes whose walls are thin, than in tubes whose walls are thick, and more readily in large than in small tubes.

3. That these bruits are more readily produced by water than by milk; more readily by milk than by a mixture of water and blood; more readily by diluted than by pure blood.

4. That the production of these bruits is favored by any constriction of the tube, because this constriction necessitates a quickened current at the part.

5. That a certain velocity in the moving current is necessary to the production of these bruits.

6. That these bruits are principally propagated by the parietes of the tubes.

Among other remarks, the author is disposed to refer the placentary murmur to pressure upon the large arteries in the neighborhood of the uterus—the external iliac, the common iliac, the hypogastric, or the abdominal aorta: and, occasionally, to pressure on the large veins. He found in each case examined by him, that the murmur disappeared when the patient inclined slightly forwards.

ART. 47.—*On Capillary Emboli.* By Professor RUDOLPH VIRCHOW.

(*Virchow's Archiv,* bd. ix, 1856, p. 307 ; and *Dublin Quarterly,* Aug., 1856.)

"After I had, in my first Essay on Acute Inflammation of the Arteries (Archiv, i, p. 272), established the theory of the obstruction of the larger class of vessels, by means of the entrance of plugs (emboli), a great void still remained in reference to the smaller arteries, and our apprehension of metastasis, as dependent on such obstructions of the more minute vessels, continued more or less obscure. Some later cases, which I have observed, point out the way in this direction also ; and I will, therefore, now give a short notice on the subject.

"The first case was that of an individual, æt. 55, affected with very decided albuminuria, who had latterly been rather soporous, and, seven days before death, which ensued on the 24th of December of last year, had suddenly become amaurotic. On post-mortem examination, the so-called metastatic, or pyemic ophthalmia, which has been recently and very faithfully described by H. Meckel ('Ann. des Charité-Krankenh.,' ii, 276), was found to exist in a very remarkable degree. The choroid, the retina, the vitreous humor, the zonula, and the lens, were filled with white opacities ; the retina, besides, was studded with numerous ecchymoses, partly resolved and softened. Microscopic examination gave the same result as Meckel had obtained, namely, partly young purulent elements, partly granular and fibrillar infiltrations of the tissues.

"Similar conditions also existed in the kidneys, and were found of older standing in the spleen. But nowhere was a primary purulent or ichorous spot found ; only in the heart were there considerable changes in the auriculo-ventricular and aortic valves, as well as of the endocardium on the septum, with very extensive degeneration of the arteries. The diseased portions of the left ventricle, especially those on the septum, were rough, swollen, superficially softened, and covered with brittle masses, which, under the microscope, were seen to consist of dense, amorphous, highly granular, yellowish-looking lumps. To what then, could the metastases be owing ? After long investigation, I at last succeeded in discovering, in the capillary vessels of the retina, the same amorphous, granular yellowish masses, of similar chemical constitution, too, as I have mentioned as having been found in the heart.

"Still more conclusive was the same condition, as it existed in a woman æt. 27, who died in childbed, of endocarditis, on the 10th of January of the present year, and in whom similar changes had taken place on the mitral valve. In this case my attention was first attracted by the emboli of the fine branches of the coronary artery of the heart, which could be recognized even with the naked eye, and had produced an acute yellow softening of the muscular structure. I then found numerous hemorrhagic spots in the spleen, in which the endocarditic emboli could, with great constancy, be traced into the penicilli (arterial tufts ?) Further, I succeeded in observing, in small ecchymotic foci of the kidneys, both little arteries and isolated loops of glomeruli filled with them. Lastly, Professor H. Müller, accidentally, had the eyes cut out for demonstration, and here again was found that metastatic endophthalmia, caused by little plugs in the vessels of the retina and choroid.

"The theory of pyemia has thus again been deprived of a portion of its dominion. The hemorrhagic inflammations of the spleen, the kidneys, and the eye, are connected with emboli ; and as we have to distinguish the *apoplexia embolica* from the *apoplexia sanguinea cerebri,* so must we, in future, consider a certain number of the cases of pyemic and uremic amaurosis as embolic."

ART. 48.—*On Arterial Plugging in the Horse.* By the late Mr. JOHN BARLOW, Professor of Anatomy, and Physiology in the Veterinary College, Edinburgh.

(*Edinburgh Medical Journal,* June, 1856.)

These remarks occur in the form of a private note written to Dr. W. T. Gardner a short time before the writer's death. They were presented by Dr. Gardner to the Medical and Chirurgical Society of Edinburgh.

"I have recently met with a few instances in which arteries of considerable size have been almost entirely plugged up with fibrinous clots, firmly adherent to their walls. In these cases during life, there was sometimes visible but unexplained atrophy of certain muscles, in regions specifically supplied by such vessels; and sometimes when a main trunk, such as the aorta posterior, became thus plugged, there was palsy of the hind parts (of course I speak of the horse). At first I fancied these things to possess no material interest, and did not preserve the vessels. However, this day week, a pony greatly disabled behind, but not completely paralytic, was brought for dissection. I found a large plug of adherent fibrin in the aorta posterior just where this vessel divides into the two iliacs on each side. (In the horse, you will remember, there is no 'common iliac,' but the aorta posterior divides into the internal and external iliacs.) This plug was firmly adherent to the root of the artery, that is, to that part lying in contact with the vertebræ. It was not sufficiently large to obstruct the stream of blood completely, but it must have caused a material lessening of the stream. The internal iliacs, however, were *completely* plugged up, and the outside of the fibrinous clot was adherent to their walls—in many places all the way round. In one place especially, a calcifying process is taking place in the coagulum."

(D) CONCERNING THE ALIMENTARY SYSTEM.

ART. 49.—*On Simple Ulcer of the Stomach.* By M. CRUVEILHIER.

(*Archiv. Générales de Méd.* April, 1856.)

In this memoir, which was read before the Académie des Sciences in January last, the principal conclusions are these :

1. Simple ulcer of the stomach (true ulcerative gastritis) may always be suspected, and almost always diagnosed with certainty.

2. The diagnosis of this affection is founded upon the differences which separate it from gastralgia and the non-ulcerative form of gastritis on the one hand, and from cancer on the other hand.

3. Simple ulcer of the stomach is distinguished from idiopathic gastralgia by the permanency of the symptoms. and by the alternating exasperation and remission of these symptoms, while gastralgia will often occur suddenly, and leave suddenly and completely. Gastralgia, moreover, is quickly calmed by opium.

4. Simple ulcer of the stomach is distinguished from non-ulcerative gastritis, as well as from gastralgia, by black vomitings and stools.

5. It is certainly probable that these black vomitings and stools may be absent, and in that case it would be extremely difficult to diagnose between simple ulcer of the stomach and non-ulcerative gastritis.

6. Black vomitings are not characteristic of simple cancer of the stomach; on the contrary, they are common to this affection, and to simple ulcer.

7. A similar remark applies to the black stools, which are also common to gastrorrhœa.

8. Black vomitings and stools are in one sense more nearly connected with simple ulcer of the stomach than with cancer of the stomach; for they may happen at all periods of the history of simple ulcer, and frequently they are the first symptom. On the other hand, they are often altogether absent in cancer of the stomach, and when they do occur, it is generally towards the close of the case.

9. The diagnostic differences between simple ulcer and cancer are :

1st (*as to physical signs*), absence of tumor in simple ulcer; 2d (*as to pain*), pain is frequently absent in cancer, but never in simple ulcer of the stomach; 3d (*as to the character of the pain*), in simple ulcer there is a sensation of a raw wound, of burning or gnawing in the situation of the scaphoid cartilage; in cancer, cramps or spasmodic contractions, with hardness of the stomach.

10. The main point of diagnosis between simple ulcer and cancer of the stomach is, however, the different effects of dietetic arrangement, for these fail altogether in cancer, and answer admirably in ulcer.

11. The grand difficulty in treating ulcer of the stomach is to find the food which can be digested without pain, and when this is once found the cure is speedily accomplished.

12. In the great majority of cases a milk diet is the only diet which can be borne. This diet seems to act specifically, but its specific action is in reality dependent on its harmlessness.

13. In short, in the treatment of simple ulcer of the stomach, pharmaceutical measures, properly so called, either internal or external, can only be considered as having a secondary degree of importance.

ART. 50.—*On Obstruction of the Bowels.*
By Dr. RANKING, Physician to the Norfolk and Norwich Hospital.

(*Medical Times and Gazette*, Aug. 2, 1856.)

[The following remarks upon intestinal obstruction were made in a clinical lecture delivered at the Norfolk and Norwich Hospital, on a case of obstruction of the bowels. The obstruction in this case (which was that of a man named Giles, 64 years of age) was in the upper part of the rectum, upon a level with the promontory of the sacrum. At this point the bowel was contracted so as barely to admit a full-sized catheter. The stricture had originated apparently in the gradual contraction of an old ulceration. Ordinary treatment failed; the indications for extraordinary treatment were not sufficiently certain; and the patient sank. Using this case as a text for some general remarks on intestinal obstruction, Dr. Ranking says:]

The various forms of intestinal obstruction may be conveniently arranged under the following heads:

1. Simple enteritis.
2. Impaction by fæces, or other solid formations.
3. Narrowing of the canal from disease within the bowel.
4. Pressure of tumors external to the bowel.
5. Displacement of a portion of the bowel, causing it to twist itself upon another portion.
6. Incarceration of a portion of bowel in a loop, formed by false membrane, or adhesions, or in some abnormal opening.
7. Invagination or intussuceptio.

1. Simple enteritis, or inflammation of the bowels, is usually, but not always, attended by constipation, which purgatives, if given in ignorance of the true nature of the case, fail to overcome. In this case the obstruction is due to the inability of the inflamed bowel to propel its contents; it allows itself to become distended. The transition from inflamed to healthy bowel is in some of these instances very marked, the upper portion being distended, congested, and even gangrenous, while the lower portion is abruptly pale, empty and contracted.

2. The usual cause of obstruction from impaction is by the presence of hardened fæces, but in some instances concretions of other kinds take place, and complete obstruction has been known to be caused by a large gall-stone. Dr. Watson relates such a case in his lectures.

3. Narrowing of the bowel from internal disease is the result either of chronic inflammation, with ulceration and interstitial deposit, or of cancerous degeneration of the coats of the bowel. Giles's is an instance of the former disease. The stricture thus induced may occur in any part of the intestinal tract, but is most commonly found in the rectum, and within reach. This is specially the case with reference to cancer, for of 378 fatal cases from this cause, in 221 the disease was located in the lower bowel.

4. Obstruction from tumors pressing on the bowel from without is comparatively rare, but cases are recorded in which such a result has been induced by large malignant tumors, and by a retroverted uterus.

5. Strangulation from simple twisting of the bowel upon itself is also rare, but several cases are on record. I have myself met with two marked instances, one of which I related some years ago to the Pathological Society; the other has recently occurred. In both the descending colon had turned over upon itself, producing fatal obstruction. Two cases are also related by Mr. Mackenzie in the "Medical Gazette," in which the colon was similarly dislocated. Now and then, also, an analogous displacement takes place in the small intestine, in consequence of a preternaturally deep mesentery.

6. The sixth variety of internal strangulation of the bowel is more common. It has occurred to me to see several cases, and an instance you lately witnessed in this hospital was one. The more common appearances found are a band of false mem-

brane, the result of some former attack of partial peritonitis; an adhesion of the free extremity of the appendix vermiformis, giving rise to a noose through which the bowel slips; or a rent or congenital fissure in the mesentery or diaphragm.

7. The last form to be mentioned is intussusceptio. In this case one portion of the bowel slips into the portion below it, as may be imitated in the finger of a glove. The portion thus inverted is sometimes of considerable length, and when it gives rise to a tumor perceptible through the abdominal parietes it is called a volvulus.

There is a great difference in the relative frequency of these several causes of intestinal obstruction, as may be seen in an analysis made by Mr. Phillips in an admirable paper published in the thirty-first volume of the "Medico-Chirurgical Transactions." He has here collected 168 cases; and of these 69 were instances of invagination or intussusception; 60 of strangulation by the constriction of bands, adhesions, and abnormal openings; while 19 only were caused by disease of the coats of the bowel; by impaction of hardened fæces or concretions; and 16 from the pressure of tumors external to the bowel.

Whatever be the cause which offers impediment to defecation, a certain train of symptoms sooner or later ensues; though it must be added they do not follow any regular gradation or combination peculiar to individual lesions; hence the difficulty I have spoken of in deciding upon the exact seat and nature of intestinal obstruction. The first thing that usually attracts attention is pain; this is or is not accompanied by vomiting, and it is found on inquiry that from a certain date there has been no action of the bowels. Day after day passes without relief being obtained; and the symptoms become more severe, the pain more constant, the vomiting more urgent, and eventually stercoraceous: the abdomen also becomes more and more distended, the pulse quickens, the countenance becomes haggard, and in fatal cases sooner or later symptoms of collapse ensue, and the patient sinks, retaining his mental faculties to the last. This is a description of an average case of ileus; but great variation is manifested in particular cases in the relative urgency of the several symptoms, and in their grouping. I will briefly consider these symptoms *seriatim*, and first of the *pain*.

This symptom is usually present in greater or less intensity, but in some few it is very unimportant, and cases may prove fatal in which there is neither spontaneous pain, nor great tenderness on pressure of the abdomen. In other cases it is the first symptom which excites alarm, and occurs often during some exertion, or after an indigestible meal. In such instances it is not uncommonly found that a portion of bowel has become strangulated, and the sudden pain would seem to indicate the precise moment in which the bowel has become imprisoned. In other cases there is little or no pain for some days, but it soon declares itself in connection with distension of the abdomen, and marks the occurrence and progress of the enteritis, which seldom fails to add to the fatal tendency of the mechanical obstruction. Towards the close of life, when gangrene ensues, the pain, as in idiopathic peritoneal inflammation, often quickly and entirely subsides.

The *constipation* is, in all cases of genuine obstruction of the bowels, complete; or if any fæcal matter passes, it is merely that contained in the bowel below the constricted point. In some cases of intussusceptio, bloody mucus passes, which, in children especially, will materially assist in forming a differential diagnosis.

The *vomiting* is a symptom subject to much variety. I have recently had a case under my care in which the obstruction was of fourteen days' duration, with immense distension, but vomiting did not once occur. This case proved fatal, without the patient once vomiting. The obstruction was in the sigmoid flexure. For the most part, however, vomiting is a very distressing symptom, and adds materially to the difficulties of medical treatment. At first it is simply the ejection of the ordinary contents of the stomach, but at some variable interval it becomes fæcal.

The *abdominal distension* likewise varies, both in degree and period of occurrence. In some cases, where the obstruction is high up, as in the duodenum, there is little or no distension; on the contrary, the abdomen becomes flat, or even retracted. Generally a tympanitic condition soon declares itself, and may proceed to an enormous extent, so that distended coils of intestine become perceptible to the naked eye.

The condition of the *urine* is thought by many, and especially by Dr. Barlow, to give important evidence as to the site of the impediment. Where it is copious, it is supposed to indicate obstruction of the lower end of the tube, and the reverse when it is scanty in quantity. Further inquiries are, however, requisite to establish this as a trustworthy symptom. The state of the circulation in intestinal obstruction fluctuates. The pulse may be unaffected at first, but rarely fails to sympathize with the gravity of the disease, in a rise of frequency and subsequent loss of power.

You will see, then, from what I have said, that there is considerable diversity in the symptoms of intestinal obstruction; it may be added that this diversity is not limited to a diversity of intestinal lesions, but that the same lesion may in a series of cases manifest an equal discordance. Hence the extreme difficulty of determining in many cases, both the nature and the seat of the obstruction; but this fact will be most forcibly impressed on your minds by reading to you the remarks of Mr. Phillips, who, in reference to the possibility of correct diagnosis, has analyzed a large number of cases. He says—

" The impression which must be produced by reading cases, is this,—That, no matter what may be the cause of the obstruction, no remarkable difference is observed in the more prominent symptoms by which it is accompanied. There are in all abdominal pain, tension, constipation, and sickness; but in the mode of their occurrence, it would be difficult to point out any distinct difference.

" The constipation may have the same characters, whether the obstruction be caused by hardened fæces, by contraction depending upon ulceration or other disease, or by bands or tumors—this is certain. The same may be said of sickness; it is usually distressing, and ends in fæcal vomiting, but it may be as obstinate in a case of invagination, as in a case of tight strangulation by bands, &c."

This opinion is very disheartening, but it is nevertheless true; and indeed you have so recently had an instance of its correctness in the case under one of my colleagues, that no more is required to convince you of the uncertainty in the differential diagnosis of these cases. Still it may be asked, Are there not some broad landmarks, so to speak, by which we may arrive at an approximate diagnosis? I should answer in the affirmative, and tell you what they are, and how far they may be made available.

In reference, then, to the nature of the obstruction, I would say that, where there is sudden pain and vomiting, with complete constipation, in a person previously healthy, and where the vomiting is an urgent symptom and the pulse quickly sympathizes with the general disturbance, we are justified in presuming (in the absence of external hernia) that the cause is either intussusceptio or an internal strangulation, the result of the intrusion of a portion of a bowel into some abnormal opening in the mesentery, or into a noose produced by a band of false membrane. In such a case, our presumption would be strengthened, if there was the history of former attacks of partial peritonitis likely to have produced false membranes. This, however, is all we can say. Between intussusceptio and strangulation by bands, I know of no means of deciding, unless the occurrence of bloody stools be considered sufficient. In relative frequency of occurrence in a given number of cases they are nearly equal.

On the other hand, when we have the history of prior disease of the bowels; one or more attacks of constipation overcome with more or less difficulty; when the symptoms, so to say, do not explode with so much violence, but are more gradual in their accession, we should lean to the conviction that the cause is one which has produced gradual narrowing of the bowel, such as cancerous or other disease of its coats, or pressure by a gradually increasing external tumor. Now, reasoning thus, we should perhaps be right in many cases, but you are bound to know that in many also we should be quite wrong, so that in every instance the diagnosis of a case of obstruction cannot be approached with too much diffidence and caution.

As with regard to the cause of obstruction, so with reference also to its seat. Where you have actual tactile evidence of an obstruction, as in a stricture of the rectum within reach, there can be little difficulty in deciding the point; but where no such evidence exists, the question becomes one of the most difficult which can offer itself. We have to ask, Is the obstruction in the large or the small intestines, and in which part? Now, taken in reference to the question of operation, the right decision is everything; we may save or prolong life, or we may uselessly perform a dangerous operation, as you have recently seen, accordingly as we interpret the evidence before us correctly or the reverse. The only help I can give you in this difficulty, and it is very small and liable to numerous exceptions, is founded on the following considerations: If we find a circumscribed tumor in any part of the abdomen, we may perhaps correctly draw the inference that there is the seat of obstruction; but we shall still hesitate between small and large bowel, volvulus and impacted fæces. If a flexible tube passes ten or twelve inches into the bowel, and a considerable quantity of fluid can be injected without returning, it will perhaps be judged that there is at least no obstruction within the descending and transverse colon; but even here a fallacy may exist, and did exist in the case of Giles; the tube may appear to pass, but, in reality, double upon itself in the rectum, or even it might have passed through in his case, as the stricture was not absolutely impervious, and thus be the very means of leading us astray. Again, it might be supposed that some assistance could be derived from observing the course of the coils of intestine when these are visible through the abdominal parietes. For instance, if a marked prominence with tympanitic resonance existed transversely across the abdomen, and appeared to descend into the left loin, any one would be justified in pronouncing that there was a distended colon, and that the constriction must be below this. Yet how fallacious any deduction drawn on such premises, may be, was shown in Dr. Copeman's case. Here, as you may remember, there was precisely this transverse prominence, thought by many to be the colon; and yet it turned out to be not the colon at all which was empty, but several distended coils of small intestines.

Among other supposed data for the localization of the seat of obstruction, I may mention the early occurrence and urgency of the vomiting when the constriction is in the small intestines, the scantiness of urine under the same circumstances, and the sensation of the patient of a passage of air up to a certain point and no further, and of enemata up to the same point in the opposite direction. All these may be occasionally of use, especially the latter, when present; but the exceptions are so numerous, that, at best, but a limited amount of confidence can be placed in them.

With reference to the treatment of intestinal obstructions in general, so much has been said when speaking of the course pursued in the case of Giles, that but little need be added.

Before any measures whatever are adopted, examine the usual seats of external hernia, the inguinal canal, the femoral spaces, and in females the vagina; the rectum should also be examined carefully.

In the majority of cases, when seen early, constipation is the prominent symptom, and the one which the patient is most urgent to have relieved. Purgatives may then form the initiative treatment in almost every case, and may be continued for two or three days, but not longer, as, should they fail after so long a trial you may feel assured that the obstruction is such as they will not overcome, and is probably mechanical. Once that this conviction is justified, purgatives should be abolished, and other measures adopted of a temporising nature. Injections, carefully given, may be continued, and should be given with a tube passed as far as can be accomplished. Calomel and opium, one grain of each, may also be given every two or three hours, or opium alone. If the patient is robust, and there is marked abdominal tenderness, blood may be taken from the arm, or leeches applied to the abdomen. The strength will require sustaining as well as the vomiting will permit, and, after a few days, the exhibition of stimulus and opium comprises nearly or quite all that can be done internally. But if the case progresses unfavorably, in spite of everything, what is the next step? is the patient to be allowed to die, or are we to endeavor to save or prolong his life by operation? This is a question very difficult of decision, on account of the uncertainty of the exact seat of obstruction; and without a tolerable assurance of this point, to open the bowel will be to add one more element of fatality to those already existing. It is clear, then, that before contemplating operative interference, every precaution to insure a correct diagnosis must be taken; should this fail to enlighten us as to the precise point of obstruction, I do not think any operation is to be countenanced; but if we are certified that the constriction is at a point above which the bowel can be safely opened, we have then to decide which of the several proceedings is to be adopted.

ART. 51.—*On the use of Chloroform in Lead-colic.* By M. ARAN.

(*L'Union Médicale*, Jan., 1855.)

In M. Aran's opinion—and this opinion is supported by an experience embracing twenty-five cases, and extending over four years—chloroform is by far the most efficacious remedy in the treatment of lead-colic. In the earlier days of the severer cases, the chloroform is used topically; but it is upon the internal use of the remedy, either by the mouth or in the form of an enema, that M. Aran places his confidence. The plan is to keep the patient continually under the influence of the remedy by repeated small doses, which together, in the course of the day, mount up to from 60 to 300 minims. The quantity used in an enema varies from 30 to 50 minims. The chloroform is suspended in water by means of tragacanth. M. Aran perseveres in this treatment for several days, gradually reducing the dose, and always continuing the enemas for some time after having given up the draughts.

ART. 52.—*The cause of Hepatitis among Europeans in India.*
By Mr. WARING.

(*Indian Annals of Med. Sci.*, April, 1856.)

The comparative exemption of children and women from hepatic diseases in India affords a strong presumption as to the real cause of these affections among the men. This exemption is shown in the following table, a table which we take from a paper already referred to, entitled " Notes on the Diseases of India :"

TABLE

Showing the Admissions and Deaths from Hepatitis amongst the Europeans connected with the Madras army in seven of the largest stations, during a period of ten years, viz., 1829–38 *inclusive.*

Classes.	Strength of each Class.	Admissions with Hepatitis.	Deaths from Hepatitis.	Per cent. of Admissions to Strength.	Per cent. of Deaths to Strength.	Per cent. of Deaths to Admissions.
Privates, ..	75,121	8111	517	10·8	0·68	6·37
Officers, ..	2319	244	8	10·5	0·34	3·28
Women, ..	6559	287	13	4·3	0·19	4·52
Children, ..	9877	36	4	0·3	0·04	11·11

Nor can this frequency of hepatic affections among European male adults be ascribed to the heat of the climate primarily and principally. This is seen in a return compiled from official sources, showing the deaths from hepatic disease in the twelve largest jails in the Madras Presidency—

TABLE.

Jail.	Period of Observation.	Aggregate Strength of Prisoners.	Admissions with Hepatitis.	Deaths from Hepatitis.	Per cent. of Admissions to Strength.	Per cent. of Deaths to Admissions.
Masulipitam, .	10 years.	3863	1	0		
Rajahmundry,	10 "	1372	6	0		
Chiracole, . .	10 "	1673	1	0		
Tellicherry, .	12 "	1191	1	1		
Calicut, . .	11 "	2564	0	0		
Madras, . .	10 "	2730	6	0	0·05	20·6
Bellary, . .	9 "	*6362	2	0		
Cuddapah, . .	10 "	3905	1	0		
Nellore, . .	10 "	5168	2	0		
Guntoor, . .	10 "	5256	1	1		
Chittoor, . .	10 "	4924	5	4		
Chingleput, .	10 "	3067	4	0		
		51,775	29	6	...	...

Mr. Waring proceeds to comment upon these tables in this manner:

* This and the five following numbers include prisoners on trial as well as those convicted.

" We have seen in a former section," he says, " that children are very exempt (though not to so great a degree as the native) from this form of disease, and we should be led to infer that those conditions or circumstances which cause the exemption in the one case may operate in the other. In what respects, then, do the conditions of the native and the European child approximate? In several, it may be replied, in simplicity of diet, in the light and unrestrained style of dress, and, above all, in abstinence from stimulating and particularly from alcoholic drinks. It has repeatedly been suggested that a very high range of temperature and exposure to the direct rays of the sun operate in the production of hepatic disease in India, but the very fact of the native convict being so exempt from its invasion, tends to disprove any such idea, as, perhaps, there is no one class of persons in India who are so constantly, day after day for years together, exposed, while working on the roads, to the full influence of the sun's rays. So, likewise, with respect to sudden and great alterations of temperature, another alleged cause of hepatic disease. The Indian convict, perhaps, more than any other class of persons, is exposed to these, often working for some hours in the full heat of the sun, and, before his return to jail, deluged with rain—and yet we see not above 5 in 10,000 are attacked with hepatic disease.

" The native of India and the European child in India, as before observed, closely resemble each other in three respects: 1st, lightness, and an unrestrained style of clothing (thus allowing unchecked operation to the cutaneous function); 2d, in simplicity of diet; and 3d, in the practice of temperance. It appears to me that in the direct ratio as a person in India departs from either of these conditions, especially the third, temperance, so are the chances of his becoming affected with hepatic disease increased. Next to the native and the child, we see that women are exempt from hepatic disease. They often depart from the above conditions, particularly as far as dress and temperance are concerned, but rarely, if ever, to so great an extent as the officer and private soldier, who, for the most part, lead a life as diametrically opposed to that of the child and native as it is well possible to conceive, and these are subject to hepatitis in an extreme degree. Rigid temperance per se is, however, no absolute preservative against the invasion of disease of the liver in India, and this leads us to consider in the next place—

TABLE

Showing the Admissions and Deaths from Hepatitis among Teetotallers, the Temperate, and the Intemperate, in six European regiments serving in Madras in 1849–50.

Class.	Strength of each Class.	Admissions with Hepatitis.	Deaths from Hepatitis.	Per cent. of Admissions to Strength.	Per cent. of Deaths to Strength.	Per cent. of Deaths to Admissions.
Teetotallers,	450	26	0	5·777	...	...
Temperate,	4318	249	16	5·766	0·370	6·421
Intemperate,	942	96	2	10·191	0·212	2·083

"These figures are too small, and the data too limited, to permit us drawing conclusions of any weight or value. It is, however, worthy of remark, that double the proportionate number were admitted of those who were known to be intemperate over those who were either teetotallers or persons of known temperate habits."

ART. 53.—*On a new species of Tænia in the human body.*
By Dr. RANSOM, Physician to the General Hospital near Nottingham.

(*Medical Times and Gazette*, June 14, 1856.)

In the summer of 1852, while engaged in observations on the entozoa of domestic animals, Dr. Ransom was led to examine the fæces of cats and dogs, to ascertain if they contained any ova of nematoid worms, and whether, therefore, it was worth while to kill the animal in order to obtain the worms. A very natural suggestion sprang from this, viz.:—that he might in the same way diagnose the existence of *Ascaris lumbricoides* in man. Very few suitable cases, however, presented themselves, and, for a long time, he could not apply the idea. While examining the fæces of children, whose symptoms suggested the possibility of their being infested with that entozoon, he met with the following case in which the ova of a cestoid worm, differing from any hitherto described, were contained in the stools.

CASE.—Ann Stead, æt. 9, child of poor parents, resided all her life at Old Radford, in a low, damp situation, near a mill dam; engaged in nursing an infant. Father and mother living; natives of this neighborhood, and have never been out of England. The child has always been delicate, but never laid up with any serious illness; her diet has not differed from that of other members of the same family, or from that of other poor persons of the district; she has, however, been fond of fruit and vegetables, especially of raw cabbage. American flour has been used by the family, and a little raw bacon has been eaten in the house.

In March, 1854, she began to complain of faintness and weakness early in the morning, with an indisposition to rise. She was treated by a druggist with purgative medicines, which were intended to bring away worms, but did not. She became weaker; lost flesh, strength, and color; the appetite was capricious; and she had occasional pain in the left side. She had no vomiting or nausea, convulsions, or itching of the seat or nostril; had not a ravenous appetite, or gnawing pains in the abdomen; never passed joints of tape-worm, or any seat-worms or round worms.

July 11th.—Consulted me, complaining as above. She was a thin, pale, badly nourished child, with some congenital deformity of the thorax. I directed some of the stool to be sent for examination, and found in it a considerable number of clear, thick-shelled oval eggs, of a cestoid worm. One of these measured $\frac{8}{12}''$ by $\frac{7}{12}''$, and another $\frac{8}{16}''$ by $\frac{7}{16}''$, so that the long diameter but little exceeded the short. The shell was marked by a delicate, concentric, irregular striation, as if it were made up of fibres; in the cavity lay a rounded, nearly transparent, finely granular embryo, not quite filling the space; and in the substance of the embryo, collected to one portion of its periphery, were imbedded three pairs of hooklets, arranged as in fig. 1.

Fig. 1.

Seen with ¼ objective, drawn without a camera—Ovum of a species of Tænia from the fæces of A. S.

There could be little doubt that these were ova of a cestoid worm of the genus Tænia; but they were distinguished at once, by their greater transparency, from the ova of *Tænia solium* or *Tænia mediocannellata*, as well as from those of *Bothriocephalus latus*. The stool contained also a few ova of *Trichocephalus dispar*, very numerous spores of the *Uredo caries*, and the usual undigested residue of food.

A dose of calomel and scammony was given, and followed by half a drachm of ethereal oil of male fern. The whole of the copious evacuations which followed was examined without finding any worms. She continued, however, to pass the same ova in the stools.

August 11th.—I examined the stools of her sister Eliza, æt. 6 months, but found no similar ova: also the stools of William, æt 7 years; Mary, æt. 11 years; Sarah, æt. 13 years; and Rebecca, æt. 14 years; her brother and sisters, were examined without finding any such eggs. During the following autumn and winter she continued to pass these ova in the stools, and though turpentine and other anthelmintics were administered, no worms or fragments of worms could ever be found on careful search. Simple vegetable bitters, and careful diet were employed with the effect of improving her general health; but as the ova were still present in the stools, she was admitted into the General Hospital, Nottingham, May 19th, 1855, at which time she declared herself well in health, but the fæces still contained the peculiar ova. The diet was limited to milk and farinaceous matters. She was treated first with kousso, which was at once expelled, by vomiting, and another dose shared the same fate.

May 31st.—Oil of male fern was given, and, to prevent sickness, which had on a former occasion been excited by this remedy, it was administered in gelatine capsules. She took altogether ten capsules in six hours, said to contain each twenty minims, but probably not holding quite so much. She was freely purged, the stools being slimy, and the mucus faintly tinged with blood; but no uneasy sensations were produced. After a very careful search in all the stools passed, no worms or fragments of them could be found. For a short time she was then put on ordinary hospital diet, and left to rest.

June 10th.—She passed unexpectedly a large *Ascaris lumbricoides*, which on examination proved to be a female, but contained in its uterus only unripe ova with imperfect shells.

20th.—Having first ascertained that the ova were still present in the fæces, she was ordered an electuary of dolichos pruriens. The motions were carefully watched till June 30th, but no worm came away.

July 2d.—Having again ascertained that the ova were still present in the stools, 1½ oz. of decoction of pomegranate was given every two hours for three days, but no worm passed in the stools.

7th.—All treatment omitted.

9th.—She passed three individuals of *Ascaris vermicularis*; in the uterus of one of these numerous nearly ripe ova were found, but they could not be confounded with the cestoid ova.

July 14th.—Having again ascertained that the ova were still passed in the stool, an extract was administered, obtained by exhausting half an ounce of kousso with ether, spirit of wine, and water successively, and mixing all the results. (As the proper menstruum of the active principle of kousso is not known, at least to me, this plan was adopted to insure the activity of the extract.) A dose of castor-oil was given after the extract, which caused no sickness, but no worm was passed.

After this she lost patience, and left the hospital; but on examining the stools sent to me afterwards, September 6th, the ova were still present as before.

Remarks.—"On considering the facts here stated, it will, I think, be fair to conclude, that a tænia infested this child, and continued during fifteen months to discharge its ova into the alimentary canal; for although it might be possible to admit that, occasionally, tænia ova might find their way into the intestines with the food, and then pass away in the stools without developing themselves in the parenchymatous organs as cystic entozoa, yet it will hardly receive credence that such accidental admission of ova with the food should continue for fifteen months in one member only of a large family, and under varied circumstances as to diet and locality. This must be a new species of tænia, as proved by the characters of the ova, and rendered probable by the inefficacy of the remedies known to be effectual in the expulsion of other cestoid worms. Without expressing a very strong opinion, I am more inclined to think that it inhabits one of the glandular ducts communicating with the intestinal canal, and thus escapes the action of the vermifuges, than that it really resists their action by reason of its specific peculiarities; for it will be remembered that male fern and kousso are efficacious vermifuges for all the known species of tape-worm.

"This new species of tænia, of which I have ventured to assert the existence, from the examination of the ova alone, is peculiar in another particular, viz., that it casts off the ova separate from the segments, and they appear free in the fæces, while the *T. solium* and *T. mediocannellata* both throw off their segments entire when ripe, and but few free ova appear in the fæces. The same I believe to be true of *Bothriocephalus latus*. In the dog, the *T. serrata* cast off ripe segments, as well as free ova, in the stools."

Dr. Ransom is of opinion that the presence of the ova of worms in the stools will be found to be a valuable means of diagnosis, not only of the presence of worms, but of the kind of worms, and of the kind of treatment necessary. He is also of opinion that the peculiar bodies which have been figured as cholera corpuscles, are these ova changed by the action of the fæces.

ART. 54.—*Fatty Degeneration of the Liver, &c., as the chief cause of mortality among European soldiers in India.* By Mr. MACNAMARA.

(*Indian Annals of Med. Sci.*, Oct., 1855.)

In 23 out of 24 cases examined by him, Mr. Macnamara found the liver, kidneys, and some other organs, in a more or less marked state of fatty degeneration, and this fact he seizes upon as accounting for the high rate of mortality among the European troops in the H.E.I.C. in Bengal. In the earlier stages these organs were infiltrated with fatty matters; in the later stages this infiltration had encroached upon the normal tissues, so as to constitute degeneration.

This state of things is referred by Mr. Macnamara to the mode of living, and not to the climate; and this is rendered evident enough by what is stated of the mode of living. First of all the men have too much to eat. "The Company's allowance is to each man per diem, one pound of bread, one of beef, a quarter of a pound of rice, and half a pound of vegetables, and to this over-liberal allowance the men add themselves one pound of meat (often the common bazar pork, and the meat they buy is always of an inferior quality, as they pay no more than at the rate of two rupees for a sheep), and one pound of vegetables, and often rice also. So that each man consumes, on an average, 76 ounces of food per diem; whereas a man in the Royal Navy, during the same period of time, eats but 35 ounces, and yet he is in a service that compels him to take a large amount of muscular exercise in the open air, while the man in the 1st European Bengal Fusiliers is in a situation which, unless he be on active service, requires him to make but little muscular exertion; and he is, moreover, exposed to the influences of a climate which, from its very nature, would compel him, if he wishes to preserve his health, to live in the most moderate way possible."

Then the habits are most unsuited to persons who have too much to eat. "After sleeping through the night in the very hot close air of the barracks, he rises at gunfire and goes to parade, after which he commonly employs himself in cleaning his accoutrements till breakfast time, 8 o'clock; this meal over, he lies down on his couch, and sleeps till dinner time, and after dinner he generally retires to his bed again, and sleeps, more or less, till 5 o'clock, the temperature of the barracks being frequently as high as 104° at this period of the day. I mention this particularly, because it is after taking food that the lungs are most active; if therefore heat and sleep diminish their activity, we see at once how small an amount of carbon will be exhaled by them at the very time when their functions should be less impeded than at any other time; about 5 o'clock the private has to prepare himself for parade; this over, he saunters about till half-past 9, and then turns in for the night. Of course there are a few exceptions to this, some half-dozen or dozen men taking active exercise every day, and these few are invariably found to be the most healthy men in the regiment."

Again, the fact that a great part of the day is spent in darkened barracks, and that spirits are drunk with considerable freedom, must also favor greatly this disposition to fatty degeneration.

The memoir closes with these comments:

"It is to the eradication of this excessive eating, sleeping, and drinking, combined with want of exercise, the effects of which I have endeavored to show must, in this climate, produce disease of the liver, &c., that I wish to draw the attention of the profession, as they have indirectly the power of removing these abuses, and if they exert this power, I am sure that their exertions will be well repaid by a great improvement in the health of the men intrusted to their charge. Well did Cornaro say of the Italians some three centuries ago, 'Dost thou not see that gluttony is killing every year more people than would perish in a season of most severe pestilence, or by the fire and sword of many battles;' and this is but too truly applicable to the case of European soldiers in India. I have shown that these men are gluttons in the strictest sense of the word, being just the reverse to those who live a sober life, viz., those 'who make a moderate use of meat and drink, such as accords with the temperament, circumstances, and actual disposition of the body and mind.' Nearly half the men in the regiment are Irish or Scotch; most of whom, before they left their native shores, had never tasted fresh meat; they had also, from the force of circumstances, been obliged to live a sober life; and well would it have been for them had that necessity followed them to India. I have seen death seize its victims in many ways, and under various circumstances, but never have my feelings been so moved by it, as when watching one of these fine young fellows, miles from home and friends, carried off by disease. which I am convinced was caused by his own imprudence, or by ours, for having allowed them to act so imprudently. For instance, an Irish boy comes to India full of health and spirits, he has, as I above observed, seldom if ever tasted meat, and having been 'a poor man's son, has never had the chance of getting drink;' this lad comes up to join the regiment at Dinapore, he takes to eating three pounds and upwards of solid food in the day; and I am told by his companion that he does not remember to have seen him sober one night since he joined the regiment; the consequence is that he is seized with dysentery; perhaps he recovers, but from a continuance in the same mode of living he is quickly attacked with the disease again, and this time he is carried off. Such, I am sorry to say, is not an uncommon history.

" In this paper I have endeavored to prove that disease must result from the effects of such a mode of living in this country. The cause of the disease is simple and definite, and there can be no reason why it should not be removed, and diet surely might be restricted, and excessive drinking in a measure put a stop to, and, what would also greatly tend to keep the men in health, their food might be better cooked; —at present their culinary arrangements are sadly deficient. How much good a little care and attention would effect in this department, simple and insignificant as it may seem, no one with any knowledge of the process of digestion can for a moment doubt. We need not, however, apply to the physiologist even to prove this, for so strong does experience bear on this point, that even amidst the din of war, we find Lord Paulit, a brigadier-general, giving M. Soyer a testimonial to the effect that ' he approved of the good things that he (M. Soyer) had made out of the usual provisions for the patients in the hospital, and, he adds, I could not have believed that such a difference could have been produced only by arrangement, and a really simple art of cooking, and a proper organization of proportions.' From this we may learn that not only is management in cooking economical, but that it is feasible in a foreign country in the time of war; surely then there can be no reason to prevent a similar plan being adopted in the military stations of India. In addition then to alterations in their diet, and the sanitary arrangements of the barracks, we may assume that a change in the mode of cooking would be eminently beneficial to the health and comfort of the troops. When these changes have been made, the cause of much of the present disease among the men will have been removed, and then we may confidently expect that the lives of the men will be prolonged to as great a length as those of their officers. Vast indeed would be the improvement effected by the simple, though it might be at first expensive and troublesome process of improving the very sadly deficient sanitary condition of the barracks at Dinapore and elsewhere, as also by the general improvement of the diet roll of the troops. The lives of the men of this and other European regiments in India might be thus prolonged, and as the prolongation of human life is the aim of our profession, let us try to remedy these existing evils. We can, by so doing, aid in the prevention of a disease, which it is totally out of our power to remove when once it has taken hold of its victim."

ART. 55.—*On Suppuration in the Abdominal Parietes.*
By Dr. HABERSHON, Assistant-Physician to Guy's Hospital.

(*Medical Times and Gazette,* May 17, 1856)

Suppuration in the parietes of the abdomen is frequently presented to the physician as simulating deeper-seated mischief, and for a short time considerable obscurity may attend it—sometimes of an acute character, accompanied with considerable pain and febrile excitement, before inflammatory œdema of the skin has come on, and while the effused products are bound down by firm fascial investments closely resembling cæcal disease or local peritonitis; in fact, every region of the abdomen presents us with disease on the surface resembling deeper injury. In the hypochondriac regions suppuration connected with the costal cartilages or ribs simulates abscess of the liver, empyema, hydatids, diseased gall blader, or corresponding disease of the spleen : the right or left iliac regions, affections of cæcum or sigmoid flexure ; in the lumbar regions, renal or spinal disease; in the umbilical, strumous or cancerous disease, and pelvic cellulitis, &c., may be mistaken for ovarian or uterine disease, &c. This simple suppuration in the parietes generally tends to the surface, is opened or discharged spontaneously, and in many cases does well, unless connected with pyæmia or in cachectic subjects. The sooner it is evacuated the less likely is the pus to burrow among the flat muscles and fascia of the abdomen; and even in abscesses, fæcal or otherwise, extending secondarily to the parietes, unnecessary delay is sometimes made in discharging their contents. The correct rule is to open them very early.

CASE 1.—*Suppuration external to the sigmoid flexure of colon: communication with the intestine and the anterior abdominal parietes.*—Elizabeth R—, æt. 39, a widow, who had supported herself by dressmaking, was admitted into Guy's under Dr. Habershon's care, March, 1855. Till a fortnight before admission she had enjoyed good health, when she felt pain in the back, which extended to the shoulders and knees. The greatest pain, however, was in the course of the ilio-hypogastric nerve. These symptoms were accompanied with considerable febrile excitement.

Saline medicines, with colchicum, &c., were prescribed. In a few days the pain, which had simulated rheumatism, ceased, and she appeared to gain strength under the use of decoction of bark with carbonate of soda.

On March 26th, three weeks after admission, she complained of pain in the left iliac fossa, and a firm tumor, about the size of a hen's egg, could be felt deeply in that part. There were no tenderness in the spine, numbness in the legs, or other symptoms of disease of the spine. An examination per vaginam was made by my colleague, Dr. Oldham, but did not give any evidence of disease of the ovary. The bowels were easily acted on by Hydrarg. cum Cretâ, by castor-oil, and by enemata; but this action did not affect the size of the tumor, or alleviate the symptoms. The urine was normal, and there was no indication of renal disease. The pain gradually increased in severity, but was considerably relieved by the repeated application of leeches, by taking iodide of potassium, bichloride of mercury, and occasional doses of morphia. It was believed that the disease consisted in disease of the sigmoid flexure of the colon, with local peritonitis.

May 10th.—The pain had returned with much severity, and hectic came on. The tumor increased in size; it could be felt extending to the quadratus lumborum; and also reached the anterior abdominal parietes, which, at the left iliac fossa, were red, œdematous, and exceedingly tender.

19th.—The bowels were acted upon three times freely, and a considerable quantity of purulent mucus discharged. The examination of this discharge could detect no cancer cells. The pain and hectic continued, the patient becoming pale and exhausted; the left thigh and leg became swollen and tender, afterwards the right; and there was excessive pain in the course of the femoral veins. Nourishment and stimulants were administered as the patient could take them. Quinine and opium, or morphia, were given.

June 8th.—The inflammatory œdema of the anterior abdominal parietes had increased. My colleague, Mr. Callaway, made an incision at this part, and more than a pint of exceedingly offensive pus was evacuated. Every means were used to sustain the patient; but the discharge continued abundant, and bearing feculent odor, and her strength gave way. Her tongue remained clean and moist; but her appetite ceased, so that she became quite unable to take food. There was no pain at the scrobiculus cordis, vomiting, or thirst; but emaciation and sense of exhaustion. Bed-sores formed on the sacrum; and, a few days before her death, cough, which aggravated her distress. She gradually sank, and died June 24th. Inspection was made twenty-four hours after death. The body was blanched, and the lower extremities œdematous; the pleura was healthy, but the posterior lobes of the lungs were in a state of red hepatization; the heart and its valves were healthy. *Abdomen*—The peritoneum was healthy, except in the left iliac region, where the omentum, and several coils of intestine, were adherent. In this region was an abscess, situated behind the peritoneum and fascia, and containing offensive feculent pus; it extended to the anterior abdominal parietes in front, above to the diaphragm and kidney, and posteriorly nearly to the spine. Very careful examination could detect no disease of the ileum or vertebra, or pelvic cellular tissue. The abscess communicated with the sigmoid flexure by three small openings, in close contact the one with the other; the edges not thickened, but valvular. The small and large intestines were otherwise healthy; and the opening into the intestine was evidently secondary. The uterus, ovaries, and kidneys were normal. The stomach was of normal size; the mucous membrane pale, and had undergone degeneration. The liver was more than 5 lb. in weight, and extremely fatty. The lower portion of the vena cava, and of the common iliac and external iliac veins were filled with very firm, white, adherent fibrin, and the coats of the vein were much thickened.

The review of this case showed that the pain in the course of the ilio-hypogastric nerve arose from direct pressure upon that nerve by inflammatory effusion, that the

tumor felt in the iliac fossa consisted of this effusion pushing forward the peritoneum
and sigmoid flexure; that the subsequent symptoms arose from suppuration, and
its extention in various directions inwards into the colon, leading to some extravasation of fæces and of pus into the alimentary canal, and into the abscess forwards,
so as to reach the anterior parietes, where it was opened,—upwards to the diaphragm,
and inwards to the cava and iliac vessels, which became involved and obstructed by
fibrinous material. That it did not arise from diseased bone was proved by careful
examination; and it appeared probable that some accidental blow had led to this
suppuration, with its fatal results, or that irritation in the intestine had led to inflammation external to it, and subsequent suppuration.

After the tumor had been felt, evidence of suppuration soon arose, and the discharge of purulent mucus showed that it had formed some connecting link with the
intestine, or that there was ulceration of the coats of the intestine itself Renal,
ovarian, spinal, or parietal suppuration, or cancerous disease of the sigmoid flexure,
might give rise to many of these symptoms. The absence of all indication of diseased kidney was shown in the condition of the urine. Disease of the spine was
exceedingly doubtful, from the want of tenderness, numbness, and the course of the
suppuration. The position which the tumor assumed, and vaginal examination,
showed that the ovary was not involved. It appeared to arise from disease near to
the sigmoid flexure, either commencing in that viscus and extending outwards, or
beginning in the parietes and making its way into the intestine. It was in deciding as to which of these might be the case, that the principal difficulty consisted.
The discharge of purulent mucus from the intestine, and the feculent character of
the pus, indicated a connection between the abscess and the intestine; the inspection after death showed that the reverse was the case. Before death, I was led to
believe that the disease commenced in the sigmoid flexure, and that the suppuration external to the intestine was secondary. It was closely allied to cases of suppuration external to the rectum, but so deeply was it situated that any exploratory
incision would have been unjustifiable, till there was more certain evidence of suppuration than was presented at the commencement of the disease.

CASE 2.—*Abscess in the loins; feculent-smelling discharge; pleuro-pneumonia,
with feculent-smelling sputum; recovery.*—T. H—, æt. 34, was admitted into the
Clinical Ward, under Dr. Habershon's care, June, 1855. He was a man of steady,
industrious habits. His health was good till an attack of rheumatic fever, two years
before; and at Christmas last, six months before admission, had a very severe fall
while at work; he fell upon his head, and it was believed that the skull was fractured. He remained for some time in the hospital, under the care of Mr. Birkett.
His present illness commenced three weeks before admission, when, in the middle
of the night, he awoke with great difficulty of breathing, respiration being accompanied with considerable distress and pain. These symptoms increased much in
severity, and presented the signs of pleuro-pneumonia on the right side.

On admission he was exceedingly ill; his countenance pale, his eyes glistening,
lips and nostrils contracted, the teeth covered with sordes, the tongue brown at the
base and edges, the skin hot and clammy. In the chest there was found to be increased roundness on the right side at the base, imperfect mobility, increased dulness on percussion, loss of tactile vibration, and in front, below the nipple, was a
pleuritic rub. On the left side, the respiration was puerile, and, at the apices, the
expiratory murmur was prolonged and coarse. The position of the heart was normal; its sounds healthy; but the præcordial dulness was somewhat increased; the
respiration was 26 per minute; the pulse 95, feeble and compressible; the urine
was high-colored, acid, sp. gr. 1025. His position, on lying in bed, was midway
between the right side and the back, with knees drawn up and the head thrown
forward.

The prostration and typhoid state increased till June 14th, when deep-seated fluctuation below the ribs on the right side could be detected, beneath the lumbar fascia
about the quadratus lumborum muscle. An exploring needle was passed, and
afterwards a director, and the wound enlarged: about a pint of pus, having a strong
fæcal odor was discharged, the abscess continuing to discharge freely. After the
opening of the abscess, the respiration became more free, and he coughed up a considerable quantity of frothy mucus, having the same odor as the pus. His strength

was sustained by nourishing food and stimulants—by quinine and opium; diarrhœa was occasionally troublesome, and the offensive expectoration exceedingly distressing.

On July 3d he had so much improved as to be able to be carried out into the open air for half an hour. The offensive character of the breath and respiration gradually subsided; healthy respiration became audible nearly to the base of the lung, and he continued to gain flesh.

In October he returned to his work, and now appears a stout, hale man; but a fistulous opening remains up to the present time, which occasionally discharges freely. In this case deep-seated suppuration took place near the quadratus lumborum muscle, acute pleuro-pneumonia on the right side, and the most severe constitutional symptoms followed. The pus which was evacuated, and the mucus expectorated, were of a most offensive and feculent odor; but microscopical examination of the pus could not detect decided fæcal elements. Diarrhœa came on; the feculent character of the discharges slowly subsided; but the expectorated matters tried the patient much. Several facts render it probable, that the abscess was in close contact with the ascending colon; mere contact with the intestine would probably be sufficient to explain the fæcal odor; and it may be, that the contents of the abscess were partially discharged into the colon.

In the investigation of the case several modes of explanation were suggested— 1. An abscess, the result of the blow. 2. Caries of the vertebra or its processes. 3. Abscess of the liver. 4. Empyema. 5. Suppuration external to the kidney, from disease of that organ.

Although there was evidence of acute disease of the chest, the abscess was evidently below the diaphragm, and probably in contact with it; there was no evidence that the kidney was affected. The character of the pus, and the absence of the elements of bile, indicate freedom from hepatic disease. It is probable that disease of the vertebra or its process had been set up by the blow.

The principal interest arises from the difficulty in forming a correct diagnosis, especially at the earlier stages of this deeply seated inflammatory disease.

(E) CONCERNING THE GENITO-URINARY SYSTEM.

ART. 56.—*The influence of Atmospheric Conditions upon the Urine.* By Dr. THOMAS MOFFATT, of Hawarden.

(*Assoc. Med. Journ.*, Aug. 30, 1856.)

From meteorological observations taken at Hawarden during five years, in connection with the phenomena of disease, it would appear that the maximum of diseases takes place with decreasing readings of the barometer and thermometer, and with directions of the wind from points between S.E. and N.W. by way of south; that the maximum of deaths occurs with similar readings of the barometer, but with directions of the wind from points between N.W. and S. E. by way of north; and that the maximum of ozone corresponds with the atmospheric conditions which give the maximum of diseases, and the minimum with those which give the maximum of deaths.

Seeing these results, it was thought highly important, both in a scientific and practical sense, to ascertain whether any changes in the animal functions could be discovered during atmospheric variations; and, if so, to conduct a series of observations on such functional changes, in connection with meteorological phenomena. Believing that variations in the physical character of the urine are sure and certain indications of functional derangement in the animal economy, I commenced examinations of the density and quantity of that fluid daily, and continued them for a time. On applying these to my meteorological register, the results were so encouraging that I determined upon conducting a regular series of investigations. The observations from which the results are deduced extend over a period of eighteen months.

The person whose urine was examined is a healthy man, of bilious temperament. He was actively employed, both in body and mind, in and out of doors, during the whole period of investigation. His time out of doors, freely exposed to the weather, was on an average six hours daily, namely, from 11 A.M. to 5 P.M.; and the quantity and character of his urine, for these hours, and for twenty-four hours, were daily ascertained. As the density of urine, like that of all other fluids, varies with its temperature, it was necessary to fix a standard temperature, and to apply a correction, plus or minus, as the case might be; and, as 62° Fahr. is the standard heat of water by which the specific gravity of liquids is compared, I took that number for the standard temperature of urine, and reduced all observations in this inquiry to that degree.

From frequent examinations of urine, while passing from higher to lower, and from lower to higher degrees of temperature, I found that the mean increase of density of the liquid, in passing from 95° to 65° Fahr., is 0·001 for every ten degrees; and that, in increasing the temperature from 40° to 60°, the decrease of density is about the same value; so, if the density of urine be increased 0·001 for every ten degrees of Fahrenheit above 62°, and reduced 0·001 for every ten degrees between 40° and 62°, it will be found that the correction is sufficiently accurate for all practical purposes.

In conducting examinations of the urine, it must be borne in mind, that the quantity of *liquid* evacuated is no measure of the quantity of urine secreted. The *solids* excreted are the " real urine;" and it is by ascertaining the amount of these, that the depurating power of the kidneys can be estimated.

In calculating the quantity of solids, I used the formulæ of Drs. Christison and Golding Bird.

The following table shows the percentage of diseases, with variations in the readings of the barometer, with the quantity of ozone, and directions of the wind, for a period of four years; and it also gives the mean daily quantity of solids in the urine, with similar variations, for a period of eighteen months.

	Percentage of disease.	Mean daily quantity of solids in urine. grs.
Barometer :—Increasing readings, ...	26·8	1386
" Decreasing readings, . . .	73·2	1460
Thermometer :—Increasing readings, . . .	37·7	1366
" Decreasing readings, . . .	61·8	1439
Ozone :—Absent, ...	28·1	1395
" Present, ...	71·1	1450
Winds :—North points of compass, . . .	47·1	1284
" South points of compass, . . .	59·3	1368
Calms, ...	49.5	
Calms and variable breezes, ...		1427

By this table it appears, then, that the maximum of solids in the urine corresponds with those atmospheric conditions which give the maximum of diseases. The quantity is greater in dry than in moist air; the numbers being, on days of decreasing degree of humidity, 1506 grains, while there are 1354 grains on days with increase of humidity.

Believing that the animal economy adapts itself to existing atmospheric conditions, and that it is owing to frequent changes of the weather that functional derangement and diseased action are produced, I ascertained the quantity of solid urinary products on all the days on which periods of increasing readings of the barometer commenced and on those on which periods of decreasing reading began. The following are the mean quantities for these two sets of days:

grs.
Mean at commencement of increasing periods, . . . 1413·5
Mean at commencement of decreasing periods, . . . 1547·7

giving a mean daily quantity of 134·7 grains greater on days at the commencement of periods of decreasing readings, than on days on which periods of increasing readings commence.

Taking the mean quantity of solids on days on which diseases occur, and on days of no disease; and on days on which deaths take place, and on days on which there are no deaths; we find that the mean quantity is 29 grs. greater on days of disease than on days of no disease; and 74 grs. less on days of deaths than on days of no deaths. Thus we find that the maximum of solids in the urine corresponds with the atmospheric conditions which give the maximum of ozone and disease; and the minimum with those which afford the minimum of ozone and the maximum of deaths. The quantity of solids is 69 grs. greater than the mean daily quantity on days on which attacks of rheumatism and gout take place.

The mean daily quantity of urine from which the above results are deduced is 72 oz., and a mean daily density 1·019; which, according to Golding Bird's formula, gives the mean daily quantity of solids 1418·4 grs.

The mean daily quantity of urine evacuated from 11 A.M. to 5 P.M. was 11 oz., the mean density of the same 1·020; which gives for six hours a mean quantity of solids 227 grs.

The mean quantity of liquid for one hour in twenty-four hours is 3 oz.; and the mean quantity of solids for one hour in the same period is 59·1 grs. The mean quantity of liquid for one hour from 11 A.M.* to 5 P.M. is 2 oz. (1·8): and the mean quantity of solids for the same period in six hours is 37·8 grs.; giving a mean of 21·3 grs. less per hour daily, while a person is exposed to the open air, than the mean per hour for twenty-four hours.

According to these results, a man evacuates by the action of his kidneys, in round numbers, three and a half ounces of solids daily; or seventy-three pounds avoirdupois annually. Assuming that these numbers represent the mean quantities evacuated by the inhabitants of these islands, and taking the adult population of twenty millions, we find that they excrete 660,165 tons of solids annually; and by referring to the figures in the table, we find that they evacuate during the year 35,714 tons more on days of decreasing readings of the barometer and thermometer, than on days of increasing readings; 7142 tons more when the humidity of the air is decreasing than when it is increasing; 26,785 tons more on days when there is ozone than on days of no ozone; 35,714 tons more with directions of the wind from south than from north points of the compass; and 276,785 tons more during calms and gentle variable breezes than when there is a moderate current of air.

Taking the adult population of London as two millions, and assuming that all the solids secreted by their kidneys are carried into the Thames, that river must hold in solution, or have suspended in its waters, a mean daily supply of 181 tons of solid urinary products. The quantity, however, varies with the weather; for, according to the above results, the Thames will contain ten tons more on days when the reading of the barometer and thermometer are decreasing than when they are increasing; a daily mean of three tons more when the humidity of the air is decreasing than when it is increasing; seven tons more on ozone days than when there is no ozone; about ten tons more with south than with north winds; and a daily mean of seventy tons more during calms and gentle breezes than when there is a current of air. Let agriculturalists bear in mind, that from the action of the kidneys alone of a London population, 66,016 tons of British guano are annually swept into the Thames.

The quantity of solids excreted in twenty-four hours ranges between 650 and 1381 grains, giving a range of 1181 grains. The greatest quantity of liquid evacuated in twenty-four hours were 115 ounces, and the smallest 20, giving a range of 95 ounces. On the day on which the greatest quantity of solids occurred, the reading of the barometer, which was decreasing, was 29·764 in. The wind was southeast; and ozone was perceived on the previous and following days. On the day on which the smallest quantity of solids was observed, the barometer reading (the commencement of a period of increasing readings) was 30·040 in.; the wind veered from southeast to northwest. There was a trace of ozone, which had not been detected for two days, and it was not again perceived for a week. It then re-appeared with the commencement of a period of decreasing readings of the barometer, and an increase of the quantity of solids in the urine from 650 to 1379 grains.

The mean quantity and density of the urine I have given is above that of Drs. Prout and Golding Bird, and M. Becquerel. By the former, from 30 to 40 ounces are given as the mean daily quantity of fluid, at a mean density of 1017; by the latter, the average quantity is stated at 45 ounces. I do not know from what number of observations these results were arrived at; but I do not hesitate to say that if they did not extend over a period of at least one year, very little dependence can

---

* The urine examined between 11 h. and 5 h., was that of two meals, viz., breakfast and dinner.

be placed in them; *for the physical character of the urine is as variable as the wind.* To show how much the quantity of solid urinary products varies at different seasons, I may mention that the mean daily quantity for the three months, April, May, and June, 1855, was 1427 grains; while that for the three months ending September was 1192 grains, giving a difference of 235 grains. I may also state that the extreme quantities occurred once only in twelve months. To arrive at anything like accuracy, the urine of several persons should be examined daily for a period of two years at least.

The period over which this investigation extends is too short to allow of anything like reliable conclusions; but it may be stated that there is a greater quantity of solids excreted by the kidneys during decreasing readings of the barometer and thermometer than when the readings are increasing; that the quantity is greater during ozone than during no ozone periods, and with directions of the wind from south than from north points of the compass; and that it is greater during calms than when there are atmospheric currents.

It also appears that the quantity is greater with dry than with moist air, which may be owing to the cutaneous exosmosis being increased by the moisture in the atmosphere. We observe, then, that warmth and moisture of the air diminish the quantity of solids in the urine; and it is worthy of remark that Mr. Copland Hutchinson attributed the rarity of calculus among sailors to their sleeping in the lower decks, where the *temperature* and *moisture* of the air are increased to that degree, that the place becomes a vapor bath. The smaller quantity of liquids and solids in the period of the day between 11 A.M., and 5 P.M. may be attributed to the free action of the skin while the body was exposed to the open air.

It also appears that the quantity of solids is greater at the commencement of periods of decreasing readings than at the period of increasing readings; and it is with the former class of readings that the maximum of diseases takes place.

It also appears that while the urine of one person gives signs of functional derangement, without any apparent disease, under certain atmospheric changes, another person may be seriously ill under similar conditions of the air.

ART. 57.—*Peroxide of Iron in the treatment of Lithic Acid Deposits.*
By M. CANTILENA.

(*Giornali Veneto d. Sci. Med.;* and *Gaz. Méd. de Paris,* March 8, 1856.)

The case which is here related has a very important therapeutical significancy. It shows very clearly that the presence of these lithic acid deposits may depend upon deficient oxygenation, as well as upon a superabundance of proteine articles in the diet; and that in treating these deposits, it is not enough to restrict the proteine articles. It shows, indeed, that in some instances the real fault may be entirely and exclusively in the want of a proper degree of oxygenation in the system.

CASE.—A lady, æt. 32, suffering under marked symptoms of chlorosis, had been troubled with lithic acid deposits in the urine for two or three years. A vegetable diet and alkaline medicines had been tried, and failed. Peroxide of iron was then tried in moderate doses, and this with a view to its direct oxygenating effects, as well as with a view to the multiplication of the natural oxygen-carriers—the blood corpuscles. Five days after this treatment was commenced, the quantity of lithic acid was sensibly diminished; twelve days later, scarcely a trace of this acid remained; a week later, and the last trace had disappeared. The treatment was then suspended, in order to see whether the acid would again make its appearance. In three days there were traces; in three or four days added to these, these traces were still more marked. Then the treatment was resumed, and the urine again became quickly normal. The treatment was persevered in for two months, and the last report is, that the patient got well, and had been well for seven months.

ART. 58.—*On the treatment of Diabetes.*
By JOSEPH BELL, Physician to the Royal Infirmary at Glasgow.

(*Glasgow Med. Journal,* July, 1856.)

In some remarks on the treatment of the cases of diabetes admitted into the Glasgow Royal Infirmary, from November, 1854, to April, 1856, Dr. Bell concludes that—

" 1. Opium has a most powerful effect in diminishing the quantity of urine, but does not cure the disease.

" 2. Ammonia seems to possess, at least in some cases, the power of reducing the amount of urine, the specific gravity, and quantity of sugar.

" 3. Opium and ammonia combined have a most beneficial effect.

" 4. Cod-liver oil alone is beneficial,—it improves the general condition of the patient, reduces the quantity of urine, and lessens its specific gravity.

" 5. Cod-liver oil, combined with opium, rapidly improves the strength of the patient, and reduces the urine.

" 6. The combined use of cod-liver oil, opium, and ammonia, effects the most prompt and permanent benefit.

" 7. Blisters to the hepatic region are useful.

" 8. The restriction of diet is rather baneful than beneficial. A mixed generous diet is the best.

" 9. In the present state of our knowledge, we can only expect to improve the general condition of the patient, restrain the waste of tissues, maintain the vigor, and reduce the amount of urine. In this way we can mitigate the disease, and protract the life of the patient. We are bound to confess that we have no cure for diabetes. It is not the only disease which defies the efforts of our art. In many other affections, we can only palliate suffering and prolong existence. These objects we can very satisfactorily accomplish in diabetes, by the judicious use of cod-liver oil, opium, and ammonia.

" But it may be asked, how are we to explain the instances of reported cures that from time to time are published, ever and anon exciting our hope that an agent has been placed in our power, by which we can secure an easy victory over the disease? My answer is twofold. 1st. That such cases may have been of a mere temporary nature; a character under which diabetes is sometimes presented. 2dly. That in many of the published cures, an erroneous diagnosis may have been made in consequence of the use of Moore's or Trommer's tests, both of which are deceptive, a brown precipitate being produced by the presence of other organic matters as well as by sugar. I would admit no case as genuine diabetes unless the yeast test had been employed. I do not speak from conjecture on this point; but from experience. Indeed, I fell into this very mistake some years ago, in consequence of this brown deposit. The fallacy was pointed out to me by the late Dr. M'Gregor. I have reason to suspect that many of the cases that have been published regarding the presence of sugar in the urine of old persons, especially when laboring under disease of the lungs, the deoxidation of the copper is effected by some other organic matter, and not by sugar. I have often, in such cases, been able to produce a brown sediment, but I have always failed to effect fermentation."

Art. 59.—*On Diabetes Mellitus.* By Dr. Gray.

(*Glasgow Med. Journal*, Oct., 1856.)

The following remarks upon the pathology and treatment of diabetes occur in a paper recently read before the Medical and Chirurgical Society of Glasgow. Dr. Gray is still confident as to the advantages of this treatment. "Experience" (an experience now extending to twenty-eight cases of decided diabetes), he says, " warrants me in pronouncing it superior to any yet adopted."

Dr. Gray proceeds:

" The rational basis on which I build my theory is that, if rennet out of the body converts a solution of sugar into lactic acid, it may possess a similar property within the body. Bearing in mind, too, that lactic acid is found in the juice of flesh, and, according to Liebig, is a supporter of the respiratory process, I conceived that if sugar formed in the body of a diabetic patient could be converted by the rennet into lactic acid, it would be burned in the lungs; and that, if a larger quantity were formed than could be consumed in that way, it would be excreted by the kidneys. In this I was not mistaken, for lactic acid was more than once detected in the urine of my first two patients. To say that rennet is an infallible remedy in any or every case of diabetes, would be overrating its virtues. Where this complaint is complicated with organic disease in any organ, the organic disease must be removed before we can look for a cure. It will, at least, in such cases, ameliorate the symptoms, mitigate suffering, and tend to lengthen life—the greatest desiderata after an effectual cure. I have been led, from my own personal experience, to classify diabetes under three heads:

" 1. Where the stomach is primarily affected, as has been shown by the experiments of M'Gregor (to whom I am indebted for my first clear views on this disease), and since by Bouchardat, who, as already stated, discovered a substance similar to diastase, and possessing the power of converting starch into sugar.

" 2. Where the liver is primarily affected, as has been prominently brought out by the experiments of Bernard. He has shown that, besides its use in the economy as an eliminator of bile, the liver is a sugar-forming agent, and that this power rests with the tissue of the organ, which seems to act the part of a ferment on the nitrogenous fluid circulating in the body, and from which sugar is eliminated; thus one equivalent of protein, fifty-two of oxygen, and four of water, may be represented by two equivalents of grape sugar, three of urea, and eighteen of carbonic acid.

" In support of such a doctrine, I may state that I have kept patients for weeks on a strictly animal diet, where not a single atom of starch or sugar was taken, and where not a particle of sugar could be detected in the fæces, and yet sugar was excreted with the urine in large quantities.

" 3. Where both stomach and liver are simultaneously affected.

" I am inclined to term the first diabetes gastricus, the second diabetes hepaticus, and the third diabetes gastro-hepaticus; and have adopted such a division the more, that it does not locate the disease in one special organ, believing, as I do, that something of truth may be found on either side.

" In diabetes gastricus, where the hydrocarbons come into play, and where uncomplicated, I believe the rennet treatment will be found eminently successful. The mode I adopt and recommend of preparing the rennet is the following: the stomach of a calf (and the younger it is the better) is gently washed with water, taking care not to injure the mucous membrane; it is then well salted, tied up, allowed to dry. After this, it is cut up into small pieces, macerated in a pint and a half or two pints of water, according to the size of the stomach, for four days, or longer in the winter, shaking it at intervals; the fluid is then poured off and bottled; and to test its power, a spoonful may be added to a pint of warm milk, which if it curdles, it is now fit for use. Some stomachs are better than others, in which case the preparation is much stronger and more efficacious. This depends materially upon the honesty of the party from whom the bag may be procured; for I have been told by a respectable butcher, that the parties who are in the habit of selling bags for this purpose, not unfrequently take a dozen or so of stomachs, macerate them with salt and water, pour off the fluid, and dispose of it to farmers for dairy purposes; the stomachs are then tied up, and passed off as genuine first-hand articles. I may also call attention to a fact, well known to dairymaids, that after a thunderstorm rennet is useless to curdle milk—thus showing that a certain electric condition of the atmosphere exerts an influence upon the fluid. A little spirits, or decoction of sparrowgrass, may be added to make it keep. The dose of rennet thus prepared is a tablespoonful, three, four, or six times a day, usually about half an hour after each meal, and during the process of digestion—followed shortly after by an alkali, to neutralize the lactic acid formed. That which I recommend is the alkaline tribasic phosphate of soda; but the carbonate of potash will answer very well, either alone, or combined with the tincture of nux vomica, in five or ten drop doses. The nervous system in these cases seems at fault, and the nux vomica here serves as a stimulant and valuable tonic. In many of the cases treated, I have further recommended the inhalation of chlorine, from the power it possesses of destroying putrefaction, and arresting the fermenting process. In all, I have now treated twenty-eight cases of diabetes by rennet, of which nineteen were males and nine females. Of the males were five gentlemen following no profession, two youths, one chandler, one laborer, one engineer, one wright, one ploughman, one policeman, and six farmers; females—one mill-girl, three maid servants, and five domestic married females. Of these, seventeen were, more or less, connected with agricultural pursuits. The ages varied from 11 to 65 years; with three exceptions all were in comfortable circumstances; eleven were in the habit of smoking, or using tobacco in the form of snuff; and although a few occasionally indulged to excess in alcoholic liquors, this was not by any means a general feature.

"The complications of most frequent occurrence I found to be phthisis; next, dysentery; and, lastly, anasarca, depending upon remote disease of the kidneys. The diet which I advise at first is strictly animal; and where the poverty of the patient does not permit of the free and generous use of the better quality of butcher's meat or eggs, I recommend the heart, lung, liver, and kidneys to be substituted, as many good and savory dishes can be made from these organs; a soup made from the liver answers admirably in the troublesome constipation which accompanies this disease. Bread free from starch may be made as follows, according to the recommendation of Prout and Christison: six eggs beat up, to which are added four ounces of butter; make into cakes with finely ground bran. An excellent pudding is also made with curds, well washed, dried, and powered—butter and eggs—which is salted and spiced to taste. Salted fish makes a good change, and does not increase the thirst so much as might be supposed. A variety of vegetables may be also given, as greens, kidney and French beans, and nettles even make an excellent dish, lettuce, artichokes, &c. As it is impossible to keep a patient for any length of time on a strictly animal diet without doing injury, I therefore add, after a little while, bran bread as found in the baker's, which I think quite equal to the gluten bread as it is made in this city, and much less expensive.

"If we consider the slow and insidious approach of diabetes, and that it generally has a firm footing before the patient is alarmed into taking advice upon his increasing symptoms, and that for weeks or months the true nature of his complaint may remain undetected even by the physician, we will not be surprised that it should take a considerable time to be entirely removed. The shortest period in which I have found sugar to disappear has been two weeks, the average from that to nine months. The importance of air and exercise cannot be over-estimated, as they are indispensably necessary to improve the general health. Hence, I do not consider an infirmary a proper place for treating a diabetic patient. Attention to the functions of the skin is no less requisite, for which purpose the tepid bath, followed by friction, should be used, as also anointing the body with oil. The patient being usually melancholy, and a prey to gloomy apprehensions, it is of paramount importance to gain his confidence, and if possible infuse hope into his desponding heart This the physician should know how and when to do in each respective case. In a word, nothing should be left untried which might tend either to improve or invigorate the body, or restore serenity and hope to the mind.

"Where diabetes is complicated with phthisis, I prescribe cod oil and morphine, and although I have never known such a case to recover, I have found such much benefited. I have also seen this disease follow as well as precede consumption. The preparation I have used with most success in such cases was a solution of phosphorus in chloroform, with the tincture of benzoin. Of the twenty-eight persons treated, seven have recovered; that is to say, they have regained the weight lost, their urine was diminished in quantity to about the usual standard, and contained no sugar, and they expressed themselves as being 'fit for their work, and in as good health as they ever were.' Three died; two from disease of the chest, and the other from dysentery, complicated with effusion of pus in the left pleura, and seven still remain under treatment. Of the remaining eleven, while I have lost sight of several from the fact that they were at considerable distance from town, I hold letters from others, expressing their thanks for benefit derived from the treatment. In thirteen of those cases, organic disease, and chiefly of the lungs, could be detected. I may finally remark, that only a few of those cases had not been previously under the treatment of other medical men, so that there could be no mistake in the diagnosis."

ART. 60.—*On the action of Digitalis in affections of the Genital Organs.*
By M. BRUGHMANS.

(*Journ. des Conn. Méd.-Chir.; and Révue Med.-Chir. de Paris,* Dec. 1855.)

The action of digitalis upon the generative organs is very little known; but, according to M. Brughmans, it is very marked and powerful. In order to be convinced of this, it is only necessary to take thirty-five or forty-five centigrammes of the powdered leaves daily, for five or six days, when complete flaccidity and loss of all virile desires will be the result. Indeed, so marked is this action said to be, that the person experimented upon will almost disbelieve in the existence of his genital organs.

Acting in this manner, M. Brughmans conjectured that digitalis would be of great use in all inflammatory affections of the genital organs; and experience, he tells us, fully verified his conjectures. Heat, congestion, erethism, irritation, inflammation even, are always obliged to succumb to the influence of this drug. Six cases are given in corroboration.

CASE 1.—A countryman suffering from epididymitis and blennorrhœa. The scrotum was enormously distended. Low diet, rest, and digitalis were prescribed, 40 centigrammes on the first day, 35 on the second day, 30 on the third day. On the third day the swelling had almost entirely disappeared. A smaller dose of digitalis was then given. Two days later every trace of the epididymitis had disappeared, and the discharge was greatly diminished in quantity. On the fifteenth day from the commencement of the treatment the discharge had ceased.

CASE 2.—A patient suffering from chronic articular rheumatism. Digitalis in small doses was prescribed. When the patient was nearly well of the rheumatism, he mentioned a gonorrhœa from which he had suffered for a long time, and for which he had tried many remedies in vain. He was ordered to continue the digitalis, and in four days this discharge ceased.

CASE 3.—A patient suffering from engorgement of the epididymis of six years' duration. This engorgement had resisted the influence of both mercury and iodine; but it yielded to low diet and rest, and digitalis, in about fifteen days.

CASE 4.—A patient suffering from a thick and abundant urethral discharge, with inflammatory stricture, for six months, became cured, both of the discharge and stricture, in sixteen days, under the influence of the digitalis.

CASE 5.—A patient suffering from symptoms somewhat similar to the last, became cured in four weeks under the same treatment.

CASE 6.—A young man subject to nightly pertes séminales, who had tried many modes of treatment without relief, had digitalis given him in doses of 35 centigrammes. The next night passed without a perte. The dose was diminished by 5 centigrammes. The night following there was no perte. The same treatment was continued for fifteen days, and during the whole of this time there was no perte. Then the treatment was discontinued. A week later there was a perte. After this the digitalis was continued for a time in diminished doses for two months, and at the end of this time the patient was entirely well.

It is not easy to know what to say about these cases. We should be glad to think that the digitalis was half as efficacious in such cases as M. Brughmans supposes. At any rate, the question is worthy of consideration.

(F) CONCERNING THE CUTANEOUS SYSTEM.

ART. 61.—*On the Classification of Skin Diseases.* By Dr. GULL, Assistant Physician to Guy's Hospital.

(*Assoc. Med. Journ.*, May 31, 1856.)

"A classification I would be inclined to adopt myself," says Dr. Gull in a clinical lecture, " is founded on the pathological facts of *common* inflammations of the skin, and *specific* inflammations, in the first place. Next, hyperæmia of the skin, as roseola or rubeola, pure congestion, but no inflammation; and hyperæmia passing into hemorrhage, as the familiar disease purpura; and lastly, *epiphytes* and *ectozoa*, one well demonstrated in porrigo lupinosa and porrigo scutalata—ectozoa by the insect in scabies. It is the common inflammations of the skin that puzzle the student, not the ectozoa with the long names, such as *microsporon furfur*, the new name for the sporules of dandriff, *trichophyton tonsurans*, the sporules of porrigo, or another, *microsporon* in the bulb of the hair in porrigo decalvans. Common inflammations puzzle the student, because in such a puzzling variety of constitutions met with; such a variety of applications, also, are used by patients themselves, that the appearances of the disease are changed. The student is seldom at a loss to recognize at once syphilitic lepra, small-pox, purpura, or porrigo; but in common inflammations (and these are the varieties of skin diseases to which I would more particularly direct your attention), he will be constantly at sea.

"Now, in conclusion, there are some diseases apparently of the skin, but not skin diseases at all, such as erythema leve, so common in young women, or the skin disease apparently of varicose veins in older people; or take *lichen circumscriptus*, where you have itching and papules. A young woman, perhaps, sitting up at night with a sick friend, watching, bowels neglected, &c., gets covered with lichen, but the disease is in the general system; let her rest forty-eight hours, and have a little opening or other medicine, and it disappears. I was consulted the other day in such a case; another practitioner sent her away, and said he did not pretend to understand skin diseases; but it was neither a skin disease, nor one difficult to cure. Then there is the 'Barbadoes leg,' thought to be a skin disease, but it is a disease of the areolar tissue, with permanent deposit under the skin. Prurigo pudendi, again, arises from a varicose condition of the veins of the vagina; but, though classified as such, is not a skin disease, and so of a few others, as ephelis, the scorched leg of people who sit much at the fire, freckles, spots of epidermis not bleached, &c. I think the greatest improvements of late years are those few new facts of a microscopic character added to Bateman and Willan, and the fact of recognizing the causes of some disease as *non-inflammatory*. No doubt this is the direction in which further improvement lies: for, as Bacon well says,— *Per causas scire, vere scire.*"

ART. 62.—*On Purpura.* By Mr. Hunt.

(*Medical Times and Gazette,* May 3, 1856.)

In this paper (which was read before the Medical Society of London, April 19th, 1856), Mr. Hunt considers purpura as having no better claim to be considered as a cutaneous disease than jaundice or cholera. He objects to regard it as necessarily a disease of debility, though so described by Willan and others, and he views it as simply a tendency to extravasation of blood, either beneath the epidermis, or in other parts of the body, producing hemorrhage, and as existing in two forms, the congenital and the acquired. For the former, he suggests no remedy. The treatment of the latter should depend upon its cause and the circumstances attending its development. Mr. Hunt cannot agree with Dr. Salter and others, that the existence of purpura necessarily demonstrated any special and necessary pathological condition of the capillaries; but he maintains, that in all cases there must be a disproportion between the momentum of the circulation and the resisting power of the capillaries; and whether the one or the other was in fault, or most in fault, was the question to be inquired into in every case. He has seen the disease arising from debility, and from insufficient nourishment, just as its analogue, sea-scurvy, arises from improper food. In these cases, the indications were nourishing food, astringents, and tonics. But it frequently occurs under widely different circumstances. One prominent form of the hemorrhagic diathesis he has frequently seen connected with hepatic congestion and obstruction of the vena porta system, with well-marked symptoms, and occasionally complicated with jaundice. In these cases, if the patient were treated with astringents, tonics, and a nourishing diet, he would certainly die; the only available treatment being active purgation, with repeated doses of calomel and jalap, with a view to unload the intestines of the black, tenacious, pitch-like fæcal matter with which they are always loaded. The author also describes another form, in which, without any apparent cause, in robust and healthy subjects, purple spots, ecchymosis, and vibices appeared, together with hemorrhage from the mouth, nose, eyes, or ears, and from the internal organs likewise, from which the patient often sank. The remedy, and the only remedy, in these cases, is frequent vomiting, artificially induced. The petechiæ which appeared in severe cases of typhus and the eruptive fevers, presented again another form of purpura, which required the mineral acids, quinine, and nourishment. The author concludes by expressing his conviction that purpura, or the hemorrhagic diathesis, presents, *per se*, no proof of the existence of any particular or invariable lesion; that it does not necessarily indicate debility, nor a friability of cell-wall, nor a diseased condition of the blood, nor a gorged liver, nor the approach of collapse in fever, nor an increased momentum of blood in a robust or healthy subject; but that yet it may occur as a result of any one of these conditions, and perhaps many more ; in short, that it was in fact no disease at all, nor even a symptom necessarily of any one diseased condition, but that it was simply an accidental complication, and that the thing to be avoided in its treatment was the error of assigning to it a pathological character, and thus treating it as itself the disease, instead of inquiring most carefully into the circumstances of the individual case, and thus ascertaining correctly what is the thing signified by this most alarming, yet most equivocal sign.

ART. 63.—*Rapid Cure of Itch.* By Dr. E. SMITH.

(*Assoc. Med. Journal*, March 15, 1856.)

At a meeting of the Medical Society of London, Dr. E. Smith called attention to an article in the "Gazette Hebdomadaire," by Dr. Bourguignon, in which is a confirmation of the value of the treatment of itch, in Belgium, by sulphur, combined with lime, in a liquid form. The remedy is prepared by boiling one part of quick lime with two parts of sublimed sulphur, in ten parts of water, until the two parts are perfectly united. During the boiling it must be constantly stirred with a piece of wood, and, when the sulphur and lime have combined, the fluid is to be decanted and kept in a well-stopped bottle. A pint of the liquid is sufficient for the cure of several cases. It is sufficient to wash the body well with warm water, and then to rub the liquid into the skin for half an hour. As the fluid evaporates, a layer of sulphur is left upon the skin. During the half hour the acarus is killed, and the patient is cured. It is only needful then to wash the body well, and to use clean clothes. In Belgium the treatment is introduced by first rubbing the body for half an hour with black soap; but this does not appear to be necessary. The only essential act is that of the careful application of the fluid sulphur. The lime is of no importance in the treatment, except to render the sulphur soluble, and such would probably be the case if potass or soda were employed. The chief point in the plan thus employed, which is an improvement upon the mode of application of sulphur in substance with lard, is the more ready absorption of the remedy, and consequently the more certain and quick destruction of the insect, by using sulphur in a fluid form. In so disgusting a disease, it must be of great moment to be able to cure it in half an hour.

ART. 64.—*On the Keloid of Alibert.* By Dr. LUDWG BENJAMIN.

(*Virchow's Archiv.* Bd. viii, Ht. 4, 1855; and *Dublin Quart. Journ. of Med.*, May, 1856.)

As among the few descriptions which exist of Alibert's keloid, not one, so far as I am aware, enters upon its microscopic characters,—probably because its comparatively rare occurrence affords but little opportunity for investigation,—it has occurred to me that the following report might prove interesting :

A practitioner in this city attempted, by means of the application of caustic, to remove a small congenital mark situated on the buttock of a girl; but as during six weeks' treatment the affection appeared rather to increase in circumference, the parents lost confidence in the very painful remedy, and gave it up.

At the age of two years they brought the child, who was then very strong, to me, their apprehensions being excited by a tumor which had arisen out of the spot, and was steadily increasing and extremely itchy. On examination, I found in the situation indicated a keloid, almost as large as the palm of the hand, projecting three or four millimetres (·11811 or ·15748 inch) above the cuticle, with a very irregular border, and numerous processes of various lengths and forms, which extended, some triangularly pointed, for two or three centimetres (·7874 or 1·1811 inch), others rounded at the end, for one and a half or two centimetres into the surrounding healthy cutis. Clearly defined from these by its elevation, the tumor was also distinguished by a pale red coloration and some deep furrows, while the fine depressions and hairs of the healthy skin were absent; it resembled a very prominent cicatrix, but in hardness considerably exceeded the latter. Little hemorrhage attended the extirpation, which was effected in the healthy skin.

The tumor, examined while fresh, was found to be everywhere as distinct from the surrounding healthy adipose mass as it was inseparably connected with the cutis. In two opposite places near the edge, a number of small vessels, not extending far, penetrating a capsule, which adhered to the tumor with tolerable firmness, and was thick and hard, consisting of areolar tissue, with scarcely any admixture of elastic fibres. The tumor contained no other vessels. On the surface of section it was of a silvery white appearance, and of cartilaginous hardness, and consisted of areolar tissue and corpuscles of the same; the former does not constitute curly bundles, but thick trunks, the firmly compressed fibres of which run at first in an almost straight direction, gradually separate from one another, and finally fall into several distinct bundles, which, vibrating in curls after repeated subdivision, are at last in nothing distinguishable from normal areolar tissue. The trunks of areolar tissue (sit venia verbo) are so closely compressed that no free space is left between them, whence the great hardness of the tumor; they do not run a parallel course, but interlace in various directions, giving the field of vision the aspect of containing a number of trees jumbled together. The meshes which are formed by the bundles separating and leaving little chasms between the fibres are almost completely filled with numerous corpuscles of areolar tissue; this part of the tumor forms, nevertheless, a firm tissue, which is, however, of much looser texture than the basis is, and replaces the normal cutis otherwise occupying its place.

The structure and development of the tumor thus appear to be very simple: a few vessels passing at the basis through a capsule of areolar tissue supply the plasma, from which a fibrous layer, little differing in structure from normal areolar tissue is formed; between the fibres lie corpuscles of areolar tissue, as they are found in almost all tumors consisting of this tissue which are still in process of growth. The keloid is, consequently, only a modification of the subcutaneous areolar tissue, and is to be classed with warts, condylomata, &c.; it is probably more frequently connected with varices; as in this case in two places it proceeds from the cutis, or draws the latter into its circle of formation; is free from pain, but excites violent itching; does not always grow so quickly as in the present instance, in which within two years it attained so considerable an extent as to occupy a space equal to that of the palm of the hand, and has probably no defined limit to its extension, unless this be artificially effected. The general health does not suffer by it, at least it did not in my case; the wound, too, healed without any interruption, so that the theory that keloid is a product of a dyscrasia certainly does not hold good in every instance.

Finally, I may mention, that the tumor, in its interior, in one place contained striated muscular bundles, precisely as earlier observers (Rokitansky, Virchow, Weber, and Billroth) have seen. I suspect that these occur much more frequently in tumors than has hitherto been found to be the case, and that they shall be discovered more commonly in proportion as the use of the microscope gains ground among surgeons, and as the number of more minute investigations shall consequently increase.

ART. 65.—On a vesicular disease contracted from Sheep.
By Dr. BURROWS, Physician to St. Bartholomew's Hospital.
(Medical Times and Gazette, June, 14, 1856.)

In its general characters this disease is very similar to acute pemphigus, but it differs apparently in the circumstance that we have vesicles mixed with bullæ. It further seems to differ from pemphigus in the fact that the mucous membrane of the eye, the nostrils, the mouth, the tongue, and the pharynx, are all implicated at the same time.

Dr. Burrows' remarks occur in a clinical lecture:

"I am about to describe a peculiar disease, which I believe to be derived from the sheep,—a disease, as far as I know, not hitherto described or adverted to by systematic writers. I have myself only seen two examples of this disease; they both occurred in young butchers, who had wounded themselves while cutting up sheep's heads, or dressing them for sale. The disease consists essentially of an abundant eruption of successive crops of vesicles and bullæ, of various sizes. These vesicles and bullæ are in some parts isolated from each other, and in other parts more numerous, and congregated together,—what we call confluent. These vesicles and bullæ appeared principally upon the finer and more delicate portions of the skin and body, about the cheeks, the lips, beneath the chin, on the throat, the breast, upon the upper and lower extremities. These vesicles, or bullæ, however, are not confined simply to the cutaneous surface; they are found also upon the conjunctiva, upon the mucous membrane covering the tongue, the membrane lining the lips, upon the soft palate, and perhaps, also, similar vesicles might be found on the lining membrane of the nostrils and of the pharynx. During the continuance of the disease, a discharge of mucus exudes from these parts, the nostrils and pharynx. The external appearance of this eruption generally resembles that of acute pemphigus, but not altogether; for we observe, that in some parts this vesicular eruption resembled the aggravated form of herpes, the vesicles being small and congregated together, with inflamed margins. In other parts the vesicles are larger, and isolated, the eruption more closely resembling pemphigus; in other parts the surface appears blistered, as by the action of boiling water. The whole of the cuticle of a certain portion, one of the extremities (for example), is raised in continuous blisters, running into one another, as if the surface had been irritated by the action of boiling water.

" This is the general character of the eruption of the peculiar disease in question. Now, I will proceed to detail the symptoms of the particular case to which I have adverted.

" On the 8th of April there was admitted into Matthew Ward a young man, named Charles Handsdale. The following is the account which he gave of himself:

" He is a single man, in good circumstances, of healthy parents, living at Barnet. He states that five weeks ago, while cutting a fresh sheep's head, the knife slipped and cut his left thumb. He remembers the sheep's lung was full of ' white knobs;' but he remained perfectly well (with the exception of the thumb being incised, and subsequently discharging), till Saturday, April the 5th, without any symptoms of fever. He then noticed a spot upon his lip, which he states was like a scald; then a discharge from the eyes came on, but no headache and no shivering; and these spots gradually increased about his face and hands, till the disease had the appearance that it presented on admission. On April 8th, when admitted, his condition was as follows:

" On his face, more especially about the chin, was a crop of small bullæ, about the size of split peas. There were also similar spots on the mucous lining of the lip, as well as on the edge of the tongue, and on the soft palate and uvula. There was also a purulent discharge from the left eyelids. On the back of the hands there were some red elevated spots commencing to be papular. There were also about his abdomen and back and the upper part of his thighs, many red elevated spots.

" When I saw him on the following morning, his expression was anxious; face flushed; eyes suffused; accompanied with a purulent discharge from the inner canthus of the left eye and the outer canthus of the right. There was also a purulent discharge from the right nostril. Lips dry. About his face, below the chin, there was an abundant crop of bullæ, which to-day seem to be of a more pustular character. They are also increased in size, some being larger than a fourpenny-piece. Around each of the bullæ the cutis seemed inflamed. A few were now observed on the hairy scalp. The eruption was seen about the hands, around the wrists, extending up the inner aspect of the forearms. A similar eruption was also detected in each iliac region, the inner aspect of the thighs, upon the scrotum, upon the penis, and upon the back of the trunk; also upon each foot, about the ankle, and along the tarsus. Some of these bullæ were very minute, and others larger, about the size of split peas. As I have already said, the eruption was confined to the finer parts of the skin; in those parts where the cuticle was thickened,— on the outer aspect of the arm and thigh, the palms of the hands and soles of the feet,—this vesicular eruption was absent. The wound in the thumb was open, and discharging. The constitutional disturbance was much less than might have been expected to accompany such an extensive eruption. He was evidently a youth of great courage, and made light of his pains. His breathing was easy. There was slight cough, and sore throat. Skin hot and dry. Tongue coated on the dorsum with a thickish white fur, the edges presenting an appearance of having small pimples upon them. Has a tolerable appetite; is not sick; no headache, and no thirst; bowels not open; urine free.

" Now, I shall not pursue this case day by day, through its progress, but I will read you the note of the day after his admission, and then I will tell you generally the progress of the case for the ensuing fortnight. We found, on the following morning, that he had slept but little, in consequence of the discharge from his eyes, which had been constant all night. His expression was anxious. He was lying on his back, with his mouth open. Lips and teeth dry. On the internal lining of the lower lip we observed a number of these minute vesicles, and some were to be seen on the soft palate, which had the appearance of being covered with patches of slough. About his face there were numerous bullæ, especially below the chin, and these had now begun to desiccate. About the upper extremities—on the inner aspect where the skin was soft—there was an appearance of these bullæ and vesicles; they were so numerous, and congregated so closely together, as to have become completely confluent. You could have fancied that the skin had been scalded with boiling water. About the thorax, also, the spots were more numerous, some of them containing fluid, which on the previous day they did not contain. They were more numerous about the trunk, about the axillæ and back, and in the iliac regions, the groins, the inner aspect of the thigh, and over the scrotum. Some of them were ruptured, and a copious discharge was taking place from the surfaces. The eruption was more abundant, also, over the lower extremities, ankle-joints, and over the footsteps. The constitutional disturbance was greater than on the previous day. He had a very restless night, having been kept awake by the discharge from the eyes, and a soreness over the surface of the body. The pulse was accelerated—108—small and sharp, but compressible. The dorsum of the tongue was still covered with fur. His appetite began to fail. He stated that he was very thirsty, but had no headache. The bowels were opened once in the morning, the motion being confined. Urine free. He complained of some sore throat. There was slight cough, and scanty mucous expectoration.

"Such was the condition on the second day. The disease was obviously a very peculiar one, such as is not usually presented to our notice in this hospital, or, I believe, elsewhere. The moment I saw this young man, I recognized a disease which had been under my notice about two years ago. In the month of March, 1854, a young man, named George Richardson, about the same age as this patient, was admitted into John Ward, and he presented over the surface of his body an eruption of a precisely similar character to the one I have just described. I learned, on inquiring into his history, that he was employed as a shopman at a butcher's, and had been engaged in skinning, cutting-up, and dressing sheep's heads for sale, and that he had wounded himself. An erruption succeeded, and he came into the hospital at a more advanced stage of the disease, remaining there about a fortnight. He gradually sank, and died, worn out by the continual irritation, and the copious discharge from the surface. The body was not examined. From the moment I saw the present case I recognized it as a fellow-case to that which fell under my observation two years ago."

ART. 66.—A new solution of Iodine in Skin Diseases.
By Dr. Max Richter.

(Wochenbl. der Zeitschr. der k. k. Gesellsch. der Aertze zu Wien, No. 51, 1855; and Medico-Chir. Review, July, 1856.)

The solution is made thus: half an ounce of iodine is to be dissolved in an ounce of glycerine, and subsequently half an ounce of iodine is to be added, which completely dissolves in a few hours. In the experiments made with this solution, it was applied to the surface by means of a hair pencil; the part was then covered with gutta percha paper, fixed at the edges with strips of plaster, so as to prevent the volatilization of the iodine. This was removed after twenty-four hours; and for a similar time, cold pledgets were applied. Burning pain, more or less intense, but rarely of more than two hours' duration, was produced. The repetition of the painting depends on the appearance of the part and the amount of disease. The conclusions of the author are—1. That the iodine thus applied acts as a caustic. 2. That while it possesses considerable curative powers in respect of scrofulous and syphilitic affections, it is especially useful in lupus. 3. That the solution dissipates even deeply seated tubercles of lupus, and may be applied for this purpose to the most tender surface without fear of eroding it. 4. That when the solution was applied only to a part of a diseased surface, the remainder was, nevertheless, influenced. 5. That it is particularly serviceable to large and superficial sores. 6. That after a series of paintings, and when the sore was almost healed, the local pains greatly increased in intensity.

PART II.—SURGERY.

SECT. I.—GENERAL QUESTIONS IN SURGERY.

(A) CONCERNING TUMORS.

ART. 67.—*On the spreading of Cancer cells into the neighborhood of the Tumor.*
By M. SCHRŒDER VAN DER KOLK.

(Archiv. Gén. de Méd., Jan. 1856.)

IT is not only in epithelial and scirrhous tumors that we find nucleoli, nuclei, and the characteristic cells of cancer; on the contrary, the neighboring parts, although healthy in appearance, present manifest alterations under the microscope,—alterations consisting in small cells, nuclei, granular matter, and fatty molecules, and which are more abundant in the immediate neighborhood of the tumor.

The cause of this contamination of the neighboring parts is ascribed principally to the infiltration of the intercellular fluid of the heterologous mass.

In M. Schrœder van der Kolk's opinion, the pain of cancer is always due to the invasion of the surrounding nerves by the cancerous elements.

The practical consequence is that in extirpating a tumor of the character in question, it is necessary to carry the incision far beyond the extent of apparent mischief.

ART. 68.—*On M. Landolfi's method of treating Cancer.*
By M. BROCA and others.

(Gaz. Hebdom. de Méd. et Chir., May 9, 1856.)

The commission appointed by the Académie des Sciences, consisting of MM. Broca, Cazolis, Furnari, Manec, Mounier, and Moissenet, have just reported most unfavorably upon M. Landolfi's method of treating cancer (*vide* "Abstract," XXII). According to the report, there is nothing new in this method, and the caustic employed is only the caustic of M. Canquoin disguised by the addition of a coloring and strongly smelling substance, and rendered more unmanageable and less certain in its action by the addition. The report also condemns M. Landolfi's plan of attacking only small portions of the tumor at a time. Nor is there anything of a practical character to recommend this plan,—for of 9 cases of cancer of the breast, and 3 cases of cancroid disease, which were treated by M. Landolfi at the Salpetrière, under the eyes of the commissioners, the results were as follows :—among the 9 cases of cancer of the breast, there were 2 deaths, 4 decided aggravations of the symptoms, and 3 cicatrizations with immediate *repullulation,* consequently no cure; and among the 3 cases of cancroid disease, there was 1 in which cicatrization was followed by immediate *repullulation,* 1 in which the symptoms were so aggravated as to require amputation of a limb, and only 1 cure. In a word, the report stigmatizes the plan under consideration as more painful and more uncertain than other modes of cauterization.

ART. 69.—*An unusual and obstinate form of Swelling.*
By Mr. J. L. MILTON.

(Medical Times and Gazette, June 28, 1856.)

The author (who described his own case at the meeting of the Royal Medical and

Chirurgical Society, held June 10th, 1856) had long suffered from eczema of the scalp, to which, in June, 1855, were added most severe colicky pains, and neuralgia of the face. For this complication of maladies, the inhalation of chloroform was frequently used, combined with quinine, steel, croton oil, and galbanum internally, and the application of counter-irritants, and a strong astringent lotion containing a large amount of hydrocyanic acid and zinc, externally. Under this treatment the neuralgia disappeared, while the eczema was slightly remedied. One morning in September, 1855, a large pyriform swelling, firm and painless, of the color of the skin, was observed, extending from the inner to the outer side of the left thigh, just below Poupart's ligament. It had disappeared before night. On the following morning a swelling, five or six inches in length by two in breadth, of the same character in every respect, save that it was red, appeared just below the crest of the left ilium; this travelled slowly down the left side of the sacrum, and then across to the right side of the pelvis, where it gradually faded away in a few days; that portion of the tumor which had been first formed having, however, disappeared much earlier. For three weeks, similar tumors formed daily about the pelvis and thighs; sometimes two or three formed simultaneously; after that time they were scattered, and less frequent. About the end of October the face was first attacked; a hard swelling, which ran its course in about eight hours, passed slowly over both eyes, from right to left, completely excluding light while the attack was at its height. On the 11th of December a most severe attack occurred in the face, the mouth and parts about it being the first seat of the swelling. Three times the throat was affected, the swelling reaching its maximum in that situation in half an hour, and giving rise to great alarm from the interference with respiration. One or two appeared at different times on the legs and arms. The number and severity of the attacks steadily declined from the last-named date, and finally disappeared in the March following. The swellings were never painful, nor did they yield, though firmly pressed. Stiffness and distension were the only sensations remarked in connection with them, the integument over them being generally raised half an inch, and unaltered in color. No desquamation or itching followed their subsidence, nor did any constitutional disturbance accompany either their outbreak or decline; the eczematous eruption was neither aggravated nor improved by their appearance; they never formed in the afternoon or evening, all which were noticed having commenced between four and ten o'clock A.M.; and, with one exception, all reached their utmost height in four hours. Those on the face were generally a week in subsiding; the others disappeared almost as rapidly as they arose. Colchicum and bichloride of mercury appeared to hasten the disappearance of an affection, of which the author, after diligent search, could discover no previous description.

(B) CONCERNING WOUNDS AND ULCERS.

ART. 70.—*A new method of treating Phagedæna.* By Mr. COCK.

(*Medical Times and Gazette*, April 12, 1856.)

Mr. Cock has recently been trying, in Guy's Hospital, a plan of treating phagedænic ulcers by constant irrigation. The method is, to have the sore well exposed, and the affected limb placed on some waterproof material; a reservoir above the bed is then filled with lukewarm water, and, by means of an elastic tube, a stream is kept continually flowing over the surface of the sore. By this means all particles of discharge, &c., are washed away as soon as formed, and the ulcer assumes the clean, pale appearance of a piece of meat which has been long soaked. In all the cases in which it has been practicable to employ the irrigation efficiently, a speedy arrest of morbid action has been secured, and the number has included several in which the disease was extensive and severe. The theory of the treatment is, that phagedænic action is a process of local contagion, the *materies morbi* by which the ulcer spreads being its own pus. Admitting this supposition—which there is every reason for doing—to be true, the object to be kept in view in curative measures is either to decompose or to remove the local virus. This end is accomplished somewhat clumsily by such remedies as the nitric acid, which, unless so freely used as not only to char up all the fluid matters, but to destroy the whole surface of the ulcer to some depth, fails to prevent a recurrence. Mr. Cock's plan of subjecting the ulcer to a perpetual washing attempts the accomplishment of the same end by a more simple and direct method. It involves no pain to the patient, and does not destroy any healthy tissues. Its one disadvantage seems to be, that, excepting on the extremities, its use would be attended with some inconvenience, from the diffi- culty of preventing the water from running into the patient's bed. Should, how- ever, further trials confirm the very favorable opinion which has been formed at Guy's as to its value, these difficulties might no doubt be surmounted by the con- trivance of suitable apparatus. The directions as to temperature of the water are that it should be as warm as comfortable to the feelings of the patient; and, as preventive of smell, Mr. Cook advises the addition of a small quantity of the chlo- ride of lime or of soda.

ART. 71.—On Hemorrhage following Gunshot Wounds.
By Dr. G. H. B. MACLEOD.

(Edinburgh Medical Journal, May, 1856.)

" Hemorrhage following gunshot wounds is not now so dreaded as it used to be, because it is known to be by no means so frequent in occurrence as it was formerly believed to be. I have heard surgeons declare that tourniquets might have been left at home, so far as any use they were of at the battles of the Alma and Inker- mann, but I suspect, though cases did not often require them when seen by the medical man, that hemorrhage is in reality the chief immediate cause of death in the case of the majority of men killed in the field. It would be a dangerous experi- ment to make, but withal a very interesting one, to go over a field of battle imme- diately after a fight, and record the apparent causes of death in each case.

" The returns fail to inform us of the numbers of cases in which secondary hemor- rhage succeeded gunshot wounds in the course of this war, and though I have no figures to which I might refer in corroboration of the statement, I am inclined to think that the proportion is higher than that set down by Mr. Guthrie. The period of its occurrence has appeared to range, on an average, between the fifth and the twenty-fifth day, without drawing any minute distinction, as is done by Dr. John Thomson, between hemorrhage due to sloughing, ulceration, or simply excited arterial action at different stages of the process of cure. The fifteenth day has, curiously enough, been that on which it has taken place in the vast majority of the cases of which I have retained notes. One instance, the particulars of which I failed to learn, was said to have occurred as late as the seventh week, when the wound—a gunshot wound of the thigh—was nearly cicatrized. Hemorrhage occur- ring early has been almost universally treated on the principle laid down by Bell, and so well supported and elucidated by Guthrie, of tying both ends of the wounded vessel; but when the limb is much swollen, the parts infiltrated matted together and disorganized, it is all very well to say the same principles must be carried out not- withstanding the additional risk that the coats of the vessels may be diseased, but any one who has tried it a few times will know that to do so is no easy task. With a vessel like the posterior tibial, which has repeatedly bled and infiltrated the tissues of a large muscular calf, changing their appearance and matting them together, and with a large irregular wound, into which the blood from the vessel does not seem to be poured in a collected form, but to well out from a large sloughing surface, so as to afford no guide to its exact position, the undertaking is one of the most difficult that can be imagined. The rules and precepts laid down in books about passing probes from the surface towards the seat of the bleeding, the appearance assumed by the vessel, and the dissecting-room directions to find it, are all utterly useless in actual practice; and the knowledge of them is often more a hindrance than an assistance. Watchful eyes and careful cutting are the only reliable guides.

" I believe that pressure so carefully applied over a long tract of the main vessel above, as will diminish, without arresting, the stream passing through it, will, in many cases, be sufficient to allow such coagulation to take place in the open mouths of the vessels as will prevent any future annoyance—that is always supposing a very large extent of an artery be not ripped open, as it were, and as I have seen it, by a rifle-ball. The French do not seemingly act so unreservedly on the principle of putting a ligature on both ends of a bleeding vessel as we do. They perform Anel's operation in not a few cases. The interesting and instructive nature of the following case is evident:—A Russian boy, wounded at Inkermann, was received into the French hospital at Pera. He had sustained a compound fracture of the leg from gunshot. On the fifteenth day after injury profuse hemorrhage took place from both openings. Pressure failed to arrest it. The popliteal was tied the same day according to the method of deligation recommended by M. Jobert, viz., on the inner side of the limb, between the vastus and hamstring muscles. The foot remained very cold for four days, and then violent reaction set in; and on the eighth day from the ligature of the main vessel hemorrhage recurred both from the original wound and incision of ligature. Pressure was tried in vain. The superficial femoral was then ligatured on the tenth day from the deligation of the popliteal. Four days afterwards the bleeding returned from the wound, and pressure then seemed to check it. The ligature separated from the femoral on the twelfth day after its being tied, and the third day after, *i. e.*, the twenty-fifth day from the first occurrence of hemorrhage, bleeding again set in from the wound, the limb was amputated in the thigh, and the unfortunate patient ultimately recovered. Would Mr. Guthrie not have saved this man's limb, and the surgeons much trouble? It was a matter of common conversation in the hospitals at Constantinople, that when the weather was close and sultry, with little wind, there was certain to be a large number of cases of secondary hemorrhage.

"A soldier, resting his right hand on his musket, was struck by a ball on the web between the thumb and forefinger. The wound seemed trivial, but the whole hand swelled exceedingly. On the fourteenth day arterial hemorrhage occurred, and pressure was applied. The bleeding repeatedly recurred, and still pressure was persevered in. Finally the radial, and then the ulnar, was ligatured before the hemorrhage was commanded. An early search in the wound, and a thread applied to the orifices of the vessel, would have saved much annoyance and risk. The following occurred under my own notice.

"M'Garthland, a soldier of the 38th regiment, an unhealthy man, who still suffered from the effects of scurvy, which had been followed by fever, was shot through the left leg from behind, and externally forwards and inwards, on the 18th of June. The fibula was broken and the edge of the tibia was injured. He walked to the rear without assistance. On admission the limb was greatly swollen. This swelling very much diminished in a few days. On the fifth day arterial bleeding, to a limited extent, took place from both openings. Recalling a case put on record by Mr. Butcher, of Dublin, the wound of the post-tibial, I determined on trying the effects of well-applied pressure along the course of the popliteal and in the wound, and employed cold, while the limb was raised and fixed on a splint. The object of the pressure on the main vessel was to diminish, not arrest, the flow of blood through it. On the eighth day there was again some oozing. Pus had accumulated among the muscles of the calf (one great objection to using pressure on the orifices of gunshot wounds), and required incision for its evacuation. On the ninth day a pulsating tumor was observed on the external aspect of the leg, and the next day the bleeding returned from both wounds.

"I wished then to cut down and tie the vessel in the wound, but consultation decided on waiting a little longer, in the hope that the bleeding might not return. On the night of the eleventh day most profuse hemorrhage recurred. The attendant, though strictly enjoined, failed to tighten the tourniquet, but the necessary steps to arrest the bleeding were taken by the officer on duty. Next morning, when I first heard of the occurrence, I found the patient blanched, cold, and nearly pulseless. A consultation decided that the state of the parts made the securing of the vessel in the wound very problematical, and that as the limb would not recover if the main artery was taken up, amputation must be performed so soon as he had sufficiently rallied. When reaction had fairly taken place, I amputated the limb. The removed parts were much engorged, sloughed, and disorganized. The anterior tibial was found to have been opened for about an inch shortly after its origin, and on it was formed the aneurism, which had a communication with both orifices of the wound. The artery should have been tied in the wound on the occurrence of the second bleeding. I say the second bleeding, as it very often happens that even when hemorrhage has taken place, to a considerable extent, and evidently from a vessel of large calibre, it never recurs. Many most striking instances of this have come under my notice. But though more than even this is true, and that frequently blood thrown out repeatedly is spontaneously arrested, still the great preponderance of cases in which it recurs in dangerous repetitions and quantities, as in the above instance, should cause us, I believe, to interfere on its second appearance, if it be in any quantity more particularly, and that we should not delay, so as to run the risk of such a return as will cause exhaustion. Not to interfere unless the vessel is bleeding, must not always be understood too literally, or we will often be prevented from performing a necessary operation till our patient is beyond our help. The hemorrhage recurs over and over again, and the surgeon, though as near as is practicable, arrives only in time to see the bed drenched, and the patient and attendant intensely alarmed. There is at the moment no bleeding, and he vainly hopes there will be no return ; and so on goes the game between ebbing life and approaching death, the loss not great at each time, but mighty in its sum, till all assistance is useless.

" The use of acetate of lead, or gallic acid, though often trusted to in these hemorrhages, are surgical farces—mesmeric passes along the vessels would be of infinitely more service."

ART. 72.—*On the diagnosis of certain forms of infecting and non-infecting Syphilitic Sores.* By Mr. HENRY LEE, Surgeon of King's College Hospital.

(*Medical Times and Gazette,* June 7, 1856.)

In this paper (which was read before the Royal Medical and Chirurgical Society, May 13th, 1856), the author observes that Jenner regarded a peculiar kind of inflammation as essential to the production of the effects of the vaccine poison on the patient's constitution ; and Willan made similar observations respecting the inoculation of the poison of smallpox. Unless the morbid process peculiar to each poison were gone through, although other constitutional effects might follow, yet that which constituted the peculiar action of the poison upon the patients would not. It was the same with respect to the syphilitic poison ; the peculiar morbid process which indicated its introduction into the system was attended with inflammation of the adhesive character, as in the case of the cow-pox. The application of the syphilitic poison often gave rise to true suppuration in the inoculated part, but this was essentially a different morbid process to that by which the poison was introduced into the patient's system. Where a syphilitic sore at an early stage produced well-formed pus globules, that affection would not infect the patient's constitution ; the virus from such a sore might be readily enough inoculated ; much more certainly, indeed, than that from a genuine infecting sore. Inoculation, therefore, was no test of the necessity of treating a patient by mercury, since these suppurating sores, most readily inoculable, were not, if left to themselves, followed by secondary symptoms. Induration, the author regarded as affording no invariable evidence of the adhesive inflammation ; for, in the first place, the product of the inflammatory action might be poured out upon the surface of the affected part, without infiltrating its tissue, which was as true of the adhesive as of the suppurative inflammation, and in neither case would there be any induration of the inflamed part ; and, in the second, the presence of induration gave no invariable indication of the nature of the inflammation which produced it. The sense of touch alone would not invariably indicate whether the effused lymph would remain such until absorbed, or whether, in fact, the inflammation was of the adhesive or suppurative character. The information which the sense of touch failed to give, the examination of the secretion from the infected part would often supply. Examined under the microscope, fresh from the different sores, the globules in the discharges would often appear very similar ; but if acetic acid were added before examination, a clear distinction might be drawn between those cases in which true pus globules were formed, and those in which they were not. When true pus globules were formed at an early period, and were not produced by artificial irritation, the author maintained that no constitutional syphilitic disease would result. The various points mentioned in the paper were illustrated by cases.

(O) CONCERNING DISEASES OF BONES AND JOINTS.

ART. 73.—*On Incisions into Joints.* By Mr. GAY.

(*Lancet*, Oct. 25, 1856.)

Mr. Gay commences his paper (which was read before the Medical Society of London, 18th October, 1856), by observing that three years ago he had brought before the profession, through the same medium, a method of treating certain forms of articular disease by free incisions into the affected cavities ; but that, since that period, his experience of this treatment had led him somewhat to modify his views, and had enabled him with more distinctness to define the particular forms and stages of disease for which it is more especially adapted. His object in making incisions was not merely to evacuate matter, as in the case of an ordinary abscess, and as this proceeding has been adopted and recommended by others, but as well, and even chiefly, for the purposes of allowing the more ready escape of cartilaginous or bony *débris*—often a cause of destructive irritation to a joint—and of setting up reparative action by making a closed or partially closed and diseased sac a part of a large and externally communicating wound. The results of his experience, as of that of many of his professional brethren who had adopted his views, had been still more to convince him that free incisions were of the greatest value in those forms of disease to which they were appropriate, inasmuch as they bring the diseased processes to an equally speedy termination as after resection of the joint, and have the greater merit of leaving the limb less mutilated, and the joint often almost as useful as before. Moreover, the incisions are comparatively harmless, and, in case of failure, do not lessen the chance of restoring the limb that resection, or other measures of a graver nature, might afterwards afford.

The first case, that of a lady aged 43, who had suffered for three years from all the symptoms of disease of the cartilage and bony structures of the knee-joint, and had come to town to have the limb amputated. On making an incision into the joint, over the seat of the principal pain, a small quantity of sero-purulent fluid trickled out with the blood. On examining the interior of the joint carefully, the cartilage was found to be entire, but slightly uneven, leading to the conclusion that the affection commenced in the synovial capsule, and had not seriously implicated other structures. The intense pain from which this lady suffered, especially at night, prior to the operation, was completely relieved by it ; and, with the exception of a rigor on the day following, succeeded by a slight fever, which soon yielded to treatment, not a bad symptom followed. The capsule soon healed, and in a month the patient began to walk about. She has since (three years having elapsed) enjoyed the perfect use of her limb.

The second was a case of hip-joint disease of three years' standing. A sinus, having two external openings, led into the joint. The limb was bent upon the trunk, and the joint still flexible, but with great pain. The discharge had almost ceased, and the diseased action appeared to be almost stationary, and had been so for several months. The joint was fairly opened by enlarging the sinus ; the head of the bone had been partially removed, and was bare. The joint recovered completely after fourteen weeks, with considerable mobility, quite enough to make the limb useful.

The third case, of "strumous" disease of the articular cartilages of the knee-joint of long standing, in a boy 9 years old ; the pain was severe, and the discharge profuse. The incision did not answer in this case, the disease making progress subsequently, as though pursuing its natural course, with the addition of a severe wound, which refused to heal.

The fourth case, of "strumous" disease of the knee-joint of three years' standing, in a girl 12 years of age. The joint was greatly distended, and has been so for more than six months. It was opened, a considerable quantity of sero-purulent fluid exuded, and, in defiance of every attempt to keep it open, the wound healed in three weeks, leaving the joint in the same condition as before. It was opened again after six weeks, and from this time the course of the disease was onwards ; and removal of cartilages, caries of the ends of the bones, with profuse discharge, and failure of health and strength followed. The treatment in this was of no avail ; at last, amputation of the limb was resorted to. The articular ends of both bones were carious, and the spongy texture of the bones intensely inflamed for some distance along their respective shafts. No traces of tubercle were found, but small deposits of pus in those parts of the bone where the inflammation was most severe.

The fifth case, a woman, aged 62, for disease of the joint belonging to the phalanx of the forefinger. It had existed six months, and remained stationary. The joint was quite loose, and grated when moved, also painful. A free incision on each side, and keeping the wounds plugged, led to speedy anchylosis.

The sixth and seventh cases were of hip-joint disease in children, of 7 and 8 years of age respectively. The disease in both cases was in its early stages, and in one only had a sinus been formed. The joints were opened freely, but with somewhat varied results. In both, fresh abscesses formed, and burst on the front of the thigh. In one, severe pain in the knee-joint followed, which could only be palliated by blisters, mustard poultices, and opium; in the other, symptoms of rapid pulmonary phthisis. These, however, subsequently yielded, and in both cases, after some weeks, the joint disease relapsed into its ordinary forms, the discharge in each being profuse, and the health bad. The incisions in these cases were useless.

The last case was of a lad, aged 12, who had symptoms of subacute inflammation of the knee-joint. After three weeks of severe pain, a small opening was made into the joint, and some matter passed away. This did not give much relief. The wound ulcerated, and soon after an opening formed spontaneously, nearly two inches from the first, which also led into the joint. Very little matter exuded, and the joint continued extremely painful. Some white (apparently) sloughy matter could be seen through these openings. Chloroform was given, and the joint laid open by an incision which passed through the two sinuses, and a large "pus-clot" was removed, which appeared to have filled the joint to painful distension. Suppuration followed, and the joint rapidly recovered, the lad being able, in six weeks, to move about by means of a stick, the joint being entire. There were no indications of bone disease in this case.

After making comparisons between these several cases, the author drew the following practical conclusions: That joints might be opened with advantage—1st. In cases of chronic inflammation of the synovial capsule of a joint, with effusion into its cavity, and pain; especially if these symptoms shall have been of long standing, have resisted ordinary remedies, and are associated with marks of declining health, as in the first case. 2d. In cases of acute or subacute synovitis, where the symptoms are unusually severe, and the external coverings of the joint indicate a tendency to ulceration; or where, after a reasonable period, the symptoms do not remit, but indicate the existence within the joint of matter, which, from its becoming a source of irritation, threatens to produce more serious mischief, as in the eighth case. 3d. In cases where the joint is occupied by bony or cartilaginous *debris*, which, from the small size of existing sinuses, cannot find exit: and 4th. In cases of carious disease of the bones, in which, from diminution of pain and secretion, as well as from other confirmatory symptoms, the disease in which the local affection has originated, shall appear to have exhausted itself, as in the second and fifth cases. He condemned the practice (except for the purpose of relieving severe pain) in all cases in which a chance remains that the joint will recover without; and especially in what are termed "strumous" affections of the joints, so long as the continuance of profuse discharge indicates that the constitutional disorder, in which it is presumed to have originated, has not burnt out; and in the event of this becoming exhausted, only when the persistence of sinuses but slightly discharging beyond a reasonable time, might lead the surgeon to suspect either the existence within the joint of some dead and irritant matter, or the want of some general stimulus to final and reparative action, which, connecting a diseased sac with an external wound would supply.

ART. 74.—*On Hyperæsthesia in Rickets.* By Dr. BETZ.

(*Froriep's Notizen*, Bd. i, p. 231, 1856; and *Medical Times and Gazette*, Oct. 25, 1856.)

Dr. Betz calls attention to those cases in which young children often whine and cry without any obvious reason, and shrink from all contact, while those who are old enough complain of tenderness and sensibility of the entire surface. This condition he agrees with Wunderlich in attributing to rachitis. This hyperæsthesia has its seat in part in the cutaneous nerves, and in part in the nerves of the bones and periosteum, those of the latter organs being especially concerned both in the pain resulting from pressure, and in the paroxysm of spontaneous exaggerated sensibility. This condition is an early accompaniment of the rickety state, existing in different amounts of severity, but not entirely disappearing, unless the rickets have become cured. A catarrhal condition is also always present, manifested by increased discharges from the bronchi, nose, mouth, stomach, or intestinal canal, just as the hyperæsthesia of adults, e. g. odontalgia, is followed by abundant secretions. With the increase of sensibility is sometimes conjoined an increased hyperæmia of the enlarged ends of the bones, for in minute examination of rickety children, we find that there are slight variations in the volume of those bones, corresponding to the state of the sensibility.

This hyperæsthesia is made known to us by the following signs. Both older as well as young children begin crying without apparent reason, and cry both much and often. Even gentle handling gives them more or less pain, and especially at the parts where the bones are but slightly covered, as the wrists and sides of the thorax, particularly at the swollen points of contact of the ribs with their cartilages. The pain induced by pressure on the hypochondria is due to this hyperæsthetic state, and not, as is often believed, to enlarged mesenteric glands or pleuritis, although this last sometimes gives rise to similar sensibility there. Not only are the superficial bones thus painful, but also others that are covered with muscles, as the femur. The cranial bones may also suffer, and the children be unable to bear any contact, such as combing or pommading the hair, or the pressure of a cap. Hyperæsthesia of the jaws is often accompanied by discharge from the mouth, and is attributed to toothache when no carious teeth exist. The mouth is hot and irritable, and sensitive to the temperature of food and drink; and the children use the incisor teeth so as to avoid bringing the food in contact with the sensitive periosteum of the toothless portion of the jaws. Rickety children are fond of crossing the legs while sitting, as this relieves them of a painful weariness of the limbs, and this is also one of the signs of hyperæsthesia. Although this hyperæsthesia principally affects the nerves of the bones and periosteum, increasing or diminishing according to the amount of hyperæmia, the cutaneous nerves may also suffer from it. The author is not certain whether or not spontaneous increased sensibility to pain be present in these, but he has remarked their greater excitability, as shown in the increased ticklishness of these children.

Art. 75.—*On a new method of treating False Joint.* By Mr. Jordan, Surgeon to the Royal Manchester Infirmary.

(*Medical Times and Gazette,* Sept. 13, 1856.)

The following remarks are reported by Mr. W. H. Bellot, as having been made, not by Mr. Jordan himself, but by M. Nélaton, in one of his clinical lectures:

"Mr. Jordan, Surgeon of the Manchester Royal Infirmary, is the inventor of this method, and he has taken advantage of his sojourn in Paris to propose to M. Nélaton the application of this happy invention. Mr. Jordan has already been able to obtain a cure in a desperate case, treated in vain by many other surgeons. Observe, in a few words, in what this method consists. In the first place, the bone must be uncovered, as in the cases where it is intended to practise the resection of the two ununited fragments. When the bones are reached, a vertical incision must be made upon the periosteum, commencing higher or lower upon the shaft of the bone, and terminating where the fracture ends. Each fragment is treated alike; the periosteum is dissected from every part, that is to say, separated from the bone. This dissection ought to be made with the handle of the scalpel, and by little blows; it is a little tedious, but we must not employ the blade of a bistoury, because then we infallibly cut the vessels of the periosteum, which often perforate at the same time this nourishing membrane, and thus expose us to fail in our object. We must not forget that, when there is a diseased condition in a bone, as in a false joint, the periosteum is thickened, more turgid, more vascular, and more easily separated from the osseous substance. After this dissection, a kind of periostic flap is left, like the sleeves of our coats or our shirts. For the other fragment a similar operation must be performed, taking care to push the dissection to a rather less extent. Secondly, the ends of the broken bones must be cut off, and here the same instruments are employed as in an ordinary resection—the saw, &c. Every portion of bone which is covered with bony stalactites ought, as much as possible, to be removed: and it is known that these stalactites appear precisely at the point where the periosteum has been destroyed or altered from the injury, at the time of the fracture in general. One centimetre (which is not half an inch) and a half, or two centimetres of each fragment, ought to be cut off. Thirdly, one of the ends of the bone is to be inserted into the periostic sheath of the other, and then a suture at the free extremity of the flap, and the periosteum is disposed in such a way as the union of the bones allows. The edges of the incisions of the soft parts are then brought together, the limb supported in a suitable dressing, and the operation is completed as in an ordinary case.

"In the case where a complete dissection of all the periosteum cannot be made, Mr. Jordan has proposed another plan. In this case the bone is denuded of two little periostic flaps, which answer to the little flaps of skin in the amputation of M. Senoir: the other fragment is denuded upon the side opposed to that of the first fragment. In the second place, the two fragments must be cut diamond-shaped; there are thus, as it were, two beaks of a flute opposed one to the other; they are faced (or, as we should say, dovetailed together), and they fold the periosteum all round. It is evident that this last proceeding gives the same result as the preceding one; it would, perhaps, be more difficult to maintain the ends of the bones in immediate contact.

"Does not this proceeding offer something new? Authors, or rather surgeons, have employed friction, needles, the seton, the ligature, resection, abrasion, scraping the ends of the bones, and, lastly, cauterization. White, and other surgeons, have spoken well of scraping the periosteum, but they have not formed a clear idea upon the point. Have they shown, what Mr. Jordan has truly made a happy invention, and which may admit of numerous applications, that is, the autoplastic plan applied to the periosteum? When we reflect that we often see in the hospitals patients having pseudarthrosis, undergoing a great number of surgical operations, without any benefit, we ought to hail with delight a plan which is based upon sound physiological data, and upon a clinical fact, followed by success. Finally, we must not omit to say that Professor Nélaton has accorded it his approbation, and that it was with great regret that he was not able to employ it upon the patient with respect to whom he had shown to his auditory the plan of Mr. Jordan."

ART. 76.—*On Plaster of Paris Bandages in Fractures.* By Dr. WEBER.

(*New York Journal of Medicine,* May, 1856.)

Dr. Weber calls attention in this paper to the practice of the celebrated Russian surgeon, Prof. Pirogoff, of using bandages soaked in plaster of Paris solution, in the treatment of fracture. Dr. Weber gains his information from the "Deutsche Klinik," for 1854, and from a few cases in which he has tried the plan in his own practice. He says—

"The following articles for bandages are wanted:—long, old, hospital stockings, opened at the seam—old drawers, jackets, or waistcoats of linen. For fractures of the thigh,—belts which can go round the pelvis one and a half time: old linen, cotton, and cushions filled with lint or flax (to fill up depressions round the ankles, &c., &c); splints of different lengths, out of two or three layers of the coarsest linen, and strips of the same material.

"The splints must be two to eight fingers broad, and a little longer than the injured limb;—the strips ought to be two to ten inches broad, and reach two to three times round the limb.

"At last a quantity of plaster of Paris, perfectly dry and finely pulverized, and cold water, with brushes, are to be kept in readiness.

"It takes some practice to make the solution not too thin nor too thick, so that it dries neither too slowly nor too fast. Equal parts of water and plaster will be the best proportion. When the application of the bandage takes up more than ten minutes, a few drops of carpenter's glue will retard the process of hardening, for a quarter of an hour and longer. On application of the plaster of Paris bandage, the injured limb is first covered with dry linen; the depressions and projections are filled with cotton; extension and coaptation are made *lege artis;* and then the splints, soaked in the solution, are applied lengthways close to the limb, and fastened crossways by the strips. Instead of the strips, a roller can be used, which has to be covered with the solution by means of a brush, gradually, throughout the time that it is applied.

"At the exterior margin of the limb the splints are applied ; so that a small space of an eighth in width is left open. A piece of tape soaked in oil marks this space. The strips are also oiled crossways, in their middle, so that the solution is not taken up there—the oiled parts must fit the line of the tape; in this way, a small space is left open, and uncovered by the plaster of Paris, so that the bandage can either be made tighter, by application of a new roller, or easily cut open, to be removed. The plaster of Paris bandage is well adapted to the quick construction of capsules, for the transportation of the injured."

ART. 77.—*On the influence of Phosphate of Lime in the formation of Callus.*
By M. MILNE EDWARDS.

(*Comptes Rendus*, xlii, p. 631 ; and *Med.-Chir. Rev.*, July, 1856.)

The question of aiding the formation of callus by the administration of phosphate of lime has recently been revived in Paris, and the author of this paper alludes to some experiments tried by M. Gosselin at the Hôpital Cochin, especially in cases of fracture of the arm, which are sometimes so long in uniting. In the six cases observed by him the result seemed satisfactory, inasmuch as the apparatus could be removed in from twenty-seven to thirty days, the fracture appearing quite consolidated. As, however, in these cases, the condition of the callus could not be verified, M. Edwards undertook a series of comparative experiments on animals. Fractures, as nearly as possible alike, were executed upon dogs and rabbits of the same size and strength, to some only of which the lime was administered. The phosphate employed was prepared by the calcination of bones, and consequently was combined with carbonate. The results were decidedly favorable ; and the author believes that the phosphate may be usefully employed as an adjuvant, expediting the union in ordinary fractures, and tending to prevent the non-consolidation of others.

From another communication,* it appears that in one of M. Gosselin's cases of fracture of the lower third of the humerus, complete consolidation occurred in thirty days. He administers as a minimum dose half a gramme per diem.

ART. 78.—*A case of universal Anchylosis.* By Dr. H. P. C. WILSON, of Baltimore.

(*The Philadelphia Examiner*, June, 1856.)

This case is described as a rigid, anchylosed human skeleton, the result of rheumatism.

"E. E— was admitted to the almshouse in May, 1846. Was then 21 years old. Was a native of Germany, and had come to this country some three years previously. Had been married twice. By first husband had two children, both dead. By last husband had one child, still living. Two years before admission, was attacked with rheumatism, with which she suffered uninterruptedly with greater or less severity up to the time she came in. Was a laboring woman, and had to undergo much exposure, and endure many privations to obtain a support for herself and child. Her second husband being dead, and her disease, from having been acute, becoming chronic, so that her joints began to stiffen and incapacitate her for labor, she was compelled to take refuge in the Baltimore City and County Almshouse.

"When admitted, could help herself in various ways ; could feed herself, turn in bed, walk, and perform most of the other motions of which the joints are capable, but most of them with difficulty, and none with the facility belonging to healthy, uncomplicated joints.

"She went on from bad to worse; and when I took charge of the hospital, in March, 1855, I found her lying on her back, without the ability to move a single joint in the body, save a very partial motion of the lower jaw, and the costo-vertebral articulations. Her hands were pronated, and her forearms flexed upon the arms, and resting upon the upper part of the abdomen. The soles of her feet were applied one to another. Her legs were flexed upon her thighs, and her thighs upon

* "Gazette des Hopitaux," No. 150, 1856.

the pelvis. This, I am told, has been her position, from soon after the date of admission until the date of death, a period of nine years, during which time she has remained a rigid, motionless being. Dry gangrene had taken place in many of her fingers and toes; and in this dry parched state were twisted upon themselves in various ways, so as to resemble more the talons of birds of prey, than what they were.

"The various functions of animal life were performed well. Slept well, appetite good, circulation, defecation, and urination all good. Was a picture of patience, and seemed not to suffer a great deal, except at certain periods, as during stormy weather. Was fed on liquids, being incapable of mastication.

"She died of typhoid fever, supervening on scurvy, July 9th, 1856.

"By inspecting the skeleton of the above subject, now in my possession, the inter-articular cartilages of the upper and lower jaw will be found completely ossified; with such an amount of bony matter thrown out in and around the joint as to allow but very partial motion. The history of the case substantiated the same during life.

"The occipito-atloid articulation is so anchylosed, as to blot out all evidences of a joint having ever existed.

"The inter-vertebral substances are converted into bone, and the spinal column thus changed into a rigid inflexible pillar.

"The sterno-clavicular, and scapulo-clavicular articulations are completely obliterated, the three bones being united into one, without the trace of a joint.

"The xiphoid and costal cartilages are all changed into bone.

"Each humerus is anchylosed to its scapula. Each radius and ulna to its humerus, and to each other. Each carpus is as a single bone, firmly anchylosed at the wrist-joint. Each metacarpal bone, with its phalanges, is as one firm inflexible bone. Similar to the wrist, and hand, and fingers, is the anchylosed condition of the ankle, foot, and toes; and as for the radius, ulna, and humerus, so for the tibia, fibula, and femur.

"No joint in the body then was capable of the slightest motion, save the two above mentioned, and in these motion was but very partial. The bones were exceedingly light, not weighing one-third as much as their counterparts in the healthy subject. The earthy matter was apparently wholly removed from the cancellated structure.

"It is to be regretted that circumstances prevented me from making a careful autopsy of this subject. No doubt ossific matter would have been found extensively deposited in and about various organs (especially the circulatory system), to add additional wonder to this truly anomalous case."

(D) CONCERNING OPERATIONS.

ART. 79.—*Is it always necessary to resort to amputation when a limb is attacked with Sphacelus?* By M. BARDINET, of Limoges.

(*Presse Méd. Belge*, March 23; and *Dublin Medical Press*, April 9, 1856.)

The following is a *résumé* of M. Bardinet's memoir:

1. In this memoir I report eight new cases of sphacelus (two of the finger, three of the forearm, and three of the leg), in none of which amputation was performed. The task of eliminating the dead parts was intrusted to Nature, except that her operations have been actively aided by the employment of the ordinary disinfectants, and especially by the early resection of the dead parts near the eliminatory circle. In these eight cases recovery took place.

Had amputation been performed, it is, on the one hand, extremely probable that a certain number of patients would have died; on the other, several of them would have been deprived, in consequence of the necessity of amputating above the eliminatory circle, of a portion of their limbs (the knee, for example, or the upper part of the forearm), which they are fortunate in having been able to preserve.

It is, therefore, not always necessary to amputate in cases of sphacelus.

2. We should, above all, be extremely cautious in having recourse to amputation in cases of spontaneous gangrene—first, because in such cases, whatever we do,

and even after the establishment of the eliminatory circle, we can never be sure that the gangrene will not reappear, and that we shall not thus needlessly add the pain and dangers of a serious operation to those of the original disease.

3. Because the fear of amputating the parts whose vessels are diseased obliges us to carry the section up to a considerable height, and thus involves, and sometimes very uselessly, the sacrifices of parts which might have been preserved, and the loss of which is to be lamented.

4. Because the gangrene may attack several limbs in succession, and even all the limbs, of which I have quoted two examples, and we should then find ourselves compelled to perform a series of sad mutilations.

5. Because, on the contrary, in confining ourselves to cutting away the dead parts near the circle of elimination, we perform an operation which is always practicable and always useful, as it liberates the patient from a focus of infection.

6. Because we avoid the risk of performing an amputation, all the benefits of which will be lost if the gangrene makes fresh advances.

7. Because, in adopting the new mode, we do not unnecessarily remove parts which the patient is much interested in preserving.

8. Because we have still the power of performing amputation if it should become necessary.

ART. 80.—*Some account of the "écraseur" of M. Chassaignac.* By Mr. T. SPENCER WELLS, Lecturer on Surgery at the Grosvenor Place School.

(*Medical Times and Gazette*, Oct. 11, 1856.)

" The instrument which M. Chassaignac uses, says Mr. Wells, after some introductory remarks, "is made by an instrument-maker named Mathieu, and costs 48 francs. M. Luer has contrived one on the same principle, but of superior construction, for which he charges 80 francs. Both these instruments, however, appear to me to be inferior to the one here figured, which is made by M. Charrière, and costs only 30 francs. In all these instruments the essential part is a sort of blunt chain-saw, which is tightened in M. Charrière's instrument by a screw, in the others by a rack and pinion. The great objections to both the latter are, that the chain passes through a closed channel which is difficult to clean or keep dry, and it is not passed through very easily, or fastened readily. Comparatively clumsy, more complicated, and dearer, I cannot doubt their inferiority.

Fig. 2.

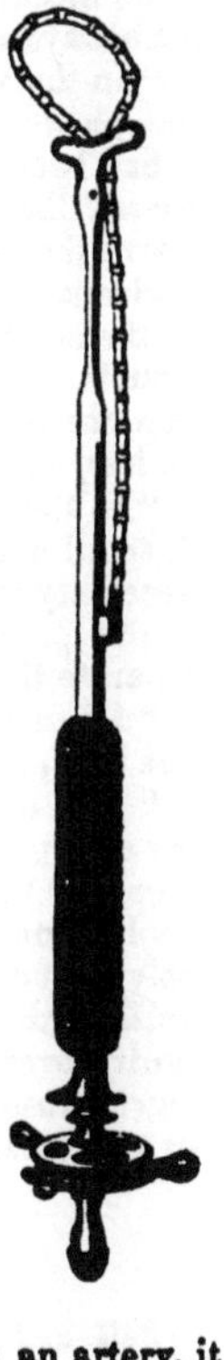

" If it were wished to give this instrument a Greek instead of a French name, it might be called sarcotrite or histotrite, flesh or tissue breaker or crusher. It is intended to replace the knife on the one hand, and caustics and ligatures on the other, when we have to remove parts of the body or morbid growths, where considerable hemorrhage may be looked for. In a word, it is intended to prevent the loss of blood in surgical operations. The tongue has been removed; the neck of the uterus amputated; a number of erectile polypi, naso-pharyngeal, uterine, and rectal, have been taken away, we are assured, without the loss of a drop of blood. A full account of these operations, of the origin of the method in 1850, and its advance to the present time, with detailed directions for the use of the instrument in its various applications, will be found in M. Chassaignac's 'Traité de l'écrasement linéaire,' a book of 560 pages, with 40 wood-cuts, which has been published this year by Baillière, of Paris, for 6 francs. There is a copy in the library of the Royal College of Surgeons.

" The action of the instrument, though slower than that of the knife, is much more rapid than that of the ligature, and its action is direct; not indirect like the ligature, which only divides tissues by the process of gangrene it induces. The *écraseur* first condenses the tissues it acts on, and then divides them with extreme regularity. The wound does not appear at all bruised or torn. When it acts on an artery, it first divides the two internal coats, which are folded up in such a manner as to plug the vessel. The closure is assisted by the agglutination of the outer coats, before they are divided, and after separation has been effected, the closure is so perfect that the channel cannot be opened by blowing forcibly through it. Experiments have been made at the Veterinary School near Paris, and the carotids of sheep have been divided without loss of blood. There is nothing surprising in this, when we remember how seldom severe gunshot, lacerated, or contused wounds bleed; that a limb may be torn off by machinery, and no blood be lost; and that *bites* are very rarely attended by hemorrhage. The lower animals have no occasion to apply a ligature upon the umbilical cord of their young. They simply bite it through, and the action of the *écraseur* is much more like that of biting than of crushing.

"My personal experience of the use of this instrument in the living human body amounts only to three operations I saw M. Chassaignac perform—the removal of a portion of the tongue, the testicle, and a mammary tumor. In the first case, about a third of the tongue was removed, on account of supposed malignant disease. The man was not under the influence of chloroform, and the operation occupied twenty minutes. It appeared to be very painful, although we are informed that the pain is not in general complained of after the first tightening of the instrument benumbs the parts. There was some bleeding, which was explained by the dresser who had continued to tighten the chain, having done so too fast, and by the patient having jerked his head at the conclusion of the operation, and separated the last shreds of the tongue suddenly. A quarter of an hour afterwards I followed the man to the ward, and found him bleeding profusely. I could see a small artery jetting freely at the lower part of the wound. A Sister of Charity was supplying the man with lumps of ice to keep in his mouth; and she told me that, expecting what would happen, she had the ice all ready by the time the man returned from the theatre. She said she had seen a great many of these operations on the tongue, perhaps fifty; that they occurred almost every week, and that there was troublesome bleeding in a large proportion, perhaps about half or rather more; but that ice always succeeded in stopping it.

"In the second case a testicle was removed, and not a drachm of blood was lost, though we could see the spermatic artery pulsating very distinctly at the spot where it had been divided. Two *écraseurs* were used in this operation, the chains being passed through an opening made by a trocar in the upper part of the scrotum, above the testis and behind the chord. One divided the chord and integuments horizontally, the other divided the scrotum vertically. Thus a very large portion of the scrotum was removed, and there was not enough left to cover the remaining testicle. It appeared to me that if the *écraseur* were used at all in such an operation, the scrotum should certainly be first divided with the knife, so that none should be lost, and the *écraseur* be merely used to divide the cord.

"In the third case I could not understand why the instrument was used at all. A small mammary tumor was to be removed, and to get the chain around it, it was necessary to lay it bare with the knife. Of course the principal vessels were divided in this process, and a very few more touches of the knife would have sufficed to separate the tumor when the *ecraseur* was applied.

"I found that of upwards of a hundred operations on piles with this instrument, one had proved fatal. The man was suffering at the time from secondary syphilis.

"The impression left on my mind from what I have seen and heard, and from my own trial of the instrument on the dead body and on the arteries of sheep and a calf, is that, if slowly and properly used, hemorrhage will very rarely follow its application, but that its use will most likely be restricted to the removal of piles, polypi, and such erectile or malignant growths as could not be removed by the knife without a probability of dangerous hemorrhage. In such cases the superiority over the ligature in the time gained, and the non-liability to purulent or putrid absorption is self-evident. Whether it will answer as well as a wire heated by galvanism experience alone can decide."

ART. 81.—*On the employment of Setons.*
By M. BOUVIER and others.

(*Bull. de l'Académie*, t. xxi, pp. 52–249; and *Med. Times and Gazette*, Aug. 2, 1856.)

This not long since formed the subject of an animated and prolonged discussion at the Academie de Medecine. It led to learned dissertations on the antiquity of the doctrine of revulsion and various other topics to which we cannot advert; but we may sift out from the wordy mass the few practical observations that were made upon the subject.

M. Bouvier introduced it by adverting to the objections to the employment of setons entertained by many modern practitioners, and attributing any ill effects they may have observed to the mode of operating. That which he himself employs is much less painful and quite as efficacious as the old mode. He uses a very narrow needle, with a lance-shaped point, which, in place of a skein of silk, carries only a small thread, covered with some impermeable substance, such as that which forms the gum-elastic bougies, but somewhat more supple. It is let in at a slit at the end of a needle. The passage of this small thread causes little or no pain, and its polished surface allows of its being kept very clean. If an insufficient amount of irritation be induced, another thread, or even two or three, may be placed in juxta-position with the first, and in this way we are able to dose or regulate the amount of irritation. In this way the filiform seton may, in a great number of cases, be employed as a substitute for the ordinary painful seton, while it leaves far less considerable cicatrices. Gutta percha is found to be too hard a material, but flexible chains of gold, silver, or platinum may be advantageously employed, especially as precautionary setons in relapsing ophthalmia. As in the case of earrings, the suppuration ceases around the foreign body, and no inconvenience, beyond the necessity of attention to cleanliness, is caused to the patient. M. Bouvier presented several children to the Academy who had suffered from ophthalmia, and had derived benefit from the employment of filiform setons.

M. Gerdy observed that the employment of the seton is so convenient that it is frequently had recourse to; but in his own experience he has found it not only giving rise to circumvicinal inflammation, but also augmenting the original mischief, as, for example, in ophthalmia and amaurosis—so that the result following its employment has sometimes proved quite opposite to the one proposed. For these reasons he has abandoned the use of the seton. M. Malgaigne observed that, originally a believer in the efficacy of exutories, he had recourse to them very many times under the form of seton, moxa, or issue; but he has come to the conclusion that their beneficial effects are very doubtful indeed—the success seeming due to their prolonged employment having been really due in many cases to mere expectation. He has long studied the action of setons and moxas on diseased joints, and has arrived at the conviction that if good effects do not result from their employment during the first few days, they are of no service. For years he has now left off employing setons, the moxa, or prolonged issues. He has been long struck with the great abuses that result from the retention of issues. He particularizes their retention, for he is far from denying the utility of the moxa or cautery in inducing the cessation of pain. But we must not confound the influence of a sudden irritation, or of one even prolonged for some days, with that of setons or issues remaining *in situ* for months or years, and to which nature becomes so habituated that patients are compelled to retain them, their operation becoming, however, as inert as that of earrings. Since he has held the doctrine of the inutility of exutories, he has in vain requested numbers of practitioners and pupils to see whether they could tax their memory with a well-authenticated example of their successful employment in one case in ten, or even one in twenty.

M. Velpeau observed that without being a great partisan of the seton, he admits its therapeutical power; but he regards the filiform suture now recommended as of very questionable efficacy, and approaching the fallacies of homœopathy. Like the homœopathic remedies, these setons are employed in chronic affections, the various phases of which are little known beforehand; which are sometimes cured spontaneously, and which are successively treated by a crowd of remedies, the last given, if it happen to have arrived at an opportune time, reaping the whole credit of the case. M. Velpeau cannot, however, join with M. Malgaigne in his wholesale reprobation of setons and issues. As regards their employment in diseases of the eye, the following are the conclusions he has arrived at: " All revulsives cannot be indiscriminately resorted to, each being more fitted for certain forms of disease. Blisters are of special use in acute and superficial ophthalmias, such as conjunctivitis; issues in the chronic affections which engage the ball of the eye; while the seton should be reserved for some of the diseases belonging to the latter category, but especially for affections of the cornea, and those of undefined seat. In these even they are rarely to be used at first. I usually employ them only in obstinate cases, and especially in amaurosis, complex forms of disease, the precise anatomical characters of which can hardly be ascertained. It is in such cases, when the amaurosis is not dependent upon deep-seated disorganization of the eye, but upon some unseizable modification of the membranes, that I apply setous to the nape, and, I add, with indubitable advantage, after the failure of numerous other remedies." To sum up, M. Velpeau employs the seton in amaurosis when it is not sympathetic of organic lesion or visceral disturbance, depending upon certain little-known modifications of the eye, or the nerve or brain; and in keratitis, tending to chronicity and resisting bleeding, blisters, collyria, calomel, and purgatives. When perforation has been threatened, he has found very remarkable effects result from the seton. In vascular keratitis, though still sometimes proper, it is in general less useful; and in conjunctivitis it is still less indicated. M. Clot-Bey stated that the Arabs from time immemorial had employed small setons in their treatment of diseases of the eye. They are placed at the external angle of the eye, over the eyelids themselves, or in their vicinity. For several days there is a considerable fluxion around the suture, and this is followed by moderate suppuration. He has frequently followed the practice with advantage both in Egypt and in France. A noose of black silk is passed into a fold of the skin, and may be easily hid by the hair, its presence not preventing the patient following his occupation.

M. Bouley observed that the seton is much used and abused in veterinary practice. The horse offering a remarkable predisposition to suppuration, this follows in a few hours after the application. By a coincidence, the explanation of which is not attempted, the production of artificial suppuration is attended with a cessation of that which may elsewhere exist, and this may give rise to the abuse of the seton; but it has also its intelligent use. One point M. Bouley insisted upon, viz., the different mode of action of the seton according to the degree of gravity of the disease. If the affection is simple and of regular course, a suppurating phlegmon is formed around the seton in a few hours, while, when a grave condition is present, likely to prove fatal to the organism, there is complete absence of all reaction. The seton also indicates other general conditions, e. g., medicinal saturation. Absorption of mercury never induces salivation in the horse, and the seton becomes a precious means for indicating saturation—the suppuration becoming grayish and very fetid. It also facilitates the exploration of medical constitutions. At certain periods the most simple wounds of operations have a tendency to become gangrenous, so that the operation of castration has sometimes acted like a true epidemic, while the condition of the wound resulting from a seton would have warned against our undertaking any operations. M. Bouvier has stated that a seton acts more by the irritation it produces than by reason of the suppuration that results; but certainly this is not the case in the horse. A seton of three metres long yields about 48 grammes of pus per diem; and six such, which are not uncommonly applied, would yield 288 grammes; or for the six days, which constitutes the medium time of application, 1728 grammes. A horse losing this quantity is in an analogous condition to that of a cow, from whose udders a similar quantity of the elements of the blood are abstracted. Such cows, though their appetite and digestive powers are so active, do not become fat; and so too the seton is a true spoliative agent, and an exutory in the truest sense of the word, removing from the blood a notable portion of its constituent elements, and operating as a resolvent. By the activity it imparts to interstitial absorption it may cause the disappearance of morbid products that have not acquired a too great tenacity.

M. Piorry, during the first twenty years of his practice, habitually employed setons and the other means of inducing permanent secretions; but he now believes that he never obtained in such cases any other results than were derivable from regimen, repose, and the other means simultaneously employed, and he has now wellnigh renounced their use. He never has found any inconvenience to result from their removal from the numerous patients who come to him bearing them. Not only does he regard means of artificially inducing suppuration as useless, but he believes that they may often act mischievously upon the fluids of the body. Thus persons who have long retained them, and who have become pale and cachectic, resume their color and good looks when the suppurating surfaces are dried up.

SECT. II.—SPECIAL QUESTIONS IN SURGERY.

(A) CONCERNING THE HEAD AND NECK.

ART. 82.—*Extensive Absorption of the Bones of the Head.*
By Mr. CÆSAR H. HAWKINS, Surgeon to St. George's Hospital.

(*Lancet*, June 21, 1856.)

The two cases which are here reported were narrated at the meeting of the Royal Medical and Chirurgical Society, held 27th May, 1856. In one of them the absorption was followed by hernia cerebri.

The first case narrated was one of scrofulous caries, in a young man aged 24, in which, quite contrary to the usual chronic character of that disease, most extensive destruction of the bones and soft parts of the head took place in a very brief period. Within the space of ten weeks from the first sensation of pain over the lower part of the right parietal bone, more than half the cranium became affected on both surfaces, in some parts the bone being entirely absorbed, having large openings. The entire parietal bone, the right half of the occipital, the squamous and mastoid portions of the temporal bone, and a considerable part of the frontal, with a part of the greater wing of the sphenoid, were thus affected in the short period mentioned.

The second case related was that of a man, aged 36, who was admitted into St. George's Hospital, under the late Mr. Keate, February 2d, 1832, with a pulsating tumor, nearly five inches in diameter, on the upper and posterior part of the right side of the head. It was soft and elastic, with a well-defined boundary; in its centre a round fungus projected, through an opening in the scalp, of the size of a small walnut, in which pulsation was also evident, and the apex of it looked like layers of coagulated blood. On the opposite side of the head was a similar depression, about three inches in circumference, which was soft and elastic, and pulsated strongly, the edges of the bone not being abrupt or well marked round the aperture; and pulsation could also be felt in another smaller depression near this large one. He had lived freely, had been in tropical climates, had been twice salivated for syphilis, had a tendency to rheumatism, but otherwise enjoyed good health. Two years and a half before his admission, after sleeping on the grass in the sun, he suddenly felt acute pain in the head, which continued some days, and was followed after some time by a depression in the situation of the present tumor, of sufficient size to admit the end of the little finger. This depression increased in size during the next six months, and at length the tumor took its place. Eighteen months before his admission pulsation was first observed in the tumor; at that period the pain and general symptoms were so severe as to lay him up. Poultices were applied, and the tumor was punctured with a lancet, the effect being to let out a little blood simply. The puncture healed, and a month afterwards the same thing was repeated with the like result. Eight weeks previous to his admission, some severe head symptoms occurred, and after being bled from the arm, and having leeches applied to the tumor, it was again punctured, and from that time the present fungus began to protrude. On his admission, some difference of opinion existed as to the seat and nature of the tumor; it was twice ligatured. On the twenty-fifth day after his admission, numbness of the extremities and dimness of sight came on, with giddiness and sickness; on the thirty-third day the left side was more or less paralysed; on the thirty-ninth completely so, and the sphincters were relaxed; on the forty-third he was comatose, and died on the forty-seventh. Examination after death showed the anterior part of the calvarium to be much thickened, in some places to the extent of half an inch, the bony tissue being firm and dense, like ivory, the diploe being obliterated; while towards the posterior parts of the head the bones were very thin and presented large apertures, where, during life, pulsation could be readily felt. The external surface of these bones was rough and mammillated, and the internal more porous than natural. The dura mater adhered completely to the integuments around the opening in the scalp, and the arachnoid and pia mater were also adherent to the inner surface of the former. An opening conducted from the centre of the fungus into a large abscess in the right hemisphere, almost as deep as the lateral ventricle; this abscess had discharged itself during life. It was evident that the disease commenced in the bone, and not in the brain, from the fact that the depressions preceded the protrusion, from the extensive disease of the bones in other parts, and from the fact that below the smaller apertures in which the pulsation of the brain was seen without protrusion, the dura mater and the brain were quite unchanged. The narration of the cases was accompanied with many valuable practical comments upon the rarity of these two affections, their modes of production, and, in the latter case especially, the probable nature of the exciting constitutional cause. The communication was illustrated by many pathological preparations of the parts involved.

ART. 83.—*Extensive injury of the Brain, with remarkable absence of the usual symptoms.* By M. CARMINATI.

(*Il Raccogl. Med. de Fano ;* and *Gaz. Méd. de Paris*, March 15, 1856.)

The remarkable feature in this case is that the patient lived six months in the full enjoyment of his several functions, although two-thirds of one of his cerebral hemispheres was entirely disorganized.

CASE.—A man, æt. 38, strong, and the father of five children, was struck on the head with a pitchfork on the 4th of October, 1854. All consciousness and sensibility was destroyed at the time. On examination the scalp was divided to the extent of about two inches towards the posterior part of the right parietal bone ; the bone was fractured ; and a considerable portion of the cerebral substance, medullary as well as cortical, was exuding from the wound.

Some hours later, the consciousness returned, correct answers were given to questions addressed to him, and objects were distinguished, though indistinctly. The bone was elevated, ice was applied to the head, a purgative given, and a considerable quantity of blood abstracted.

5th.—Some fresh portions of brain came away. No fever.

6th.—Complete apyrexia.

The patient continued to progress favorably until the middle of November, when he was seized with pemphigoid erysipelas of the face, with general symptoms.

December 22d.—The last-mentioned symptoms have entirely disappeared, and the patient now appears to be well in every respect, except that he experiences a degree of feebleness in the lower extremities when walking. The wound in the head, however, has not healed entirely, and a probe may be introduced to a considerable depth into the substance of the brain. He returns to-day to his usual occupation.

April 4th, 1855.—After some months of malaise, for which he sought no treatment, and which was always aggravated by errors of diet, he became comatose and died.

On opening the head, the meninges were found to be deeply injected, particularly on the left side, and a considerable amount of yellowish serum was lodged at the base of the brain and in the ventricles. The posterior two-thirds of the right hemisphere were entirely disorganized, being of a tawny yellow color, and in a semi-fluid state. In the anterior third of the same hemisphere there was an abscess containing from five to six ounces of pus. The rest of the brain was healthy.

ART. 84.—*A case of Encephalocele, with a tabular analysis of seventy-five cases.* By Mr. JOHN Z. LAURENCE.

(*Medical Times and Gazette*, Aug. 2, 1856.)

Congenital hernia of the brain is a rare malformation, and it is a still rarer circumstance for the subject of it to live for any length of time, especially when the protrusion was large. In the present case (which was read before the Medical and Chirurgical Society, 24th June, 1856), the tumor equalled in size the child's head, yet life was prolonged for 144 days, and in that respect it formed a more remarkable case than any which the author had met with in his researches for his table. The mother was healthy, and had previously given birth to five healthy children. The labor was natural; the child a female. At birth the tumor was not quite so large as the head. When first seen by Mr. Laurence, two months and a half after its birth, it presented a conical tumor as large as its head, apparently originating from the occiput and nucha, and measuring five inches and a quarter in length and three inches and a half from side to side. The walls of the tumor were very thin; it fluctuated freely to the touch, was very transparent, but there was no pulsation perceptible. The child had a vacant, idiotic aspect, was to all appearance blind, but was startled by any sudden noise; the limbs were not paralysed; it was found dead in bed beside its mother. On examination after death, the tumor was found to contain the entire cerebellum and a portion of the cerebrum; these parts had been protruded through an opening in the occipital bone, which was oval in form, continuous with the foramen magnum, and measured (including this latter) two inches and a quarter from before backwards, and one inch and a quarter across. The paper was accompanied with a valuable analysis of seventy-five cases of this malformation, divided into three tables—the first, containing an analysis of fifty-three cases of encephalocele occurring in the occipital region; the second, an analysis of seventeen cases occurring in the frontal region; the third, an analysis of five cases occurring in the parietal and temporal regions. The dates of the cases ranged from 1677 to 1853.

ART. 85.—*The condition of Vision the best test of the Squinting Eye.*
By Mr. HOLTHOUSE, Assist.-Surg. to the Westminster Hospital.

(*Medical Times and Gazette*, June 28, 1856.)

"It is remarkable," says Mr. Holthouse, "that among the numerous writers on the subject of strabismus, there should be so little accordance as to the best test for discovering the faulty eye in those cases in which the squint shifts from one to the other. To be convinced of this, one has only to refer to the works of the three latest English writers on the subject. Walton observes, ' It is not an easy matter to determine which is the defective eye, and the sound eye is sometimes operated on. When this cannot be readily ascertained, I place the patient in front of me, at the distance of two or three yards, and direct him to cover one eye,—say the left,—and look at me with the other, keeping the head straight: the right eye will be in the centre of the orbit; I then direct him to uncover the left. Now, if the right, which has not been closed, is normal, it will keep its central position, while the left eye is turned inwards; but if it be deformed it will turn in, while the left will become straight. The experiment should be reversed.' Again : ' When a patient is under examination, he is generally excited, and exerts the orbital muscles unnaturally ; and then it is out of the question to obtain a sight of the squinting eye even in a moderately quiescent state: and hence I have sometimes been obliged to wait until a second visit to detect the faulty eye.' Mackenzie follows Lucas's rule for discovering whether one or both eyes are affected. ' We are able readily to detect non-alternating as well as alternating strabismus, by desiring the patient to look steadily with either of his eyes at any object straight before him, while with one hand we hide the object from his other eye, but keep the hand sufficiently raised towards the temple to allow us to watch the movements of the eye which is thus shaded. Whether the strabismus is alternating or non-alternating, the shaded eye is distorted. If in such a case we close both eyes, and then suddenly raise the upper lid of either while the other remains closed, the one which is opened is seen to be distorted. If both eyes are suddenly opened, the pupil of the worse eye is discovered to be more distorted than that of the better eye. If, on trying these experiments, the eye which is shaded, or either of them, on being opened suddenly showed no obliquity, we would pronounce that eye to be sound.'

"Dixon observes, ' When both eyes appear to be affected with strabismus and to turn inwards, it becomes a question which eye ought to be operated on. Various optical tests have been suggested to enable the surgeon to decide this point; but it usually happens that a patient, when subjected to any of these tests, is so anxious and embarrassed, that he becomes very liable to a sudden increase of strabismus in the eye, which, on ordinary occasions, would be affected in the slighter degree; and from this cause the experiment may fail to infallibly determine the question. I believe the best rule is, to watch attentively which eye squints in the more decided manner when the patient uses both eyes in his ordinary way, and to operate on that in which the distortion predominates.'

"In my lectures on strabismus, published two years ago, I pointed out the law which determines the alternation of the squint; and since then I have had abundant opportunities of testing its value, as well as proving the inutility of all other tests. This law may be thus expressed:—The less the difference in the visual power of the two eyes, the greater the tendency of the squint to alternate; and, conversely, the greater the difference in the visual power of each eye, the less the tendency to shift.

"The visual power, then, is the only test that can be depended on, and the rule of practice would appear to be this:—In true alternating squint, where the power of the two eyes is alike, it is immaterial which eye is operated on; while in the false, and by far the most frequent variety of alternating squint, that eye should be selected for operation the visual power of which is inferior.

"Shortly before my return from the East, I was requested by Dr. M'Craith, of Smyrna, to operate on a young Greek lady, who squinted very decidedly, though with which eye it was difficult to determine, as it continually shifted from one to the other; it seemed, however, to have a preference for the left. Walton's test failed completely; but vision was most perfect in the left; that is, in the eye apparently most affected; it was not bad in either, the patient being able to read with both, though a smaller type with the left than with the right. Notwithstanding the right eye seemed to be the straight one. I operated on it rather than on the other, owing to its less perfect vision. The correctness of the diagnosis was at once made manifest, by the extraordinary size and toughness of the tendon of the internal rectus, as well as by the rectification of the deformity in the other eye. The preference (if I may so use the term) of a squint for the better eye is a curious phenomenon that was noticed many years ago by Dr. Radcliff Hall, and is occasionally due to certain extraneous and sometimes appreciable causes. A little boy, 10 years of age, was brought to the public dispensary for a stye on the outer part of the left upper lid; the eye on the same side was also considerably inverted. At first sight, I considered that this was a case of single couvergent strabismus of the left eye; but on placing a book before it, I found its vision quite perfect; while, on placing it opposite the other, or straight eye, he could with difficulty decipher the letters. This fact at once assured me that the latter was really the strabismic organ, and that the inversion of the opposite one was only temporary. In the course of a few days the stye had disappeared; and, as I anticipated, the squint had disappeared with it, and had been transferred to the opposite eye. I think there can be little doubt that the inflammatory condition of the eyelid in this case determined the strabismus to the good eye; for the movement of the lids, being in great measure regulated by that of the eyeball, the quiescent condition of the latter in the inner canthus would entail a corresponding condition of the former, and thus the pain arising from their movements be avoided. The bad eye was thus instinctively called into requisition, so that a superficial observer would readily have mistaken it for the good one."

ART. 86.—*On operations for Convergent Strabismus.* By Mr. HOLTHOUSE.

(*Medical Times and Gazette,* May 17, 1856.)

"Shortly before my departure for the East," writes Mr. Holthouse, "I was consulted by a gentleman who had been operated on some time previously for convergent strabismus, but who now was affected with a slight divergence of the eye operated on; this, together with the retraction of the caruncle, gave to this eye an appearance of rotundity and fulness not possessed by its fellow, and the symmetry of the two was thus impaired. The patient could bring the cornea into a position equidistant from the two canthi, and could even invert it slightly; and the eversion appeared to be due rather to the new insertion of the internal rectus having taken place too far backwards, than to any hypertrophy, or overaction of its antagonist. Under these circumstances, I was unwilling to run the risk of increasing the fulness of the eye by dividing its abductor muscle, and was even doubtful how far such an operation would rectify the eversion. I accordingly pinched up a fold of conjunctiva with the subjacent fascia, internal to the cornea, and snipped it off with a pair of scissors, trusting that the contraction which would ensue from the healing of the wound might be sufficient to rectify the slight divergence. In this hope I was not disappointed, the greater fulness of the eye disappeared, the caruncula lachrymalis was drawn more towards the cornea, and the power of inverting the eye was increased. A small granulation made its appearance in the course of treatment, which required touching three or four times with the nitrate of silver. A month after the operation none but an ophthalmologist would have discovered any difference between the two eyes, and the patient took leave of me, highly gratified with the result.

"It is seldom one is called upon to remedy so slight a defect as that for which this patient consulted me. In more marked cases of abduction, following a too free division of the contracted parts in convergent strabismus, some such operation as that so ingeniously devised by Mr. Critchett, must be performed; but I am of opinion that many cases, even of primary strabismus, where slight, might be remedied by such an operation as that described in this paper."

ART. 87.—*On a special point connected with the diagnosis of Hard Cataract.* By Mr. HAYNES WALTON.

(*Medical Times and Gazette,* June 28, 1856.)

Under adult age the pupil is usually so black that any opacity is quickly recognized, and the existence of cataract at once detected; but later in life, if the power of vision be interfered with from any cause, the crystalline coloration which is then developed may deceive and induce the suspicion, if not the conviction, of the existence of cataract. Again, at the latter period, when cataract is quite incipient, and the central part of the lens is first affected, as it sometimes is, although not by any means so frequently as surgeons suppose, it may be impossible, in our present state of knowledge, to detect it, because of the "coloration," and, at best, only a broad guess can be made according to the subjective symptoms. The introduction of a case will serve as illustration. A lady, aged 75, desired Mr. Walton to examine her eyes, as an optician, to whom she had applied to have her spectacles repaired, pronounced, from the appearance of her pupils, that there was cataract. Certainly, if a brownish-gray color may be taken as indicative of this much-dreaded disease, the tradesman was justified in his supposition, as this was very apparent; but, being well aware of the possibility of deception, and the absolute necessity of a careful examination of a person who, with such eyes, could walk readily into the consulting-room, and, in front of a large window, on a bright day, take a seat without blundering, Mr. Walton reserved his opinion till after the necessary inquiry. He asked her to read with the eyes alternately, and putting on her glasses, a pair of 48-inch focus, the same very low power that she had used since such aid was required; she read rapidly, with the left eye, diamond type, and the still smaller characters on the dial-plate of my watch, while, with the other, only large print could be made out. A close inspection of the eyes did not discover any very marked difference in the crystalline lenses, till the pupils were dilated, when he perceived the disparity, which was not great, but yet unmistakable. The remark of the optician induced her to compare the power of her eyes, and until this time she was ignorant of the existing defect, an occurrence not at all uncommon. It was evident, therefore, that in both eyes "coloration" was very marked. In the left there was nothing more. In the right was added the commencement of lenticular degeneration. It is difficult to account for the fact that an amount of color so decided as to be apparent to an unprofessional bystander, and according to our notions of the physiology of the eye, more than enough to affect sight materially, did not produce a more decided result. That it has an effect by absorbing light, there can be no question; and its chief consequence is, the necessity for convex glasses in advancing life. From a very extensive examination of lenses extracted soon after death, Mr. Walton has found that the "coloration" is not uniformly in a ratio with the age of the individual, as in some persons it may be more marked at 50 than in others at 80, and he has even met with a difference in the eyes of the same individual. But this is only a confirmation of what may be observed in life, and with which he has been acquainted for years. A practical inference, therefore, is, that coloration is not a disease, not a progressive affection that destroys sight, but a slight natural change, incidental to age, and that cataract is a degeneration, a decay that progresses. It is well, however, to give some substantial proofs of the correctness of these views, and, in order to this, Mr. Walton refers to that which has been afforded by the labor of his colleague, Mr. R. Taylor, who has been investigating the matter microscopically. He writes: "In elderly people, without an exception, so far as I have observed, the lens assumes an amber color, more or less deep. The age at which this change commences varies exceedingly. I have seen it distinctly present at 30, and very strongly marked at 35, while, again, it has been but slight in a person of 60. Generally speaking, it will be found at the age of 40; I have never failed to find it at 45. It appears to be more easily developed in the colored races, and in persons with any admixture of black blood; but my opportunities of observation on this point have been very limited. The color pervades the whole of the lens, but is most intense in the nucleus, and fades off gradually in the cortical layers. When the 'coloration' is very intense, it impedes the transmission of light, so as to impair the sight, though the lens remains perfectly clear and free from opacity. Such persons see best in a bright light, and are frequently benefited by convex glasses, which concentrate the light. Notwithstanding the depth of color, I have never heard any complaint of a yellow hue being thrown over objects, as is the case in looking through a piece of yellow glass, nor is there any difficulty in distinguishing different shades, even of blue and green. The coloring matter, which is said to be iron, is in solution. There are not any pigment-cells or granules; which last, it is said, are found in black cataracts.

"The coloration does not appear to interfere in any way with the healthy condition of the lens; in the oldest which I have examined, from a woman, 93 years of age, the lens tubes, both nuclear and cortical, were perfectly healthy; though they, as well as the superficial cells, were tinged of a bright amber color. In cataract, on the contrary, the lens is disorganized; the superficial layers are softened and broken up, so as, in advanced cases, to be reduced almost to the condition of a pulp, which renders the drop of water, in which it is examined, turbid and milky. The opacity is due chiefly to a quantity of fine molecular matter, the result of the coagulation of the albuminous blastema of the lens, which is found partly aggregated in masses, and partly studding the exterior, perhaps also the interior of the tubes, as well as, in many instances, filling the large globular cells which lie immediately within the capsule. Occasionally, in cases of long duration, crystals of cholesterine are found interspersed among the lenticular débris. The nucleus also undergoes a very remarkable change, becoming hard and dry to an extent very far from anything that is ever seen in the healthy lens of the oldest persons. The tubes are withered, atrophied, and brittle, and fall asunder and in fragments on the slightest touch of the dissecting needle. Their outlines are disfigured by deep, transverse, and longitudinal cracks and fissures, and by irregular nodules, probably of coagulated albumen, and in many instances they show a tendency to split into minute fibrillæ." It is evident, therefore, that on the recognition of these data, and the practical application of them, much error may be avoided, and the absence or existence of cataract rendered more certain, not to speak of the assistance that they offer in unravelling other ophthalmic disease; for lenticular "coloration" has been described as an objective symptom of other affections, "amaurosis" being one of these. It would answer no good purpose to tell of any of the many cases of "coloration" and impaired vision, not due to opacity of the lens, that have been sent by surgeons for operation, under the supposition that cataract existed, nor of other mistakes connected with the subject that have come under the author's notice, such as the extraction of lenses, not cataractous, but merely colored. Mistakes are frequently made. In the case detailed, it is easy to understand that there had been defective sight in the left eye, from disease at the posterior part of the eyeball, how readily it might have been supposed that cataract was present. It may be received as a rule, that, if a person can see to read the smallest type with or without glasses, and discern distant objects clearly, the pupil being undilated, no matter how clouded the lenses may appear, cataract does not exist. After this is understood, the only point on which there can be difficulty is to pronounce whether, in any given case of defective sight, cataract is present or absent; and the solution of which, so far as it can be told, depends on the proper discrimination of physical appearances, the distinction between "coloration" and lenticular degeneration rather than on any subjective symptoms, although these may greatly assist. With undilated pupils it is difficult, if not often impossible, to recognize the difference. Surgeons of the first eminence in this metropolis err respecting it; hence the necessity, whenever doubt exists, for dilatation. Then, in the expanded pupil, the presence of striæ or opaque bundles of fibres, which so commonly exist in the early stage of cataract, at the circumference of the lens, can at once be detected. "Coloration" is more central and browner, the light penetrates the lens, and the concentration of it is perceptible in the direction in which it falls. The opacity of cataract is more diffused and opaque, and reflects the light. In the first, vision is made worse by dilatation of the pupil, while in the other it is almost always improved, certainly always when the opacity is marked. Indeed, when the pupil is dilated, it is seldom that a correct conclusion cannot be arrived at. The exception is this: when the lenticular degeneration is yet slight, and has commenced in the centre, it may be impossible to detect it, that is, to be able to say with certainty that cataract is present, and the lapse of time only can decide. The late Mr. Dalrymple treated a gentleman for amaurosis. He had prescribed an arsenical preparation for some time without benefit. Mr. Walton was then consulted, and, after a long investigation, he decided that cataract was present, at least in one eye. This disease soon became palpable, and in time he operated on both eyes with the best success. There had never appeared the slightest amaurotic symptom. Can there be a stronger proof that there may be uncertainty in the matter? When vision is much affected by loss of transparency in the lens, the opacity must be palpable; therefore, when this is not readily detected, any material loss of visual power must be attributed to some other cause, and this applies especially to defective vision in the very aged, in whom the "coloration" is most marked, and when the eye, in obedience to the laws of mortality, which allows an exception, perhaps, only in the prostate gland, is apt to get shrunken, and also becomes, so to speak, vitally impaired. Several times, under these circumstances, Mr. Walton prevented the performance of a needless operation, and proved that a feeble retina was the defective cause. Mr. Walton has not found the ophthalmoscope of any service in this matter.

ART. 88.—*On the Treatment of Traumatic Cataract.*
By J. H. SOLOMON.

(*Assoc. Med. Journ.*, March 15, 1856.)

In a paper read before the Birmingham and Midland Counties Branch of the Prov. Med. and Surg. Association, Mr. Solomon, after giving an outline of the physiological anatomy of the lens and its capsule, which, he said, was of interest, by throwing light upon some of the nutritional changes of which the lens is the subject, and as affording a *rationale* of certain operations which are performed for their cure, defined traumatic cataract as an opacity of the lens or its capsule, in consequence of a blow upon, or penetrating wound of the eyeball. Mr. Solomon then considered the subject under three heads.

a. In cases of traumatic cataract, attended by little or no inflammation, and where the capsule having been ruptured accidentally the lens is undergoing absorption, his practice is to break it up ten or fourteen days after the accident, and clear the pupil of capsule, and so prevent the formation of a capsular cataract within the area of the pupil. The operation is performed by penetrating the cornea with a fine needle, &c. (Keratonyxis). Where the case is complicated by an ununited wound of the cornea, his first care is to obtain union by closing the eyelids with strips of plaster, and enjoining rest of the organ. Prior to which any portion of recently protruding iris is returned within the anterior chamber by gently pressing upon it with the spoon end of the "curette," whilst the patient is under the influence of chloroform; but when that drug is contraindicated, or lymph covers the irident tumor, it must be snipped off, unless it should happen to be very small, with a pair of sharp-cutting eye scissors. When the wound is central, belladonna is to be immediately applied to the brow and a drop of atropine to the conjunctiva; but when such is not the case, the application must be delayed until cicatrization has taken place.

b. In cases where the cataract is dislocated against the back of the iris, or is pushing its way through the pupil, and is attended by severe ocular pain and inflammation, Mr. Solomon's invariable practice is to extract the lens by Gibson's operation, which, by removing a cause of irritation, alleviates suffering and accelerates recovery. In the event of these cases being treated only by the ordinary means applicable to internal inflammation of the eyeball, all the symptoms are protracted, and the pupil remains small and obstructed by thickened opaque capsule or organized lymph. Moreover, the deep-seated structures are prone to be affected by inflammatory disorganization. In a word, the eye is left, on the subsidence of the ophthalmia, in a very unfavorable condition for any operation that may be at any time undertaken with the intention of clearing the pupillary aperture, unless the canula scissors can be made of use. It is in this class of cases that chalky or bony material forms within the capsule.

c. With regard to cases of single traumatic cataract, occurring in an organ in other respects, as far as can be judged, healthy, the author advocates the operation of solution (Keratonyxis), on the grounds that it (1) removes a deformity which, to many persons, is a serious obstacle to their comfort and well-being in life; and that (2) it tends, if the patient occasionally exercise the eye by wearing a suitable cataract spectacle, to preserve a healthy condition of the retina. Deprive an organ, he said, of its natural stimulus, and its nutrition will become either feeble or perverted; in illustration of which might be cited those cases where amblyopia or amaurosis is persistent after the removal of a congenital cataract from an adult.

The primary effect of the removal of a single cataract, as respects vision, is in many instances to render it double or confused; the patient, however, soon ceases to regard the impressions conveyed through the retina of the eye which has lost its lens, and recovers single and clear vision. In illustration of this, the cases recorded by Dr. Andrew Smith, in the "Edinburgh Medical and Surgical Journal," No. 74, are most apposite and conclusive. Three saw objects double when the bandage was first removed, and for nearly twenty-four hours, and then singly. Two saw double about three hours; and one of them, two days afterwards, upon being surprised, and opening his eyelids suddenly, experienced, for a few seconds, the same imperfection. A sixth saw constantly double for four days, and after that, as distinctly as ever he did; and the other three cases, as above remarked, always single.

ART. 89.—*On extraction of Cataract by a single stroke.* By M. CHASSAIGNAC.

(*Mon. des Hôp.*, No. 74, 1856; *Med.-Chir. Rev.* Oct., p. 550.)

M. Chassaignac observes that several oculists, and especially Wenzel, have extracted cataracts at a single stroke: opening the capsule as the knife traversed the anterior chamber on its way out. This procedure, which has hitherto been justly considered as an exhibition of a somewhat dangerous dexterity, may be very well accomplished by the aid of chloroform. It offers, indeed, great advantages; for, whatever may be the dilatation at the moment of commencing the operation, it contracts immediately after the escape of the aqueous humor, and the knife introduced subsequently may easily wound the iris. In this operation, the pupil remaining wide open, the accident is not to be feared. In other respects, however, Wenzel's operation was really dangerous, and presented difficulties well-nigh insurmountable without the aid of chloroform.

M. Chassaignac habitually employs chloroform in his operations for cataract, and the advantages he has derived from it he thinks are due to the observance of the proper principles that should regulate its employment. No patient can be operated upon with security if he has not been brought to the stage of tolerance, that he sleeps deeply and placidly, without irregular movements, restlessness, cries, or delirium. His respiration is normal, his *facies* excellent, his pulse large and full—presenting, in a word, an assemblage of conditions not only well suited to tranquillize the surgeon, but also eminently fitted to facilitate the execution of the operation. Vastly different is it to operate upon an eye rendered quite immovable, and to act upon one essentially mobile, and incessantly seeking to escape from the action of the instruments. Among the accidents thus avoided, is wounding the hyaloid membrane. It is in fact almost always to this accident, and not to the pressure exerted upon the globe of the eye, that is due the escape of more or less of the vitreous humor after cataract operations. This almost inevitable accident, when operating without chloroform, is easily avoided in the immovable state of the eye. The same may be said of wounds of the iris, and most of the accidents consequent on extraction. The possibility of producing vomiting has been urged as an objection to the use of chloroform in this operation, but, by waiting before commencing the operation until the period of tolerance has been reached, M. Chassaignac has never met with vomiting or struggling.

ART. 90.—*On the operation of extraction in certain cases of Artificial and Closed Pupil.* By Mr. CRITCHETT, Surgeon to the Royal London Ophthalmic Hospital, &c.

(*Lancet*, June 21, 1856.)

In this paper Mr. Critchett notices some cases of ophthalmic disease that afford types of certain conditions that have hitherto been peculiarly embarrassing and unsuccessful in their treatment, and he founds upon these cases suggestions for a method of operating that is at variance with rules hitherto laid down by the best authorities on diseases of the eye.

"There are two morbid conditions to which I desire especially to draw attention. The first is where an artificial pupil has been made, and the lens or its capsule, or both, are found to be opaque at the time of the operation, or to have become so at a subsequent period. The second is where, in consequence of some form of iritis, the pupil is small, irregular, and more or less adherent, and the small portion of the capsule that is visible presents a white opacity, with a fringe of uveal deposit, the amount of both varying much in different cases. In the first of these conditions, one of two complications exists: if it be a case of penetrating ulcer or wound of the cornea, with a dense opacity of a portion of the cornea, in which an artificial pupil has been made opposite to the most transparent part of the cornea, under these circumstances, the anterior chamber is small and shallow, and the amount of aqueous humor is of necessity very limited, and far below the normal average; if, again, it has been a case in which the disease has been in the iris and lens, there will be a morbid condition of the aqueous chamber, and a proneness to the lighting up of a slow form of inflammation of the deeper textures of the eye. In the second of these conditions, in which the pupil is small, irregular, and adherent to an opaque lens, the sight is often seriously damaged, and it is difficult to determine how far this is due to visible changes in the lens and its capsule and the iris, and how far to changes in the deeper textures consequent upon the former iritis. The previous history, and the appearance of the eye, are our only guides in determining this.

"In both classes of cases, where an artificial pupil has been made, and the lens is found to be opaque, or has become so at a subsequent period, it is a most important point to determine what is the safest and most successful method of getting the cataract out of the field of vision. The best and more recent authorities seem to be very meagre and unsatisfactory upon this point. In the last edition of Mackenzie's work, I have not found any allusion to the complication of cataract with artificial pupil. He merely states generally, that extraction should never be attempted where any adhesion exists between the iris and the capsule of the lens. Mr. Haynes Walton writes as follows: ' When the pupil is adherent to a capsulolenticular cataract, and the cornea is sufficiently clear in the centre to allow it to be seen, the cataract must be first attended to. This has been fully dwelt on under the head of Drilling.' 'When the opacity of the cornea precludes the application of instruments to the centre of the iris, or when adhesion of the iris to the cornea renders it impossible that the cataract can be operated upon without transfixing the iris, the pupil should first be made, and the opaque lens be disposed of afterwards—that is, by a subsequent operation for *solution* or *displacement.*' Mr. Dixon does not, as far as I can perceive, lay down any rules upon this point in the body of his work on the Eye, but in the appendix he mentions a case which is so applicable to this subject that I beg to quote it.

"'John R—, æt. 67, presented himself in June, 1852, in the following condition: both pupils were very small and irregular, and closed by a whitish membrane, evidently the product of old iritis. I made an artificial pupil. I was sorry to find the lens opaque, and presenting the ordinary appearance of a firm senile cataract. To extract or to depress this seemed equally out of the question, on account of its firm adhesion to the iris—to say nothing of the objections which, to my mind, always exist against ' depression' as an unscientific and destructive operation. I had therefore no alternative but to get rid of the lens by solution. The needle was first used about the beginning of August, again at the end of September, and again early in December. Early in March the edge of the cataract opposite to the artificial pupil was absorbed, the bulk remaining unacted upon. With a convex glass, the patient could read large type.'

" The above quotations from these modern authors tend to show that but little attention has been given to this point, and the few hints that are thrown out suggest the operation of solution or of depression as the only alternatives. *A priori* reasoning would lead to the conclusion that these two operations offer but faint prospects of success. Solution is not a very prosperous operation even in a normal condition, unless the cataract is soft; but when the anterior chamber is diminished in size, and the aqueous humor is lessened in quantity, the very conditions upon which absorption depends are very materially curtailed, the space in which the fragments of the broken lens lodge is too small, and the old disease to which the change in the eye has owed its existence, is prone to be aroused. These form serious objections to this operation under such circumstances; and, I may add, that the unfavorable results which have seemed theoretically probable, I have found, in several instances, practically true. It was the occurrence of an unsuccessful case, in which, after making an artificial pupil, and carefully breaking up the cataract, destructive inflammation ensued, that led me to the conclusion that it is an unsuitable and dangerous operation. As regards 'depression,' I quite agree with Mr. Dixon, that it is always an unscientific operation, and, under the conditions I am now considering, peculiarly so. If the cataract be soft, it is impracticable; and, if hard, the adhesions very much increase the probability of its rising again into the axis of vision, and the previously diseased state of the eye renders the presence of a cataract floating in the vitreous humor a most undesirable and dangerous complication.

" These very serious, and even fatal, objections to these two modes of operating in cases of artificial pupil, complicated with cataract, led me carefully to reconsider the whole subject, and to examine into the force and validity of the objections to extraction through an artificial pupil. They may be stated as follows : First. The adhesions that exist between the capsule and the iris. Secondly. The unyielding character of the artificial pupil preventing the escape of the cataract. Thirdly. The risk that, in cases where an opacity of the cornea already exists, the flap that is made for the removal of the cataract may not unite, or, if it does unite, may lose its transparency.

" The more I reflected on this subject, the more I felt inclined to doubt the validity of these objections. The adhesions, which are always considered by ophthalmic surgeons as entirely prohibiting extraction, only exist between the capsule of the lens and the iris. The cataract itself lies as loose as ever within its capsule, and will as readily escape when the capsule is freely opened; so that this, which has always been regarded as the principal objection, is quite fallacious and unsubstantial.

" The other two objections have not been found of any weight when put to the test of experiment. I am, therefore, of opinion, that in all cases where opacity of the lens coexists with an artificial pupil, the opaque lens should be extracted through the artificial pupil. If it occur in a young person, and the cataract is soft, it may be removed through a small opening, just sufficient to admit the spoon of the curette, with which it may be gradually but effectually removed. When the cataract is firm, and of the usual size, a section must be made close to the junction of the cornea with the sclerotic, and in such a position that the flap corresponds with the artificial pupil; the capsule must be opened in the usual way, and the cataract may be gradually pressed out just as readily as in an ordinary case of cataract. One inconvenience that frequently attends the operation of extraction in a normal eye—I mean prolapse of the iris—never can occur in consequence of the artificial pupil. I have had several cases illustrative of these points, out of which I propose to select the following :

CASE 1.—Mary Anne A—, æt. 28, came under my care, at the London Hospital, early last June. About a year previously she had entirely lost the right eye, the globe of which was shrunk. In the left eye there had been a penetrating ulcer, with complete adhesion of the pupillary margin of the iris to the corneal cicatrix; the anterior chamber was consequently diminished both in depth and circumference; about half the cornea retained its transparency; the iris also appeared healthy, with its fibres tightly drawn towards the cicatrix, to which it was firmly adherent. The patient could just distinguish light from dark; and had been in that condition about nine months when she first came under my care. The first step towards the restoration of sight was the formation of an artificial pupil, which was made in the following manner: a small opening was made in the cornea, close to its junction with the sclerotic; the canular forceps were introduced, and a strip of iris was drawn away from its attachments to the scar in the cornea, and having been brought through the opening, was cut off. A well-defined, narrow, oblong pupil, was thus formed obliquely upwards and outwards, opposite the largest clear surface of the cornea. It was then found that the lens was opaque. About three weeks after the first operation, I made a small section in the cornea, about a line and a half in extent; and after opening the capsule with a needle, with the aid of the spoon of the curette, the cataract, which was soft, was gradually and completely removed, good union took place, and the patient recovered her sight so far as to be able to read with a suitable lens.

CASE 2.—James B—, æt. 54, first applied to me at the Ophthalmic Hospital about eight years ago, in the following condition: the left globe was shrunk, and had been destroyed some years previously from inflammation. In the right eye the lower half of the cornea was densely opaque, and the pupil was partially adherent, and drawn down behind the opacity so that there was no useful vision. I succeeded, with Tyrrell's blunt hook, in making a well-defined oblong pupil directly upwards opposite the transparent part of the cornea; the lens was not injured. For above seven years he enjoyed useful vision, and earned his living. At the end of that time his sight began gradually to fail, and when he again applied to me, being about eight years after the first operation, he was once more nearly blind. On examination, I found a dense amber cataract occupying the pupil. After much deliberation, I determined to attempt extraction. I had never tried such an operation, nor had I ever heard of its being done, and I could not help fearing that a hard fully formed cataract might refuse to pass through an artificial pupil, and even if that difficulty were overcome that the flap might become opaque. I was, however, agreeably surprised to find that the operation was as easy and as successful as an ordinary case of extraction. I made the upper section close to the sclerotic, and very nearly of the usual size. Everything progressed favorably, and in a few weeks after the operation my patient was able, with a suitable lens, to see as well as after the first operation.

CASE 3.—William L—, æt. 31, came under the care of my colleague, Mr. Wordsworth, in January last. The left eye was irretrievably lost; in the right eye there was a faint perception of objects; the pupil was small, irregular, and adherent to the capsule of the lens, which was opaque. Mr. Wordsworth made the man an artificial pupil downwards and outwards, with a pair of canular forceps, so as not to injure the lens or its capsule—a method that was, I believe, suggested and first executed by my friend Mr. White Cooper. Soon after this, the man came under my care. Very little improvement of sight followed this operation. On examination, an opaque lens, with its defined sharp edge, could be plainly seen through the artificial pupil. I extracted this very readily through a moderate-sized section; good union took place, and the artificial pupil closed again. A few weeks after, I opened this with two needles in such a way that I once more succeeded in getting a small and nearly central pupil, through which he has now very useful vision. These cases, at least, prove the possibility of extracting a cataract, even when hard and fully formed, through an artificial pupil of average size, and the fair prospect of success with which such an operation may be undertaken. It is one which I should always perform in future, and I feel assured that, as contrasted with former methods, it enormously increases the patient's prospect of recovering sight. There is another class of cases equally important and more numerous, to which I have applied the same principle. I allude to cases, the result of old and neglected iritis of a chronic character, in which the pupil is small, irregular, and adherent, and the capsule of the lens, and sometimes the lens itself, are opaque, and in which, as a consequence, there is no useful vision, and to which I propose to direct attention in another paper.

ART. 91.—*On anæmic protrusion of the Eyeball.*
By Mr. R. TAYLOR, Surgeon to the London Ophthalmic Hospital.
(*Medical Times and Gazette,* May 24, 1856.)

A key to the pathology of this obscure affection, Mr. Taylor thinks, "has been given by Dr. Marshall Hall in his valuable writings on the subject of convulsive and paroxysmal diseases. He has shown that, in such diseases, there is a tendency to spasm of the muscles of the neck; and that the seizures are the direct result of impeded return of blood from the head, the deep-seated veins being compressed by the irregular muscular action. Now, the subjects of anæmic protrusion of the eyeball are eminently of the class to which Dr. Hall's remarks apply. Some of them are subject to fits, hysterical or epileptic; in all, the nervous system is in a state of extreme excitability, so that the slightest agitation produces starting and trembling, sometimes so violent as almost to resemble convulsion in a minor degree. Is it not probable that, as in the confirmed epileptics, there may in these cases also be an impediment to the free return of blood from the head, only to a less amount, and perhaps more continuously? In the only two post-mortem examinations that have been made, the internal jugular veins were found to be greatly dilated, as though they had long been subject to distension by some obstructing cause towards the lower part of their course; and, as in neither case was there any solid growth by which they could have been compressed, it does not seem unreasonable to suppose that the obstacle was due to muscular spasm. The same explanation would account for the enlargement of the thyroid gland, which, as has been already stated, is due to simple hypertrophy of its normal structures, and would be a probable result of long-continued hyperæmia. The palpitation of the heart does not require any explanation here, as it is common to all cases of anæmia, whether accompanied or not with protrusion of the eyes.

"The different stages of the disease, then, may be stated as follow: First, some debilitating disease, or exhausting discharge, producing—secondly, anæmia; thirdly, that peculiar state of the nervous system, in which there is a tendency to spasm of the muscles of the neck; fourthly, as the result of such spasm, and consequent impeded return of blood from the head, hyperæmia and hypertrophy of the thyroid gland, and dilatation of the veins of the orbit, causing exophthalmia."

These remarks are offered suggestively, but at the same time it is necessary to say that they have arisen out of a careful consideration of the cases which have fallen under Mr. Taylor's own notice, as well as of the cases recorded by others. Mr. Taylor's cases are three in number.

"Case 1.—Mrs. T., aged 26, has been married eight years, but has never been pregnant. Her menstrual periods have been regular; but the discharge has always been in excess, and she had several attacks of menorrhagia, losing much blood on each occasion. She has long been subject to leucorrhœa, which, six months ago, became very profuse, and shortly after this she was attacked with palpitation of the heart. About the same time she observed a swelling in her throat, and her eyes became so prominent as to attract the attention of her friends. These symptoms, which appeared as nearly as possible simultaneously, have gone on increasing slowly but steadily. Leeches and tincture of iodine have been applied to the throat, but without producing any diminution in the swelling.

"Present State.—She is very pale and feeble. She suffers from spinal tenderness, intercostal neuralgia, ringing in the ears, œdema of the ankles, and other symptoms of anæmia. She is exceedingly nervous, starting and trembling violently when suddenly addressed; she has occasional hysteric fits. The pulsations of the heart averaged 134 per minute, and are very distressing; the carotid arteries also throb violently. The thyroid gland is enlarged to about three times its natural size, its surface being smooth and regular; several of its enlarged arteries can be felt pulsating near the surface. The eyeballs protrude so as to expose a broad rim of the sclerotica around the margin of the cornea, giving her a wild and staring appearance, which attracts attention and exposes her to annoyance in the streets. The amount of protrusion varies, within certain limits, with the degree of nervous excitement, being always much greater when she is agitated. The eyeballs can be readily replaced by gentle pressure, but they speedily resume their prominence when the pressure is remitted. There is some congestion of the conjunctival vessels, and slight increase of the meibomian and mucous secretions; in other respects the eyes have a healthy appearance; their movements are perfect in every direction, and the sight is unimpaired. The eyelids, which are of a dusky color, cannot be closed without a slight muscular effort.

"The treatment, which extended over a period of three months, consisted in the administration of iron in several forms; astringent injections, per vaginam, to check the leucorrhœa; and belladonna plasters over the region of the heart, which afforded great relief by diminishing the violence of the palpitation. As her general health improved, the heart's action approached more and more to the natural standard, and the prominence of the eyeballs was reduced, until they ultimately resumed their proper position: but no change took place in the size of the thyroid gland so long as she remained under observation. She subsequently had a slight relapse, brought on apparently by mental agitation, but a similar plan of treatment again proved successful in a few weeks.

"Case 2.—Mrs. C., aged 40, has had eight children, the last two of whom were twins, and were born four years ago. One of these she suckled for twelve, and the other for sixteen months; during which time, as on previous similar occasions, she menstruated regularly and abundantly. When she had suckled both infants for a year, she first observed an enlargement of her throat, and the swelling increased slowly for about two years, since which it has remained stationary. Some months after she first observed this enlargement her eyes began to protrude, so as to attract the attention of her friends. She then applied to a surgeon, who told her that she had disease of the heart—a fact which she then learned for the first time, as she had never felt the slightest uneasiness in that region; how long the palpitation may have existed it is impossible to say, as even now, although it is very violent, she is quite unconscious of it, unless when much excited.

"*Present State.*—Pale, anæmic, and highly excitable. The eyeballs protrude so as to expose a narrow rim of sclerotica around the cornea. They can be readily replaced by gentle pressure; their movements are perfect in every direction, and the vision is unimpaired. The protrusion varies with the amount of nervous excitement. The conjunctivæ are slightly injected, but in other respects the eyes appear to be perfectly healthy. The heart beats violently and rapidly, the pulsations being 142 per minute; but it is probable that this exceeds the usual standard, and is partly due to excitement, consequent on a stethoscopic examination. The carotid arteries pulsate strongly and visibly. The thyroid gland is enlarged, chiefly in a lateral direction, to more than thrice its natural size; its surface is smooth and regular.

"The treatment was conducted upon the same general plan as in the preceding case, and extended, with one or two interruptions, over a period of five months. The general health was restored, and the eyes resumed their natural position; but there was not any diminution in the size of the goitre.

"In each of the above cases, a careful stethoscopic examination of the chest was made by my friend Dr. Hare, who has kindly permitted me to condense and make use of his report.

"In the first, there was some hypertrophy, with a little dilatation of the heart, but no valvular disease. In the second, the condition of the heart was almost exactly similar, but there was a doubtful murmur with the first sound, the exact nature of which could not be clearly ascertained, on account of the excited state of the circulation at the time.

"Case 3.—I have reserved this case for the last, although it is the first entered in my case-book, as I am desirous of calling attention to a very striking peculiarity which it presented, in the sudden appearance of the exophthalmia.

"Letitia M., aged 21, was subject to fits, probably epileptic, in childhood. These gradually ceased as she attained the period of puberty, but she remained excessively nervous and hysterical, and has long suffered from spinal tenderness, intercostal neuralgia, coldness of the extremities, and other symptoms of nervous debility. Three years ago, after a fall by which she severely bruised her right side, she began to suffer from palpitation of the heart; this has continued ever since, being constant and annoying, interrupting her sleep, and greatly aggravated by the slightest agitation or exertion. One year after this, the thyroid gland began to enlarge, and gradually increased until it attained its present volume, about four times that of the healthy gland. She was for some time under hospital treatment for this as well as for the palpitation, but without receiving any benefit. About a week before I first saw her, she felt an unusual sensation in the brows one morning on awaking, and on looking in the mirror she found that her eyes, which had been perfectly natural in appearance when she retired to rest, were protruded to such an extent that she could scarcely close the eyelids.

"*Present State.*—The eyeballs protrude as above described; their movements are perfect; the sight is not impaired, and they appear to be perfectly healthy. They can be readily replaced by gentle pressure, but resume their abnormal position when the hand is removed. She says that the prominence varies very much, and that at times it is scarcely perceptible. The action of the heart is very violent; the pulsations, under the excitement of being examined, are 140 per minute. There is a slight blowing murmur with the first sound; on percussion, the dulness over the heart is rather more extensive than natural. The carotid arteries throb violently. The enlarged thyroid gland is smooth and regular, and several of its dilated arteries can be felt near the surface.

"Under treatment of a similar character to that adopted in the preceding cases, and extending over rather more than two months, the eyes had very nearly resumed their normal position, and the general health was very much improved, but there was no diminution in the size of the thyroid gland. She then left town, and I have not had an opportunity of seeing her since."

ART. 92.—*Speculum Oculi and Ophthalmostat.* By Dr. J. RITCHIE BROWN.

(*Medical Times and Gazette*, Oct. 18, 1856.)

To the already long list of inventions for retracting the eyelids and fixing the eyeball, Dr. Brown adds another, which combines, to a certain extent, the properties

Fig. 3.

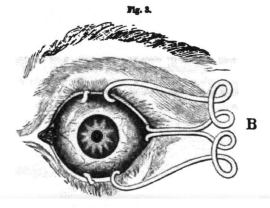

of each. It is a combination of the old and much approved wire speculum of Pellier, with the fixateur of Nelaton. The diagram will at once explain its construction. It is made of one piece of German silver wire.

Fig. 4.

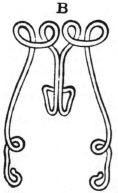

The intermediate part, B, is first placed in the fold of the conjunctiva, which connects the external angle of the lids with the globe of the eye; the retractors are then adapted to the lids. By the pressure of the part B on the cul-de-sac of the conjunctiva, the eyeball is completely prevented from turning inwards.

To persons who have no assistant it will prove useful, as it leaves both hands free for such operations as artificial pupil, strabismus, snipping off small tumors, &c.; and this advantage is gained without any additional risk or pain to the patient, which can hardly be said of the ophthalmostats of Jaegar, Gräfe, or Rothmund.

The part B might also be adapted, by means of a tube soldered to the spring, in which it may slide, so as to be regulated to avoid pressure on the eyeball, or be removed altogether at pleasure.

ART. 93.—*A new plan of treating Obstruction of the Nasal Duct.*
By Mr. T. WESTROPP, of Clifton.

(*Medical Times and Gazette*, June 7, 1856.)

"I have long thought," says Mr. Westropp, "that by carefully and frequently passing up from the nostril a catheter of very small calibre, we might be able to cure those cases without the disagreeable necessity of making a deforming incision at the angle of the eye, which patients much object to. I propose that a fine wire of silver or gold, or a fine bit of catgut, be passed down through the puncta and brought out at the nostril; on this let a No. 1 catheter be passed up to the lachrymal sac, in the same way that a catheter, with its point cut off, is passed along a piece of gut previously pushed through a stricture into the bladder.

"The various measures already practised for improving the general health and removing local vascularity, should be first had recourse to. In addition to the lotions in common use, I would recommend a collyrium composed of iodide and bromide of potassium dissolved in water, a few grains of each to the ounce; this may tend to produce absorption of the effused lymph, or correct the thickened state of the lining membrane. I have used such a lotion with benefit in opacities of the cornea. In addition, the power of the tensor tarsi, or Horner's muscle, might be restored from its long distension by a lotion containing strychnia, or by the endermic application of strychnia over the sac.

"I have been on the point of putting this mechanical contrivance to the test in two appropriate cases, but, unfortunately, the patients ceased to attend when they were relieved of the inflammatory symptoms."

ART. 94.—*A new method of reducing Dislocation of the lower Jaw.*
By Dr. LEO.

(*Deutshe Klinik;* and *Gaz. Méd. de Paris*, June 7, 1856.)

The method here described consists in reducing each condyle *separately*. The patient being seated in a chair, the surgeon places himself behind him towards the right side, and fixes his head against his chest, and having done this he introduces the thumb of the right hand into the patient's mouth and presses upon the posterior molars, until he feels the jaw move downwards, when he pushes the condyle into its cavity by a backward motion. After this he repeats this operation with the left hand on the other side.

An experimental trial of this method, in two cases, has convinced the author that the reduction is more easily accomplished in this way than in the ordinary way.

(B) CONCERNING THE CHEST, ABDOMEN, AND PELVIS.

ART. 95.—*Statistics of the operation for tying the Brachio-cephalic Artery.*
By Drs. PAUL and EVE.

(*Philadelphia Medical Examiner*, Aug., 1856.)

These statistics are from a paper containing the history of the different cases in which this operation has been performed. They require no comment.

Statistics of attempts to obliterate the Brachio-cephalic.

Surgeon.	Year.	Age.	Sex.	Result and Cause of Death.
1. Mott, . .	1818	57	Male	Death on the 26th day, from repeated hemorrhage.
2. Graefe, . .	1822	Adult	"	Death on the 65th day, from hemorrhage.
3. Norman, .	1824	"	—	Death.
4. Arendt, .	1826	—	—	Death on the 8th day, from inflammation of sac, pleura, and lung.
5. Hall, . .	1830	Adult	Male	Death on the 6th day, from dyspnœa and hemorrhage.
6. Bland, . .	1832	31	"	Death on the 18th day, from repeated hemorrhage.
7. Bujalski, .	before 1840	—	—	Death on the 2d or 3d day.
8. Bujalski, .	1840	—	—	Death on the 2d or 3d day.
9. Lizars, . .	1836	30	Male	Death on the 21st day, from repeated hemorrhage.
10. Dupuytren,	—	—	"	
11. Hutin, . .	1842	Adult	"	Death on the 11th hour; antecedent hemorrhage and exhaustion.
12. Porter, . .	1831	—	—	No ligature; patient recovered.
13. Kuhl, . .	1836	43	—	Death on the 3d day, of hemorrhage.
14. Liston, . .	1838	Adult	Male	Death on the 13th day.
15. Key, . .	1844	"	Female	Failed, yet patient died of pulmonary distress and exhaustion.
16. Hoffman, .	about 1840	—	—	Died.

In reality the ligature was tied around the innominata in only ten of these cases, viz.: Mott's, Graefe's, Norman's, Arendt's, Bland's, Bujalski's, Bujalski's, Lizars' Dupuytren's, and Hutin's. In Hall's the ligature was passed through the artery; in Kuhl's and Liston's the carotid and subclavian were tied just beyond the bifurcation; and in Porter's, Key's, and Hoffmann's the operation was abandoned and no ligature employed.

In every case where a ligature was applied, either to the brachio-cephalic or near its division into right subclavian and right carotid, namely, in 13 cases, death has followed; even in 2 where the operation was abandoned there was a fatal result in 1; and in the sixteen cases 1 alone recovered, and in that no ligature was used, the vessel having been simply exposed; the cure in this case was spontaneous, and in all probability entirely independent of the operation.

ART. 96.—*Practical deductions from a clinical record of twenty-six cases of Strangulated Hernia.* By MR. BIRKETT.

(*Medical Times and Gazette*, May 3, 1856.)

The object of this paper (which was read before the Medical Society of London, 26th April, 1856) is, first to bring prominently into the foreground the causes of death; secondly, the circumstances by which those causes are brought about; and, thirdly, the means by which they may be avoided. It is shown, by means of a table of the cases, that a certain number of unfavorable circumstances occurred in each case, and that in proportion to the aggregate, as a general rule, the case was cured, or terminated fatally. But in some of the cases only two, three, or four unfavorable circumstances existed, and yet the patients died; and in these, as well as others with a large number, the causes of death are sought for and demonstrated. Of the 26 cases, all of whom were operated upon by the author, one half terminated fatally. In the fatal cases, death resulted from causes over which the operation could have but little influence; and it was undertaken only with the view to place the patient in a condition more favorable to recovery. The causes inducing the fatal result may be thus enumerated:

1. The consequences of a journey performed while the patient was suffering with strangulated hernia.
2. The defective constitutional nutrition of the patients generally.
3. Irrecoverable prostration, the result of long-continued vomiting and strangulation of the bowel in aged women.
4. Violence inflicted on the hernia. To this cause the death of not less than 5 out of the 13 is to be attributed.
5. The administration of purgatives before the operation.

The author unhesitatingly preferred to reduce the hernia without opening the peritoneal sac in those cases in which the surgeon would be justified in returning the protrusion by the taxis, if it could be accomplished.

In the 26 cases the peritoneal sac was opened in 12, and the causes which prevented the reduction of the hernia without so operating were the three following:

1. The contents of the sac.
2. The morbid condition of the contents of the sac.
3. The dimensions of the neck of the sac, and the unyielding state of its tissue.

Six cases were related in which the author had reduced the hernia by a simple division of the fibrous tissues about the neck of the sac, and external to that covering of the hernia known as the fascia propria. To this simple method of relieving the constriction around the bowel the author gave the name of "The Minimum Operation." The causes of death in the fatal cases were shown, by post-mortem examination, to be referable to peritonitis; injury of the bowel inflicted in the taxis; exhaustion after fæcal fistula; phlegmonous inflammation; collapse; acute bronchitis; and perforation of the bowel. Of the cured cases, the minimum of time during which the bowel was strangulated, was three hours; the maximum seventy-seven hours. Of the fatal cases, the minimum period of strangulation of the bowel was eleven hours; the maximum seventy-nine hours. Of the cured cases, the average number of hours during which the bowel was strangulated amounted to thirty-three. Of the fatal cases, the average period of strangulation of the bowel was forty-six hours. The causes of death were primary and secondary: 1. Prostration; peritonitis; gangrene of the intestine; perforation. 2. Bronchitis; abscess behind the peritoneum; phlegmatous inflammation, and suppuration. The circumstances by which they were brought about: Age; a journey; the defective constitutional nutrition of the patient; the morbid state of the canal above the strangulated piece of bowel; injury of the hernia caused by the constriction of the ring, and by manual violence inflicted on it; the duration of the sufferings; the intensity of the constitutional sympathies; fæcal fistula; neglect of the tumor; the administration of purgatives; the warm bath. The means by which they may be avoided are: By care in manipulation; the early relief of the bowel from constriction; the reduction of the hernia without opening the peritoneal sac; the exhibition of opium; and the avoidance of all causes likely to induce exhaustion.

ART. 97.—On the "expiratory method" of performing the Taxis in Hernia. By Dr. ANDREW BUCHANAN.

(Glasgow Medical Journal, July, 1856.)

"This method is a modification of the ordinary manual operation for the reduction of hernia, commonly named the 'taxis.' The patient is placed in the position usually recommended, or which may be deemed most suitable in the various forms of hernia, and the compressing force is applied in the usual way. The peculiarity of the method consists in this, that just before the force is applied, the patient is directed to make a very full expiration, and thereafter to refrain as long as possible from making a fresh inspiration; or, as it is more intelligibly expressed to the uninitiated, he is directed to blow as much air out of his mouth as he possibly can, and to continue thereafter as long as he can without drawing a fresh breath. While this is going on, the operator, having made all necessary preliminary arrangements, attempts to return the hernia, beginning as soon as the expiration is a little advanced, and continuing his efforts gently but steadily during the whole period of suspended respiration.   When the patient is at length compelled to draw a fresh breath, the pressure should be relaxed, so as not to oppose the force of the muscles of inspiration; but it should not be altogether given up, and as soon as the patient is a little recruited from his exhaustion, he is made to perform another expiration; and so the operation is continued as long as may be required.   The first indication of success, consisting in a slight internal motion or gurgling noise of the tumor, almost universally occurs during the suspension of the breathing, and it is during the same period that the complete return of the hernia is usually effected.

"There are some important minor details in the operation, which depend on the intelligence and strength of mind of the patient. If he possess both those mental qualities in a sufficient degree, he will be able, after making the full expiration, to refrain from inspiring by a voluntary effort. Such cases are the most favorable for the success of the operation. In other cases, and these cases occur more especially among females, the patient understands and acts fully upon the direction of blowing out the breath, but wants strength of mind for the subsequent control over the inspiratory muscles. In all such cases it is indispensable to have an assistant, whose duty is, as soon as the expiration is completed, to apply his hands over the mouth and nose of the patient, so as to prevent inspiration for as long a period as may be deemed safe and advisable. If, however, the lungs can be sufficiently emptied, such cases are little less favorable than the former. Last of all, there are persons who, whether from natural stupidity or from fright and confusion of mind arising from the condition in which they are placed, cannot be made to comprehend and follow out the directions given them. In those cases the lungs are never emptied to the necessary degree, and the success of the operation is proportionally uncertain.

"The theory of this operation is simple. In the first place, it disassociates the diaphragm from the abdominal muscles, and by preventing them from acting in concert, removes the chief obstacle to the reduction of hernia. Secondly, it weakens the muscular power of the body, and diverts it from the act of resistance.

"It is the simultaneous contraction of the diaphragm and abdominal muscles which enables the patient to press down and resist the efforts made to return the hernia. This is one of the most important combinations of muscular action in the whole animal economy. It constitutes the *nixus* of physiologists. Acting in the natural way, it forces out the contents of the bowels, of the urinary bladder, and of the uterus, according to the direction given it; and when misdirected, it becomes the principal cause of the production of hernia, forcing out the bowels themselves where the walls of the abdomen are least able to resist the pressure; while it becomes also, after the disease has been once produced, the force which opposes the return of the hernia into the cavity of the abdomen. Now, it is quite indispensable to the existence of this force that the diaphragm act as well as the abdominal muscles, and the moment the diaphragm is relaxed the force is necessarily destroyed. The intention of the instructions given to the patient before proceeding to taxis will therefore be at once apparent. Expressed in other terms, those instructions just amount to this—'relax your diaphragm, and keep it in a state of relaxation;' for there is no mode of relaxing the diaphragm but by making an expiration, nor any mode of keeping the diaphragm relaxed, but by refraining thereafter from breathing.

"In so far as the general muscular system is concerned, the mode of proceeding here recommended is not confined to the application made of it, but might be successfully employed in facilitating the reduction of dislocations, or counteracting any other muscular resistance. The state of expiration and the suspended breathing which follows it, produce rapidly an overwhelming sense of debility over the whole body, which paralyses all muscular exertion. These conditions of the respiratory organs not only produce a positive but also a negative effect of a useful kind; for they prevent full inspiration, and the *nixus* of which it constitutes a part. Now that act, by giving fixity to the trunk of the body, and a firm point of support to the muscles thence arising, is an indispensable preliminary to every vigorous muscular effort, and of course to every act of resistance. Last of all, there is no feeling more absorbing than that produced by a want of breath, whether kept up voluntary or enforced, and the diversion of the patient's mind from the hernia so produced, operates just like the well-known expedients employed in cases of dislocation to facilitate reduction."

Dr. Buchanan has practised this mode of reducing hernia for several years.

ART. 98.—*A new mode of reducing Strangulated Hernia.*
By Baron SEUTIN.

(*Bull. de Thérap.*, tome i, pp. 161–206; and *Med. Chir. Rev.*, July, 1856.)

Baron Seutin declares, that with his mode of reducing strangulated hernia, which he has now practised for twenty years, he hardly ever in his large practice finds it necessary to have recourse to an operation.

The patient is laid upon his back, with the pelvis raised much higher than the shoulders, in order that the intestinal mass may exert traction upon the herniated portion. The knees are flexed, and the body is slightly turned to the opposite side to that on which the hernia exists. The surgeon ascertains that the hernia, habitually reducible, cannot be returned by continuous and moderate taxis. He next seeks with his index finger for the aperture that has given issue to the hernia, pushing up the skin sufficiently from below, in order not to be arrested by its resistance. The extremity of the finger is passed slowly in between the viscera and the herniary orifice, depressing the intestine or omentum with the pulp of the finger. This stage of the procedure demands perseverance, for at first it seems impossible to succeed. The finger is next to be curved as a hook, and sufficient traction exerted on the ring to rupture some of the fibres, giving rise to a cracking very sensible to the finger, and sometimes to the ear. When this characteristic crack is not produced, the fibres must be submitted to a continuous forced extension, which, by distending them beyond the agency of their natural elasticity, generally terminates the strangulation. This mode of procedure is more applicable to Gimbernat's ligament, the hooking and tearing of which are more difficult than in the case of the inguinal ring. Considerable strength has sometimes to be exerted, and the index finger becomes much fatigued. When, in consequence of the narrowness of the ring, the finger does not at once penetrate, it is to be pressed firmly against the fibrous edge, and inclined towards the hernia. After a time the fibres yield and the finger passes. When the finger becomes fatigued it is not to be withdrawn, but it should be supported by the fingers of an intelligent assistant, who seconds the action it is desired to produce. In inguinal hernia, the traction should not be exerted with the finger upon Poupart's ligament, but in a direction from within outwards, and from below upwards, by which the aponeurotic layers between the two ligamentous pillars constituting the inguinal aperture are easily torn through.

The ring is then enlarged by this tearing, just as if it had been divided by a cutting instrument, or largely dilated, and reduction takes place easily, by performing the taxis in a suitable direction. The mobility of the skin, its laxity in parts where hernia prevails, and its extensibility, greater in proportion to its thinness and to the absence of a lining of fatty cellular tissue—by allowing the sliding and the thrusting of this membrane in front of the finger it cushions, affords protection to the intestine from all immediate contusion. When the strangulation is induced by the issue of a considerable mass of intestine, or an accumulation of fæcal matters, it is desirable first to disengage one of the extremities of the noose, and to seek to expel the gas or fæcal matters by moderate pressure, in order to facilitate the reduction of the tumor. In the few cases in which the finger cannot be introduced, a small incision may be practised in the skin, and the handle of a spatula or any blunt instrument may be passed in by separating the cellular tissue. Pressing this against the border of the ring, while avoiding the intestine, this orifice may be eroded or dilated without danger. The greater the resistance offered by the aponeurotic fibres, the greater will be their tension, and the more easily will their laceration be produced.

As a general conclusion, it may be laid down, that the facility and promptitude of this procedure, and the immunity that attends it, ought to diminish the gravity of the prognosis of strangulated hernia, by rendering the circumstances under which recourse need be had to an operation quite exceptional. Such exceptional cases will be found (1) in old, irreducible herniæ. (2) When the strangulation in inguinal hernia occurs at the internal ring. Generally the external ring and inguinal canal are large, and allow of the easy penetration of the finger; and then the new method is applicable, and the rupturing or dilatation of the internal ring should be attempted, and the manœuvre is rendered easier by the fact, that in these cases the canal is much shortened, and the two rings much approximated. If, however, the exernal ring is too narrow to admit the finger, an operation is required. (3) When there are general symptoms of a gangrenous state of the intestine.

ART. 99.—*On Prolapsus Ani.* By Mr. SYME, Professor of Clinical Surgery in the University of Edinburgh.

(*Edinburgh Medical Journal,* Aug., 1856.)

There is no better illustration of the evils which may result from the improper naming of a disease, than in the case of prolapsus ani. This title being understood to comprehend all protrusions beyond the orifice of the bowel, includes conditions entirely different in regard to their nature and remedy. It also suggests the idea of weakness in the sphincter, and leads this to be regarded as the cause of derangement, when, in truth, it hardly ever is so. Under the erroneous impression thus produced, mechanical support has been most improperly employed, and, if the frequency of advertisements, in respect to contrivances for this purpose, may be taken as a measure of the extent to which they are used, the amount of suffering, thus unnecessarily endured, must be very great.

In nearly all the cases of what is called prolapsus, there is no displacement of the bowel, and merely a protrusion of its lining membrane in the thickened vascular condition, which constitutes internal hemorrhoids. When pain or bleeding is the predominant symptom of this disease, it generally retains its proper designation; but when the patient is chiefly annoyed by descent of the tumor, through the effect of exertion in the erect posture, the morbid state of the texture concerned is apt to be overlooked, so that the evil is attributed solely to relaxation of the sphincter. Many unhappy people pass through life in perpetual misery, from this source, to which peculiarities of conduct and manner might often be more correctly ascribed than to original disposition.

Whatever may be the symptoms proceeding from them, the treatment of internal hemorrhoids should be always the same. It is necessary (these principles were laid down by Mr. Syme thirty years ago, when the subject was little known):— First. That the whole of the existing enlargement within the sphincter should be removed by ligatures. Second. That each of the tumors of which it is composed should be transfixed at its root by a double ligature. Third. That the ligatures should be tied with the utmost possible tightness; and Fourth. That any enlargement exterior to the sphincter should be removed by scissors. Morbid growths, whether within or without the anus, being thus taken away, the sphincter is allowed to resume its proper action, and the patient is relieved from prolapsus, no less effectually than from pain and bleeding.

But in other cases, comparatively rare, the coats of the rectum descend so as to constitute a tumor independently of any morbid growth beyond mere thickening, or engorgement of their texture. In children, this usually depends on the straining caused by irritation, as that of a stone in the bladder, and in old people it may proceed from a paralytic state of the sphincter. It may also, as in the case about to be related, depend upon a condition of the anus, remediable through proper management. For this purpose it is requisite that the whole of the pendulous folds of skin should be removed by incisions radiating from the centre of the orifice— that the patient should be confined to the horizontal posture for several weeks, even when the bowels are evacuated—and that the diet should be restricted, so as to prevent distension by feculent matters.

The case in illustration of these remarks is of peculiar interest.

"About three years ago, Dr. Dick, of Mid-Calder, called upon me with a gentleman suffering from an enormous protrusion of the rectum, which he had been led to regard as irremediable, and which at first sight certainly appeared to be so. A slight expulsive effort brought into view the tumor, which in size and form resembled a large cocoa-nut. It had a firm consistence, rough irregular surface, dark brown color, and coating of bloody mucus, so as to be more like a malignant growth than a simple descent of the bowel. Nevertheless, being satisfied from the history of the case, that the disease was of the latter kind, I held out the prospect of beneficial treatment, and the patient readily promised submission to whatever I should propose.

"The integuments round the anus being greatly relaxed and thickened, so as to constitute a number of pendulous folds, I removed all this redundant texture by repeated applications of the scissors, not in a circular direction, but pointed from the circumference towards the centre of the orifice. This would have been a painful operation if performed on a conscious patient, but being executed under the influence of chloroform, was accomplished without suffering, and also the difficulties attendant upon involuntary straining. I then enjoined the necessity of strictly maintaining the horizontal posture, and of abstaining from food beyond what was absolutely requisite. The bowels were not disturbed for several days, and at the end of this time were evacuated without any protrusion or difficulty, in consequence, no doubt, of the intestinal coats regaining their natural condition, while the sphincter was no longer impeded in the discharge of its duty. In the course of a few weeks, the patient felt able to resume his service in an office of the government in London, where he has ever since been employed, and felt so well as to enter into the matrimonial state. He lately sent me the following account of his case, which contains some details that may prove instructive as well as interesting.

"'My earliest recollection of having prolapsus ani is, that after every stool the nurse had to push up the rectum. I remember that I always used to throw myself forward on my knees, with my face almost touching the floor, and while in this attitude she pushed in what I (as a child) then called "the bone," having an idea that a bone always came out when I went to stool. I am told that the origin of my misfortune was caused by my receiving a severe blow on the back, after which I ran to the nursery, and on attempting to go to stool the gut immediately fell. This must have occurred between the age of three and four. I have no recollection of it whatever, but I believe that from that time I never evacuated the bowels without the gut coming down.

"'At the age of six, I was able to replace it myself, and having at that time left home, and entered a boarding-school, I was of course obliged to make the best of it. Then, and afterwards, I thought it a matter of course that I should suffer as I did. I always felt very keenly the difference betwixt myself and other boys. I could neither jump, run, nor play in any way like them, and was a poor hand at most games, from a strong fear of "receiving a blow on the back." I have frequently been struck on the back with a hand ball, after which I felt overcome for the rest of the day. I always felt ashamed to speak to any one about the gut, and spent my years at school in silent suffering. Many a time have I felt cut to the heart by the boys calling me "heavy bottom!" knowing that justly I did not deserve the name, but that my want of agility was caused by what I then began to call "my weakness in the back." I was quite uncared for at school, with respect to this weakness, and the teachers have frequently joined in the laugh against "poor heavy bottom!" During my first two or three years at school, this hurt me very much, and my spirits, already overcome by my complaint, were increasingly depressed by frequent shedding of tears in secret. I mention this merely to show what a poor child may suffer when neglected.

"'After the age of nine, I had sufficient sense to refrain from joining in any but very quiet games, where there was no running, pushing about, or any danger of rough movements. Being obliged always to accompany the other boys, I used to sit a solitary spectator of their games, and I well remember, that when any boy happened to come rushing near me, I had a standing cry of terror—"I'm not playing, I'm not playing!"

"'I always considered myself a most unfortunate boy as I advanced in years, and I had no one to whom I could communicate any feelings, excepting during my yearly holidays of five or six weeks, which I spent at home. On these occasions, both my father and mother were always very anxious about me, and tried to get me to do many things, with a view to effect a cure, but I was then too glad to enjoy the short opportunity I had of joining in all the pleasures of home, and used to tell them that "I did not mind it." The only thing they got me to do, was to sit in water which had been boiled with oak bark.

" 'On my return to school, matters always went on as usual, and thus I passed my early years. I never could undergo the same amount of fatigue as others of my own age and apparent strength. In severe cold weather, I was generally in a state of shivering, except when leaning over a fire—skating being almost the only exercise at which I could get thoroughly warm.

" 'In December, 1845, I sailed from this country for Ceylon, and during the voyage was more troubled than I had ever been before with indigestion and constipation, which caused great straining of the bowels.

" 'In April, 1846, I arrived at Ceylon, and was for a long time under a strong impression that the climate suited me well. Towards the end of my first year's stay in the island, the bowels became more slackened than usual, and the gut protruded further than formerly, but I did not take any particular notice of this at the time. Towards the end of 1848, I was obliged to go more frequently to the water-closet, and the straining became more and more severe, so much so, that I had often to stay half an hour, and sometimes longer, before I could push up the rectum.

" 'In the beginning of 1849, blood and mucus began to pass so freely, that I took medical advice. Simple diet and the use of the enema were recommended, but the malady increased. In the month of March, my medical friend told me that my only chance of recovery was to return to England.

" 'Up to this time the anus retained its usual natural appearance; but I now found an excrescence on the sphincter like a long wart, the top of which was open, and discharged a sticky waxy sort of matter. To this I was advised to apply caustic, which I did, but one trial was quite enough. I never touched it a second time.

" 'During former years, the appearance of the rectum was a healthy red, but it now began to look dark and inflamed, and towards its outer edge was covered with little growths like the tops of a cocks-comb.

" 'In the month of May I sailed for England. The first circumstance which alarmed me in connection with my illness, occurred on the morning I left the island. On getting out of bed, I had hardly stood upright, when a quantity of stuff fell from me (without my feeling anything of it); it was a jelly-like substance, and looked very much like prepared arrow-root, colored with port wine. During my voyage, I was constantly passing this bloody mucus; and, as I lived almost entirely on arrow-root and sago, I passed but little fæces.

" 'The discharging excrescences on the anus, like the one above described, increased in number, and I was tortured by the sea-doctor, with an application of strong pepper to the affected parts. Like the caustic, however, I never applied it a second time.

" 'Several times during the voyage, I almost lost entire control over the rectum, and felt as if it would fall out, and remain so in spite of me.

" 'I reached London in the end of June, in a state of great exhaustion. I was almost helpless as a child, and, had it not been for the kindness of some of my fellow-passengers, and the strangers who took care of my luggage, and found lodgings for me, &c., I know not what I should have done.

" 'After a stay at Richmond, my strength began to increase, so that I could walk without assistance, and was soon able to undertake the journey, by sea, to the North of Scotland, without a protector.

" 'During the winter of 1849–50, I had kind medical advice, but the rectum and anus continued in an inflamed and shattered state, and my life was still a misery and burden. Constant running to the water-closet—continued straining—rectum bleeding, and the constant flow of discharge made me think that I was to remain for life unfit for any of its duties.

" 'In 1851, I was placed under the care of Dr. Macleod, of Benrhydding. The use of the sitz-bath, and spouting water on the lower part of the back, were the principal items of treatment, with occasional slipper and such like baths. This treatment was the first from which I derived benefit—the rectum and its vicinity resumed a healthy red appearance; the straining was not so great, the discharge and bleeding lessened, my strength greatly increased, I could often walk a mile without much inconvenience, the stomach and digestive powers restored to action (indeed they seemed entirely renewed), and the whole system changed from a diseased to a healthy condition.

" 'The prolapsus still remained, and, during a residence in London with sedentary employment and confinement in 1852, and beginning of 1853, it became very much worse. Its size increased, and it bled very profusely. I had more difficulty in replacing it, and frequently could not do so until I had soaked it for fifteen or twenty minutes in a basin of water. I have had this to do three, four, and five times a day. The attitude in which I had to place myself over the basin was so awkward, that it aided in exhausting my strength, and I had invariably to lie down for half an hour, or longer, after having succeeded in pushing up the rectum.

" 'Since the beginning of 1849, I had always bled more or less when straining with the rectum, but the flow of blood was now greater than ever. It often ran in a perfect jet, as if a vein had been opened with a lancet, and when occasionally I have raised the rectum out of the basin, in the act of straining, the blood has spurted six or seven feet across the floor.

" 'One other feature of the case I will mention, which made me very miserable. I do not know that I can describe it correctly, but I will try. When the large ball of the rectum came down, the heart or centre of it frequently filled with fæces, and so distended it, that in this state it was impossible to replace it. Occasionally it would empty itself slowly, after I had soaked the rectum for some time in warm water; but I frequently had to introduce my finger, and take them out piece by piece, before it could be pushed up, and then it was always accomplished with difficulty.

" 'In February, 1853, I had a severe attack of diarrhœa, which reduced me very much in strength, and increased the diseased state of the rectum. In the month following I visited Mid-Calder, with a view to recover my strength, and there met my kind friend, Dr. Dick, through whose friendly interest, in the month of April, I received from your hands that act of kindness which relieved me from the troubles of the prolapsus, and which I ever remember with a sense of the deepest gratitude.' "

ART. 100.—*A new method of Puncturing the Bladder.* By M. SANTOPADRE.

(Bull delle Scienzi Med.; and Gaz. Méd. de Paris, March 7, 1856.)

The instrument employed in the following case may be described as a trocar of the same length and form as the lithotrite of Heurteloup. The central stem was made flexible, so as to allow the necessary backward and forward motion through the curved portion of the sheath by the insertion of a spiral spring. When the instrument was being introduced the pointed stem was drawn back within the sheath. This instrument was suggested and tested by the following case :

CASE.—A man, æt. 65, hemiplegic, was admitted into hospital on the 2d of December, 1854, for retention of urine depending upon an enlarged condition of the prostate. This retention had existed four days. The bladder was distended to the umbilicus, and the constitutional distress was extreme.

The patient was placed in the ordinary position for catheterism, and the sheath of the instrument already described was introduced up to the point of obstruction, its course being under the guidance of a finger introduced into the rectum. Then the pointed stem was pushed forwards in the direction of the prostatic portion of the bladder. The bladder was penetrated without any difficulty, and with very little pain. There was hardly any bleeding at the time, and there was no constitutional disturbance afterwards. Twenty days later, the patient was well enough to leave the hospital.

Three months after this time the patient died of apoplexy, and an opportunity was thus given of examining the parts. The report is that the urethra was perfectly whole, and of sufficient capacity to allow the passage of an ordinary sound, and that the prostate was of double the natural size. The course of the instrument through it could not be traced.

ART. 101.—*Lupulin in Spermatorrhœa.* By Dr. PESCHECK.

(Buchner's Repert. für Pharm., No. 1, 1856 ; and Med.-Chir. Rev., July, 1856.)

"Dr. Pescheck has employed lupulin for several years in a great number of cases in which spermatorrhœa seemed to depend upon no mechanical cause. At first he used to give two grains night and morning; but finding such doses of no avail, he prescribed from ten to fifteen grains to be taken just before bedtime, prohibiting the drinking of water after it. From such doses, even continued for a long time, he has found no inconvenience to arise, while they have acted beneficially on the disease. In some cases he combined with it one or two grains of pulv. digitalis. A valuable peculiarity in the operation of the lupulin, is the beneficial action it exerts upon the digestive process, which so often suffers in these cases. It is also very useful in mitigating the urethral irritation and discharges consequent on former excesses, and, in many cases, more so than iron or quinine. Its especial utility in the chordee of gonorrhœa, Dr. Pescheck has had many opportunities of witnessing. It is best administered without any additions that might diminish its bitterness, as its effects are very proportionate to the intensity of this property. Old lupulin deprived of its oil and bitter taste is almost always useless."

ART. 102.—*A simple method of reducing Dislocation of the Humerus into the Axilla.* By Mr. BIRKETT, Surgeon to Guy's Hospital.

(*Lancet*, Feb. 2, 1856.)

In this mode all the conditions required for the reduction of such a dislocation were easily obtained.

1. Perfect loss of voluntary muscular contraction from the chloroform.
2. Counter-extension, made by fixing the scapula with the index finger and thumb of the right hand.
3. Extension by the operator at the most desirable part of the injury.
4. And lastly, a fulcrum, formed also by the operator's hand, upon which the head of the humerus was thrust outwards from the axilla.

The whole arrangement was thus under the control of a single operator, which must be considered of the greatest practical importance.

This plan is much more neat and delicate than that of placing the heel into the axilla, or of having two or more individuals to effect that which in this individual was so easily accomplished by one.

CASE.—A healthy, robust, agricultural laborer was admitted into the Cornelius Ward on January 11th, 1856. He stated that on the 7th ultimo, whilst in a state of intoxication, he fell down and injured his right shoulder. He did not apply to any surgeon until three weeks after the accident, when an attempt at reduction was unsuccessfully made. After admission into the hospital there was found, on examination, an exceedingly well-marked case of dislocation of the head of the humerus completely into the axilla. The head of the bone was directly beneath the glenoid cavity, neither in front of it nor behind it. There was considerable swelling of the shoulder. Chloroform was administered, and the man was placed on his back. Then, under the direction of Mr. Birkett, Mr. Valentine (the dresser, from whose notes the history of the case is taken), standing at the side of the patient, placed his right hand against the axillary region of his chest, pressing his index finger against the coracoid process of the scapula, and his thumb against the inferior costa of the same bone, when the arm of the patient almost formed a right angle with his body. The head of the dislocated humerus was then lodged against, or in the fossa formed by the heads of the metacarpal bones of the dresser's index finger and thumb, which thus formed a fulcrum upon which the caput humeri necessarily impinged. By this disposition of the right hand of the dresser, the counter-extension upon the scapula was made, and that bone firmly fixed. Extension was then made upon the dislocated humerus by grasping the arm with the left hand; and in this way as much force as the operator was capable of exerting was freely employed. Immediately after all voluntary muscular contraction ceased, Mr. Valentine performed extension on the patient's arm for a few seconds, and then, on his bringing it down from its position at right angles with the body to the chest on the fulcrum formed by his right hand, the head of the humerus was replaced in the glenoid cavity, the replacement being indicated by a jerk.

(c) CONCERNING THE UPPER EXTREMITY.

ART. 103.—*On a simple mode of reducing a Dislocated Elbow.*
By M. BIDARD, of Arras.

(*Gaz. Hebdom. de Méd. et Chir.*, Aug. 15, 1856.)

In a recent communication to the Société de Chirurgie de Paris, M. Bidard relates a case in which a dislocated elbow was reduced in a very simple manner, after the ordinary means had failed. A child, æt. 13, had dislocated his elbow, and the dislocation had been reduced in the ordinary way. A month later the elbow was again dislocated. On this occasion the child said nothing about the accident, and five weeks passed before the mischief was discovered, and the attempts at reduction repeated. These attempts failed. It then occurred to M. Bidard to persuade the child to swing himself by both his hands from a cross beam of wood, and to allow his hands to be held in this position by another person when he became tired. These swingings were continued for fifteen or twenty minutes at a time, and repeated every morning and evening; and the result was, that the displacement had entirely disappeared on the seventh day. It appears from the account, that the displacement diminished progressing between the first and ninth suspension; and that the rest of the deformity disappeared suddenly during the fourteenth suspension.

This method, as M. Larrey observed afterwards, possesses some analogy to that of the *door*, as formerly practised by some surgeons, but with this difference, that the reduction is effected gradually in this case and suddenly in that.

As to the rest, we are disposed to think that there need have been no difficulty if chloroform had been employed; for, unquestionably, dislocations of much older standing are easily reducible with the help of this agent.

ART. 104.—*On Sub-arterial Cysts of the Wrist.* By M. CHASSAIGNAC.

(*Mon. des Hôp.*, No. 78, 1856 ; and *Med.-Chir. Rev.*, Oct., 1856.)

M. Chassaignac calls attention to a form of ganglion which, placed beneath the radial artery, unless properly understood, may give rise to very serious errors. From excess of labor, or the exertions necessary to raise heavy burdens, the small tumor may acquire considerable development. The fingers of the surgeons, when applied over the cyst, are raised by the pulsations, which are remarkable for their energy and the breadth of space they extend over. This extent of pulsatile surface immediately suggests the idea of radial aneurism, and if the examination be continued with the limb remaining in its ordinary attitude, an error can scarcely be avoided. The differential diagnosis may be established by bringing the wrist into a state of forced flexion, when—whether it is that the artery is displaced, or that it ceases to be stretched over the eminence formed by the cyst—the pulsations no longer exist, and it is evident that no aneurism is present. In treating these cases, M. Chassaignac employs the iodide of potash ointment, rubbing it in every two hours during a week. On the dorsal surface we may treat ganglia with advantage by crushing them, by subcutaneous puncture, seton, or iodine injection; but in the case of these sub-arterial cysts of the wrist, which are in communication with the radio-carpal articulation, these means of treatment are not applicable. The iodine frictions give rise to no accident, and seemed possessed of all desirable efficacy.

On one occasion, M. Chassaignac had the opportunity of examining one of these cysts in a subject brought for dissection. The tumor resembled an almond in form and size, and occupied the space between the tendons of the *supinator longus* and the *palmaris longus*, lying on the anterior portion of the *pronator quadratus*. The radial artery in its downward progress having reached the upper part of the tumor, was at first so intimately connected with its front part as to seem to form a portion of its walls. Very soon, however, it deviated obliquely on its external side, and reaching the fossette called the anatomical snuff-box. With the object of ascertaining the anatomical origin of the tumor, it was dissected with the greatest care, and separated from all parts with which it had not contracted fixed adhesions. In this way it was circumscribed for four-fifths of its extent, but posteriorly and below it was firmly fixed to the bone by a kind of pedicle proceeding from the anterior part of the lower radio-cubital articulation. It was only, in fact, a diverticulum of the synovial membrane of this joint, and it had raised up the lower fibres of the *pronator quadratus*, which, forming a kind of arc, produced a sort of strangulation of the pedicle at its upper part. The continuity of the cyst with the articulation was completely demonstrated, a probe freely passing from one to the other.

ART. 105.—*On Dislocation of the Thumb at the metacarpo-phalangeal articulation.* By Dr. BATCHELDER.

(*New York Journal of Medicine*, May, 1856.)

The mode of reduction described below is very similar to that which was recently described by Dr. John Doe (*v.* "Abstract," XVIII). Dr. Batchelder informs us that this mode has been publicly practised by him for several years:

"The uniform failure of the ordinary mode and means of reduction prevailed on Blandin to invent a pair of forceps (known in all our shops as Blandin's forceps), for making the extension more effectual; but, so far as I have had an opportunity of knowing, these and all the other methods have generally failed, unless the lateral ligaments of the joint were divided by a subcutaneous incision, as suggested by Sir Charles Bell. Most surgeons, among whom are Sir Charles Bell and Mr. Hey, impute the difficulty to these ligaments, between which the head of the bone is forced, and by which, being put thus on the stretch, it is steadfastly retained; they seem, however, to have forgotten or overlooked the fact that there are two sesamoid bones, lodged one on each side of this joint in the tendons of the flexor brevis pollicis, between which the inferior extremity of the metacarpal bone is forced forward and ' projects very much inward, towards the palm of the hand, and the extremity of the phalanx projects backward.' In this displacement, parts of the flexor brevis are put on the stretch, which, acting like extensors, draw the proximal extremity of the phalanx upward along the posterior surface of the metacarpal bone, and fix it there; hence, every attempt at extension only makes the matter worse. How, then, is this difficulty to be overcome, and the reduction accomplished? Not by extension, of course; but in the following manner. The surgeon should take the metacarpal portion of the dislocated thumb between the thumb and finger of one hand, and flex or force it as far as may be into the palm of the hand, for the purpose of relaxing the muscles connected with the proximal end of the phalanx, particularly the flexor brevis pollicis. He should then apply the end of the thumb of this hand against the displaced extremity of the dislocated phalanx, for the purpose of forcing it downwards, and at the same time grasp the displaced thumb with his other hand, and move it forcibly backwards and forwards, as in strongly forced flexion and extension, the pressure against the upper extremity of the first phalanx being kept up. In this way the dislocated bone may be made to descend, so as to be almost or quite on a line with the articulating surface of the metacarpal bone, when the thumb may be forcibly flexed, and, if it be not reduced, as forcibly extended, and brought backward to a right angle with the metacarpal bone, when, if the downward pressure, with the thumb placed as before directed for that purpose, has been continued (which thumb, by maintaining its position, acts as a fulcrum, as well as by its pressure), the bone will slip into its place, and the reduction be effected in less time than has been spent in describing the process. I derived the first hint of this procedure from hearing an empiric, somewhat noted as a bone-setter, describe the process by which he had succeeded, in a similar case. This occurred about the time I commenced the study of medicine, and from the manner in which it was told, the relation has never escaped my memory; but from his being considered somewhat of a quack, and moreover, a professional braggart, it was not subsequently analyzed or acted on, until after I had failed in a case of the kind. That failure induced me to investigate its causes in the dissecting room, which brought up a vivid recollection of the statements of the bone-setter; and the consequent analysis of the anatomical relations of the parts involved, resulted in the adoption of the method just described, which I believe will always be attended with prompt success, especially in recent cases; and also in those of considerable standing, say a week or two."

ART. 106.—*On the desirability of removing part of the Metacarpal Bone in amputating a finger.* By Mr. HILTON, Surgeon to Guy's Hospital.

(*Assoc. Med Journ.*, June 7, 1856.)

At a recent operation in Guy's Hospital, Mr. Hilton dwelt on the desirability of removing part of the metacarpal bone in amputating a finger. A V-shaped incision was made in the back of the hand, and the head of the metacarpal bone, as well as the finger, were removed. A much more shapely and useful hand is left by this mode of operating.

(D) CONCERNING THE INFERIOR EXTREMITY.

ART. 107.—*Internal derangement of the Knee-joint.*
By Dr. GORDON BUCK, Surgeon to the New York Hospital.

(*Philadelphia Medical Examiner*, Aug., 1856.)

The following case corresponds with great exactness to the description of this rare and perplexing accident, as given by the late Mr. Hey, of Leeds, in his "Observations on Surgery:"

CASE.—"On the morning of May 24th, 1856, Mr. S—, of Lowell, Massachusetts, called on account of a lameness of his left knee that had suddenly occurred the evening before, at the moment of rising up from a position in which his knee was sharply flexed under him. He could now no longer apply the sole of his foot to the floor in walking, but was obliged to bear his weight on his toes, with the knee maintained in a slightly flexed position, and as if anchylosed. Any attempt to straighten the knee to its full extent was resisted on account of the pain it produced, which was referred to the anterior space between the inner condyle of the femur and the corresponding head of the tibia. At this point *alone*, pressure gave pain when applied with the end of the thumb forced deep into the space between the bones. It was thought too, that the end of the thumb did not penetrate as deep into this space as in the other knee. There was no tenderness on pressure of any other part of the joint. There was no swelling or any change in the form of the joint. The same accident had occurred to him on several previous occasions; but Mr. S. had been able to get prompt relief without surgical aid, by having the limb stretched and repeatedly flexed and extended. In this instance, however, his efforts had been unsuccessful. Regarding a displacement of the inner semilunar cartilage forwards, as the cause of this derangement of the joint, the reduction of it was attempted in the following manner, as advised by Mr. Hey: the patient being placed in a chair, the limb was raised above a horizontal position and the leg flexed on the thigh to its full extent, and then extended in like manner, at the same time pressure being applied over the advanced cartilage with the end of the thumb. This latter movement of extension and pressure gave severe pain, while flexion caused none. This manœuvre was repeated several times, till, at length, while urging the extension to its full degree, the patient suddenly grasped the knee with both hands, and begged we would proceed gradually, as he felt the cartilage slowly slipping back to its place. In another moment he sprang upon the floor, and stamping with his lame foot, exclaimed with delight, 'I am all right again.' "

ART. 108.—*A case of unusual Dislocation of the Patella.* By Dr. WRAGG.

(*Charleston Medical Journal and Review*, May, 1856.)

This case is one of considerable interest. It is described as one of *complete* revolution of the bone on its long axis; but in reality only half a revolution upon this axis was accomplished.

CASE.—On the 29th June, 1855, a black man was engaged in loading lumber upon a boat. It was conveyed by means of a car running on rails. He carelessly allowed himself to be caught by the loaded car, while it was in motion, and jammed against the cross sticks on which the piles of lumber rested. The accident occurred about 5 o'clock P.M., and I saw him in half an hour. He was lying on his back, and his right leg was stretched stiffly out. The knee was entirely changed in form. A sharp and prominent edge was apparent on the outer part of the joint, projecting about half an inch forward of the normal plane of the anterior face of the patella, and about the same distance over the outer edge of the joint. Beneath this edge there was a depression into which the ends of the fingers could be readily passed, and at the bottom of which the outer edge of the articulating surface of the outer condyle of the femur could be felt. The inner part of the joint was flattened and depressed, and the fingers could readily detect the inner edge of the inner condyle of the femur, over which no portion of the patella rested. Passing the fingers from this point outwards, and pressing well upon the surface of the bone, a depressed edge was plainly felt, about half an inch or less from the rough elevation which borders the articulating surface of the inner condyle of the femur, on its inner edge. Above and below the patella an evident twist was discovered in the tendinous insertion of the extensor muscles, and in the ligament of the patella. The joint was stiff, and allowed but limited motion.

From these appearances I recognized a dislocation of the patella, by which the bone was twisted completely round on its longitudinal axis, so that its outer edge corresponded nearly to the inner edge of the articulating surface of the femur; its anterior face was turned backwards, and rested on the same articulating surface; its inner edge looked outwards and a little forwards, forming the projecting edge in front and on the outside of the joint; and its posterior or articulating face was under the skin, looking forwards with slight inclination inwards.

To remedy this displacement the indication was evident. It was, to untwist the part. But before attempting anything, it was necessary to determine the exact nature of the twist, whether in coming to its new position the projecting (inner) edge of the bone had passed forwards and then outwards, or backwards and outwards. An inspection of the parts, and a consideration of the manner in which the accident had happened, showed that the former was the true mechanism of the dislocation. The inspection showed this by the evident direction in the twist of the ligaments; and the manner in which the accident occurred proved the same state of things. Thus: the man was standing in front of the car, so placed against the pile of boards that his thigh was firmly fixed on its inner side, the outer and anterior part of the leg presenting to the approaching car. The projecting edge of the car, or the end of one of the boards with which it was loaded, struck the outer edge of the patella; and as the car moved on (the limb being firmly fixed), the force applied to the bone on its outer edge acted in such a way as to press this edge backwards and inwards, causing it to slip along the large articulating face of the external condyle, while the inner edge of the patella, following a converse direction, was tilted forwards. Had the force ceased to act at this point, there would have been a dislocation to the extent of that already described by several authors, only that instead of the outer edge of the patella presenting forwards, the inner edge backwards, the posterior or articulating face outwards, and the anterior face inwards, the positions would have been just the reverse. But as the force did not cease to act, nor the bone to yield to it, the outer edge of the patella was driven onwards and made to mount the small articulating face of the inner condyle. Here it rested; and as the inner edge of the bone was performing a counter movement under the skin, the result was a complete revolution of the patella on its long axis.

An inspection of the two bones concerned in this dislocation will show that when their relative positions have been changed in the manner and to the extent described, the appearances given to the joint must necessarily be such as were seen in this case. The articulating surfaces of the bones are both divided into two parts: that of the patella by an elevated ridge, and that of the femur by a deep depression. In both the bones the outer of these surfaces are large, the inner small; the outer surface of the patella being larger than that of the femur, so that the outer edge of the former bone overlaps the outer edge of the latter. From this arrangement of the parts it follows, that when the patella is displaced in the manner now under consideration, its inner border must project slightly beyond the outer border of the external condyle of the femur, and thus give rise to one of the most striking symptoms of the luxation, viz., the well-defined prominence which was given to the outer part of the knee-joint in the case before us, and also to other symptoms described by authors, viz., the perceptible ridge under the skin due to the ridge on the posterior face of the patella.

Again: of the two surfaces of the femur the outer is much the most prominent, while of the two edges of the patella the inner is much the thicker; hence in the new position of the bone an unnatural prominence must be given to the outer part of the joint. This alteration in the shape of the knee was another striking symptom in the dislocation.

From a consideration of all these points there could be no doubt that the bone had come into its new position by an entire revolution, in which its outer edge (which received the force) revolved from before backwards, and from without inwards, the inner edge performing a counter movement in correspondence with that of the outer. In a thin-skinned subject there will probably be no difficulty in discriminating the surface which is presenting under the skin by the prominent ridge which divides the articulating faces; for if this be detected with the fingers, it must remove all uncertainty as to which face of the bones is forward.

*   *   *   *   *   *   *   *

The reduction was effected without difficulty. The thumbs of both hands being placed on the outer and under edge of the projecting border of the patella, while the index and middle fingers were pressed against the other border in a direction outwards and backwards, force was applied with a view to roll the bone over into its place. The first efforts failing, a bystander was directed to pass his hands under the knee-joint, and make forcible and intermittent flexion of the leg. In a moment the bone performed its evolution, slipped into its place, and the man rose up and walked. He experienced no further inconvenience, the ligaments, cartilages, and investing membranes of the joint having received no injury whatever from this extensive displacement.

ART. 109.—*On the treatment of Inverted Toe-nail.* By Mr. LOVEGROVE, of Brighton.

:(*Lancet,* Aug. 30, 1856.)

The idea here carried out is borrowed, Mr. Lovegrove tells us, from some forgotten surgical work. At any rate it is a very good one.

CASE.—"A young person, about 26 years of age, had been under a surgeon of some renown in London for three or four months, and in spite of all the means usually adopted in such cases, continued to get worse. She visited Brighton, and consequently the case came under my notice; I saw at once it was a fair opportunity of trying this new idea, which is as follows: The nail, which is usually very thick on the great toe, was scraped moderately thin with a piece of glass, and then the whole surface covered with a good coating of nitrate of silver, which was accomplished by rubbing the stick of silver carefully over the whole of the nail, moistened with a little water; after which a linseed-meal poultice (hot) was applied, and the next morning nearly the whole of the nail was separated from the flesh, and another milder application divided it entirely. The nail was then removed without the least pain, and the patient assured me she had not suffered at all during the whole operation. In less than a fortnight after the operation was completed, the patient wore her usual boots with comfort, and before leaving Brighton, a new nail was rapidly growing."

PART III.

MIDWIFERY AND DISEASES OF WOMEN AND CHILDREN.

(A) CONCERNING PREGNANCY AND PARTURITION.

ART. 110.—*On Sterility in relation to the Vaginal Secretions.*
By Dr. KUCHENMEISTER.

(*Wien Wochenschrift*, No. 6, 1856; and *Med. Times and Gaz.*, Sept. 13th, 1856.)

SCANZONI, Tyler Smith, and others, have shown, that while the mucus of the vagina is acid, that of the cervix uteri is alkaline. If we compare these observations with those made by Moleschott and Kölliker, on the movements of spermatozoa in diluted alkaline fluids, we must perceive that these spermatozoa find a very favorable soil in the cervix uteri or the uterus itself, and a highly unfavorable one amidst the acid mucus of the vagina. One of the causes of sterility has long been known to be the deviation of the os uteri from the axis of the pelvis, the semen being unable to enter at once into the cervix. We can expect in such cases few living spermatozoa to reach the os by the laws of capillarity, and none at all if the vaginal secretions are very acid. That motionless spermatozoa, will not fructify is well known ; but whether motionless spermatozoa, brought by capillary action into contact with the uterus, are susceptible of being revivified by means of its alkaline mucus, is a point we are unable to reply to, though the probability is that they are not. Scanzoni and Kölliker have further shown, that when the vaginal discharge is abundant, the acid reaction is increased, and irritation extends to the outer edges and commencement of the cervix of the uterus, and the alkaline mucus then becomes converted into neutral—such neutral condition being a more unfavorable condition for the vivacity of the spermatozoa than the alkaline condition of the secretion. Another point, in relation to sterility, is the complete temporary and periodical closure of the os uteri, shown by Kölliker and Scanzoni to take place. In the ordinary state of things, when no abnormal irritation or secretion of the canal of the cervix is present, this canal is closed from one menstrual period to another, by means of mucus, either in the form of an arterial plug, or of a drop projecting from the external os. About the menstrual period, however, the secretory power of the canal is aroused, the plug is cast out, and the passage becomes free. In most women, this issue of the cervical mucus continues for a short time after menstruation, when the canal again becomes closed : and we see the importance of this, in relation to the advice often usefully given to sterile women, to admit of coitus just before or just after the period.

In treating a patient for sterility, the practitioner should first of all make an examination with the speculum, to ascertain if any abnormal position or physical obstacle exists, and whether this last depends upon atresia, or plugging of the canal with mucus. He must repeat his examination at the menstrual periods, to ascertain when this plug becomes loosened and the canal free, and how long a time elapses after the period before it becomes again closed. Thus, suppose the plug is only separated during or soon after the period, having connection just prior to it will be of no avail. As the introduction of the semen into the uterus shortly before the occurrence of the period seems to favor impregnation, the canal of the cervix should be cleared out a day or two before this time, and coition then accomplished. In obstinate cases, the practitioner or a midwife acquainted with the use of the speculum, should clean out the cervical canal, by means of a pencil of charpie, and then inject a solution of the basic phosphates of soda, or the alkaline carbonates, in the proportions employed by Moleschott and Kölliker, in their experiments upon the spermatozoa. Coitus should take place as soon after as possible. In many cases, the injection of the alkalies would suffice for rendering the canal free. In the most obstinate cases, where much depends upon the removal of the sterility, and when the canal first opens at the middle of the period, or towards its end, coitus should be recommended during the period itself, when, therapeutically and physiologically speaking, the canal is more certainly open, when the spermatozoa can most easily gain admission to the uterine cavity, when the ova have descended into it, and when the salts of the serum of the menstrual blood may confer upon the spermatozoa a more active and more prolonged vivacity.

ART. 111.—*On a cause of Vomiting in Pregnancy.* By M. BRIAU.

(*Gaz. Hebdom. de Méd. et Chir.*, July 18, 1856.)

The conclusions arising from the following case are—First, that unmanageable vomitings may be caused by the confinement of the gravid uterus in the hollow of the sacrum; and secondly, that these vomitings may immediately cease upon the correction of this irregular condition. M. Briau mentions that several cases of the kind have occurred in the practice of M. Moreau.

CASE.—Madame X—, æt. 25, of lymphatic temperament, well formed, and healthy. Six years ago she was confined of her first child, and everything went on perfectly well. Three years afterwards she was confined again, and on this occasion also she went on well, with the exception of some feelings of malaise and vomiting during the first months. A few weeks afterwards, however, she was gently startled by an accident, and from this time she suffered more or less from leucorrhœal symptoms. Madame X— again became pregnant in March, 1856. About the middle of the month following she began to vomit, and these vomitings progressively became more and more unmanageable until nothing would remain on the stomach. Throughout the whole month of May she was affected with severe gastralgia, with constipation and continual thirst. Then she began to suffer from frequent cramps and convulsive movements, with sleeplessness and great depression of spirits.

M. Briau was called to the case on the 2d of May, and all the usual means were tried without success. Then an experiment in homœopathy was tried, and with the same result. M. Briau was recalled on the 2d of June, and on this occasion he suspected that the vomiting might depend upon some uterine displacement. He did this partly on account of the continuance of the leucorrhœal symptoms, and partly from the fact that the uterus could not be felt in the proper position. Two days later M. Moreau was called in consultation, and an examination made, when it was found that the uterus was in a state of incomplete retroversion, as well as in a state of incarceration in the hollow of the sacrum. This malposition was corrected without causing any pain to the patient, and immediately her former sufferings began to subside. On the same day the vomitings ceased, and some food remained on the stomach. On the night following she slept comfortably. In less than forty-eight hours the belly acquired the usual development belonging to the third month of pregnancy; and, in a word, the patient recovered rapidly, without another bad symptom.

ART. 112.—*Tincture of Iodine in the Vomiting of Pregnancy.*
By Dr. EULENBERG, of Koblenz.

(*Preuss. Ver. Zeitung*, 25, 1856; and *Edinburgh Medical Journal*, Oct., 1856)

Dr. Eulenberg, of Koblenz, says that this remedy, even in very small doses, is a most efficacious agent in arresting the troublesome vomiting which so often occurs in pregnant women. He orders the tincture in a very dilute form (Tinct. Iodin., ℈j; Spir. Vini. Rect., ℨiij; M.), and in small doses, three drops several times a day in water. The cardialgia which accompanies this morbid condition is also relieved by it. Dr. Eulenberg alleges that other sympathetic irritations, and neuroses of the nerves of the stomach, are alleviated by similar treatment. The author has not found iodide of potassium equally serviceable in the affections alluded to.

ART. 113.—*Carbonic Acid as a means of procuring Abortion.*
By Professor SCANZONI, of Wurzburg.

(*Weiner Med. Wochenschr.*, No. 1856.)

M. Scanzoni was led to employ carbonic acid in this manner, partly by the marked congestion of the genital organs which resulted from a prolonged exposure to a stream of this gas, and partly by the experiments in which M. Brown-Séquard has shown that carbonic acid will provoke contraction in the muscles of organic life. The carbonic acid was generated in the ordinary way, in a Wolff's bottle, and carried to the uterus by an elastic tube, the end of which was fitted, by means of a cork, into an ordinary glass uterine speculum. The quantity of gas was regulated by the amount of acid added to the bottle.

CASE.—D. S—, æt. 26, a primipara, menstruating for the last time on the 26th of May, 1855, was received into the Maternity at Wurzburg on the 29th of January, 1856. The antero-posterior diameter of the pelvis, which ought to be from four to four and a half inches, was not more than three and a quarter or three and a half, so that delivery at the full term was impossible.

On the 2d of February, at 8 P. M., the carbonic acid was applied for twenty minutes, but without any marked results.

On the day following, at 8 A. M., and again at 8 P. M., the gas was applied for about half an hour, and during the application the patient complained of disagreeable pricking sensations in the vagina. These sensations were followed in the course of the day by gripes around the navel. In the evening, the vaginal portion of the neck of the uterus was sensibly moistened.

On the 4th of February, the apparatus was applied morning and evening for about the same time as yesterday, and the former pricking sensations were produced. In the course of the day the neck of the uterus became dilated so as to allow the introduction of the tip of the finger. During the night, the patient suffered from sharp pains in the region of the uterus, and, towards the morning, distinct uterine contractions were felt by the hand placed over the organ. These contractions, however, passed off very speedily.

On the 5th of February, the gas was applied for half an hour, with the same local effects as previously. At this time the os uteri had dilated to the size of a two-franc piece, and was easily dilatable under the finger. The vaginal secretion, moreover, was sensibly increased. In the afternoon, the uterus again began to contract in a very decided manner. At 6·30 the membranes were ruptured, and the infant, weighing 1350 grammes, was expelled an hour later. There was some little hemorrhage during the delivery, which rendered it necessary to remove the placenta a quarter of an hour after the birth of the child. After this everything went on well.

ART. 114.—*On Cranial Presentations.* By Dr. R. U. WEST.

(*Glasgow Med. Journal*, Oct., 1856.)

The chief points to which Dr. R. U. West is desirous of directing attention in this memoir are:

1. A more correct appreciation of the diagnostic value of the presence of the ear at the symphysis pubis; the ear in the great majority of cranial presentations lying in that situation during the whole progress of the head into the pelvis.

2. That in *vertex* positions, the presence of the ear at the pubes proves that the head is already in a favorable oblique occipito-anterior position, becoming more and more so as the os occipitis comes more and more within contact, although the ear may not have left the symphysis.

3. When the occiput is fairly under the arch of the pubes in the last stage, the long diameter of the head will be found to be accurately in the long diameter of the outlet; the two lambdoidal sutures being evenly one on each side of the symphysis,

and the anterior fontanelle exactly on the raphe of the perineum, as described by all writers except Nägele, and those who follow him.

4. That in this last position the ears are at each acetabulum, rather than at each ilium, as taught in books.

5. That the first and second most frequent positions of the vertex are, in the majority of cases, the converse of each other, as taught by nearly all writers, except Nägele.

6. That in his grand discovery of the universality of *bregmato-cotyloid* positions in the second position, he has deceived himself, by not reversing all the conditions, both of the patient in her position, and of the examining hand of the accoucheur.

7. That Nägele, in maintaining that his predecessors are all wrong in this matter, has deliberately confounded mere bregmoto-cotyloid with *fronto*-cotyloid positions, the latter being always intended by writers, though they may have loosely denominated them presentations or positions of the *vertex*.

8. And that, therefore, Nägele is right in maintaining that the normal progress of the labor in bregmato-cotyloid positions, as in all true *vertex* ones, is for the occiput to make its way to the arch; and that quite as easily, *cæteris paribus*, as when the occiput lies originally most forward.

9. That there are only *two* positions of the *vertex;* that is, only two ways in which, in *vertex* presentations, the head enters the pelvis, and makes its way to the outlet.

10. That in all, or nearly all, presentations of the *vertex*, the occiput will surely come to the arch of the pubes by a natural and necessary process; and that whether the vertex presentation be bregmato-anterior or bregmato-posterior originally.

11. That the cases which terminate with the face or forehead at the pubes, are originally positions in which the uterine efforts are so perversely directed, that the forehead gets down into the pelvis during the first stage.

12. That, in that first stage, the ear is usually at the symphysis, as it is also in vertex presentations.

13. That in these perverse cases, which are usually *bregma* presentations, the ears will really occupy opposite parts of the pelvis, the head lying at first with its long diameter in a transverse position across the pelvis.

14. So that some of them may terminate with the occiput at the arch, after a very hard labor.

15. But the original perverseness in the direction of the uterine efforts, which has placed the head in this unfavorable position, continuing, the anterior or frontal end of the head will frequently pass first to the floor of the pelvis, and then come forward to the arch of the pubes.

16. That Nägele, on his own showing, had never seen a genuine case of true *fronto*-anterior position, incredible though it may seem; at any rate, such a case as is described by nearly all writers, and as is met with continually in practice. He decidedly ignores all such cases.

17. That Nägele is quite as wrong in maintaining that all first positions are originally *occipito-cotyloid*, as that all second positions are originally *bregmato-cotyloid;* bregmato-cotyloid positions, in the former class of cases, being common enough, and having been overlooked through the method of examination.

18. But that most of the bregmato-cotyloid positions met with are merely instances of a kind of *deceptio factus.*

19. For it is only necessary to place the patient on her other side, and to use the other hand in examining, in order to be convinced that the first and second positions of the vertex are the converse of each other in *every respect.*

20. And that, although there may be quite sufficient in the patient's position to account for this *deceptio*, we may be justified in taking into consideration, also, the deceptive impression conveyed to the finger, when it is passed *blindfold* from one point to another of a globular surface, along a line ordinarily looked upon as a straight one, lying over that *globular* surface.

21. That it is no wonder that disputes and discrepancies should have arisen among authors, when we find one set speaking of presentations of the "vertex," and meaning presentations of *any part of the whole cranium;* while another set, like Nägele, speak of " *cranial* positions," meaning positions of the *vertex* exclusively.

22. And finally, that the dispute between Nägele, and those whom he so utterly condemns as guilty of *ignorance* ("Unkunde der Art und Weise," &c.), is something like the quarrel between the two knights about the shield which was gold on one side and silver on the other.

ART. 115.—*Rules for the performance of the Cæsarian Section.* By Dr. GENTH, of Schwalbach.

(*Verhandl. der Ges. für Geburtsh. in Berlin,* viii, 1855; and *Edinburgh Medical Journal,* Nov., 1856.)

This formidable operation (to judge from the frequency with which we meet cases of its performance in the medical journals) seems becoming a favorite operation in Germany. Dr. Genth, of Schwalbach, has published an interesting case, which he read to the Berlin Obstetric Society, in which he performed it successfully in the case of a rachitic woman with contracted pelvis. He believes that, for the favorable performance of the operation, in addition to the careful application of cold to the abdomen (in the form of ice-water dressings), for the first three days, the following points should be attended to: 1st. The timely performance of the operation, without having previously exhausted the patient by trying other modes of artificial delivery. 2d. The obtaining, in good time, copious alvine evacuations. 3d. The exhibition, for some weeks, of medicines which soothe the nervous system, especially of opium. 4th. The wearing of a plaster to afford efficient and permanent support to the abdomen. 5th. The allowing the lower angle of the abdominal wound to remain open for six weeks.

ART. 116.—*Statistics of Operative Midwifery.* By Dr. RICKER.

(*Monatshr. für Geburts.,* Bd. vi, pp. 81-101 ; and *Med. Times and Gazette,* Oct. 11, 1856.)

This interesting contribution is derived from midwifery practice in the Grand Duchy of Nassau. This contains 429,341 inhabitants, and there are 100 civil practitioners, besides 20 others who practise while holding military or other appointments. These practitioners are required to make half-yearly returns, stating the characters of prevalent disease, the most remarkable of the surgical cases, and all the midwifery cases. The author has had access to the midwifery returns, and furnishes here an account of the results of his examination, as far as operative midwifery is concerned. Between 1821 and 1842 inclusive, *i.e.* 22 years, 304,150 births were recorded.

1. *Forceps.*—These were employed in 4223 cases, or about 1 in 72 cases. As. however, the earlier returns were somewhat incomplete, Dr. Ricker believes that 1 in 70 would be nearer the mark. The results were that 93 of the mothers died either during or soon after the operation, and that 684 children were born dead; being 1 death in 45 of the mothers, and 1 in 6 of the children. The indications for the employment of forceps are noted in 708 of the cases only, viz.:

Disproportion of size in the head and pelvis,	287
Absence or feebleness of pains,	269
Weakness or exhaustion of patient,	33
Prolapsus of funis,	29
Spasmodic or violent pains,	22
Face presentation,	20
Convulsions,	12
Descent of parts with head,	8
Placenta prævia,	3
Faulty presentation of head,	7
Rigidity,	4
Tumefaction of pudenda,	4
Erysipelas pudendi,	7
Putrescency,	1

2. *Turning.*—There were 10 cases of cephalic version, and 2473 of turning by the foot, or 1 in 123. The results were 176 deaths on the part of the mother, or 1

in 14, while 1431 children were born dead, or died soon after, or nearly 1 in 2. The indication for turning is recorded in 530 cases, viz.:

Transverse presentation, ... 388
Placenta prævia, ... 82
Prolapse of funis, ... 28
Narrow pelvis, ... 18
Hemorrhage, ... 5
Other dangerous affections, ... 4
Face presentation, ... 2
Faulty presentation of head, ... 2
Convulsions, ... 1

3. *Perforation* was resorted to in 143 instances, or 1 in 2126. There were recorded 88 recoveries and 35 deaths, while in 20 cases no results are given.

4. *Dismemberment* was effected in 22 cases, 16 mothers recovering, and 6 dying.

5. *Cæsarian section.*—Between 1821 and 1843, with 311,409 births, this operation was performed 12 times, 2 mothers and seven children being saved. This gives about one Cæsarian operation in 26,000 births. The operation was performed 33 times after the death of the mother, but none of the children were saved.

The author compares these results with the statistical accounts of the authors; but these being well known we have not quoted them.

ART. 117.—*On Chloroform in Labor.* By Prof. SCANZONI.

(*Monaschr. fur Geburts.*, Bd. vi, p. 461; and *Medical Times and Gasette*, Sept. 13, 1856.)

1. *In normal labor.*—Notwithstanding the flattering accounts from Britain, Professor Scanzoni has found so many disadvantages result from its use, that he is averse to the employment of chloroform in entirely natural labor. The uterine contractions are at all events temporarily diminished in both force and frequency, while the adjuvatory action of the abdominal muscles is weakened. Lying in women require much larger doses to induce narcosis than others, apparently because the inspiration is often interrupted by the pains, while the entire nervous system is more blunted, as is seen from the feeble action of other medicinal agents, as opium, &c. Perhaps, too, the more watery state of the blood admits, as in the chlorotic or hysterical, of an increased employment of these. This diminished sensibility explains the harmlessness of the means, and the fact that no death has hitherto been recorded consequent upon its obstetrical application. Nor are the after consequences, such as delirium, headache, convulsions, &c., that so often occur under other circumstances, met with here. On the other hand, however, chloroform imparts a decided inclination to hemorrhage during or after the fifth stage of labor, against which the administration of ergot, shortly prior to the expulsion of the child, does not offer any certain security.

2. *In abnormal labor.*—(*a*) In too precipitate labors, the chloroform is well suited to effect a decided weakening and delay of the pains. (*b*) In spasmodic pains, when the patient suffers much from their severity, and is very restless, and when warm applications, opium, or venesection have been employed in vain, chloroform is indicated. (*c*) In spastic stricture of the os uteri, chloroform always leads to a relaxation of the tense, unyielding edges; but as such spastic contractions are known to be conjoined with relaxation of the body and fundus of the organ, we should not continue its use too long (at most half an hour), and should try other means before resorting to it at all. As soon as the strictured condition is relieved also, we must endeavor to induce strong labor-pains by means of warm injections, &c. Stricture occurring during the last stage of labor is easily subdued by chloroform; but here it must be very carefully employed, in consequence of the danger of hemorrhage. (*d*) In tetanus of the uterus chloroform is always admissible and useful, and its employment much facilitates turning, so often required in these cases—these tetanic spasms usually only occurring when some mechanical impediment irritates the uterus into increased action. (*e*) In threatened abortion, the author has found chloroform very useful in calming pains that menaced this occurrence. (*f*) In eclampsia, Professor Scanzoni has employed it eight times, and has arrived at the conviction that, if not infallible, it is one of the most certain

means of subduing the attacks. Sometimes it is difficult to effect the narcosis, but
this can always be done by perseverance. When the disease is obstinate and long,
and the inhalations have to be often repeated, these are the best employed on the
very first appearance of each attack. (g) In excessively severe pains, whatever
may be their cause, chloroform does good service. (h) In after-pains it is also to
be recommended. In a case, however, that occurred to M. Scanzoni, the child,
put to the breast three hours after the mother had been narcotized, fell into a deep
sleep that lasted eight hours, and caused uneasiness respecting it for two days
after.

3. *In Obstetrical Operations.*—Here the chloroform is always indicated, and so
great are its advantages, that it is incredible that several practitioners still neglect
its employment. In pelvic presentations it should not be resorted to, as the delay
of the labor that may follow might prove dangerous to the child.

ART. 118.—*On irregular Contraction of the Uterus.*
BY DR. CHANNING.

(*Boston Journal,* Vol. liv, pp. 309–318; and *Medical Times and Gazette,* Aug. 23, 1856.)

Dr. Channing observes, that he never now meets with the hour-glass contractions
he supposed to occur in his earlier practice. The following is his account of the
nature and cause of these irregular contractions. "In these cases referred to, the
following facts have been observed: They have most generally occurred in first labors. Everything has proceeded naturally, it may be, through all its stages. The
after-birth has been expelled, and the patient may have been arranged in her bed.
Sometimes, however, before this, pain may have been complained of. This increases
until it amounts to agony, with expulsive efforts. The abdomen is examined externally. In about its middle, or higher, a hard ball-like tumor is felt, very sensitive,
and easily distinguished from everything about it. Below this the abdomen feels
soft, and bears pressure without any complaint. Not a sign of hemorrhage is present. We think of after-pains and of their accidental exaggerations. But it isa
first labor—a perfectly natural one—and after-pains are rare under such circumstances. We examine per vaginam. Severe suffering is complained of. We have
scarcely entered it when a firm obstruction is encountered. We proceed along one
of its sides, and discover a very large coagulum. We go on, and at length feel the
firm contracted portion of the womb above. The open hand is now passed above
the coagulum, and slowly presses it downwards and out. Relief is instantaneous.
Slowly the hard tumor descends, under regular but insensible contraction, and gets
its natural place above the symphysis. Rarely is relief expressed so completely as
after this operation; not even when the head is passing the external organs. These
cases strikingly resemble each other, and, when once seen, they will always afterwards be easily recognized."

This condition may be confounded with retained placenta, inverted uterus, severe
after-pains, and internal hemorrhage. Of the first of these the author gives instances,
and the characters of inversion of the uterus are sufficiently obvious to prevent
error. After-pains do not usually follow first labors, and when present in severity,
they probably depend on irregular contraction, with retention of coagula in the un-
contracted portion; while, in other cases, when retention of urine has been present,
the uterus takes on pseudo-expulsive action. The internal hemorrhage met with in
this case differs from that usually so designated. Thus there is sudden and severe
pain, and faintness is very rare, and rather due to prior exhaustion than to the loss
of blood, which is much less than in ordinary hemorrhage. There is not the enlargement of the abdomen, and it has not the same firmness, except at the spots,
where the contraction exists, where, indeed, it is much firmer. Elsewhere it is soft
and is not tumid. The flow is slight at first, and the blood coagulates as it takes
place. It is forced down into a solid mass through the dilated os into the vagina,
becoming firmer and firmer, until at last it gives rise to strong painful contractions,
for the purpose of obtaining its expulsion. The diagnosis is still further aided by
the perfect relief that follows the removal of the coagulum. In none of the cases
has secondary hemorrhage, so common in ordinary hemorrhage, been met with;
and there is here a feeling of safety which does not attach to ordinary cases.

ART. 119.—*On the Treatment of Cracked Nipple.* By M. LEGROUX, Physician to the Hotel Dieu, Paris.

(*Gaz. Hebdom. de Méd. et Chir.* Aug. 22, 1856.)

M. Legroux proposes to cover the affected nipple with an artificial epidermis, and he thinks that the "baudruche" will answer this purpose very conveniently. This "baudruche," first pricked with a few pin-holes to allow the milk to pass through, is drawn over the nipple, and then fixed to the skin of the breast by a varnish consisting of collodion, 30 grammes; castor oil, 50 centigrammes; and turpentine, 1 gramme 50 centigrammes. In applying this varnish, it is necessary to avoid the nipple itself, or much inconvenience and pain may be caused by the subsequent contraction of the drying film. When the infant is applied to the breast the "baudruche" is first made soft and supple by the application of a little sugar and water. With care one of these sacs may last for several days—until, in fact, the cracks may have healed.

ART. 120.—*On the differences in the composition of Milk at different times of the day.* By Professor BÖDEKER.

(*Zeitsch. für rat. Med.*, vol. vi, part 2, 1856.)

The very careful analyses of Dr. Bödeker lead to the following results:

1. The quantity of fatty matter increases continually from morning until evening, and in the evening it is nearly doubled. In sixteen ounces of milk drawn in the morning the infant received three-eighths of an ounce of butter, while in the same quantity of milk drawn in the evening it received from five-eighths to three-fourths of an ounce of the same substance.

2. This augmentation in the quantity of fatty matter is accompanied by a trifling augmentation in the quantity of caseine. In sixteen ounces of milk drawn in the morning, there were three-eighths of an ounce of dried caseine; and in the same quantity drawn in the evening, about nine-twentieths of an ounce.

3. As the caseine increases in quantity the albumen diminishes, and almost in the same proportion.

4. The sugar of milk undergoes little variation. It is, however, somewhat more abundant in the morning than in the afternoon.

5. The quantity of the saline constituents of the milk remains constant.

ART. 121.—*On the effect of Belladonna in arresting the Secretion of Milk.* By Dr. GOOLDEN, Physician to St. Thomas's Hospital.

(*Lancet*, Aug. 9, 1856.)

The two cases here detailed are not sufficient to prove that belladonna will always be either successful or safe, but they render it highly probable that it will be so. Dr. Goolden writes:

"E. J—, æt. 28, was admitted into Anne's Ward, St. Thomas's Hospital, with severe rheumatic fever, and with a child at the breast four months old. She had been ill four days. At the time of her admission she had swelling and acute pain in both wrists, right elbow, both knees, and left ankle. The knee-joints were distended with synovia, and erythematous patches were on the skin of the knees, ankles, and wrists. She was bathed in perspiration, and the secretion of milk was abundant. According to the regulation of the hospital the child was removed; indeed, from her helpless condition, it was necessary, considering the difficulty of attending to an infant in a ward with other patients. Soon after her admission she took eight grains of calomel and a grain and a half of opium, followed by a senna draught; and one scruple of nitrate of potassa, ten grains of bicarbonate of potassa, and half a drachm of spirit of nitric ether, in peppermint water, every four hours. The joints were covered with cotton wool.

"On the following day, at two o'clock, I found she had been freely purged; the joints were in nearly the same state. She had had no sleep. The breasts had become tumid, hard, painful, knotty, and extremely tender. The superficial veins were distended. Some milk had been drawn, but the process was attended with great pain, and we could not listen to the heart's sounds on account of the tenderness.

"A milk abscess, in complication with rheumatic fever, was of all things to be avoided, and unless the secretion could be at once arrested it appeared inevitable. In this strait I recollected that I had somewhere met with an observation (but I cannot remember whether it was in an English or foreign journal) that atropine applied externally to the breasts would dry up the milk; and thinking it reasonable, I caused the areola of the breasts to be smeared with extract of belladonna, in the same way that it is used to dilate the pupil of the eye. I likewise ordered the addition of half-drachm doses of colchicum wine, knowing that whenever milch cows eat the meadow saffron in the pasture, they immediately become dry; and though I have not much faith in colchicum as a remedy in rheumatic fever uncomplicated with gout, there could be no objection to its use, and it has the sanction of much higher authority than my own.

"On my third visit, the following day, the first inquiry was about the breasts. They were all right. But was it the colchicum or belladonna that had relieved them? The extract was used before I left the ward; before the mixture was given the secretion of milk had been arrested, and the breasts had become soft. The rest of the case has no further special interest. I will only state that there was no heart affection, and that the fever, though very severe while it lasted, was of short duration, and the patient left the hospital quite well, in fourteen days.

"The second case that occurred to me was uncomplicated with any disease, and such as would usually fall under the care of the accoucheur rather than the physician:

"A lady, the wife of a clergyman, was travelling with her husband, and in order to accompany him, had weaned her baby (then seven months old). Happening to be at Oxford at the commemoration festival, he came to me in great trouble, telling me that his wife had done a foolish thing in weaning the child, and that they were now arrested in their progress in consequence of the state of her breasts. They were tumid, very tender, painful, and hard, with large superficial veins, and the milk had been drawn with difficulty several times, with temporary relief. I recommended the application of the extract of belladonna to the areolæ, desiring them to send for a medical practitioner if the inconvenience did not immediately subside, or unless she felt quite well. A few days brought me a letter, giving a very satisfactory account, and thanking me for what she was pleased to call my wonderful prescription. Within two hours she was perfectly relieved, the milk absorbed, and (what is very important) there was no fever or other inconvenience attending the sudden suppression of the milk; and instead of taking the opening medicine I had prescribed for her, she continued her journey the next morning.

"I have not been able to discover that the fact that belladonna is available for the purpose of arresting the milk secretion is at all generally known—certainly it was not to several accoucheurs in large practice of whom I have inquired. The fact is important, if true, for then milk abscesses will become a matter of past history, and probably many diseases of the breast may be rendered less complicated by its use."

(B) CONCERNING THE DISEASES OF WOMEN.

ART. 122.—*The Contagiousness of Puerperal Fever.* By Dr. CREDE.

(*Verhandl. der Ges. für Geb.*, 1855; and *Br. and For. Med. Chir. Rev.*, April, 1856.)

"Dr. Credé, in a report on puerperal fever, confirms the conclusions arrived at in Vienna, as to the contagiousness of that disease. He relates that for nearly two years puerperal fever had raged with but little intermission in the Charite Hospital in Berlin. He refers to a statistical account by Dr. Quincke, to show that of about 650 women delivered there in the last year, 139 had been removed for illness to the inner station; all of these, with the exception of 15, were affected by puerperal fever, and 68 died. All the apartments used for the labor patients were twice changed, and once every utensil and all the attendants were changed. All had little or no influence. In the new room, as in the old, puerperal fever continued. Upon this, the physicians of the outer station made the observation that the contagion of hospital gangrene and of pyæmia, which also had not ceased within that time, was in close relationship with the puerperal fever contagion. It was therefore weighed by the committee whether it would not be desirable to remove the lying-in institution altogether from the Charite. Dr. Crede added, that it appeared manifest that whenever hospitals were connected with lying-in wards, puerperal fever contagion assumed far greater development and intensity, as in Vienna, Prague, Stuttgard."

ART. 123.—*On Phlebitis of the great venous trunks of the Neck subsequent to Labor.* By Dr. M'CLINTOCK, Master of the Lying-in Hospital, Dublin.

(*Dublin Quarterly Journal of Medical Science,* Aug., 1856.)

The two nearly related subjects—phlebitis and pyæmia—both still require close investigation, and offer for solution many important problems. Every new fact, therefore, in their history—every novel aspect under which either disease is seen—should be placed upon record for the purposes of future generalization. Accordingly, the following case is brought forward by Dr. M'Clintock, as presenting some features of peculiar interest:

CASE.—S. D—, æt. 22, was confined of her first child, a boy, on March 8th, after a labor of twenty-eight hours' duration. The consumption of time chiefly took place in the first stage, and in consequence of rigidity of the os uteri. For several days previously to the setting in of true labor, she suffered much from spurious pains; and very considerable hemorrhage occurred immediately on the expulsion of the after-birth. From the time of delivery her pulse was remarked to be quick, above 100; and this rate of frequency did not subsequently diminish. During the ensuing week she remained in a very unsatisfactory state. She had no rigor, nor anything like a distinct accession of fever or inflammation; but the pulse was constantly 110, or upwards; the belly was tumid; the uterus large, and tender on deep pressure; and she was troubled with painful tenesmus, and frequent dysenteric stools. Nevertheless, she was cheerful, and made no complaint of uneasiness in any particular situation. On her ninth day there was an apparent improvement in every respect, the pulse falling to 96, the belly becoming soft, and bowels being moved only five or six times in the twenty-four hours. On her tenth day she drew our attention to a fulness and tenderness immediately above the inner end of the right clavicle. There was a slight tumefaction in this situation, such as might be caused by a simple glandular enlargement. About this time she began to complain of a short, irritating, dry cough, which used to annoy her in the evening, and for which no satisfactory cause could be discovered A few days later a similar swelling appeared in the corresponding situation on the left side of the neck. She did not seem to experience any serious uneasiness from these tumors, and beyond fomenting them with warm water, and painting with tincture of iodine, no decisive treatment was employed. Some days later, namely, on the 22d of March, her fifteenth day, I detected the existence of considerable œdema at the root of the neck, and across the upper and anterior part of the chest, but more so at the left side. The diarrhœa still continued, though with greatly diminished severity; her pulse was usually about 108; and the abdomen was flaccid, and entirely free from pain or fulness.

On the 26th of March the œdematous swelling of her neck was decidedly less, though her face seemed somewhat puffy, and the tenderness still remained. As she was now eighteen days confined, and seemed better, we yielded to her own urgent request for leave to be dressed, and to lie on the outside of the bed. Before she was dressed, however, she got an indistinct rigor, and had to be put back into bed.

From this time forward her symptoms underwent a striking change; and she progressively became worse and worse. There was a marked exacerbation of all the febrile symptoms; with hurried respiration and occasional vomiting. In addition to these it was noticed, that the superficial veins, beneath the clavicles, and on the fore part of the chest, had manifestly become varicose.

From a careful review of her history, and an attentive consideration of her present symptoms, there seemed little room to doubt the existence of inflammation of some of the deep veins of the neck; and though not aware that such a diagnosis had

ever been made, still we conceived that no other lesion could satisfactorily explain
the peculiar features of her case.

On March 28th she is reported to have slept tolerably well; pulse 120; a deep
flush on each cheek; the rest of the face is puffy, and of a chlorotic hue; the belly
is soft and relaxed, and everywhere free from tenderness; the network of enlarged
veins is still more apparent than heretofore, and includes some branches of the
upper arm. The tongue is dry, and has a brown streak down the centre. Her
breathing is somewhat oppressed; and she continues to have towards evening a
short, teasing cough; this seems to be her chief source of discomfort; for, unless
she moves her head, she experiences no pain in the neck. A slight rigor occurred
to-day; in the evening it was remarked that her hearing was somewhat impaired.
A rough bruit was detected with the first sound of the heart.

Her condition on the next day was, in every respect, more alarming; the pulse
128, and weak; tongue dry, brown, and crusted; slight subsultus of hands; frequent sickness of stomach; face much swollen; eyes prominent and pupils dilated;
deafness increased towards evening; she complained of indistinctness of vision.
Her mind continues clear and undisturbed.

On the 30th it was plain that her dissolution could not be far off. The respirations were frequent and labored; the pulse scarcely countable, and very weak, though
the heart was beating strongly; a thick brown crust on the tongue; pupils very
much dilated. She was drowsy, and towards evening lapsed into a comatose state,
which ended in death, at 9 P.M.

Autopsy, twelve hours after death.—The enlarged veins in the neck and chest
still very distinct, though changed in color. The abdomen, when laid open, presented no morbid appearance; the liver was healthy. The *uterus* was rather large for
this period—twenty-two days—after delivery; its structure was remarkably soft and
friable. Behind this organ, and deep in the pelvis, existed a small abscess. The
mucous membrane of the large intestines seemed thickened, and was of a very dark
color, apparently from intense congestion. The *kidneys* were in an advanced stage
of fatty degeneration. On dissecting back the integuments of the neck, and exposing the great venous trunks in this region, it was at once apparent that phlebitis,
in its most marked form, had existed here. The deep jugulars, both subclavians,
the upper part of each axillary, the right vena innominata, and superior portion of
left, were the vessels engaged. In calibre they seemed enlarged, their coats were
thickened, and internally they contained firm plugs of coagula and lymph, the latter
being the more external, and adhering very closely to the wall of the vessel. These
formations extended down to near the superior cava, the lining membrane of which
was redder than natural. The pulmonary valves were intensely red, as was the
interior of the pulmonary artery, contrasting strongly with the aorta, which presented
its natural color. In the right auricular appendix was a small incipient abscess.
The tricuspid and mitral valves were intensely injected, so as to present a bright
scarlet color. The aortic valves contained some calcareous matter, but otherwise
presented no abnormal appearance. The lining membrane of the heart itself was
pale, and showed no traces of inflammation.*

" Such," proceeds Dr M'Clintock, " is a very brief history of the symptoms and
morbid appearances which this case presented. It will be remarked that, at an
early period after parturition, the patient became affected with symptoms of low
puerperal fever, the gastro-intestinal mucous membrane being the part on which
the action of the poison seemed to be chiefly expended, though it is possible this
diarrhœa may have had some connection with the renal disease. A variety of circumstances concurred in this case to favor the development of puerperal fever. The
kidneys were far advanced in fatty degeneration : she had spurious pains for a considerable time before the setting-in of true parturient action; her labor was tedious
(twenty-seven hours), and was followed by severe hemórrhage. Another circumstance there was in her case, yet more influential than all these together, in predisposing to the invasion of puerperal fever : she had been seduced, and was laboring
under intense mental depression, from the conjoint influence of bitter disappointment, and the cheerless prospect of a life of irretrievable disgrace and shame.

" The attack of puerperal fever seemed partially to yield to treatment; there
was some mitigation in the local and general symptoms. In the middle of the

* The preparation showing these morbid alterations is now in the museum of the Lying-in Hospital.

second week, however, the first indication of phlebitis of the neck showed itself. Now, in most cases of crural phlebitis, we find the course of events to be much the same as that just described. Thus, of sixty cases of puerperal phlegmasia dolens, collected by Dr. Mackenzie, the attack followed upon some form of puerperal fever in thirty-three instances, and even this proportion I believe to be much under the mark.

" The local effects of phlebitis were present, for some days, without being attended with any remarkable constitutional symptoms; and I freely confess that no suspicion crossed my mind, at this period, of the real nature of this swelling in the neck. To this localized tumefaction œdema succeeded; then came a rigor, and after it a sudden explosion of alarming symptoms, which too plainly revealed that the very fountain of life itself was poisoned. At a later period the dilated condition of the superficial veins on the front of the chest attracted our attention, and first suggested the possible existence of phlebitis of the deep veins of the neck. But little reflection was required for this conjecture to settle down into absolute conviction; in fact, for the establishment of this diagnosis, no symptom was now wanting: there were local swelling and tenderness, œdema, unequivocal signs of venous obstruction, and the constitutional disturbance ordinarily attendant upon phlebitis. Mark, also, the sequence in which the symptoms appeared: first, puerperal fever, and apparently partial recovery; next, localized pain and tumefaction; then œdema; and, some days later, a rigor, with increased constitutional disturbance; and, lastly, varicose enlargement of the superficial veins.

" The condition in which the deep jugular veins were found after death, plainly showed that they had become wholly impervious, so that the return of blood from the head must have been entirely effected through the vertebral and superficial jugular veins. That great obstruction existed in the venous circulation, was manifest during the last few days of her life, and caused the aspect and expression of her face to bear a very close resemblance to those cases in which heart-disease, and enlargement of the thyroid gland, coexist. I regret exceedingly that an examination of the head could not be obtained.

" The subclavian vein on each side was more or less obstructed by firm coagula and lymph; yet there was no œdema on either hand or either arm. It is, perhaps, impossible to say, with certainty, in what particular spot the phlebitis began, or in what direction it spread; that is, whether in a direction towards or from the heart. My own opinion is, that it extended along the veins *contrary* to the course of the circulation, as is generally observed in crural phlebitis. This opinion is founded on observation of the situation of the tumor during life, and of the morbid appearances in the veins, the apparently more recent inflammatory deposits being at the remote point from the heart.

" The existence of fatty degeneration of the kidneys is a feature in this case that should not be overlooked, particularly at the present time, when so much attention is being directed to the influence which this organic lesion exercises over the progress and results of intercurrent diseases. The urine was not at any time tested, as, owing to the constant presence of diarrhœa, it was not procured free from the admixture of fæcal matter.

" I believe it will not be an exaggeration to assert, that the case just detailed, in so far as relates to the phlebitis of the venæ innominatæ, is almost unique in medical literature. I know of but one similar instance; it was exhibited at the Pathological Society, in November, 1851, by Dr. Mayne, and the account of it is published in the thirteenth volume of the 'Dublin Quarterly Journal,' new series."

ART. 124.—*On the Cramps of Nurses.* By M. VERDIER.

(*Bull. de Thér.*, tom. 1, p. 201.)

In this communication M. Verdier directs attention to the cramps which occasionally occur in enfeebled and ill-fed nurses. These cramps occur more frequently in the upper extremities than in the lower, and occasionally they are confined to the muscles of the neck. The pain is often very severe and continued. Most generally the cramps were accompanied by evidence of scrofula or hysteria. Weaning, an improved diet, with opium and ether for the pain, were the remedies.

ART. 125.—*On the treatment of Milk Abscess.*   By Dr. JAMES GILMOUR.

(*Lancet*, June 7, 1856.)

After some prefatory remarks, Dr. Gilmour says, "I beg to reintroduce to the notice of the medical profession the treatment of milk abscess by *compression*, as advocated by Trousseau and Contour; the compression being made with very long strips of adhesive plaster.   I give their own words: 'The compression is to be accomplished by strips of plaster, broad, and sufficiently long to go several times round the body.   The surgeon, standing by the side of the patient, must first fix one of the extremities of the slip at about the middle of the back; then carry it towards the side of the chest; then pass it over the breast, beginning from the lowest part; then obliquely from below upwards to the outer third of the clavicle on the healthy side; and then obliquely downwards across the back, so as to cover the extremity of the slip already fixed.   Following this course several times, he must take care that the portion of the band applied each time covers the two upper thirds of the preceding turn.   But it is easy to see that if the bandage is always carried in the same direction, the breast cannot be completely covered; and that, on the other hand, as its several turns go across the clavicle of the healthy side, the movements of the shoulders would tend to displace it, and the lower part of the breast might soon be uncovered.   Other strips of plaster are therefore applied, which, proceeding from the anterior and upper part of the abdomen, ascend, crossing the first obliquely; then pass under the axilla, and return, after passing over the posterior part of the chest to the part where they were first applied, and then are carried again along the same track, covering each time the two upper thirds of the strip last applied.   The breast is thus completely covered by the bandage, which is prevented from rising by this last described, which ought to cover only the upper part of the breast.'

"And what advantages did the authors attribute to this plan?   They found that it immediately relieved pain, and diminished the inflammatory engorgement.   When applied, after the abscess was opened, it favored the evacuation of matter and shortened the suppurative period.   I have considerably modified Trousseau's method in my practice: I use bands of plaster about 14 inches long and 1 inch broad; occasionally they may be required rather longer.   The extremities of the strips are attached to the ribs behind, pass over the tumefied mamma, and fastened on or about the sternum: whilst a second set pass from the anterior part of the abdomen to the clavicle, covering the first layer, and *vice versa*.   I am satisfied this answers as well as the longer bands, the amount of compression is nearly as great, and the benefits very satisfactory, as will be seen by the recital of only three cases selected from a large number."

CASE 1.—Mrs. H—, æt. 27, confined May 4th, 1854, of her first child; breech presented; still-born.   Forty-eight hours afterwards, and when the breasts were tumefied and painful, the adhesive strapping was applied, as above described, *the nipple being entirely covered.*   Saline aperients were freely administered.   On the second day after compression, the breasts felt full, and attended with considerable pain.   She says that the strapping slightly interferes with her breathing, but objects to have it taken off.   Next day feels more comfortable; the swelling and tension gradually subsided until the plaster became loose, when it was removed.   She was quite well in ten days.

CASE 2.—Mrs. E—, æt. 29, confined June 4th, 1855, of her second child, which was very delicate and strumous.   She had witnessed the good effect of the strapping in Case 1; she also told me that at her first confinement both the breasts suppurated, and did not heal until after two months of great suffering.   Two days after delivery I applied the strapping, but *the nipples were not covered.*   The lacteal secretion was not entirely suppressed; the baby sucked at regular intervals; and when I considered the breasts sufficiently prepared for a larger flow of milk to enter, I removed the plaster, and she also was well in ten days.   However, three weeks afterwards, from exposure to cold, the left mamma became swollen and painful; a hard tumor formed in the superior part of the organ, next the clavicle.   The compression was again applied for four days, and removed; the swelling had disappeared.   Saline purgatives were taken during both periods of compression.   Since that time she has had no return of any inflammatory engorgement.

Case 3.—Mrs. S——, æt. 24, delivered on December 2d, 1855, of a strong healthy infant, a *primipara*. On the third day afterwards, when the breasts were very full and painful, owing to the baby refusing the nipple, which was small and flattened, the strapping was applied in the usual manner, *leaving the nipples uncovered*. The lacteal secretion was abundant, and ran from the nipples. She says she has had no pain since the compression was commenced. One week afterwards she removed the strapping, owing to its getting loose, and she continued quite well. Aperients were given as usual.

"In cases where the plaster was applied too late to prevent suppuration, I was astonished at the relief afforded from pain, tension, and throbbing, though the abscess gradually proceeds to complete maturation. After suppuration has taken place, and the abscess having naturally burst before the surgeon had been called in, the greatest benefit will be found from the application of this mode of compression; and amongst the many advantages arising from the strapping, not the least important is the prevention of the pyogenic action from extending through the lax tissue of the organ.

"Again, when suppuration has gone on unchecked, and after one or more sinuses have formed, marked benefit will be derived from this mode of compression. In such cases great attention and perseverance are requisite, because the plaster will have to be repeatedly changed, for it becomes loose, as the chronic engorgement and tissue infiltration disappear. I prefer the preliminary trial of this method in sinuous abscess to others recommended—to laying open the sinuses, at first practised by Hey, and still followed by others; or to the injection of the sinuses with iodine, as pursued by Mr. Birkett at Guy's Hospital. At the same time that local strapping is employed in these cases, we must resort to constitutional treatment by tonics and alteratives, for the system is generally weakened and debilitated, owing to the continual drain kept up from the sinuses. Hectic may exist; many women are greatly emaciated, so much so that Ramsbotham states that 'the body has been known to dwindle almost to a shadow.' I have a patient under my care at present, aged 23, with sinuses in one breast, of six weeks' duration, who presents all the appearances of a person far advanced in phthisis. If the compression be employed in these cases without a generous diet, fresh air, and tonic medicines, we shall assuredly fail in causing the sinuses to heal up; but when all are conjoined, the improvement of the patient is gradually manifested."

Art. 126.—*Glycerine and Tannin in Vaginitis.* By M. Demarquay.

(*Bull. de Therap.*, t. l, p. 541; and *Med. Chir. Rev.*, Oct. p. 549.)

In the treatment of this affection, M. Demarquay has found a composition, consisting of eighty parts of glycerine and twenty of tannin, of great service. When the vaginitis first appears, the inflammatory symptoms should be calmed by appropriate regimen, baths, and frequent emollient injections. When the first stage of the inflammation has passed away, and the careful introduction of the speculum has become possible, abundant injections of water are to be thrown in, so as to remove all the muco-pus which lines the walls of the vagina, and these are then dried by a plug of charpie placed at the end of a long forceps. Then, three plugs of wadding, well soaked in glycerine and tannin, are to be introduced. Next day, after a bath, the plugs are removed, new injections made, and the dressing repeated. M. Demarquay has never had to have recourse to more than four or five such dressings. After discontinuing them, astringent injections, consisting of infusion of walnut leaves, in which one drachm of alum to the quart has been dissolved, are employed two or three times a day for a week or ten days.

Art. 127.—*On some of the injurious effects of Prolapsus Uteri.* By Professor A. Retzius, of Stockholm.

(*Anatomiska iakttagelser;* and *Edinburgh Medical Journal*, July, 1856.)

On a previous occasion, a case was communicated by Professor Duben, where, in an individual suffering from prolapsus uteri, one of the kidneys was found atrophied, with dilatation of its pelvis and ureter, in consequence of pressure by the tumefied lower portion of the uterus. Shortly afterwards, Professor Retzius had an opportunity, in the anatomical rooms, of examining a subject affected with an extensive prolapsus. He found here both kidneys atrophied, forming, as it were, thin caps over the greatly dilated pelves; the calyces and the papillæ renales being obliterated. The ureters were also dilated, and lengthened to more than twice the normal dimension. They lay flattened, of the breadth of half an inch, and presented many windings. The urinary bladder was also remarkably large, and in its lower part considerably thickened. The place where the ureters enter into the posterior wall of the bladder was pushed down into the lower opening of the pelvis. The under portion of the bladder lay thrust forward, between the arch of the pubis and the prolapsed and swollen uterus. The urethra, which, in its natural condition, has a straight direction between the vagina and the arch of the pubis, through the fascia profunda of the pelvis, was here compressed towards the arch, by the prolapsus, and had a greatly bent course upwards, around and beneath the arch, almost in the form of a loop. The canal was at the same time widened and lengthened; and from its orifice depended a flat, lancet-shaped flap, a prolongation of the mucous membrane.

It is obvious that the prolapsus had proved here a source of pressure, as well posteriorly on the corpus trigonum, into which the ureters open, as towards the arch of the pubis, and upon the prolonged and thickened neck of the bladder itself. Hence ensued an obstruction of the flow of the urine, which had evidently, as the case of Professor Duben had already demonstrated, led to the atrophy of the kidneys, and to the lengthening and distension of the urinary passages; which again, in their turn, must have conducted to a deleterious influence upon the condition of the blood, and upon the whole organism.

ART. 128.—*Inversion of the Uterus replaced on the third day.* By Dr. ISAAC G. PORTER.

(*American Journal of Med. Science,* July, 1856.)

The point especially inviting attention, in the following case, is the length of time that elapsed before the replacement of the inverted uterus.

CASE.—A lady, 30 years of age, of delicate organization, though of uniformly good health, was confined in the country, at 4 o'clock A.M., Tuesday, March 18th, under the care of a neighboring practitioner. The labor was not severe, lasting but little over four hours, but the delivery of the placenta was delayed one or two hours, doubtless owing to atony of the uterus. It came away somewhat disrupted, although the physician disclaimed having used any undue interference. Previous, and subsequent to its delivery, there was much flooding, attended with great faintness, prostration, nausea, &c. Some hours after, she partly arose in the bed to urinate, when the uterus made a complete descent, through the external parts, forming a tumor the size of "two fists." Increased prostration, and much alarm and distress followed the shock which the system sustained from the abnormal displacement and the downward pressure of the contents of the abdomen, as well as from an entire inability to pass water. This function was not performed after the accident, until the reinversion of the uterus, except as the mass was crowded upwards by manual assistance, thus relieving the pressure on the urethra; and, on my arrival, I found the protruded body partially returned, within the vagina, where it was supported by a pessary, or tampon, resting externally on the bed. The physician and patient both informed me, that great relief followed this partial reposition, she being enabled thereby to pass water, yet with difficulty, while, by the same means, the traction of the uterus on its ligaments, was considerably lessened.

The patient resided about twenty miles distant, and I did not see her until Thursday eve, at 8 o'clock, almost three days after the accident. The foregoing account I received from the physician in attendance. At this time moderate reaction had come on; countenance anxious and deadly pale; pulse 120, and irritable. There was much distress and tenderness in the abdomen, flooding not severe, since the complete inversion, and immediate danger to life did not appear imminent. An examination confirmed the suspicion of inversion. The vagina was filled with a firm, yet compressible, globular, and sensitive mass, answering the usual description of books—no os tincæ was discovered, but there was a marked fold of the vagina encircling the tumor, which is mentioned in this place as being confirmatory of the opinion that this constitutes a valuable diagnostic between inversion of the uterus and polypus. Gentle but gradually increasing force with the back of the flexed fingers caused the mass to diminish in size, and slowly to ascend in the direction of the superior strait. As it grew less in dimensions it was more easily grasped, and ultimately, the uterus, with the hand encircling and compressing it, was used as a *stem*, with which upward pressure was exerted. Under this compound action of compression and elevation, the restoration became much more rapid. Owing to the extensibility of the soft parts, considerable counter-pressure on the abdomen became necessary. The sensation communicated to the hand was very different, when the parts were returned as far as the os tincæ and the uterus, in which latter the regular process of involution had evidently commenced. There was less resiliency in the uterus at the last stage of the operation than is common immediately after delivery—but rather a spontaneous yielding to a slight force, with one or two fingers; these were retained in the cavity for some minutes after the completion of the operation, which occupied about twenty-five minutes. Immediate relief followed, the uterus resumed its place in the hypogastrium, and the abdomen became much less tender on pressure. Under the influence of a stimulant, and an opiate, the patient enjoyed her first sleep since her confinement. The horizontal position for a week was strictly observed, and there being incontinence of urine for a few days, the catheter was uncalled for. Some febrile excitement existed in the form of thirst, frequent pulse, and much pain in the back. The lochia was sparing, and the secretion of milk never occurred. The countenance was blanched and leucophlegmatic, and there was anæmic headache.

On the thirteenth day, while attempting to sit in a chair for the first time, a severe pain in her right leg and hip seized her, which was the commencement of a mild attack of phlegmasia dolens. For two days the disease was extreme, as was the tenderness in the tract of the femoral vessels. The case, however, speedily yielded, verifying the principle, that the later the attack after parturition, the more amenable to remedies.

ART. 129.—*On the surgical treatment of Uterine Polypi.* By Dr. SPAETH.
(*Zeitsch f. prac. Heilkunde*, June 6, 1856.)

How is it that there are such discrepancies in the experience of surgeons with respect to the ligature and knife? How is it that the ligature has succeeded so admirably in some hands, and failed so completely in the hands of others? The explanation, M. Spaeth thinks, is to be found, not in the operator, but in the circumstances under which the operation is undertaken. M. Spaeth is of opinion that *the operation ought to be deferred until the polypus is liberated from the neck of the uterus*, unless there are some special reasons to the contrary; and he says that it is of little moment how we operate, if the operation be thus deferred.

ART. 130.—*On Carbonic Acid as a local anæsthetic in uterine diseases, &c.*
By (1) Professor SIMPSON, and (2) Dr. WM. WILLIAMSON.

1. (*Edinburgh Medical Journal*, July, 1856.)
2. (*Ibid.*, Aug., 1856.)

1. At a recent meeting of the Obstetrical Society of Edinburgh, Dr. Simpson said that he had used carbonic acid successfully as a local anæsthetic, in neuralgia of the vagina and uterus, and in various morbid states and displacements of the pelvic organs accompanied with pain and spasms. He had found it also sometimes of use in irritable states of the neighboring organs. Two years ago he had under his care, from Canada, the wife of a medical gentleman, who was suffering much from that most distressing disease—dysuria and irritability of the bladder. Many modes of treatment had been tried in vain. The injection of carbonic acid gas into the vaginal canal several times a day at once produced relief, and ultimately effected a perfect cure. She has remained well since her return to America, and lately became a mother. Occasionally, relief follows immediately. In two or three instances, he stated he had seen the use of the gas continued daily for months, and that he had notes of one case where the patient was invalided, and almost entirely kept to the supine posture for years, from feelings of pain and bearing-down in the uterus and neighboring parts, particularly on attempting to sit or walk. Many

modes of treatment were tried by himself and others, with little or no benefit. She has, however, at last regained in a great measure the power of progression, and freedom from suffering in the erect posture—a result which she herself ascribes to the local application of carbonic acid gas.

In practice, he generally used a common wine-bottle for the formation of the carbonic acid gas, and formed the gas by mixing in the bottle six drachms of crystallized tartaric acid with a solution of eight drachms of bicarbonate of soda, in six or seven ounces of water. A long flexible caoutchouc tube conducts the gas from the bottle into the vagina. The cork fixing this tube into the mouth of the bottle should be adapted so as to prevent any escape of the gas by its sides. With this view the cork should be perforated by a metallic tube, and covered externally with a layer of caoutchouc. In a case in which the two preceding children were both lost, he had successfully brought on premature labor at the eighth month, by the repeated application of carbonic acid gas to the vaginal canal with this apparatus—the carbonic acid not acting directly as a specific oxytocic or excitor of uterine contraction, but indirectly only by distending greatly and mechanically (as examination with the finger proved it to do) the vaginal canal, and ultimately separating, like the injection of water, the membranes from the cervix uteri.

The application of carbonic acid as a local anæsthetic to the uterine mucous surfaces and to other parts of the body is not a discovery of late times. He had found that in this, as in many other examples, that what appeared at first novel, was, when fully investigated, a practice known previously in its essence, and perhaps in its more minute details also. Besides here, as elsewhere, when once a principle is detected, such as the anæsthetic power of carbonic acid gas when applied topically, we can explain by it the good effects of modes of practice which, previously perhaps, we were inclined to ridicule and reject. The fact that carbonic acid, when locally applied to a mucous surface, acts as a sedative or anæsthetic, explains a practice common among the ancients, viz., Hippocrates, Paulus Ægineta, Rueff, Pare, &c., all of whom used to burn herbs, aromatic and medicinal, and convey the fumes by means of tubes and appropriate apparatus to the interior of the vagina; and such vapor being loaded with carbonic acid, it is more than probable that if such treatment was effectual, it was through the anæsthetic properties of the gas here alluded to. Again, there is a modern practice much in vogue on the Continent, of injecting the vagina, &c., with the German waters of Nuheim, Marienbad, &c.; the utility of the practice, which Dr. Simpson has been assured by his friend, Dr. Funck, of Frankford, is most marked in some diseased states, will find its true explanation in the local anæsthetic effect of carbonic acid, as these waters contain a large quantity of the gas. A knowledge of the topical effects of carbonic acid serves, perhaps, also to afford an explanation of other points in common therapeutics; as, for example, its action in subduing gastric and intestinal irritation. Hence the use of effervescing draughts, aerated waters, &c., in gastric irritability and nausea; perhaps the antacid action of the alkali may have some effect, but most likely it is the anæsthetic properties of the carbonic acid gas. The sedative and curative effects of injections into the rectum of carbonic acid gas in dysentery have a similar explanation, and serve to corroborate this view of its action. As an example of its use as a local anæsthetic to a cutaneous surface, Dr. Simpson alluded to the *cataplasma cerevisiæ*, or yeast poultice, which exhales from its surface a quantity of the gas. It was commonly applied to irritable and sloughing sores, and its soothing, healing, and antiseptic properties were doubtless owing to the carbonic acid gas. As an anæsthetic application to cancerous ulcers, the effects of carbonic acid gas are excellent. Dr. Ewart of Bath, says, "he has kept a person in ease and comfort, who, for so great a length of time before, had known only agony and torture." "What," he elsewhere observes, "strikes us in the two preceding cases with the greatest astonishment, is the *almost instantaneous relief of pain*, which *never failed to follow the application of the gas*." In reference to the effects of carbonic acid upon raw surfaces and wounds, Dr. Ingenhouz mentioned to Beddoes the following experiment: "Blister your finger, so as to lay bare the naked and sensible skin. The contact of air will produce pain; put your finger into vital air (oxygene), and this will produce more pain; introduce it into fixed or azotic air (carbonic acid or nitrogen), and the pain will diminish or cease." In relation to this statement, Dr. Beddoes informs us that he made the following experiments on three different persons : First. The raised epidermis of a blistered finger, after all action from the cantharides had ceased, was cut away in carbonic acid gas. No pain was felt. Secondly. A second blister being opened in common air, smarting pain came on. In a bladder of fixed air, this pain soon went off. Thirdly. After opening a third blister, the finger was instantly plunged into oxygene. It felt as when salt is sprinkled on a cut. In carbonic acid gas, the pain in two minutes quite subsided ; but returned when the denuded skin was again exposed to the atmosphere. If there be no source of fallacy in these experiments, they certainly point to one kind of improvement in the treatment of some painful burns, wounds, &c. For they appear to suggest the possibility of the suffering which is attendant on such injuries being controlled and cancelled by keeping the pained parts in contact with carbonic acid, or with some other gas or fluid, capable of acting as a local anæsthetic. If the reports of Ewart, Beddoes, and Fourcroy are correct, we ought also, indeed, to find carbonic acid an excellent application even as far as the mere healing and cicatrization of the broken surfaces are concerned.

2. Dr. Williamson confirms the previous statement of Dr. Simpson. He believes, moreover, that carbonic acid acts peculiarly and specifically upon the organs of generation as a sedative and stimulant. Dr. Williamson also gives some interesting particulars about the "gas-bath" of Marienbad.

"In 1845," he says, "I spent some time in Marienbad, where carbonic acid, in various forms, plays a very important part among the curative agents in use there ; and where I had an opportunity of becoming acquainted with its various therapeutic applications, and, in particular, with its use in the form of bath, under the name of '*the Gas Bath*,' which was at this time in great repute throughout Germany ; and to these I shall confine the following remarks.

"The 'Guide Books' abound with accounts of its therapeutic properties, many of which my friend, Dr. Hirzig, resident practitioner there, corroborated, with other additional details, particularly of its use in uterine affections, which induced me to follow up the subject more fully.

"The carbonic acid employed there has a small admixture of sulphuretted hydrogen, sufficient to render it very disagreeable to the sense of smell, and to injure the polish of your gold watch or pencil-case (should you expose them to its influence, which I was thoughtless enough to do), but which is not believed to exert any therapeutic effect, that being entirely owing to the carbonic acid.

"The gas is obtained from the surface of an extensive natural mud deposit, which abounds in the neighborhood of the establishment. This is constantly boiling and bubbling forth immense volumes of this gas from its miry depths, and a portion of it is covered by a large funnel, which collects and confines the gas as it rises, and which is thence conveyed by a tube into the bath compartment.

"This compartment is barrel-shaped, and provided with a seat, and a lid or cover, which fits closely around the neck of the patient, whose trunk and extremities are thus alone exposed to the vapor, which rushes with great force into the compartment against his person, but without being in any way directed to any particular part thereof. While undergoing the operation, therefore, the patient is immersed in a powerful current of the gas, which plays freely over his whole trunk and extremities.

"The therapeutic influence, however, is said to be confined to the pelvic viscera, or more particularly to the organs of generation ; and the bath has an extensive reputation for the cure of diseases seated in those parts, and in particular, for the removal of certain kinds of sterility, of which many interesting, or perhaps fabulous instances, are related in the ephemeral publications which abound at all such establishments. Much of this must, no doubt, be put down to the spirit of exaggeration too frequently indulged in by the interested writers of those local Guides and Hand-books ; although I have reason to believe, that in this instance they contain a certain amount of truth and fact.

"I was, of course, rather sceptical as to its powers of removing sterility, as well as to the more specific effects it was said to exert upon the generative organs in particular, and resolved to put the matter to some simple test ; for I was told that its physiological effects even, were marked and palpable to the senses, and of which I could easily persuade myself by experiment. Still, knowing how apt peculiar sensations, and even vascular changes, are to be set up in the human organism, and particularly in these organs, through the medium of suggestion, or by concentrating the attention on them for a given time, I was careful to prevent this source of error, and arranged that two young men of our party, who were entirely ignorant of the reputed effects of the bath, should subject themselves to its influence, requesting them to attend carefully to any peculiar sensations or effects it might produce on them.

" After remaining in the bath about fifteen minutes, they described their sensations to be almost identical, viz., that a prickling heat extended over the genital organs, followed by free perspiration and moist exudation from the mucous surfaces. Finding such result from this simple experiment, I was quite prepared to believe that very important therapeutic effects might be obtained by properly guiding and directing the application of this agent in many cases of uterine disease, as well as of many other diseases affecting the organs of generation."

ART. 131.—*A very large Ovarian Tumor.* By Dr. GEO. D. GIBB.
(*Trans. of the Pathological Soc. of London*, vol. vii.)

This tumor is probably the largest ever removed entire from the dead body, its weight being no less than 106 pounds. It was obtained from a young unmarried woman, æt. 31, and, so far as could be ascertained, it had occupied about seven years in its growth. As might be expected from its extreme size, the displacement of the viscera was very remarkable, the stomach and the greater part of the bowels occupying the position of the left lung, which was completely shrunk and carnified, the cervix uteri and vagina being remarkably elongated, &c. The tumor itself was composed of simple fibro-cellular tissue, with some cysts—a large one, containing forty four pints of homogeneous puriform fluid, and several minute ones, containing a yellowish-red, serous-looking fluid,—but none of these cysts appeared to be proliferous.

ART. 132.—*Vesical Calculus in the Female removed by a new method of Dilatation.* By Dr. R. T. CORBETT, Surgeon to the Royal Glasgow Infirmary.
(*Glasgow Med. Journal*, Oct. 1856.)

" Mrs. M'K—, æt. 42, admitted June 25th, 1856, into the Glasgow Royal Infirmary, under my care. About ten months ago patient gave birth to a still-born child. About a week afterwards the desire to evacuate the contents of the bladder became very frequent, sudden, irresistible, and attended with considerable pain, which was rather increased when the urine had been expelled. Mere change of position frequently induced the desire, and sometimes, when the urine was passing in full stream, the flow would suddenly stop, to begin again when the posture was changed. On admission the above symptoms continued.

" On passing a sound into the bladder, a stone was readily detected. There was considerable mucous deposit in the urine, and the sleep was much disturbed.

" June 27th.—The patient having been put under the influence of chloroform, a fine specimen of the common 'fusible calculus,' measuring fully one inch and an eighth in length by one inch in breadth, was extracted by means of the following simple apparatus. A piece of vulcanized india-rubber tubing, half an inch in diameter and six inches in length, was tied at the one end to a metallic rod fourteen inches long, slightly bent, and the size of a No. 10 sound. The elastic tube was then stretched along the rod, till the four inches of its extremity were scarcely thicker than the rod itself; and having been oiled, the apparatus was introduced into the bladder for three or four inches, and the tubing allowed to contract itself, which readily took place, when the hand that held it extended was gradually relaxed. By this means, general and equable dilatation was in two or three minutes accomplished to the extent of the diameter of the tube, and the instrument was allowed to remain for a few minutes longer, when it was withdrawn, and the forefinger of my left hand, previously oiled, introduced into the bladder, which was easily done, and the stone brought to its neck, from which it was readily extracted by a small pair of lithotomy forceps. The calculus was unusually rough, weighed 166 grains, and a section of it presented a uniform appearance. An analysis of it by Dr. Penny gave the following as its composition : 'A mixture of the phosphate of ammonia and magnesia, or triple phosphate, and bone-phosphate of lime; also a small quantity of lithic acid, with a little animal matter.'

"The patient was ordered an anodyne draught at bedtime. The report next morning was, that she had slept well and suffered no pain. She could now retain her urine for two hours, whereas, before the operation, she could only retain it for five or ten minutes. On account of the mucous discharge from the bladder, which continued, but in a slighter degree than before the operation, I ordered the following:

R Pulv. Uvæ Ursi, gr. xii, ter in die, ex Cyatho Aquæ.
    Tinct. Hyoscyami, ʒj;
    Aquæ Menth. Pip., ʒss. Misce.
Fiat haustus, hora somni sumendus.

"From this date till her dismissal, about the 25th of July, she continued to improve, never having had the slightest incontinence of urine.

"It will be remarked, that upon this occasion I used half-inch tubing; but in any case in which I expected to find as large a stone, I should now employ three-quarter inch, take more time to dilate, and allow the instrument to remain a little longer in the bladder, when, having withdrawn the apparatus, I should proceed as already described.

"The above is the description of my original instrument, the construction of which was the work of a few minutes; but I expect soon to have an opportunity of testing a more perfect apparatus, adapted for the removal of all the varieties of stone that are likely to be met with in the female bladder—an instrument which, when introduced, will permit small stones to be removed through its cylinder by means of long, slender forceps, and also the fragments of very large stones, previously broken down by a pair of cutting pliers carried into the bladder in the same way as the forceps. From the success which attended this case, I should feel disposed, in all instances of vesical calculus in the female, to remove the source of irritation, by dilatation, by lithotripsy, or by both, in preference to lithotomy; and this I fondly hope will not only be practicable, but easily accomplished by the method just described, and that without the drawback of incontinence of urine, which hitherto has too often followed the best performed cutting operations.

"Dr. South, in his translation of Chelius's System of Surgery, observes, in a note:

"'In all the previously described operations (i. e. lithotomy in the female), incontinence of urine is a very troublesome consequence, and often incurable. Astley Cooper, indeed, says: "In all cases of this operation which I have performed or witnessed, the urine has not been afterwards retained; but I would not deny that a patient might recover the retentive power. As the loss of retention is a greater evil than I can describe, producing excoriation and a very offensive state, I shall, in any future operation for lithotomy, try what may be effected by employing a suture to bring the divided parts together." Brodie's operation seems to have been partially successful; but Liston seems to think that his mode causes only a temporary incontinence. Most surgeons, however, are, I believe, sadly perplexed with this tiresome result; and the patient necessarily still more so. Very recently I have seen a woman who was cut with the gorget about twenty years ago. She cannot retain her water at all; but it is constantly dribbling away, and she is in a very pitiable condition.'

"I differ from the opinion commonly entertained, viz., that incontinence of urine is more likely to follow rapid than slow dilatation of the urethra. I believe the converse will be proved to be true, and I think that in those cases which have turned out so unfortunate, a more general and equable dilatation, performed by the means I have mentioned, and whilst the patients were under the influence of chloroform, would have been followed by opposite results; and dilatation may be made as rapid as can be wished, provided always care be taken not to destroy the muscular structure of the part, which could only follow if the tubing was allowed to contract itself with great celerity.

"This dilatating agent may be made available for many similar purposes, which will at once suggest themselves to the mind of the reader; such as stricture of the rectum and œsophagus, for dilatation of the os uteri, and the prepuce in phymosis, &c.

" With regard to the other methods of dilating the urethra, such as by the use of prepared sponge and by metallic instruments, I consider them very objectionable."

(C) CONCERNING THE DISEASES OF CHILDREN.

ART. 133.—*On the good effects of Pepsine in the diarrhœa of young Infants.*
By M. CORVISART.
(*Révue Medico-Chir. de Paris,* Dec., 1856.)

In this communication M. Corvisart relates two cases of diarrhœa depending upon the presence of undigested food—the *diarrhœa stomacalis* of Hoffmann, the *diarrhœa ac ventriculo et cibis corruptis* of Sennert—in which the administration of pepsine was productive of the highest benefit.

CASE 1.—M. X—, æt. 4, was admitted into the Hospital of Ste. Eugenie on the 23d of November, 1854, under the care of M. Barthez. For many months this child had suffered from frequent diarrhœa, until it was emaciated and debilitated to the last degree. The appetite was voracious, and the stools contained much undigested food. In the first instance, M. Barthez tried the effect of a properly adjusted diet, with small doses of the trisnitrate of bismuth, but without avail. He then tried the pepsine, giving a "demi-paquet" (the quantity is not stated), at the commencement of a meal composed of the ordinary food of the hospital. On the following day (the 1st of December) the stools were of a better color, and in other respects more natural than they had been before; and, encouraged with this result, the same quantity of pepsine was ordered to be given before each meal.

December 3d.—No stool. This was the first day without a motion for many months.

4th.—Still no stool. The pepsine discontinued.

5th.—Two somewhat fluid motions, although there was no change in the diet. There was, however, no undigested matter in the motions. The child was much better in every respect.

Three weeks afterwards, the child was discharged cured. M. Barthez, however, did not return to the pepsine, but contented himself with small doses of the trisnitrate of bismuth.

This case led M. Corvisart to try the effects of this remedy in the diarrhœa of very young children.

CASE 2.—Alexandrine Lang, born on the 2d of August, 1855, was seized, on the 25th of October, with diarrhœa, after a very obstinate attack of erythema and eczema. This diarrhœa was accompanied with frequent hiccup and vomiting. On the 3d of November, fifty centigrammes of pepsine were given night and morning. On the 4th, the same treatment was continued; and now the vomiting and purging have disappeared, the stools have become natural, and the child takes the breast with avidity. The pepsine discontinued.

November 22d.—The vomiting and purging have returned, M. Corvisart has again had recourse to the pepsine.

23d.—The vomiting and purging have ceased, and the stools are natural. From this time the little patient went on well.

M. Corvisart adds, that many cases of the kind have fallen under his notice, and that the acidified form of the pepsine, which he himself tried, was quite as efficacious in these cases as the neutral form proved to be in the hands of M. Barthez.

ART. 134.—*On the Treatment of Eczema Infantile.*
By Mr. ERASMUS WILSON.
(*Assoc. Med. Journ.,* July 31, 1856.)

After an excellent account of the disease itself, Mr. Wilson thus writes upon the subject of treatment:

" In the treatment of eczema infantile, the three great principles which I have on every occasion advocated as the *law of treatment* of cutaneous disease, namely, *elimination, restoration of power,* and *alleviation of local distress,* are to be put in force, but with a change in their order. Elimination must always go first; but in eczema infantile, I would place alleviation of local distress second; and restoration of power third. Thus the principles of treatment, the indications for treatment being settled, let us consider the means.

"For *elimination*, the remedy is calomel or gray powder: I prefer the former; one grain of calomel rubbed down with one grain of white sugar, or sugar of milk, is the dose for the youngest infant; for a child a year old, a grain and a half; for a child two years old, two grains. Of course this dose is modified according to the apparent strength of the child in the first instance, and in accordance with the action of the medicine in the second; the object to be attained being such a dose as will produce an efficient relief to the alimentary canal, and moreover such an amount of relief as shall act as a diversion to the morbid secreting action taking place in the skin—in other words, as shall divert the morbid secretions of the skin into their more natural and proper channel, the alimentary canal. For this purpose, calomel excels every other medicine; from its small bulk it is convenient for exhibition, merely requiring to be dropped into the child's mouth. It stimulates the liver to an increased flow of bile, and in children it always acts most kindly on the alimentary canal. Again, a free action of the alimentary canal being secured, all probability of *repulsion* of the eruption by the remedies required for the second indication is at an end, and the mother's and nurse's alarms lest the disease should be *driven in* are set at rest. A free clearance of the stomach and bowels is therefore a primary, a necessary step, at the very commencement of the treatment. After the first dose, the calomel may be repeated according to circumstances; once a week, twice a week, every other night for a few times, even every night for two or three nights if it be absolutely necessary. In my own practice, I usually find once a week sufficient; and I am guided to the repetition of the dose by the state of the little patient. If there be any feverishness, fractiousness, irritability of temper, any increase of pruritus, inaction of the bowels, morbid secretion of the bowels, or threatened congestion of the mucous membrane of the air-tubes, then the calomel powder is to be administered at once without hesitation and without delay. The mother or nurse soon learns the moment for a powder, and, whatever prejudices they may have to the *name* of calomel, they are always ready to resort to it after they have once seen its action in this disease. As I have already said, I have no objection to the mercury with chalk, beyond the fact of its being more bulky and less agreeable to swallow, while it certainly possesses no recommendation which can render it superior to calomel. Sometimes I find one or two grains of nitrate of potash a useful addition to the calomel and sugar.

"Having disposed of the first indication, and cleared out of the system any acrid matters that might be rebellious and capable of exciting irritation and feverishness; having moreover unloaded the bloodvessels of some of their watery and solvent elements by the same remedy; we may now have recourse to our means of *alleviating the local distress*, in other words, of soothing and healing the eruption, subduing the pruritus, and arresting the morbid discharge. We can do all this by the benzoated oxide of zinc ointment rubbed down with spirits of wine, in the proportion of a drachm to the ounce. This ointment should be applied abundantly, and gently distributed upon the surface, until every part of the eruption has a complete coating. The ointment should be applied morning and night, and if accidentally rubbed off, or used upon parts exposed to the air and friction, it may be repeated more frequently. When once applied, the ointment should be considered as a permanent dressing to the inflamed skin, and never removed until the skin is healed, unless special conditions arise which render such a process necessary. To insure undisturbed possession to the ointment, a piece of linen rag should be laid over it and maintained in position in any convenient manner. Thus, when the eruption covers more or less of the entire body, I have a little shirt made of old linen, with sleeves for the arms and legs, and with means of being fastened closely around the legs, and, if necessary, closed over the hands and feet. This little dress is to be worn constantly, night and day, and for a week together, if necessary. It is intended as a mere envelope or dressing to the inflamed and irritated skin; and its saturation with ointment which necessarily ensues, only contributes to its greater utility in that capacity. Where the eruption is chiefly confined to the arms or legs, linen sleeves will be sufficient for the purpose. On the face, no other covering than the ointment is necessary, but the latter should therefore be used the more largely.

" Where the oxide of zinc ointment is employed in the manner now described, the formation of crusts on the eruption is prevented, in consequence of the exclusion of the atmosphere and the consequent absence of desiccation. And when crusts are already formed, the object to be obtained is to soften the crusts by saturating them thoroughly with the ointment, and then by gentle friction to displace them and substitute a thin stratum of the ointment in their place. When the eruption passes from the acute into the chronic state, and the process of exfoliation of the cuticle is active, gentle friction of the skin with the ointment is even more desirable than in the acute stage of the disease, and, at the same time, very grateful to the little patient. On the scalp, the ointment should be applied in the direction of the hair, to avoid matting; and as soon as the oozing of ichorous discharge has somewhat subsided, the hair should be gently brushed. I am rigorous in enforcing the non-disturbance of the ointment; but sometimes my *aides* carry their instructions beyond the proper point, and accumulate the ointment too thickly over a given part, retaining thereby the secretions, and interfering with the cure. In this case, if the finger be pressed upon such an accumulated plate of the ointment, the morbid fluids will be seen to ooze up between its chinks or around its edges, and the source of evil is detected. When such an occurrence takes place, the whole of the ointment should be carefully washed off the part with the yolk of egg, and after drying the skin, fresh ointment should be applied. This excessive accumulation of the ointment takes place most frequently on the scalp, and is encouraged by the matting of the hair: a reason for keeping the hair brushed whenever the nature of the eruption permits.

" Another of my instructions is to avoid washing the inflamed skin; it may be wiped with a soft napkin to remove exudations or secretions; but washing is unnecessary, indeed injurious, as tending to irritate the skin, and to increase the pruritus and inflammation afterwards. While the washing lasts and the irritated skin is softened by the water, the part is relieved and comforted, by the drying which follows, more than avenges the temporary solace of the ablution. On the same principle, I never order or recommend lotions in this eruption.

" In cases of *chronic eczema infantile*, that is, pityriasis capitis and psoriasis partium aliarum, the stimulant properties of the nitric oxide and nitrate of mercury ointments may be brought into operation. The former is specific for pityriasis capitis, in the proportion of one part to three of lard; and the latter, variously diluted, from one part in eight, to equal parts, may be used for the chronic eczema or psoriasis of other parts, particularly of the eyelids. But even in the chronic state of the disease, the benzoated zinc ointment will be found to be an invaluable and indispensable remedy. In the parched state of the skin left by the chronic disease, glycerine may be found of use, as an emollient; but when any inflammation exists, it generally proves irritant, as compared with the zinc ointment.

" We now come to the remaining indication in the treatment of eczema infantile, namely, *restoration of power;* in other words to correct malassimilation and restore the blood to its normal and healthy condition. For this purpose, the great remedy is that admirable alterative tonic, *arsenic.* It is remarkable how well infants of the earliest age bear this medicine, and how rapidly in them it exerts its tonic and assimilative effects. As an effective harmless tonic, arsenic stands alone and without its peer in this vexatious disease. Indeed, in eczema infantile it is specific; it cures rapidly, perfectly, unfailingly. It would be difficult to say as much for any other medicine in relation to any other disease; and I pronounce this eulogium on arsenic after a large experience. The preparation of arsenic which I select is Fowler's solution, the dose two minims to an infant from a month to a year old, repeated three times in the day with, or directly after meals; and as malassimilation is always attended with anæmia in a greater or less degree, I conjoin with the two minims of Fowler's solution fifteen of Vinum Ferri, my formula being as follows:

" ℞   Vini Ferri, Syrupi Tolutani, āā ℥ss;
       Liquoris Potassæ Arsenitis, ℳxxxij;
       Aquæ Anethi, ℥j.
             M.   Fiat mistura.

The dose of this medicine is one drachm, with or directly after meals, three times a day.

"With these three remedies, namely, the calomel powder, the benzoated oxide of zinc ointment, and the ferro-arsenical mixture, representing, as they do, the three indications for treatment of eczema infantile, I regard the cure as certain and rapid, and failure impossible; and if success were not complete, I should seek for the cause, not in the remedies, but in the mode of administering them. So confident am I of success, that I have often undertaken the treatment of this disease, without seeing the patient, and at hundreds of miles distance; being satisfied for my only *aide*, with the vigilance of an intelligent mother or nurse. I have never known any evil effects, present or future, result from this treatment; but I never fail to give strict injunctions that *if the medicine appear to disagree with the child it should be given less frequently*, say twice instead of three times a day, or *suspended instantly* if the child appear ill; moreover, that, in the event of such an occurence, the calomel powder should be immediately resorted to. The period of continuance of the remedies must be left to the judgment of the medical man; the treatment sometimes occupies three weeks and sometimes more; and if a recurrence of the eruption should take place, the treatment should be recommenced, and conducted on the same principle, and with the like precautions.

"The *diet* of the child, while under this treatment, must be carefully inquired into; it should be good, wholesome, and nutritious. The leading constitutional indication is to nourish properly, and this idea should be carried out in the food as well as in the medicine. I find the juice of meat of great value in these cases, and it may be given either alone, as beef or mutton tea, or mixed with the other food.

"The consideration of diet and food brings me to an important dietetic medicine, which is of great value in this disease, when the latter is attended with emaciation, and in the chronic stage; in acute cases it is less applicable. I mean the *cod-liver oil.* The child will take the oil greedily in its natural state, and its good effects on nutrition are speedily made apparent: it may be given with safety to the youngest infant. In children somewhat older, and particularly in chronic cases, the cod-liver oil chocolate becomes a useful ingredient of diet.

"When I have wished to avail myself of the excellent properties of the cod-liver oil in conjunction with arsenic, I have often found the following formulæ a convenient vehicle for its use:

> "℞ Olei Jecoris Aselli, ℥ij;
> Vitelli Ovi, j;
> Liquoris Potassæ Arsenitis, ℳlxiv;
> Syrupi Simplicis, ℥ij;
> Aquæ Fontanæ, q. s. ad ℥iv.
> M. Fiat mistura.

The dose is a drachm three times a day, with or directly after meals.

"Where eczema infantile is complicated with diarrhœa, or congestion of the mucous membrane of the air-tubes or lungs, the arsenical remedy should be instantly suspended; the calomel powder immediately administered, and the ordinary antiphlogistic remedies adopted, magnesia and aromatic confection for diarrhœa, and ipecacuanha for the bronchitic or pulmonary congestion. Where the air-tubes are loaded with phlegm, an emetic is useful; and a poultice to the chest and abdomen will be found a useful adjuvant."

REPORTS

ON THE

PROGRESS OF THE MEDICAL SCIENCES.

July—December, 1856.

THE intention of the following Reports is to pass in review the principal additions to each department of Medical Science, which have been placed on record during the preceding six months. It is not contemplated that they should be confined exclusively to the notice of what is new; any fact or doctrine, which may be considered practically useful, will, although not strictly novel, be regarded as worthy of commemoration. It must be obvious to all who are aware of the immense mass of information which is almost daily put forth by the medical press of this and other countries, that the notice of every subject would be an impossibility. It therefore devolves upon the writers of each Report, to select only such articles for retrospection as may possess superior recommendations, either of an intrinsic character, or in relation to the main end and aim of all medical knowledge,—the alleviation of suffering and disease.

I.

REPORT ON PRACTICAL MEDICINE, ETC.

Essays on State Medicine. By HENRY WYLDBORE RUMSEY.
(8vo. London, Churchill, 1856, pp. 424.)

THE phrase *State Medicine* is sufficient of itself to arrest the attention of all Englishmen. Not, alas! that it is likely to awaken in them a desire to learn its oral significance; its effects will be rather that of causing them to erect at once those dear bristles of political, municipal, and social rights, on the muddy borders of which the true Briton loves to wallow without striking into the purer and profounder depths; and armed with which, he contrives in the most ingenious manner to confuse and baffle the best measures of the best government for his social and general welfare. Not for a moment would we depreciate those laws which set a boundary to the interference of Government with the wishes and desires of the people, and which render it necessary that they should be consulted in all things which may be deemed necessary for their benefit; but if Government is to be anything more than a mere farce, there are certain things which it is incumbent upon it to take the initiative in, and to spare no effort for carrying into effect; such, for example, as the protection of individual members, or sections of the people, or of the whole community, from dangers without or within. This is admitted in those more evident instances in which the country is liable to invasion, property is endangered, and the person is exposed to injury by accident or malevolence; but in those more deadly, but less apparent, instance of disease, it is neither admitted nor comprehended by the mass of the people.

Nor, indeed, is Government altogether free from a similar charge. Such efforts as it has directed, from time to time, towards the prevention, or, indeed, the relief of disease, have been so irregular, so contracted in scope, so incoherent in design, that they have indicated an imperfect appreciation of the necessity of measures adopted, and an ignorance, or indisposition, to make use of the methods most fitted for carrying them out; and, in consequence, these measures have in no small degree disgusted the people with the very notion of State interference for the preservation of health.

Medicine, in its relation to nations and masses of people, is a matter which it especially behooves a government to take into its own hands, for there are but few among the most intelligent nations, save those who have given particular attention to the subject, who comprehend those reasons which render other than individual exertions for the preservation of health necessary; who know, in their fullest extent, the destructive effects of the commonest diseases; who understand the degree in which those diseases are preventible; and who are acquainted with the methods of prevention. State medicine is a measure which must proceed from the educated few to the many; it is a subject which it is incumbent upon those who comprehend it to teach to those who do not, and this not only when the terrible panic of a pestilence causes the mass to ask for the means of prevention, but at all times, and at all seasons; it is a subject that it is the especial duty of a Government to take to itself, unfold, and carry out, not waiting until it is compelled to adopt lagging and abortive measures, by the devastations of wide-spreading diseases and the clamors of a terror-stricken people.

But, truly, the Government and people of England are less to blame in this matter than is generally supposed. The preservation of health and the prevention of disease might be thought the peculiar province of the physician; yet *hygiène*, properly so called, is not taught in the medical schools of Great Britain and Ireland, except as an incidental thing; neither do the representative corporations of medicine require a knowledge of it from those who seek fellowship with them. Hence, it follows, that hygiène, as a science, is almost unknown to the bulk of our medical men; hence it meets with scant attention from them; and hence, we believe, a prime source of that neglect of hygienic measures, by the people on the one hand, and the Government on the other. There have always been certain professional men, and their number rapidly increases, who have stood forward and advocated the claims of hygiène upon the profession, the public, and the State; and at no time has the State sought in vain for the aid, too often little appreciated, of men qualified in every way to advise what was best for the sanitary welfare of the people; but that wide-spread co-operation, which would arise from a correct knowledge of the scope and bearing of true hygiène,—which is necessary for its attainment, and without which it is impracticable fully to impress upon the public and the State the full value of medical polity,—has been, and is still, altogether wanting in the profession. Indeed, it is as necessary that the State should interfere for the direction of the medical corporate bodies, and medical institutions, as for the preservation of the health of the whole nation. This is a painful subject, but it is one which requires raking up from the very bottom, and exposing in all its glaring absurdity. It is time that medical corporations, and the medical profession generally, became roused to a sense of the anomalous position in which they stand with reference to the people and the State in this matter. The popular opinion that the doctor is for the *cure*, not for the prevention of disease, is an offspring of the present mode of teaching and practising medicine. We believe that until hygiène becomes an essential requirement among the regulations for examination before every examining medical board, and until it is taught in every school of medicine, medical polity will never be thoroughly respected and appreciated by the people and the state.

We hail with welcome any work which, like Mr. Rumsey's, seeks to unfold the scope and aims of state medicine; and which discusses the difficulties which impede its development in Great Britain. Such a work has long been wanted.

Mr. Rumsey, in a series of essays, gives the outline of a sanitary code; states the requirements of education in the healing and health-poisoning arts; dilates on the subject of sanitary inquiry in relation to England; gives the history, present condition, and requirements of medical relief for the poor; exposes the fetid condition of the present local sanitary administration; and describes the benefits which would arise from a health-police, in connection with a local medico-sanitary service.

To those who, like ourselves, have been victimized by corporations, magistrates, local boards of health, and boards of guardians, while they were enacting certain suppositious sanitary functions, or while they were setting themselves in opposition to all law and reason, Mr. Rumsey's work will prove most interesting, probing, as it does, the sources of those obstacles which impede or render abortive the best efforts of the medical man, for the relief of the sick poor, particularly during times of pestilence, unfolding, as it does, the methods by which those obstacles may be overcome. To those of the profession who have regarded sanitary matters indifferently, Mr. Rumsey's work may prove a means of arousing other and better feelings; and to all those, professional or unprofessional, who care for the welfare of their fellow-creatures, Mr. Rumsey's work will be invaluable, giving, as it does, a comprehensive and interesting view of the present condition, and the requirements, of sanitary reform in England.

Our notice of Mr. Rumsey's work may be fittingly confined more particularly to that Essay which contains the *sum* and result of his labors,—the "Outline of a Sanitary Code."

"The agenda of a state," he writes, "with regard to the public health, may, I believe, be advantageously comprised in three great divisions:"

DIVISION I. *Subjects concerning which the state should direct investigation.*—(A) *Statistics:* (a) of *population,* (b) of *mortality,* (c) of *reproduction,* (d) of *sickness, accidents,* and *infirmity.* It has been assumed, somewhat too hastily, the facts of this kind cannot be collected, fully and accurately, by public authority, without infringing on private rights and social proprieties. But, at all events, the census of population would show the total number of sick, the hurt, and the infirm; whilst more precise information on the subject could at all times be obtained amongst those classes of society, which owe, as it were, such information to the public. And as the numerical ratio which these classes bear to the whole population is known, some estimate, with the aid of mortality returns, might be formed respecting the sanitary state of the entire population. Moreover, by placing the members of the medical faculty in a more correct relation with the state, a still nearer approximation might readily be obtained, especially in times of unusual sickness. The public registration of diseases and injuries should include particulars respecting their connection, in different cases, with occupation, social neglect, or mismanagement, personal habits, natural and artificial peculiarities of locality; with climate, weather, and season; and with the density, grouping, and migration of the population. This department of registration should also contain full and correct details relating to epidemic visitations, noting all the circumstances connected with the origin, advent, propagation, and decline of zymotic diseases." (pp. 9, 10.) (*e*) Of *dwellings*; (*f*) of *food*; (*g*) of *animal life*.

(B) *Topographical inquiries* and *meteorological records.*—(*a*) The physical geography of a district; (*b*) the chemical analysis, at stated intervals, of its various soils, water-springs, wells, and rivers; (*c*) meteorology.

(c) *Judicial investigations—Forensic medicine.*—(*a*) Involving death-inquests; (*b*) personal disqualifications; (*c*) questions of succession, survivorship, personal identity, and pregnancy.

The subject of *mental epidemics* is, we are aware, treacherous ground to tread upon, as it so often involves phases of religious belief, but in so far as peculiar superstitions and delusions tend to foster suicide and insanity, we think that they might have found a fitting place, with proper restrictions, in the first division of Mr. Rumsey's code.

II. On those arrangements for the personal safety and health of the people which require for their enforcement direct enactments or local regulations, with the infliction of penalties for their non-observance.—(A) Measures for the prevention of disease. (*a*) In locality; (*b*) in the construction of buildings; (*c*) by the purification of buildings and towns; (1) by the removal of nuisances; (2) by drainage and sewerage; (3) by a fit ordering of pavement; and (4) by an abatement of the smoke nuisance. (*e*) By fostering healthy progeny; (1) involving the question of hereditary disease by marriage; (2) the qualification of practitioners in midwifery, and nurses; (3) lying-in hospitals, orphan asylums, and foundling institutions; and (4) private and associated efforts to these ends. "The intervention of legal authority is of the greatest importance in promoting the healthful training of the young: by checking, if not prohibiting, the employment in factories of mothers having young children; by limiting strictly the age at which children can be engaged or indentured in factories and workshops; by regulating the number of hours during which they can be employed, according to their age; by frequent and independent medical inspection and report concerning their physical condition and growth whilst so employed; by forbidding, absolutely, the employment of children in mines, chimney-sweeping, and other equally injurious occupations; by restrictions upon mental exercise, long confinement, and vehement competition in schools; by securing, under legal compulsion, the proper site, construction, ventilation, drainage, and water supply of all buildings occupied by young people of every grade; by special regulations as to the diet, clothing, education, and general management of those children who are under the immediate guardianship of the public." (pp. 21, 22.) (*f*) *By supervision of the sale of food;* (1) by inspection of manufactories, and places for the sale of articles intended for aliment; (2) by control and inspection of the production, importation, and manufacture of articles known to be injurious; (3) by a system of police for the detection of abuses (adulterations, &c.); (4) by supervision of the method of feeding animals for the butcher, and of slaughter-houses; (5) by prevention of intemperance; (6) and by checking the use of articles of food and drink injurious to health, and promoting the consumption of those articles which are known to be most conducive to the health and vigor of man. (7) "Certain notions of political economy, prevalent in some countries, seriously interfere with correct legislation on this question. But no theoretical views should be allowed to release any state from a duty incumbent on all governments—namely, to provide for the instruction of all classes, working people especially, in those maxims of health preservation which relate to the choice and preparation of food." (pp. 23, 24.) (*g*) *By supervision of the sale of medicines and poisons;* (*h*) *of other trades and occupations;* (*i*) *of locomotion;* (*j*) *and of public amusements and recreations.* "The Government should not only control popular amusements, but should take care to furnish opportunities to the people for innocent and beneficial relaxation." (p. 28.) "In order to complete administrative arrangements on the subjects mentioned in this and previous sections, it is necessary to organize a proper staff of medical officers, as sanitary visitors, as instructors of the poorer classes in all matters relating to hygiène, and as detectors of the threatenings as well as of the causes of disease." (p. 28.) To the section (*j*) Mr. Rumsey adds the surveillance of *prostitution.* (*k*) *By supervision of public establishments,*—educational, industrial, reformatory, criminal, charitable, and sanative; (*l*) and *by supervision of the burial of the dead.*

(B) *Measures for the arrest and palliation of disease.*—(*a*) *Under ordinary circumstances and at all times;* (1) by medical relief of the poor; (2) by hospitals, general and special; (3) and by medicines and dispensaries. (*b*) *On the advent and during the prevalence of any important epidemic or pestilential disease;* (1) by preparatory measures; (2) by domiciliary visitations; (3) by vaccination; (4) by quarantine, and by a supervision of *animals,* and an adoption of measures for the prevention or palliation of diseases among them.

III. On the establishment by law of an organized machinery for carrying into effect the aforesaid inquiries and regulations, for deliberation and advice in emergencies, and for the administration of existing laws.—(A) The education of medical and other technical, scientific, and administrative agents. (1) "A scheme of medical education; (2) regulations respecting license for practice and registration; (3) promotion of district faculties, to which, in connection with a central metropolitan council, might be committed the administration of local affairs requiring the attentive deliberation and action of the medical body, the promotion of medical observation and science, and particularly the power of advising the district courts of health hereafter to be proposed." (p. 43.) (4) Protection of the rights and immunities of the profession; (5) registration of those who professedly devote themselves to ailments of particular parts of the body, dentists, chiropodists, &c.; instruction, examination, and licensing of practitioners of pharmacy, bleeders, cuppers, &c.; (6) provisions for education, examination, license, registration, duties, and rights of *veterinarians.* (B) *The institution of official authorities—boards and officers for central and local superintendence and action.* (*a*) *The institution of councils and boards, central and local.* (1) A superior sanitary and medical council, presided over either by a minister of public health or connected with the ministry for home affairs. This council might consist of several *departments,* to wit, for (*a*) the vital and medical statistics of the entire population; (*b*) sanitary engineering; (*c*) direction of preventive measures relating to food, drinks, and medicines, regulation of trades, &c., locomotion, and the burial of the dead; (*d*) sanitary control of public education, pauper, criminal, and health establishments; (*e*) superintendence of medical education. The council to consist of nominees of the crown or state, of those recommended by certain learned and professional bodies, of the superior medical authorities of the war departments, and of those who may be considered by the other three portions as especially qualified to render valuable assistance in the management of public health. The section for medical education should consist wholly of the recognized heads of the medical profession. (pp. 47, 48.) "A local board to be established in every sanitary district, consisting of magistrates and rate-payers, men of science, and parochial clergy, elected by the two former portions. That the medical element of local government should be distinct, and should form a sort of auxiliary committee, or faculty, for deliberation, advice, and co-operation in each sanitary district." (*b*) *The territorial division of the country into sanitary districts;* (*c*) *the appointment of officers of various grades and functions;* to wit, (1) *medical inspectors of circuits, engineering inspectors*, and *chemical inspectors*, under the metropolitan or central council; (2) an *officer of health*, a district *chemist*, a district *veterinarian*, a district *engineer*, or *surveyor*, and in every principal seaport a *medical superintendent of quarantine*, under every district court of health; (3) a *medical officer* or *visitor* for the general superintendence of the poor in their dwellings, and for attendance upon them in sickness or accidents; *apothecaries* or *dispensers*, where necessary; a searcher for *nuisances*; a staff of *assistant visitors*; an *obstetrical officer*; one or more *mid-wives*; and educated and licensed *nurses*, in every parish, township, or sub-district.

Such are the heads of the subjects and the divisions of a code, by which Mr. Rumsey seeks to draw attention to the UNITY OF STATE MEDICINE; and to point out the connection, legislative and administrative, which ought to exist between the several departments; and in the subsequent essays in his work he more fully developes this object, and shows "the singular absence of comprehensive design which has characterized all attempts at legislation in this country, whenever circumstances or events have imposed on Government and Parliament the necessity of adopting measures, either for preserving the health and diminishing the sickness of the people, or for regulating the education and duties of the medical profession." (p. 4.)

The fourth Essay, on the "History, Present Condition, and Requirements of Medical Relief for the Poor, and its Relations to Political Economy and Sanitary Management," is peculiarly valuable and interesting.

Mr. Rumsey's work is a boon to the profession, and it ought to be in the hands of every medical man in the country. It is, moreover, a work admirably calculated to convey a correct knowledge of the scope and objects of true sanitary reform to all those who have an interest in the subject.

The influence of Tropical Climates on European Constitutions, including practical observations on the nature and treatment of the Diseases of Europeans on their return from Tropical Climates. By JAMES RANALD MARTIN, F.R.S. A New Edition. (8vo. London, John Churchill, pp. 599. 1856.)

This is not a mere reprint of the last edition of the well-known and celebrated work on the "Influence of Tropical Climates on European Constitutions," which was composed by the late Dr. James Johnson and Mr. Martin, in 1841. It is a "new edition," in which the entire work is re-cast and re-written. "Even the introductory chapter is entirely re-written—so much only of Dr. Johnson's observations being retained," says Mr. Martin, "as appeared to me proper to the subject, and all beyond is exclusively my own composition."

Mr. Martin, however, has adhered to and preserved the medico-topographic and statistical character of his original official reports, and in doing this he has been actuated by the conviction that, next to the importance of physiological investigations, stand those which relate to the external causes of disease. He has likewise continued, so far as the scope and intent of the work admits, an examination of the physiological influence of climate, both Asiatic and European, so as to give the greatest possible degree of firmness to the grounds of preventive medicine.

Mr. Martin has also reprinted from the "Lancet" certain articles published by him during the last six years, on the nature, causes, and treatment of the diseases of Europeans on their return from tropical climates; and in this way he has supplied what was obviously wanting in former editions, for a work upon the influence of tropical climates upon the European constitution could not be complete which did not comprise some description of the sequelæ to tropical diseases, and of the counter-influences which, under a European climate, affect the health of persons who have long resided in a warm region.

It is not necessary for us to say anything to secure a favorable notice of a work which has become so established a text-book upon the subject of which it treats—a work which is read by every one, both at home and abroad, who is wishful to gain a thorough knowledge of the science of medicine—for every one who has read the old, will assuredly make a point of seeing for himself wherein the new edition differs from it. For our own part, we have read the work with much additional pleasure and profit. We could have wished, however, that Mr. Martin had dilated a little more fully upon one or two subjects, and particularly upon one, and that is the treat-

ment of remittent fevers. " Very few of the author's original doctrines," Mr. Martin
quotes approvingly a remark of Dr. James Johnson, in the edition of 1841, " have
been subverted, or practices exploded, during a period of more than a quarter of a
century." Now, is it so with respect to the treatment of remittent fever? In asking this question, we have an eye particularly to a paper noticed in a former
report (" Abstract," XX), in which Mr. Hare, the surgeon to the 1st Bengal Fusiliers, endeavors to show that the practice introduced by Dr. James Johnson, of
treating remittent fever by mercury given to salivation in place of the treatment by
bark, previously in vogue, had been a very questionable improvement. He attempts
to show, moreover, that the treatment by a milder amount of mercurialization, which
had gradually crept into vogue, in consequence of the injurious effects of salivation
in many instances, is much less successful than the treatment either by bark or by
salivation; we thought at the time, and still think, that the arguments advanced
were deserving of much attention. Mr. Martin, however, does not enter into this
question, all-important though it be.

Of mercury in the treatment of remittent fever, he says:

" When bloodletting shall have produced its results on the circulation, the febrile
movement, though subdued, being still in serious progress, we have recourse to this
mineral. It is at once the best aid to the abstraction of blood, and the best preparation for the effective action of antiperiodics, such as quinine, arsenic, &c., through
its active operation on all the depurative functions. Robert Jackson, though no
favorer of mercurial treatment, admits that in fevers, complicated with abdominal
congestion, calomel is a remedy of the first importance. He says that it repairs
mischiefs which no other means with which we are acquainted are capable of touching. This is the simple truth, and it constitutes the reason why this remedy has at
all times held so high a place with the practitioners in our worst climates.

" As it is better to repeat than to leave an important subject in any doubt, I here
beg leave to transcribe from my article on Hepatitis a summary of the actions of
mercury, and especially of those of calomel: It is for the very reason that calomel
assists powerfully, both in 'drawing off' accumulations, and in promoting ' *increased
secretion*' that it proves of such value in aid of bloodletting. It is, in fact, by this
very double action of purging and increasing secretion at the same time, that calomel
relieves the loaded and inactive vessels of the diseased gland; not to speak of the
other acknowledged physiological influences of this mineral—such as its increase of
all the secretions and excretions of the body—its influence on the capillary circulation—its febrifuge effect—the peculiar specific power ascribed to it by Gooch and
others as an antagonist to inflammations, whether general or local—its stimulant
power over the absorbent function—its power of unloading, at the same time that it
gives a new impulse to the vascular system—its peculiar power in removing viscid
and tenacious intestinal secretions—its alterative, solvent, and antiplastic effects on
the blood; these are the actions and uses ascribed to mercury by the ablest of our
physicians and surgeons, and they are such as place this remedy second only in
order and importance to bloodletting, in all the more acute hepatic affections of
India. That mercury enters into intimate union with the elements of the blood is
now an ascertained fact. It must, therefore, 'modify its plasticity, and influence all the
organic functions to which it is subservient.' I have only to add here that the above
summary is quoted from the former edition of this work, with commendation, by
Dr. Copland, in his article on Diseases of the Liver.

" Dr. Billing, speaking of the treatment of disease by 'calomel and opium,' says,
justly, that, though powerful allies to the antiphlogistic treatment, they have often
failed from being employed without being supported by bleeding, or purgative, or
emetic, or diaphoretic medicines. This is equally true of tropical diseases, and I
have seen enormous quantities of calomel given with nothing but evil effect, because its action was not solicited and supported by previous depletory means.

" Robert Jackson states, that the preparation of the subject by previous abstraction of blood is indispensable to the success of mercury, in the more concentrated
fevers and more complicated dysenteries of tropical climates."

Of bark, in the treatment of remittent fever, Mr. Martin says:

" Sir James Annesley observes, that visceral disease is the necessary result of the
neglect of depletory means, including mercurial purgatives; and that congestions
often lead to inflammatory action, especially if bark or arsenic have been freely ad-

ministered during the stage of congestion, and of disturbed and impeded secretion: and this is in accordance with general experience. Here again we perceive that quina, like other powerful remedies, may not only prove of no effect, but may be administered so as actually to be injurious. It may do signal good, or even prove hurtful, according as the patient may or may not have been prepared for the actions of the bark. To apportion the dose and determine the right time for exhibiting it, so as to secure the full tonic and antiperiodic influences of the quina, we must appreciate accurately the circumstances in each individual case; the stage of the fever, and the effect of the previous antiphlogistic means. The random exhibition of quina by timid, careless, or inexperienced practitioners, does infinite harm; and, in former times, when bark alone was relied upon for the cure of all tropical fevers, the results were horrible.

" Where, with a state of general plethora, visceral congestions remain unsubdued, or only partially removed, the secretions being scanty and depraved, with the pulse full and hard, and the skin constricted, dry, and hot, the time for the exhibition of bark has not yet arrived. Robert Jackson says, that bark is not to be relied on, for the precipitate arrest of remittent fever, either in the West Indies or in other countries. Bark and the disulphate of quina are efficacious in arresting the remittent fever of Bengal, when venous congestions have been overcome by previous depletory means, when the pulse has been reduced in force and frequency, when the secretions are in free action, and the skin relaxed; when these preparatory results have been obtained, we may then be sure of establishing the antiperiodic influence of quina, with the best effect, and without risk of producing any injury. It then becomes a sovereign remedy; and the nearer the patient can be brought to the state of remission, the surer will be the operation of the antiperiodic. It must now be given in full doses, so as speedily to establish its influence. The amount of dose, and the frequency with which it is to be repeated, will depend on the nature of the fever;—where paroxysms are violent, or where the sufferer is in a malarious locality, the doses should be large, and often repeated. It is better to exhibit the quinine in five-grain doses often repeated, than to give scruple doses, as recommended by some writers; for, by the former plan, we have the advantage of observing the effects as we proceed, and we can withhold excessive doses."

Nor do we find this answer to Mr. Hare in Mr. Martin's excellent remarks upon the application of remedial means to the treatment of an individual case of remittent fever:

" Here we find, on experience," he says, " that the first and most immediate object is, to reduce the force and frequency of arterial action during the paroxysm, which if allowed to go on unrestrained, would injure or destroy some organ essential to life.

" If the patient be seen in the forenoon, on the accession of the first, second, or third paroxysm of ordinary remittent fever, if he is of a sound constitution and not beyond middle life, bloodletting from the arm, while the patient is in the recumbent posture, should be practised to the extent of relieving the sufferer from præcordial oppression, from visceral fulness and congestion, or from the intensity of headache, whichever may predominate. If along with reduced force and frequency of the pulse, and reduction of the morbid temperature, we obtain from the operation a gentle relaxation of the skin, we have the best evidence of relief from visceral congestion, whether the operation be performed for the cure of fever, dysentery, or hepatitis; the quantity of blood abstracted being regulated by the effect, and not by an arbitrary measure in ounces. It will sometimes happen, however, from peculiarity of habit, or other cause, and notwithstanding the utmost circumspection, that the relaxation of the skin will proceed to sweating, with symptoms of depression of the vital powers; then from half a grain to a grain of opium, or from fifteen to twenty minims of laudanum, with as many of chloric ether, should be administered. This will impart tone to the heart's action, and soothe the nervous excitement, while it will allay gastric and intestinal irritation. It is only in cases of depression, however, such as this, that opium is to be recommended in the very early treatment of fever; but, when requisite, it will be found to calm both mind and body. Let the physiology of the disease, and the habit and condition of the patient guide the application of remedies, and we shall approach as nearly to the correct measure of means of cure as human endeavor can compass.

"Unless the fever assume a severe form, one general bloodletting, practised as stated, in the recumbent posture, and under the studied observation of effect will, on the average, be found sufficient to relieve the patient from abdominal or cerebral oppression. Bloodletting, used as here directed, will be found to simplify the application of all the subsequent means of cure. Within an hour after bleeding a dose of calomel with compound extract of colocynth and James's powder should be exhibited, followed in two hours by a powerful cathartic, such as infusion of senna with sulphate of magnesia. After the free action of these remedies, we shall obtain in the afternoon some degree of remission; and the patient should be directed to take, at bed-time, from six to ten grains of calomel, with four of James's powder, if the skin be dry. Here, within eight or ten hours of first seeing the patient, we perceive that, of the means above generally described, bloodletting, mercury, a sudorific, and a purgative, have been used, while the patient has been allowed free recourse to cooling diluents.

"On the early morning visit of the following day the patient will probably be found in a more complete state of remission, when the sulphate of quina alone, or in combination with the purging mixture, should be freely and repeatedly administered;—given in this latter manner the quina applies itself to the whole extent of the mucous digestive surface, so as to give full effect to its tonic and antiperiodic influences; and a larger dose of it can thus be borne in the early stage of fever, than if given without the purgative. This is an important consideration; for the quina, rightly administered, will arrest the progress of a mild fever, and save the life of a patient in a severe one, by mitigating the symptoms.

"By the forenoon the paroxysm may recur in a milder degree, though to such an extent as to demand the application of leeches to the epigastric region, if any oppression or fulness exist there, or behind the ears if there be headache; while a mixture composed of antimonial wine with the acetate or nitrate of potash should be given every two hours, so as to soften the skin and determine increased action of the kidneys. It is usual in the remittent fevers of Bengal to give from five to ten grains of calomel, with or without antimonial powder, at bed-time, followed in the early morning by an active purge, and when the last is under operation quinine in solution is given freely. This is a good practice, and a sufficient means in itself to cure some of the milder forms of the fever under consideration;—preceded by an adequate abstraction of blood, this practice will even cure a severe fever. Thus, under the favorable circumstances contemplated, we witness the daily decline of the disease, and the daily diminishing occasion, therefore, for the use of active measures of cure, until towards the third, fifth, seventh, or ninth day convalescence is completely established.

"If remittent fever has existed unrestrained, however, for several days, and the patient is not seen till the accession of the third or fourth paroxysm, or even later, provided the general powers of the constitution remain uninjured, a general bloodletting is still the principal means to save life, followed by calomel, purgatives, and quinine, in the manner previously indicated. But if, on the other hand, the duration of the disease being as above, the paroxysms have become indistinct, running into each other with but brief or ill-defined intervals, while abdominal or cerebral complications arise, as indicated by epigastric fulness with anguish, or by approaching stupor or delirium, congestion now wearing the aspect of inflammation; then the time and manner of applying our more active means demand the nicest care to insure, not only their just effects, but their safety. Bloodletting may even now constitute the principal means to save life, but the blood must be guardedly abstracted, whether generally or locally; and calomel becomes indeed a remedy of necessity, as Robert Jackson would rather refuse to call it, in the treatment of the fevers of the West. To save the patient from impending dangers, in the case of unrestrained fever here contemplated, the medical attendant must be neither rash nor supine: sinking would result from the rash application of means, and effusion into one or both cavities involved in those fevers would be the result of timidity or indecision. Generally speaking the blood must here be abstracted by leeches at the accession of the paroxysm; antimonials must be used—cold must be applied to the shaved head—sinapisms and blisters must be applied; but on the influence of calomel chief reliance must be placed. It must be given every three or four hours, with an occasional mild aperient in the intervals, until the dangerous symptoms shall have yielded; and this favorable state is often observed to be coincident with the mercurial influence, as evidenced in the odor of the breath, or on the gums. Dangerous symptoms such as are here described will sometimes arise suddenly, without any loss of time, or without any neglect in the treatment; and when such conditions are associated with yellowness of the skin, in persons broken in health, or of a feeble constitution, or of dissipated habits of life, or who may have undergone much mental distress, the chances of a fatal termination are imminent.

" In the remittent, as in all forms of periodic fever, the stages of danger are those of the accession and of the decline of the paroxysm : in the first, the violence of arterial action may proceed at once, unless restrained by treatment, to destroy life by serous effusion; while, in the second, so great a prostration of the vital powers may succeed to the previous tumult of vascular action, as to terminate in a feeble and irregular pulse, a damp coldness of the surface and of the extremities, despair, and death. I have seen one paroxysm of Bengal remittent fever, and of jungle fevers, cause death in both ways, within twelve hours; and the first instance, attended with very painful circumstances, occurred within a few months of my arrival in India. A young officer was seized with fever at 11 A.M.; but nevertheless, he went into the China bazaar of Calcutta. He returned to his quarters in Fort William at 3 P.M., and placed himself under the care of a staff-surgeon there. He was bled at 4, and he was dead at 7 P.M. The same operation, practised at noon, would probably have saved his life.

" When the spleen is affected with enlargement, either of the acute or chronic nature, mercury in all forms had better be avoided in the treatment of the fever; for there is in the splenitic complication a dissolved condition of the blood, with general cachexia, that should preclude the use of this powerful mineral. Blood-letting, general or local, when found necessary, should be cautiously used, and carefully regulated in these cases; and the oozing from leech-bites should be carefully and promptly arrested.

" It is necessary to be on our guard against irregularities in the paroxysms of remittent fever, as they occasionally vary not only in their time of accession, but there may arise a double or anticipating night paroxysm, in addition to that of the forenoon. This will require a double attention, especially in respect of the time of using remedies.

"A close observation is indeed necessary as to every event and circumstance which may arise in the course of these fevers; for upon the amount and accuracy of such knowledge will depend not only the selection and application of our means of cure, but the affixing of the proper time of using them—often a vital question.

" The result of each paroxysm on the cerebral and abdominal organs should also be carefully noted, for by this knowledge we regulate both the force of our remedial means, and the frequency with which their application may be needed. Through such observations also we come to estimate aright the powers and capabilities of the patient; for the greater have been the numbers of paroxysms, the more the viscera are likely to be oppressed and congested, and the less power consequently do we find in the patient either to sustain him under further invasions of fever, or to bear him well through the operations of the necessary remedies. In such a case there will be a tendency to exhaustion, and, while we act with decision and calmness, we must be doubly watchful of effect. I have preferred a simple narrative of the treatment of remittent fever, such as is here presented, to a detail of hospital or other cases; for I have seen that, in the treatment of fevers and other acute diseases, cases are too often seized upon and followed out to the letter, by young medical officers, to the disregard of the differences of circumstances, and to the exclusion of reason and reflection on the cases before them. Cases thus become a kind of pattern in routine, and the young naval and military surgeon is injured where it was intended to afford him help. He is thrown off his reasoning powers by an array of cases, and enticed into a groove of routine, out of which it will require much exertion and firmness on his own part to extricate him. A case-book thus, while it purports to be a guide for the treatment of dangerous, varying, and violently acute diseases, carries with it, when used in the manner stated, sources of weakness, even to those whom it intends to benefit. It is otherwise in respect of chronic lesions, the results of acute tropical diseases, in which the constitution of the patient, and the symptoms are at once more subdued, brought more into a common level, rendered thus less variable, and for the management of which ample time is given to the inexperienced for consideration of means, for reflection on their effects, and for consultation with the elders of the profession.

"In chronic disease, again, no sudden changes occur, as the result of youth, constitution, influence of season, or of epidemic conditions—all which exercise powerful, immediate, and varying effects in acute disease.

"We cannot defer till to-morrow the treatment of a case of fever, dysentery, hepatitis, or cholera; duty requires that we should act on the instant; and to do so with justice to the patient requires at least a knowledge of pathology and of the principles of medicine: we should not have to rely on a guide or case-book."

The Pathology of the Diseases of the Army in the East. By R. D. LYONS, M.B.T.C.D., and WM. AITKIN, M.D., London, 1856, pp. 120.

In the spring of 1855, a commission, having at its head Dr. Lyons of Dublin, was sent out by the British Government for the purpose of elucidating the pathological history of the army in the East. Dr. Lyons went out first, and prepared the way for his assistants, Dr. Aitkin and Dr. Doyle, by making some necessary arrangements in the hospital at Scutari. After this, he proceeded to the Crimea. Dr. Aitkin, the first assistant, and formerly pathologist in the Glasgow Royal Infirmary, had the superintendence, and made all the examinations of the patients dying in the General Hospital at Scutari, and Dr. Doyle was attached to the Barrack Hospital in the same place.

The Report is the joint production of Drs. Lyons and Aitkin. It is divided into two parts,—the first part being devoted to the clinical history and morbid anatomy of the diseases of the army in the East,—the second to the pathological anatomy of these diseases, arranged in the order of organs and tissues. There is also an appendix, containing an account of meteorological observations taken at Scutari.

Great care has been expended upon the Report, and much valuable matter is contained in it, only it must ever be regretted that the labors upon which it is based were deferred until the real brunt of the war with disease was over. As it is, however, the Report is very interesting, and this we propose to show by the Report upon the Report which Dr. Lyons has added, in the form of a letter to Lord Panmure. Dr. Lyons writes as follows:

　　　　　　　　　　　　　　　　　　"LONDON, March, 1856.

"My Lord,—I have the honor to present your lordship, in this report, the results of the investigations conducted by me and my assistants, into the Pathology of the Diseases of the Army in the East.

"It may be permitted to me to state at the outset, that these results are not by any means so complete, in several respects, as I originally anticipated they would be. Various causes have concurred to this end.

"On my arrival at Scutari, at the close of April, 1855, I found that all but the expiring embers of the terrible epidemics of the past winter had disappeared. To the past no methods of pathological research are applicable; and to have been enabled to avail myself of the almost unparalleled opportunities for investigating the nature of disease, which had unhappily been presented at Scutari, I should have been in the East not less than fully two months earlier than the date at which my mission commenced.

"To prosecute with success investigations such as those intrusted to me, it requires that suitable apartments, specially adapted for the purpose, and also that instruments and other appliances, shall be in readiness. The latter it was found necessary to have made in this country; the former it was fully expected could be furnished at Scutari. Having already brought this subject under your notice, it will be merely requisite to state here briefly, that not until the expiration of more than two thirds of the period originally assigned for our inquiries, were I and my assistants put in possession of the necessary instruments and appliances for the due prosecution of our labors.

"Notwithstanding the disadvantageous position for the conduct of a scientific inquiry in which I thus found myself placed, different as it was, in all respects, from what I had been led to anticipate, I proceeded to make the best use of the materials at hand. I established for myself and my assistants a regular system of clinical visits to the hospital wards, for the purpose of determining the essential phenomena of the diseases presented in the living; and, as far as the means at our disposal allowed, we prosecuted inquiry into the pathological characters which they exhibited in the dead.

"After some time spent in the investigation of disease at Scutari, it became apparent to me, that for a due and complete appreciation of the pathological characters of the diseases of the army in the East, and for the determination of the most important medical questions connected with their nature and origin, the matériél presented by the hospitals at Scutari, at this period, did not suffice. The great morbid types which had been so fearfully illustrated a few months previously, had become all but extinct. Fevers and dysentery still continued to present themselves, it is true, but in much mitigated forms and diminished numbers.

"Having, therefore, carried my researches to a certain issue at Scutari, I thought it advisable to proceed to the front, with the object of determining, if possible, the primary nature and pathological characters of the diseases, which, in the hospitals of the Bosphorus, showed themselves, as it seemed, in more or less of a secondary form. Accordingly, having left the charge of the Pathological Department at Scutari, and the superintendence of the construction of the Mortuary and Pathological Rooms, to my first assistant, Dr. Aitkin, I proceeded to the Crimea in June.

"My anticipations were correct, for, in fact, I soon found that without a lengthened experience of both medical and surgical pathology, as presented among the troops in camp, it would not be possible to come to any just conclusions as to the nature of the diseases of the British army in the present campaign.

"In the prosecution of my observations and researches, I have held two chief objects permanently in view. First, to determine, with as much precision as possible, the primary nature and characters, and the essential phenomena of the diseases of the troops as presented during life; second, to ascertain, by careful post-mortem examination in fatal cases, the actual changes produced by disease in the various organs of the body. In dealing with these subjects, however, in an adequate and comprehensive manner, it becomes necessary to include some other considerations which bear a very close relation to the general pathology of disease. Disease is a process of great complexity, and its phenomena are influenced not only by various external circumstances, in any given series of morbid actions, but also in a marked and important manner by the type of constitution in which these morbid actions are brought to play.

"The constitution of the soldier in the Crimea had undergone the influence of agencies which, for a long period at least, sensibly depressed it below the average physiological standard, and the effects of which give a marked character to the diseases from which he suffered.

"It is not my province to investigate the causes here alluded to, which have been elsewhere as ably as fully entered into. So far only as their effects became manifested in the deterioration of the constitution of the soldier, and in the consequent modification of the diseases with which he was affected, am I concerned with them in this place.

"It seems undeniable, that the circumstances in which the British army was placed during the winter of 1854–55 were such as of themselves directly to induce the invasion of disease on a large scale and in a malignant form. Not only was this so in reality, but, even after the lapse of months, and when such causes had ceased to operate directly to any large extent, their effects were still manifest in the unstable health of the soldier, his impressionability to morbid influences, and more especially in the behavior of his constitution under the attacks of disease.

"It is also not to be forgotten that, even when to some extent relieved of the harassing and excessive duties to which the men had been exposed, when ill-clothed, ill-fed, and ill-housed in the winter months, and even when food had become both varied and abundant, and most other requisites equally so, two causes still continue in operation, capable of exercising deleterious influences on the most robust constitutions,—namely, the fatigues and night exposure of trench duty, and the singular and rapid vicissitudes of Crimean weather. Of the harassing nature of the duties of a soldier exposed in entrenched lines for twenty-four hours to every possible alternation of temperature and weather, no one can form a full estimate without some practical acquaintance with the operations of a seige. From actual observation in the French and British trenches, I can fully corroborate the statements of some of the most experienced medical officers in both these services, as to the active agency of such fatigues and exposures in the production of the gravest forms of disease.

"With regard to the second class of causes, that due to rapid meteorological changes, I doubt not that your lordship will be put in full possession of the best scientific data on this subject; yet, as directly illustrative of certain well-defined modes of the induction of disease, I may be permitted thus far to notice them. The heavy rains, not infrequent in the summer months, flooding the trenches, and often the huts and tents, caused much suffering, and I believe in many instances could be said to have been directly productive of disease. The great vicissitudes of temperature, scarcely any two successive days presenting the same conditions of the thermometer, must have largely conduced to a similar result. The effects produced by these two causes alone on the health of men unprotected by night and day, when on trench duty, have been very marked, and it is not to be wondered at, if they left lasting and almost indelible impressions, especially on the constitutions of the young and immature.

"It is, by no means, however, to be inferred from these considerations that the climate of the littoral of the Crimea on which the allied armies were encamped is naturally an unhealthy one. On the contrary, there are some very good grounds for quite an opposite opinion, as I shall have occasion hereafter to observe. Considerable immunity has been enjoyed by the allied troops from more than one form of disease, which elsewhere has caused extensive ravages amongst forces in the field. Thus ophthalmic disease has been almost unknown; lesions of the respiratory organs have been of unusual occurrence; and with the exception of certain marshy lands on the borders of the Tchernaya, intermittent fevers seemed to have no habitat within the lines occupied by the besieging armies. The more recent experience in the English camps seems very clearly to establish, that with the realization of the other necessary conditions, respecting moderate duties and fatigues, proper and abundant food, suitable clothing and protection against the weather, the climate of the southern shore of the Crimea is such as to favor the maintenance of a very excellent and satisfactory state of health, even amongst very large masses of troops. That an opposite state of things is in great part, if not wholly, due to causes which are probably *not* climatic, may be deduced from a consideration of the much less healthy condition of other troops in the same region of the Crimea.

" In treating of the various predisposing causes of disease in operation amongst her Majesty's forces in the East, there is one which may be classed amongst physiological influences, and which demands most earnest consideration at your lordship's hands. I allude to the extreme youth, incomplete physical development, and general immaturity of a very considerable proportion of the strength of several regiments; and constituting, as I have reason to believe, in the total of the army, a number sufficiently great to render the question one of vital moment, and of even national interest, as largely affecting what may be called the physiological economy of the army. Amongst even well-matured constitutions, the hardships and fatigues, trials, privations, and exposure of campaigns, such as those of the past years in the Crimea, must almost of necessity prove largely productive of disease, and induce much mortality. But on the undeveloped frames and the unripe strength of the ill-seasoned recruit, such causes operated with twofold energy, and with a more than doubly fatal effect.

" Not only does the power of resistance to morbid influences, and the consequent invasion of disease in such youths, seem inferior to that of the older soldier; but when attacked, they succumb more readily under the effects of fever or a flux. And even when such disease does not prove immediately fatal, the convalescence of the young is generally slow, constantly attended by a disposition to relapse, or to the development of those secondary enteric lesions, the almost unfailing result of such fevers as those which prevailed amongst the troops in the East. Again, should constitutional taints exist, as is not uncommonly the case, more especially in regard to the strumous diathesis so general in some of the classes from which recruits are largely raised, the fatigues and privations of active warfare, the exposure and vicissitudes of the field, and the attacks of acute disease, supply precisely the stimulus most calculated to call into active operation various low and complex forms of disease with a slow and lingering course. Such diseased processes either prove directly fatal of themselves, or so complicate other morbid states set up in the system, as to leave no expectation of aught but a fatal issue.

"Such, doubtless, is the rationale of the pathology of many of the examples of tubercular development in typhoid and dysenteric cases, which we have witnessed in the secondary hospitals of the Bosphorus, in some instances causing death by lesions peculiar to itself; in others, inducing most complex processes of disorganization in the vital parts.

"Even when the less formidable of such cases are not actually fatal, convalescence is usually so slow, lingering, and imperfect, that as soldiers, these youths cannot be, till the expiration of a long period, if ever, sound and effective men; while during such time of convalescence, they but burden the hospitals, required as they often are for the more pressing wants of the field. Thus not only does their illness cause the loss of their own services, but it encumbers the hospital staff, while their transport is an additional pressure on departments already perhaps fully worked.

"The results of surgical pathology corroborate to a large extent the observations just made, which are chiefly based on considerations arising out of the behavior of the immature constitution under the effects of disease. As a general rule, true at least in a very large part of its usual acceptance, youth forms a favorable element in the calculation of chances in surgical cases. Amongst the troops in the Crimea, however, no such favorable anticipations could be indulged on the score of youth. The constitution of the young, even independently of the presence of actual disease, seemed much impressed by the influence of the various causes already dwelt on; many succumbed almost immediately under the shock of injuries, and in the case of the graver surgical operations, no more advantageous results, but the contrary, appeared to be shown on the side of the young: in fact, youth was not to be counted on as a favorable element in determining a prognosis in such cases.

"In the statements I venture to make respecting the operation of youth and immature physical development as a predisposing cause in the production of disease, I do not rely solely on the results of my own observations. This subject has been the topic of repeated consideration with some of the most experienced and accomplished medical officers in the field, by whom my views on these physiological points have been fully concurred in. And, indeed, I do not believe that any person sufficiently acquainted with the principles of physiology could entertain opinions in the least differing from those here expressed.

"I am not in a position to prove, by actual statistical evidence, the precise proportion to strength in the entire force in the Crimea, at any given date, of those who may be considered as of immature age. I did not possess the means of determining such questions on any large scale; and I do not pretend to any such results. However, amongst a portion of the wounded of the 18th June and 8th September, I found means to make a few statistical observations. The cases may, I think, be fairly taken as a general average, and so far admit of being used to support what is stated above. The joint numbers on the occasions of the assaults on the grand Redan, received into one hospital in the field, amounting to 664, embracing all variety of gun-shot injuries, and some of the very worst kind. Of this number of men the average age was 24½. But this statement would only give an inadequate view of the actual youth of a great portion of them. Sixty-one were *under* the age of 20, of whom one was only 17, and the rest varied between 18 and 19; 75 were *of* the actual age of 20 years. Thus, of the whole, considerably more than one-fourth were actually only 20 years of age and under; 76 were found to be between 30 and 40, inclusive; two were of the actual age of 40; while one was stated to be 48, which is at least doubtful. The remainder, constituting a little more than two-thirds, were of various ages, between 20 and 30, the majority inclining to the former rather than the latter. These results show a very high proportion of immature youth, such as, I have no hesitation in saying, it is not consistent with any sound physiological principles to expose to the severe trials and hardships of actual war. Amongst them, disease finds a rich and easy harvest.

"I would not wish to be understood as implying that any objections exist to the practice of early enlistment. On the contrary, such a measure is undoubtedly of great general utility. On home service, or on secondary foreign stations in favorable climates, the training and well-regulated exercise of the young soldier conduce to the development of a vigorous frame, and in no small degree add, I am persuaded, to the natural powers of the constitution. Such training should, however, be gradual, and apportioned to the strength of the recruit, according to the earliness of the period at which he is enlisted; and under a properly regulated system, I believe it would not be necessary to fix any precise limits in this direction. Trained at home, and gradually inured to the fatigues of the soldier's life, by a suitable rotation in the selection of foreign stations, troops could, I doubt not, be slowly but steadily brought to a maximum of safe endurance of the hardships of warfare, far above the average of what is now reached. A judicious system of ' cross drafting,' or some such expedient, would enable the younger soldier and recruits of one regiment ordered to the seat of war to be replaced by the more hardy, seasoned, and service-able men of another; while in the several secondary depots on the high road to the scene of action, the former could undergo a gradual process of seasoning and acclimatization, which would ultimately add immensely to their actual strategic value and efficiency when called to the field in their turn. In this way, I believe no loss of strength or actual inconvenience to the service could result; while the increased efficiency of a large proportion, probably one-fourth of the forces in the field, would be thus almost certainly secured. I am sufficiently well aware that the employment on active service of the young and immature, prevails largely in other forces besides the English: but I have reason to know that it is with equally un-favorable results. Neither precedent nor practice, however, can be admitted as outweighing the dictates of physiology, and the results of pathological experience, in a matter of such moment. As a conviction based on these considerations, I would beg respectfully to express it as my unqualified opinion, that no soldier under 21 years of age should be sent on service to the Crimea, or any other seat of actual war; and not even then, without a previous training and gradual acclimatization in suitably chosen secondary stations. In the foregoing statements, I believe I am justified in saying, that I express views shared in by a large number of the most able and intelligent medical officers.

" Besides the class of men who, by reason of youth and immaturity of physical development, seemed to suffer peculiarly from the toils of Crimean life, it will be necessary to briefly notice another class equally unfitted to make effective troops, but from a somewhat different cause. I allude to those recruited at a rather ad-vanced age—25 to 30—from the mechanical trades in densely populated towns. Such men have seldom enjoyed a vigorous youth, and even at this age—30—the meridian of their physical development is passed. Ill fortune, or it may be a life of dissipation, has led them to take to arms as a last resource. How far any of such men are capable of becoming efficient soldiers, I know not; but it is certain that the testimony of medical officers bears me out in the observation, that they are constant and early applicants for admission into hospital, their constitution, never robust, soon giving way under exposure and fatigue. Men of such a class may add to the numerical, but never to the effective strength of an army; and it is more than doubtful if they ever repay the labor and cost of their transport, and of their maintenance in the field or secondary hospitals. One sound, seasoned, and effec-tive soldier, outweighs in value any number of immature and inefficient youths or effete adults. And in the physiological economics of an army, the maintenance of the largest number of effective men is the great problem.

" The several agencies just considered, many of them continuously in operation, and others, though ceasing to be immediately felt, leaving well-defined impressions behind them, had induced sensible modifications, as I have already said, in the con-stitution of the soldier. Some of these effects were visible to the eye. A marked characteristic of the Crimean soldier was a premature appearance of age. The veteran of 40 would be readily taken, by the inexperienced, for the old man of 60 to 65. The youth of 20 to 22 wore the settled aspect of 35 to 40. With the haggard features of disease, especially that of a chronic kind, these appearances became still more exaggerated, often to a most marked degree.

" Even with those who possessed a still robust exterior, and all the apparent physical conditions of health, the manner in which their system was observed to behave under the influences of disease, or the effects of injury or operations, showed that the force of the constitution was to a very considerable extent deteriorated.

To express this in another way, it may be stated, that the available *vis vitæ* for the resistance to, or recovery from disease, or for the resistance to, or recovery from, the effects of injury, or of great surgical operations, was below the average physiological standard. The powers of the system, and consequently the *viability*, so to speak, of the soldier, were below par. This was especially manifested in some of the prominent and distinctive characters of prevailing diseases which presented a decidedly low adynamic, and often typhous type, and such as urgently called for a generous and stimulant treatment.

"It is all but impossible to realize for the soldier in the field the same conditions of life, or the comforts he enjoys on a home station. Many peculiarities, privations, and irregularities, independently of necessary fatigues and exposure, must attend camp life. The constitution is highly impressionable, and readily acquires morbid peculiarities; and from the various concurrent causes which had prevailed in the army of the East, and from the lowered tone of constitutional powers already alluded to, the system of the soldier had become prone to the influence of certain pathological types to a greater or less extent. Some diseased constitutional states seemed to prevail, even independently of the actual development of cognizable lesions, with definite anatomical seat. Foremost and most remarkable, as well as perhaps important, amongst this class of morbid conditions, is to be reckoned the scorbutic dyscrasis.

"Well-developed cases of scorbutic and allied forms of disease, such as purpura hæmorrhagica, were, at the date of my arrival in the Crimea, of comparatively rare occurrence amongst the English troops; while, in the neighboring allied camp of the French, these affections still prevailed to a considerable extent. The continuance of these diseases in the French army at this period, did not seem to be attributable to deficiencies of vegetable diet. It is now well known that this class of affections does not recognize any such limited or exclusive cause. They are known to occur amongst masses of men, in whom the vital stamina have been impaired by any causes, as by the toils of many campaigns; and in accordance with this view, I learned that cases of scorbutus were sufficiently common amongst those veterans of the French army in the Crimea, who had served with such distinction in the campaigns of Africa.

"Uniformity of diet, when it amounts to a monotony inconsistent with the well-being of the digestive system, is perhaps, almost as fully operative in the production of scurvy, in some of its forms, as an actual deficiency of any single requisite ingredient of the soldier's food.

"Having had the fullest opportunities of becoming thoroughly acquainted with all the essential features of disease as presented in the English camp, I can safely say, that during and subsequent to the month of June of the past year, cases presenting any marked development of scorbutic lesion, as a primary and essential disease, were of the greatest rarity. Some few such I have seen, but they were, undoubtedly, exceptional. But I have not the less reason to believe that, to a considerable extent at least, a general scorbutic state was recognizable in the constitution of the soldier, which, though it seldom led to the actual development of scorbutic lesions of a primary, independent form, lent a decided influence to, and even sometimes distinctly modified, the characters of the other diseased processes which were so commonly prevalent. In more precise terms, it may be stated, that while scurvy did not, except in rare cases, exist in any form as a distinct disease—and while, from the month of June, no single fatal case came within my sphere of observation in the English hospitals, in which scorbutus was the direct cause of death, many cases of disease occurred, in which modifications attributable to a prevalent scorbutic dyscrasis could be recognized; such as various discolorations of the extremities externally, hemorrhagic effusions internally, and the very remarkable, and as yet unexplained, phenomenon of hæmeralopia. On post-mortem examination, several of such cases, besides the ordinary lesions of the dominant disease, exhibited anatomico-pathological characters, such as mucous hemorrhages, and submucous blood extravasations, which were, in all probability, referable to the scorbutic dyscrasis, as their immediate cause. Of the independent existence of scorbutic lesions at an earlier period, I wish to express no doubt; but I speak here of what came directly under my own observation.

" The next great morbid constitutional state which deserves attention is the Typhous.

" Very numerous, varied, and ill-defined significations attach to this word. I would be understood to use it at present, not in the sense in which it implies special diseases, but for the purpose of designating by it a certain generally prevailing morbid state of the constitution, which determines, in any given essential disease, or any special pathological lesion, when actually called into existence, the marked and peculiar clinical characters which, by universal concurrence of interpretation, are known as typhous. I employ the word, in its comprehensive and generic sense, to embrace as well the phenomena called *Typhoid*, as the *Typhous* proper. That some general constitutional state, brought about by various influences, did exist, and manifested its influence from time to time, in the determination of the disease, I think there is every legitimate reason to believe. Circumstances being the same, disease at one time presented acute, sthenic, inflammatory characters ; at another, and far more commonly, its phenomena tended to a low adynamic form.

" Of the diseases prevalent in the forces in the Crimea, during the period of my observations, the majority presented undoubtedly low adynamic—in other words, typhous characters ; and this will be found to have been true, not only of the essential diseases, as fevers, but to have been all but constant with regard to many other diseased processes. Acute inflammatory diseases were exceedingly uncommon. I have myself not witnessed any such, and the highest *tone* of symptoms which I have at any time determined to exist, would not, in my opinion, admit of being classed as other than *sub*-sthenic and *sub*-acute. As usually manifested, however, the *tone* of diseased action was much lower, and either verged on or actually exhibited the low typhous adynamic types ; and such, as it appears to me, was the class of diseases commonly presented. This type of disease plainly indicated, and as urgently called for, a liberal, generous, and stimulant treatment, often requiring the bold and unsparing use of wine and brandy. To the experienced clinical physician, these well-known pathological indications as clearly and unmistakably precluded the idea of antiphlogistic and depletory measures, which must be regarded under such circumstances as worse than useless ; for, in many instances, they would not have been devoid of danger to life. I have great pleasure in here offering my humble testimony to the generally just and intelligent views of the great majority of the medical officers of the army of the East on this vital point in pathology, and its immediate practical bearing. Few of those who possessed the requisite experience of disease failed to seize readily its great characteristic features, and its manifest disposition to typhous forms. It is needless to add, that their practice was most properly, and I have reason to believe, in many cases at least, as successfully regulated in accordance with these views, which indicated a generous, and often in the worst cases, a highly stimulant treatment.

" While anxious to avoid even the appearance of an approach to controversy, I cannot help, in connection with so important a subject, expressing my entire and most unqualified dissent from certain pathological views and principles, and the applications to the treatment of disease in the English forces, which necessarily and directly grew out of them, and which were as directly or forcibly urged by authorities of eminence resident in Constantinople. That the principles urged by these distinguished persons were, in all probability, true in their application to the class of disease ordinarily presented to their observation, I am free to admit. That the type of disease now and of late years prevalent in these parts of the east of Europe differs materially from that exhibited in the west, is not only possible, but likely. Furthermore, I am prepared to believe, that residence in the midst of Eastern influences will, after the lapse of even a few years, induce marked constitutional changes in the system of the western European—changes which are followed, as a natural consequence, by modifications in the types of disease when it occurs, and which both clearly indicate and require corresponding modifications in the medical treatment which they call for. It is far from improbable that types of constitution, and, as a consequence, types of disease, undergo great, varied, and extensive modifications, not only in different climates and latitudes, but even within the same climates and latitudes at different times. And, perhaps, more in this than in any of the supposed extraordinary advances in the practice of the healing art, is to be sought the explanation of the opposing views as to pathology and treatment of apparently the same disease, at different times and in different places. Certain it is, such views as to possible modifications of disease, both as to time and place, have been too much kept out of view. Be this as it may, however, to the experienced clinical physician, the characters of the typhous type were too well evidenced in the diseases of the English army during the past campaigns, to admit of doubt as to the pathological views to be entertained, or the appropriate treatment to be adopted with regard to them. What the tendency of the diseased types, and the essential pathological phenomena of the same army in subsequent campaigns, may be, I am by no means prepared to state. To the closely observant eye, an elevation, slow, gradual, but distinctly sensible, in the general type of the constitution of the soldier, with corresponding, though slight, modifications of the phenomena of disease, when induced, did not fail to make itself evident, even before the termination of the past year. And I am ready to admit it as possible, that the pathological views of the Constantinople observers may be as applicable, in their full force, to the diseases of this same army in some future campaigns, as they were in the past campaigns wholly inadmissible.

" The observations here adduced are in great measure confirmed and supported by those of several accomplished observers amongst the French and Sardinian medical officers. The latter, especially, had noticed as a result of even a comparatively short exposure of the troops of Piedmont and Savoy to the influence of the Crimean campaigns, a decided though slight depression of the constitutional tone of the men ; and not only a less urgent demand for, but a less tolerance of, antiphlogistic measures of treatment, especially the depletory. In a more general, but not less important way, the experience in the French hospitals of the field bore out the conclusions derived from the study of the characters of disease amongst the English forces in camp. The French troops had, it will be remembered, been exposed to all but the same influences as the English.

" Of the two chief pathological states which may be grouped under the head of Typhous, I must now treat somewhat more particularly. They constituted, perhaps, the gravest forms of disease which extensively affected the troops. The typhous proper and the typhoid, as essential diseases, allied as they undoubtedly are, yet presenting important differential characters, stand pre-eminent amongst the fevers which have made ravages on the armies of the East. I shall not here enter into any discussion as to differences between these types of disease. I use the terms in a sense the same as that which is a pretty general conventional recognition of their chief differential characters as assigned to them. Of the precise nature of the diseases treated of, the very full anatomico-pathological details which will be subsequently communicated will leave no doubt. Of the typhus proper, the true spotted or petechial fever, I have determined the existence in the hospitals of the East by some few but well-marked and unmistakable cases. But it would appear not to have been by any means so general, nor to me does it seem to have been of such importance, as the typhoid. This latter form of fever prevailed to a very considerable extent, and at times in a type of the gravest kind. Occurring in constitutions already depressed below the physiological standard, it is not to be wondered at that it frequently proved fatal. It is not, however, in its more immediate effects, perhaps, that its most formidable characters are to be sought.

" Fevers of this class, as it is well known, exhibit a marked tendency to secondary complications in vital parts ; and this, apparently, by reason of some cause, as it were, natural to the order of morbid actions which they embrace. Several causes foreign to such fevers likewise concurred to determine the all but constant occurrence of one class of internal lesions ; those, namely, of the abdominal organs. From both influences combined, doubtless, the secondary enteric lesions, which this order of fever induced, were of the severest kind. They were all but universally attendant upon it, and were usually of a markedly fatal character. In the typhoid fever of the Crimea, it was especially noticeable that a convalescence, more or less apparently complete, often occurred after the subsidence of the primary disease, before the development of any secondary lesion was manifested by appreciable signs. Such periods of convalescence, it must be observed, did not always occur, for the primary symptoms not infrequently passed into those of the secondary affection, with scarcely any sensible intermission. The cases assumed, it may be, a more low and lingering character, and terminated in some one of the forms of fatal issue common in this disease. Convalescent intervals, with apparent though fallacious restoration to health, did, however, sufficiently often occur, and in many instances to such an extent, as apparently to warrant a return to duty—a circumstance almost constantly fraught with increased danger to the patient. The great danger to life involved in these secondary enteric lesions, which so often lead to slow, lingering illness, with its attendant diarrhœa, wasting and gradual exhaustion of the patient, with sometimes an end of pain and misery, as when they issue by intestinal perforations, is a well-established fact in pathology. And when a fever, prevalent among masses of troops, is ascertained to present any tendency to the development of such lesions, the greatest circumspection is called for amongst those intrusted with the charge of such cases. During convalescence, however well established to all outward appearance, the utmost restrictions should be placed on the diet and drink of the patient. He should be kept under constant observation, and, if circumstances admit, transported carefully to some secondary hospital for convalescents. And till such time as he may be fairly considered beyond the danger of the possible induction of the insidious disease which he inherits, as it were, from the primary affection, he should be strictly treated as still, in all respects, in *statu ægri*. The neglect of such precautions would, I believe, be found to lead to the loss of many valuable lives. It is with regret I have to say, that it does not appear to me that the principles which furnish indications of such importance as these, are sufficiently known and properly recognized.

" Of the various causes operating in the production of disease amongst the troops in camp, the greater part tended undoubtedly to the development of morbid action in one part of the system more especially; and this almost to the exclusion of affections in other organs, at least in a primary form. The abdominal viscera were those in which disease was most commonly manifested. Physical causes from without, and irritation established within, in some measure at least, connected with peculiarities of life and diet, led to a prominent tendency to gastro-enteric derangements, and the consequent development of the diseases known as Fluxes, in their various forms. It may, indeed, be said, that the main features of the pathology of the disease, as presented in the army of the East, were embraced in the two great classes of the fevers and the fluxes; and of the latter, no inconsiderable proportion owed their origin to the former. Ample proofs will be found, in the various following sections of this report, of the extraordinary predominance of abdominal lesions. To such an extent did they prevail, that I believe I shall be warranted in stating, that in no case submitted to examination by me or my assistants, has a perfectly normal state of the digestive viscera been found to exist; while a marked absence of lesions in other parts was, in those who died in the early periods of the disease or injury, the general rule.

" Amongst the several diseased processes attended with one or other of the forms of flux, that connected with the development of enteric lesions, secondary to the variety of fever already considered under the name of typhoid, deserves most especial attention, for reasons already adduced. It seems, however, to have been not unfrequently confounded with other, and often less important affections, under the ill-defined head of 'diarrhœa.' Evidence bearing upon this point will be found throughout the body of this work. I would only further venture to remark, in reference to it at present, that this branch of diagnosis does not seem to me to be in such a position as its importance demands for it.

" As I shall subsequently have occasion to show, dysentery formed by far the greater part of the true fluxes which so largely affected this army. In its chronic forms, it was a lingering, wasting, and almost constantly fatal disease.

" When established as a chronic disease, dysentery evinced a marked tendency to the induction of other morbid states in the system. The most complicated forms of diseased action, and those presenting the most profound disorganization of vital parts, have been illustrated by dysentery in certain orders of morbid association : in one, in connection with the typhoid state, either as an antecedent or a consequent ; in another, in connection with the development of tubercle ; and in a third, with the development of both these processes in a more or less advanced degree. But the discussion of the details of such cases belongs to the domain of special pathology.

" I have before alluded to the comparative immunity from diseases of the respiratory organs enjoyed by the soldier in the Crimea. This is to be understood as referring to the primary and idiopathic forms of these affections; for, as will be evident in the details of cases subsequently given, extensive secondary diseases of the lungs have been all but constant, as the result of the typhoid and the dysenteric processes, more especially when in the chronic state.

"As a cause influencing the nature and results of disease to an important extent, I cannot omit alluding to the subject of deportation of the sick.

"Of the various diseases existing in camp, a broad practical distinction into two great classes presented itself, in a medico-economic point of view,—namely, first, into those which were characterized by a uniform determinate course, of longer or shorter duration, and with a definite primary issue in death or recovery; and secondly, into those in which, after the primary phases of morbid action had been brought to an end, the system was still under a dominant morbid influence, liable to the invasion of important, often fatal, secondary diseases, as an almost direct consequence of the primary affection, though, in many instances, periods of complete intermission occurred. In the former class were to be ranked the simple fevers, the uncomplicated forms of diarrhœa and dysentery, and such cases of acute or sub-acute idiopathic inflammatory affections of isolated organs, as, though exceptional, were found to exist from time to time. In the latter group were included, in a general way, almost all other diseases, whether fevers or fluxes, witnessed in camp. I may, however, especially mention relapsing fevers, those of the typhoid type, with tendency to the development of secondary enteric lesions, any such few independent forms of enteric disease as may have occurred, and all the forms of chronic dysentery which presented disposition to complex morbid associations, especially with the great dyscrasic types, as scorbutus, tuberculosis, and typhoid disease.

"It is not in a scientific point of view that such a broad division of disease is most worthy of attention. Certain medico-economic considerations of great practical moment arise out of it; and it is because it has seemed to me that such indications have not received that recognition which they are entitled to, that I venture to bring them into notice at present. It will need little reasoning to show that diseases having a tendency to determine issue in the primary stages should be treated *in loco*, having due regard to the place of their occurrence, and the possibility of requisite accommodation being found for their reception and cure. The same applies to the second great class during their acute stages. It is not necessary to point out the impropriety, and often even fatal effects liable to result from the deportation of disease in an acute form, either by land or sea, to any considerable distance. Yet neglect of this principle has led to very unfavorable results. With regard to the second great classes, with tendency to secondary disease subsequent to a primary attack, removal from the morbid influences in which the disease has originated, and which are capable of determining its further development, rest from all duties and fatigues, with strict attention to diet, are absolutely essential. Such conditions as are here implied can be only adequately realized in the great secondary hospitals.

"On the principles here indicated, there is good ground for believing that a large and timely extension of the system of sick and convalescent leave would be attended with marked beneficial results, and would, doubtless, restore to a state of efficiency for active service many valuable lives. It has not appeared to me that such a system has been followed to the extent that would be requisite, and which could be readily accomplished.

"I have already informed your lordship, that on the occasion of the 8th September, in the illness of some, and absence on sick leave of others of the medical staff, I had the honor of lending my services to the care of a considerable number of the surgical cases which that event produced. It is likewise, doubtless, known to you, that a large proportion of operations was performed by me on that occasion.

"The pathological phenomena exhibited in the sequence of mechanical injuries from the various forms of projectiles, or developed as a consequence of surgical operations, presented, in very many instances, features of remarkable interest. An attentive study of the pathological conditions thus brought into existence will be found of value, not only because they constitute in themselves important subjects of scientific inquiry, but also because they tend to throw light on the states of constitution in which they themselves became manifested, and to which, in all probability, they owed their origin. When elucidated themselves, they became, as it were, so far, fixed pathological standards, and then, in their turn, admitted of being used to estimate the nature and degree of the deviations from the normal physiological status of the system in which they occurred. In this manner it will be subsequently seen, that though on the whole, the general results have been satisfactory, a consideration of the pathological conditions presented as the sequence of injury or of surgical operations, leads to the estimation of very grave and important aberrations from the physiological standard in the constitution of the soldier. So far the indications furnished by surgical, corroborate those derived from the medical pathology. As a general rule, though no epidemic morbid states prevailed, low forms of diseased action attended the graver surgical cases. Destructive processes were often exhibited in limbs after the operation of amputation; and only very moderate success has been obtained in this class of operations.

"In connection with this subject, some notice must be taken of marked constitutional effects, in all probability due to the excessive and habitual use of intoxicating liquors. Testimony has been elsewhere borne, and very properly, to the general abstemiousness of the soldier during a part of the past campaigns. It was with regret, however, that I noticed, subsequent to the month of May, that the increased facilities for procuring malt and other intoxicating liquors became a means of great and general abuse. Habitually employed, even in not excessive quantity, I am far from agreeing with many that porter constitutes a perfectly healthy ration for the soldier. Immoderately used, it leads to an inflation of the system, and a plethoric state not consistent with a firm and vigorous health. Certain it is, that men presenting these fallacious appearances of strength, often presented rapid, low, and fatal forms of disease, and quickly succumbed under the effects of injury or great operations. However robust in appearance, they were far from being in a normal state. Proofs of the truth of what is here advanced will be found in a proper section hereafter.

"It will be interesting to notice here, that a tolerance of the effects of injury, and of the greater surgical operations, has been observed amongst the Russian prisoners, both in the French and English hospitals, far superior to that exhibited by the wounded amongst the allied troops, with the exception, perhaps, of the Sardinians.

"In a very considerable proportion of the Russian prisoners who came under my observation, the physical development of the frame seemed to be that best suited for the safe endurance of the hardships and fatigues of warfare. The muscular system was well developed, vigorous, and firm, with the adipose tissues at a minimum. Their frames were, in fact, 'hard,' 'firm,' and in thorough working order; and, in this respect, contrasted forcibly with the 'soft,' inflated, though apparently stalwart systems of some of her Majesty's troops. I regret extremely that my opportunities for investigating the physiological and pathological status of the Russian troops were not sufficiently extensive to enable me to communicate any definite results on these subjects.

"In the primary forms of disease, as observed in camp, lesions of the abdominal organs have been stated to have been the great characteristics; and, while in their early stages, such lesions commonly existed isolated. When, however, disease assumed the chronic form, complexity of diseased processes became manifested. This latter tendency—namely, that to multiple associations of morbid actions— was, perhaps, the greatest point of difference which existed between disease as it occurred in the hospitals of the camp and in those of Scutari. In the latter place, chronic disease was the rule, and, so far, complexity of lesions and of diseased processes was to be expected. A tendency to the development of dyscrasic states, especially that of tubercle, in association with the chronic disease, was, moreover, largely manifested in the secondary hospitals of the Bosphorus. Though I have not failed to observe some cases of similar complex affections among the sick in camp, they were undoubtedly of rare and exceptional occurrence in the hospitals in the field.

"In the several following sections, the results of the investigations undertaken by myself and my assistants, will be found detailed. I have held it in view to endeavor to give such descriptions of disease and diseased processes presented to us, as will enable them to be recognized and identified in the fullest manner at any time, or for any purpose. In some instances, it has been found necessary to go into considerable detail to furnish the requisite data for estimating the characters of the diseases observed by us. But it is not to be expected, that in a work of this nature, or within the limits of time and space properly assignable to a report, the various important pathological subjects which we shall have to pass in review could receive that complete and elaborate discussion which, under other circumstances, would be demanded for their full elucidation. To elaborate the numerous details of our investigations, and to show their full bearing on medical and surgical pathology, would have required, for its accomplishment, as many months as we have been enabled to devote weeks to this work. Such as it is, however, I trust that in this report the chief outlines of the pathology of the diseases of the army in the East will be found considered with sufficient fulness for the purposes of the inquiry.

"I cannot close this section without bringing to your lordship's notice the services of my first assistant, Dr. Wm. Aitkin. To his zeal and energy, his discretion and judgment, under circumstances of no ordinary difficulty, I am greatly indebted. And to his ability as an investigator of disease, much of the results of this inquiry are largely due.

"I have the honor to be, my lord, your lordship's obedient servant,
"ROBERT D. LYONS.

"The Right Hon. the Lord Panmure, G. C. B."

Aperçu du Système Spinal ou de la série des actions réflexes dans leurs applications à la physiologie, à la pathologie, et specialement à l'epilepsie. Par MARSHALL HALL. (Paris, Victor Masson, 1855, 12mo. pp. 246.)

The principal object of this work is to set forth tracheotomy as the remedy in laryngismus, and with this view several cases are appended in which the operation has been performed. There is nothing new for us on this side of the water; indeed, Dr. Hall tells us in his preface, "*il n'a rien à y changer,*" and as there is nothing new, we find no reason to modify the opinion we have already expressed in these matters. We greatly admire, however, the versatility of talent and the energy of character which have prompted Dr. Hall to communicate his views to our noble allies, the French, in their own language.

Outline of a Hygienic Code for the treatment of Consumption. By BENJAMIN W. RICHARDSON, M.D., Physician to the Royal Infirmary for Diseases of the Chest. ("The Journal of Public Health," October, 1856.)

In giving the following rules, Dr. Richardson presupposes their general applicability to cases of consumption in all stages of the disease : in the premonitory stage ; in the stage where the tubercular deposition is apparent ; and in the next stage, when the local mischief is much further advanced. In the last stage even, though hope is lost, many of the rules may still be rigidly followed out with advantage, for by them the course of the disease may be smoothed, and life, perhaps, prolonged.

The Rules are ten in number.

RULE 1.—*A supply of pure air for respiration is the first indication in the treatment of the consumptive patient.*

No cosy room with a temperature at 70°, with every crevice closed, and with an atmosphere in a dead calm and laden with impurities, should be permitted. A temperature from 55° to 65° Fahr. is high enough. The fire, if one be wanted, should be in an open grate, and every arrangement should be made by which the freest possible current of air should be kept circulating through the room. If the patient is cold, he must go near the fire, and, if necessary, poke it, but he must on no account make the room warm by making it close. Dr. Richardson objects very strongly to stoves of all kinds, to heated pipes, and to every other mode of supplying warmth, except an open fire, as by these means the air is made too dry. Among other disadvantages attending the inhalation of a too dry air, is hæmoptysis, and a case is mentioned in point. "A gentleman whom I knew, and whose lungs were free from tubercle and other organic disorder, was constantly annoyed and troubled with slight attacks of hacking cough and blood-spitting. He was at a loss to account for the cause. At last he detected that the attacks always commenced when he was at work in his study. With the idea of being very warm and comfortable, and ignorant of the nature of animal heat, he had introduced into a small room a large Burton's stove. To a stranger entering that room when the stove was in action, and the doors and windows snugly closed, the heat and dryness of the atmosphere would have been at once oppressive ; but he, a close student, and constantly occupying the room under such conditions, had become accustomed to it as regards external sensation, but caught the mischief effectually in the chest. The cause of the symptoms being explained, the stove was abandoned, and the open fire-grate was again resorted to: the cough and blood-spitting at once disappeared without the administration of any medicine. A few weeks afterwards, thinking that the stove and the cough might only stand in the position of coincidences, our student resumed the use of the stove; and what is more, resumed also, as an effect, the cough and the blood expectoration. This time he became assured that the stove and the cough stood in the relation of cause and effect. The cause was once more removed, and ever since he has remained free of the effect." Free ventilation is especially necessary where gas is used. The bedroom should be large—including, if practicable, not less than 1000 cubic feet of breathing space ; and, to prevent any unnecessary contamination of the air, no second person should sleep in the same room, and no light, particularly gas, should be burnt through the night. Two persons in one bed, according to Dr. Richardson, are out of the question under any circumstances. The inclemencies of the weather are not so much to be dreaded as confinement to the house. "I had occasion, some time since," says the author, "repeatedly to remark that if, from a few days' rain, the consumptives under my care were confined to their houses, instead of being able to take the daily out-door breathing always prescribed, the aggravation of symptoms was always marked and universal. The appetite fell off, the debility became greater, the mind was less buoyant, the local mischief increased." Better go out with respirators and mufflers, under ordinary circumstances, than stay in. A muffler, which a patient may make for a few pence, being as good as an expensive respirator. This is made out of a piece of fine wire gauze, cut oval, so as to cover the mouth and nose, and fixed in the centre of a handkerchief, so that it may be tied on like an ordinary comforter, with the gauze in the centre, for breathing through.

The want of pure air is thought to be an objection to hospitals for consumption. Dr. Richardson admits "that a vast deal of good is, or may be, done at these institutions by the treatment prescribed by the physicians who attend at them, and whose lives are devoted to the study of the disease, there cannot be a doubt. But that it is either physiological, or sound practical treatment, to receive into these buildings consumptive patients, is an assumption I most earnestly dispute. I know the excellent spirit in which institutions of this kind are founded. I am fully aware of the care that is bestowed on the inmates; of the attempts that are made to introduce every hygienic improvement; of the order and cleanliness that prevail; of the kindness of the attendants; of the excellence of the diet-rule; and of the skill of the physicians.

"With all this, it is to me as clear as crystal, that to bring phthisical patients into such institutions is a great charitable mistake. The very care, and waiting-servant attention, that is paid to such of the invalids as are in the first and second stages of the disease, is a cruel kindness. The remedy for them is to encourage and urge them to assist themselves and to exert themselves. Moreover, no kind of hygienic system, carried on in a large building filled with inmates, can make the air of that building in any way equal to the outer air, which it is so necessary that the consumptive person should breathe. Twenty patients, lying in one hospital ward, will throw off per minute into the air of the ward at least three and a half cubic feet of expired and impure gases, rendered in the phthisical the more impure by the pathological condition of the lungs. But the impure air thus exhaled vitiates by its diffusion twenty times its own volume of pure air ; so that, in fact, in a ward with twenty patients, there are not less than seventy cubic feet of air spoiled per minute, and rendered unfit for the purposes of life. It may be granted that during the day, when the wards are less full, and many windows are open, and the movements of the inmates are active, the expired air may be fairly disposed of. But take a winter night of twelve hours; consider that in this period of time the twenty patients would, if they exhaled even naturally, vitiate fifty thousand four hundred cubic feet of air, which ought to be removed, and to be replaced by two thousand five hundred and twenty cubic feet of *pure* air for the use of respiration ; and then reflect whether it is probable that such a ward can remain during the whole night uncontaminated. For, granting to the twenty patients a breathing-space of twenty-six thousand cubic feet, and even then it would require that the whole of the air in that space should be removed and replaced by fresh air fully twice in the one night. Against this, possibly, the artificial ventilating argumentists will urge that such a feat of ventilation is nothing at all, not worth considering, so easy to be done. M. Grouvelle would probably undertake to effect such interchange eight times in the night, or more; and if he undertook to do it eighty times, and did not succeed in doing it once, it might be difficult to prove the fact against him. But if he would take a strip of paper prepared for ozone, place it in a ward, however artificially ventilated, and place another similar paper in the open air adjoining the ward, it is a mistake if he should not find that there was a striking difference in the process of oxidation in the two localities; and that the great life supporter, oxygen, was in a condition to play a very much more active part in its outdoor than in its indoor work.

" The misfortune of a great hospital, with all its rooms communicating indirectly with each other, is, that the ventilation is always uncertain. There is, in fact, no properly ventilated space except the great vault of heaven, and no true ventilating power except in the combinations of atmospheric pressure, wind movements, and the force of diffusion.

" If special hospitals for consumptives are to be had, they should be as little colonies, situated far away from the thickly populated abodes of men, and so arranged that each patient should have a distinct dwelling-place for himself. They should be provided with pleasure-grounds of great extent, in which the patients who could walk about should pass every possible hour in the day; and with glass-covered walks overhead, where they could breathe open air, and yet be dry, even if rain were falling. Very expensive such an establishment would be, there is no doubt; but it would, I take it, be infinitely more practically advantageous to treat ten patients in this manner, than ten tens in a confined brick-and-mortar box, through which of necessity some amount of invisible impurity, some trace of transparent poison-cloud, is constantly floating.

" The strongest argument in favor of consumption hospitals is, that they receive those members of the community who could not at their own homes afford the same advantages as are supplied to them in the charity. Against this it is to be urged that the patients taken into the consumption hospitals are *not*, in this country at least, in any way to be considered as the representatives of the most needy and destitute sections of the community. These latter go to their last homes in the workhouse, or in their own poverty-stricken dwellings. The classes that fill the hospitals are often many grades above destitution ; and are sometimes comparatively wealthy. They have access to a governor, who gives them an admission-letter, and they leave their own medical adviser to enter the hospital, not because they cannot find the means to live at home and be treated at home, but because, catching at every new suggestion offered to them, they set their hearts on getting into the hospital, as though it were a certain haven of rescue. In this scramble after admission some of course succeed ; they leave their homes, they enter the hospital, and there the greater proportion of them either die or return back to their friends nearer death than before. A few recover or are relieved ; but whether the same result would have occurred, if they had been subjected to the same medical and general treatment out of the hospital—is a question which may be left very safely answered in the affirmative."

RULE 2.—*Active exercise is an essential element in the treatment of consumption.*

Next to a free exposure to air, Dr. Richardson agrees with Drs. Rush, Jackson, and Parrish, in thinking that vigorous exercise is by far the most efficient remedy in the treatment of consumption. " Walking," he say, "is the true natural exercise, and the best, for it brings into movement every part of the body more or less, and, leading to brisker circulation in every part, causes a more active nutrition generally. The extent to which exercise should be carried will vary with the stage of the disease, and temporary accidents may for the moment stop it altogether, such, for instance, as an attack of hæmoptysis. But when exercise is advisable, the general rule is to recommend that it be carried out systematically, cautiously, and courageously, and that each exercise should be continued until a gentle feeling of fatigue is felt through the whole muscular system. Violent and unequal exertion of the upper muscles of the body is unadvisable. When restored from the fatigue of one exertion, another should be undertaken, and during the day this cannot be too often repeated. If the day be wet, then the exercise should be effected by walking in a large room, or by engaging in some game, such as skittles, billiards, or tennis.

"If, in his waking hours, the consumptive patient can keep himself occupied pretty freely in muscular labor, he secures the best sudorific for his sleeping hours that can possibly be supplied; for as the cause of force is always expended in producing motion or action, so, to use the words of Dr. Metcalfe, 'the proximate cause of sleep is an expenditure of the substance and vital energy of the brain, nerves, and voluntary muscles, beyond what they receive when awake; and the specific office of sleep is the restoration of what has been wasted by exercise.' Cough is very much less frequent in the course of the night in him who has been subjected to exercise in the day; while sleep, when it falls, is more profound, and more refreshing.

"In summer time, when the temperature of the day is high, the morning and the evening time are the best adapted for the periods of outdoor exertion. In the other seasons, mid-day is preferable, as a general rule.

"I have sometimes been asked whether what are called gymnastic exercises are commendable in consumptive cases, and whether swinging is good. My idea on these points is that, in swinging, a person is much more usefully exercised when throwing the swing for his associates' pleasure, than in being himself swung. There is, in fact, but little faith to be placed in so-called scientific gymnastics. Anything that a man invents to overtop or compete with nature must needs be paltry. Brisk natural movement of the limbs is all that the consumptive requires. He need not go out of his way after a sham, in the shape of a shampooer; chopping wood is a good gymnastic feat, and playing at skittles is perfect in its way.

"The value of exercise is threefold. First, it checks waste of muscular structures, for muscles left inactive undergo a consumption, without any necessity for lung disorder. Secondly, it diverts the blood from the lungs, causes a more brisk circulation through them, and a more free distribution through the system at large. Thirdly, it induces a more free respiration; more oxygen is taken into the lungs, the body is restored to its vital purposes more surely, and, just in proportion as this restoration is effected, so is the restoration of disordered function and of disorganized tissue.

"In the performance of muscular exercise let the consumptive never encumber himself, or check the free movements of his body by strappings, loads of clothes, or carrying of weights, and the like. These are but tasks; they lead to unequal exertion in special sets of muscles, and such inequality of expenditure is that which is to be avoided. The treatment of consumption in an hospital is objectionable, again, in regard to exercise. Of what use to the consumptive is an acre or two of airing-ground confined at the back of his hospital? Let him be certain that where the gardener cannot make roses bloom, and peach-trees blossom, no doctor can give to the anæmic cheek a permanent color, to a lost function its uses, or to an impoverished body its once healthy power.

"A last consideration on the value of muscular exercise is, that it is eminently useful in keeping the respiratory muscles in a state of active nutrition. For, if to the loss of capaciousness in the lungs to receive air, there is added a daily increasing failure in the muscles by which the acts of inspiration and expiration are carried on, it is clear that a double evil is at work. Now this double evil is most actively presented in consumption. As the respiratory muscles, together with the other muscles, lose their tone, so do the general symptoms of exhaustion increase in severity; sometimes without very marked change in the pathological condition of the lungs. As a sequence, day by day, as the nutrition of these muscles decreases, and as they fail in tonic contractile power, they gain in excitability; so that the irregular spasmodic contractions to which they are subjected in the act of coughing are produced by the merest excitement, and the cough is more frequent as it becomes more feeble."

RULE 3.—*A uniform climate is an important element in the treatment of consumptives.*

No particular place is recommended for consumptives, but here is the formula for an hypothetical consumptive Atalantis. "It should be near the sea-coast, and sheltered from northerly winds; the soil should be dry; the drinking water pure; the mean temperature about 60°, with a range of not more than ten or fifteen degrees on either side. It is not easy to fix any degree of humidity; but extremes of dryness or of moisture are alike injurious. It is of importance in selecting a locality that the scenery should be enticing, so that the patient may be more encouraged to spend his time out of doors in walking or riding exercise, and a town where the residences are isolated and scattered about, and where drainage and cleanliness are attended to, is much preferable to one where the houses are closely packed, however small its population may be."

RULE 4.—*The dress of the consumptive patient should be adapted to equalize the temperature of the body.*

RULE 5.—*The hours of rest of the consumptive patient should extend from sunset to sunrise.*

This rule, in Dr. Richardson's opinion, is imperative for many reasons. "First, because in all seasons the actual amount of rest required by the natural man is pointed out with the precision of an astronomical law by the course of the sun. In midwinter men require, for physiological reasons, more sleep than they do at midsummer, and just so much more as is indicated by the difference of night in these two periods. Observe how all animals, left to their own natural instincts, obey this law. Secondly, in our present artificial mode of life, we have to extend the day by the invention of artificial lights. But whenever a man shuts himself up in his closet, and makes a little sun out of his gas-lamp or candle, he is feeding that lamp with a part of his own breathing store—the air around him. Worse still, the candle can, no more than the man, live alight without exhaling carbonic acid gas, and thus vitiating the atmosphere. A pound of oil burnt in a lamp produces, in burning, nearly three pounds; and every cubic foot of coal gas, rather more than a cubic foot of carbonic acid. The evil effects of carbonic acid on the lungs have been already described. Thirdly, as an artificial light is, by the mode in which it is produced, of necessity injurious, so, on the contrary, the pure sunlight is of the greatest worth in the acts of vitality. What sunlight does in a physiological way is undetermined; but its general influence has long been known and recognized. Plants banked up from the light become blanched, and human beings kept for a long time in dark abodes become the victims of anæmia and scrofula.

"Thus, to fulfil the natural law regulating the times of sleep, to escape from the artificial light, and to obtain the advantage of all the sunlight that can be secured, the consumptive patient should make the sun his fellow workman." But is not this going a little too far? Must the consumptive patient remain eighteen hours in bed in the shortest days of the year, and keep out of bed for the same period in the longest days? and ought the valetudinarian Laplander to remain in bed during his long winter, and to keep up throughout the entire summer? Surely not; and yet, upon this principle, he ought to have no alternative.

RULE 6.—*The occupation of the consumptive patient should be suspended if it is indoor or sedentary; but a certain amount of outdoor occupation may be advantageous.*

Among other remarks which naturally arise when speaking upon a rule such as this, is one which deserves considerable attention. It is this: "In the case of parents having children of a consumptive tendency, therefore, the greatest care should be taken to obtain for them outdoor employment. But here a serious delusion comes into play. If the child is weakly, the fond parent urges, that it is unfit for hard labor and for outdoor vicissitudes; so it is sent to a tailor or shoemaker, to a clerk's office, a draper's shop, or to some occupation of an indoor character; by this grand, ignorant, and fatal mistake, it is added to the list of the two-thirds who swell the tables of consumption cases."

RULE 7.—*Cleanliness of body is a special point in the treatment of consumption.*

RULE 8.—*Marriage of consumptive females for the sake of arresting the course of the disease by pregnancy is morally wrong, and physically mischievous.*

RULE 9.—*The diet of consumptive patients should be ample, and should contain a larger proportion of the respiratory elements of food than is required in health.*

RULE 10.—*The medicinal treatment of consumption should in the main be of the tonic class.*

There is no doubt, as Dr. Richardson says, that the public expect to be cured by pills and plasters, and not by a series of instructions tending to bring men into obedience with the laws of nature, and therefore much credit is due to him for constructing this sanitary decalogue, even though subsequent inquiry may lead him to modify some of its articles.

A practical Treatise on Disorders of the Stomach with Fermentation; the causes and treatment of Indigestion; and on Diet. By JAMES TURNBULL, M.D., Physician to the Liverpool Royal Infirmary, &c. (8vo. London, Churchill, pp. 160: 1856.)

Dr. Turnbull holds that diseases of the stomach, arising from fermentive actions, form a much larger and more important class than is generally believed, and that, in fact, fermentive actions have more or less connection with almost all the disorders, as well as the organic diseases, which occur in the digestive canal; and his object in the present volume is to establish this idea.

This object is carried out in six chapters. In the first chapter, the author considers natural digestion, and endeavors to point out how far we have reason to believe that fermentive actions are concerned in the healthy process.

In the second chapter, he examines the chemistry of eight of the different kinds of fermentation—namely, the saccharine, the vinous, the viscous or mucous, the lactic, the butyric acid, the acetous, the benzoic and caseous, and the fatty; and after this, he states the results of his researches as to the effects of certain chemical agents in arresting fermentive actions. These results are at once interesting and important. "A boiling temperature," the author proceeds, "put a complete stop to every kind of fermentive action. The ferments, being all of a nature more or less nearly allied to albumen, are coagulated at a boiling temperature; and it is believed that the change thus produced on the ferments is the cause of the complete stoppage of the fermentive action, which is not renewed so long as the atmosphere is excluded. On this principle it is that meat may be preserved from putrefaction for years, by being sealed up at a boiling temperature, so as to exclude the air perfectly. On the other hand, it has been thought by some scientific observers, and not without some apparent foundation, that boiling arrests fermentation by destroying the germs of microscopic plants and animals. To this point, however, we shall have occasion to revert. Dryness and a freezing temperature are other agencies which oppose fermentive actions.

"There are many chemical substances which have the power of checking or completely arresting fermentive actions; and as a considerable number of them are much in use as medicines, it must be obvious that it is a matter of some importance that medical men should be aware of their power of checking those actions which, we have seen, perform a part both in healthy digestion, and in producing abnormal digestion or dyspepsia. It is, however, to be regretted that this subject has not yet received the close examination from scientific and practical chemists which it merits, and that so little is yet accurately known of how most chemical agents affect the various fermentive actions. In dealing with this subject, I shall first state what is at present known in reference to it, and afterwards advert to a few facts which I have ascertained from my own researches.

"Sulphurous acid and its salts the sulphites have been regarded as amongst the most powerful agents in stopping vinous and other fermentive actions, and they are also powerfully antiseptic. The vapor of burning sulphur is not only a disinfecting agent, but it is also diffused through casks to prevent acid fermentation in cider and other kinds of fermented liquors; and it has been supposed that it acts by combining with oxygen and abstracting it from the ferment. The bisulphite of lime is a soluble salt which is a very important chemical agent in the manufacture of sugar from beet root, being used to prevent fermentation, and the formation of acid, in the sweet liquor obtained from this root. Sulphuric acid, and also the other mineral acids, have considerable power in opposing fermentation. Alcohol and wood spirit arrest fermentation and destroy the active power of yeast; the former, it has been said, acts by abstracting water from the ferment.

"We have already seen that the alkalies act chemically on some ferments, dissolving yeast; and they, as well as nitre and common salt, have antifermentive powers. Many metallic salts coagulate albumen, and most of them check fermentation, more especially the salts of mercury and copper. Tannin and alum, by coagulating the ferment of mucous fermentation, arrest this kind. Chlorine and chromate of potash oppose fermentation; and it has been stated that arsenious acid and corrosive sublimate kill fungi and infusoria, but that nux vomica destroys the latter only. The oil of turpentine, and the essential oils generally, oppose fermentation; but those more particularly which contain sulphur have decided antifermentive properties, as, for instance, the essential oils of mustard and horseradish. Creosote coagulates albumen, and is a powerful antifermentive and antiseptic agent. Pyroligneous acid, and most empyreumatic substances, seem also to have the same properties; and hence wood which has been charred is in a great measure preserved from decay. The antiseptic properties of charcoal are also well known; and in the quick vinegar-making process, by which the alcoholic vapor is oxygenated by being made to trickle through shavings of wood and twigs, any charring of these prevents the formation of the acid. The antiseptic agents which act most powerfully in preserving wood from decay, are corrosive sublimate and the sulphate and the chloride of copper.

"With the view of testing the action of some of these antifermentive chemical substances, I have made a few experiments on the effects of these and some others, used medicinally, on the vinous and on the lactic fermentations. On the vinous I have tried the effect of the following agents, viz., sulphurous acid, sulphite of soda, prussic acid, sulpho-cyanide of potassium, sulphuric, hydrochloric, and arsenious acids, common salt, chloride of lime, solution of chlorinated soda, carbonate of soda, lime-water, alum, bichloride of mercury, chloride of zinc, sulphate of copper, sulphate of iron, nitrate of silver, trisnitrate of bismuth, chromate of potass, tannin, gallic acid, mustard, horseradish, garlic, assafœtida, oil of turpentine, opium, strychnine, alcohol, wood spirst, creosote, and charcoal. Some of these agents completely put a stop to all fermentive action; others appeared to check it in a slight degree; and one or two seemed to increase it, more particularly alum. This salt also rendered the barm of lighter color; and hence its use by bakers to make the bread more spongy and of lighter color, in doing which I doubt if it has the deleterious effects so generally attributed to it, as alum is not itself deleterious, and bakers' bread is usually the lightest and most easily digested.

"The substances which arrested the fermentive action in the most decided manner were, the bichloride of mercury, nitrate of silver, sulphate of copper, chromate of potass, carbonate of soda, mustard, horseradish, wood spirit, prussic acid, and creosote. These seemed to have the power of entirely destroying all fermentive action. Turpentine, assafœtida, and chloride of lime, weakened it very much, but without so completely destroying it. Sulphurous acid and the sulphite of soda appeared to be less powerful antifermentive agents than those just mentioned; and the sulphuric and hydrochloric acids rendered the fermenting fluid clearer, without decidedly lessening the fermentive action, except when added in sufficient quantity to render the fluid decidedly acid to the taste. Tannin caused the precipitation of the ferment, and the absence of any head, but without arresting the fermentation; and gallic acid, on the other hand, caused an abundant dark-colored head. No very decided effect seemed to be produced by arsenious acid, chloride of lime, sulphate of iron, charcoal, strychnine, or opium. Garlic, the strong smell of which is due to an oil containing sulphur, did not weaken the fermentive action, as has been generally supposed, but, on the contrary, seemed rather to increase it.

"The effects of chemical agents on the lactic fermentation are not so readily judged of as those which are produced on the vinous. With the view, however, of testing the effects of some of the same agents on this kind of fermentation, I placed a saccharine solution, containing decomposing cheese, at a suitable temperature, with the following chemical substances, in separate vessels, viz., with bichloride of mercury, sulphite of copper, mustard, creosote, wood spirit, sulphate of soda, sulpho-cyanide of potassium, sulphate of iron, common salt, alum, tannin, arsenious acid, and charcoal powder. As the lactic fermentation advanced, the fluid lost the disagreeable odor of decomposing cheese; but that in the vessels containing the bichloride of mercury and sulphate of copper retained the original odor, without the development of the slightest acid reaction, showing that these agents arrest the lactic fermentation as completely as the vinous.   There was scarcely any appearance of change or formation of acid in those vessels containing mustard and creosote, and the development of acid was feeble in those with sulphite of soda and sulphate of iron, which appeared to have more power in checking lactic than vinous fermentation.   None of the other agents, except the wood spirit, seemed to have any power in checking this species of fermentive action.

"We would notice the fact proved by these experiments, that whilst three of the most powerful agents in arresting both of these two kinds of fermentive actions, viz., bichloride of mercury, sulphate of copper, and creosote, are likewise most powerfully antiseptic, there are others, equally powerful in arresting putrefaction, which exert no well-marked influence in preventing these fermentive actions.   Arsenious acid, for example, stops the putrefaction of animal substances, but has no marked influence on either kind of fermentation; and we have seen that the chloride of zinc, which is used as a disinfecting agent, has no very decided effect in checking vinous fermentation."

The third chapter is devoted to an examination of that peculiar form of disorder of the stomach in which there is vomiting of fermenting matter, containing the remarkable microscopic plant called the *sarcina ventriculi*.

In the fourth chapter, the dyspeptic disorders arising from other fermentative actions are examined, and also the conditions of the stomach and its mucous membrane which tend to induce these morbid actions, and such disorders as acidity, heartburn, pain in the stomach, and vomiting.   The fermentative actions which are actually known to take place in the stomach are pointed out as very numerous. "There can be no doubt whatever that the *vinous* fermentation occurs in the stomach, this being clearly proved by the fact that alcohol has been distilled from the matter rejected from the stomach in three cases of vomiting of sarcinæ; and as we have seen that the yeast plant has been found in fully one-third of these cases, it is probable that the vinous precedes or accompanies the acid fermentation with sarcinæ in a large number of such cases.   We know, too, that new or imperfectly fermented liquors cause much flatulent distension and uneasiness at the stomach in persons of weak digestive power, and this is owing to the heat of the stomach re-exciting the fermentive action, and causing an evolution of carbonic acid.   Dr. Beaumont had an opportunity of observing fermentation, probably of this nature, in the stomach of St. Martin after he had been in the woods all day, and had eaten nothing but whortleberries from seven in the morning to eight in the evening.   On looking into the stomach it was found full of berries and chymifying aliment, frothing and foaming like fermenting beer or cider.

"We know that several kinds of *acid* fermentation occur in the stomach, acidity after meals, especially when certain kinds of food have been taken, being one of the most common symptoms of indigestion.   *Lactic acid*, generated by fermentation of the sugar or starch contained in the food, is the most common cause of the acidity, and this kind of fermentation gives rise to less disturbance than any other, one atom of sugar being transformed into two atoms of lactic acid without the evolution of any gas.   This acid is also one of those which with pepsin produces an energetic digestive fluid, and it is so commonly present in the gastric juice, that it may in moderate quantity be considered a normal constituent.   In excess, however, we have seen that any acid weakens or stops digestion, and it is so with the lactic, whether it be, as some have supposed, a secretion from the stomach, or a product of unnatural fermentive action.   This disorder, it has been observed by Dr. Budd, is most common in nervous persons with feeble digestion, in whom it not unfrequently happens that acid collects in great quantity in the stomach after meals.   They often familiarly tell us, that almost everything they take turns to an acid.   If vomiting occur an hour or two after meals, the matter thrown up is very acid, and, on analysis, the acidity has been often found to be mainly due to lactic acid.   In the case of sarcinic fermentation observed by Professor Goodsir, a considerable quantity of lactic acid was found on analysis by Dr. George Wilson, but the chief acid in that case was the acetic.

"There is another kind of acid fermentation which often goes on along with the lactic, viz., the *butyric*, and this, being an acrid, oily acid, causes the heat and burning sensation at the stomach and in the throat, to which the name of heartburn has been given. We have already noticed the fact, that the same conditions which cause lactic fermentation will, at a higher temperature, cause the production of butyric acid. This acid has been several times found in the contents of the stomach, and its occurrence in Dr. Hassall's case of sarcinic vomiting has been already noticed.

"It has been observed that decayed cheese is the ferment which most readily causes this kind of fermentation ; and as we know that lactate of lime in contact with it yields butyric acid and tartrate of lime, and that tartrate of lime in the same circumstances yields metacetonate and acetate of lime, and as we likewise know that the pungency which some kinds of cheese acquire during maturation is due to the formation of butyric acid, and two similar volatile oily acids, the capric and caproic, we have some ground for believing that these acids, which are generated out of the body in the same circumstances, may also be formed in the stomach. The skin is the excreting organ by which butyric and other oily acids are thrown out of the system, and it is probable that the formation in the stomach and digestive organs of some of these acrid, oily matters from abnormal fermentation, is the cause of the boils and other eruptions of the skin which are so well known to derive their origin from unobserved disorders of the stomach and bowels. During butyric fermentation there is an evolution of carbonic acid and hydrogen gases, which is the cause of the flatulent distension of the stomach and bowels so generally experienced by those who suffer from heartburn.

"*Acetous* fermentation is another kind which seems to occur in the stomach, and it has been already remarked, that in Goodsir's case the acetic was the most abundant acid. In the third case of vomiting of sarcina, which I have before related, the vomited matter was distilled for me by Mr. Abraham, and two drachms and a half of fluid, obtained by the distillation of four ounces, had a vinous odor and a specific gravity of ·998, indicating nearly 2 per cent. of alcohol. It was also acid ; and as the usual tests did not indicate the presence of hydrochloric acid, we may conclude that the acidity must have been due to the presence of this volatile acid, and that in the case referred to the acetous must have accompanied the vinous fermentation.

"We may thus regard it as a matter proved beyond any doubt, that all these kinds of fermentation do occur in the stomach singly, successively, or in combination. Lehmann also states, that Frericks convinced himself that the colorless, viscid, ropy masses which are sometimes ejected in abundant quantity in gastric catarrh, possess almost entirely the same properties as the gum-like substances produced by what is called mucous fermentation. He also observes, that it appears to depend, at least in part, on the nature of the mucous secretion in gastric catarrh, whether the fermentation established in the amylacea be of the mucous, lactic, acetic, or butyric variety.

"The *saccharine* fermentation, we have seen, occurs during healthy digestion, under the influence of a ferment contained in the salivary and pancreatic fluids : but diabetes is a disease in which the stomach and other digestive organs acquire a morbid power of converting every sort of amylaceous matter, and even other kinds of aliment, into sugar. In the healthy condition, there is no sugar found in the urine ; and scarcely a trace of it in the blood, for as soon as it is absorbed into the circulation, it is, under the influence of the alkali and fibrin of the blood, rapidly oxidized, being transformed, by the oxygen absorbed at the lungs, into lactic acid, and then into carbonic acid and water. In diabetes, there is not merely the increased production of sugar, but there seems also to be a failure in the power to oxidize the sugar which is removed by the kidneys, and there is therefore a loss of an important kind of aliment required by the system, and hence the wasting and loss of flesh which sooner or later result from this disease. As there is not only the loss of power to assimilate the sugar, but also a remarkable tendency to the conversion of the food into sugar, it is obvious that there must be two great indications in the treatment of this disease, viz., to prevent the morbid tendency to the formation of sugar, and to promote the oxidation and assimilation of what is formed. The treatment of diabetes is too extensive a subject for us to enter upon fully here, and I would therefore only now observe, that, in carrying out the first indication, the attention of medical men has been chiefly directed to the use of those kinds of food which are least prone to undergo the saccharine change ; but, in examining the long list of remedies which have been found of use in this intractable disease, we find that many of them (and, amongst others that might be named, creosote) have antifermentive properties, and it is probable that, if the attention of medical men were more systematically directed to this object, and to the employment of antifermentive agents, our treatment of the disease would be improved and advanced. Astringents, both vegetable and mineral, have been found of use in the treatment of diabetes, and they, as well as opium, act probably by diminishing the mucous or albuminous ferment. The sulphite of soda appeared to be of service in one case in which I prescribed it, but it has failed in other cases, both in my practice and that of other medical men.

"The food also sometimes undergoes the *putrefactive* change in the stomach, causing eructation of offensive-smelling gas, which is sulphuretted hydrogen. This disorder is most apt to occur in children who have eaten largely of varieties of food." In this chapter, also, Dr. Turnbull shows, that similar fermentive action may take place in the bowels.

In the fifth chapter the treatment of dyspeptic disorders is considered, and the action of various remedies investigated—the main object being to show, that amongst the remedies which have been discovered to be most useful in relieving pain at the stomach, and stopping sickness and vomiting, are found several of those chemical agents which have most energetic antifermentative properties. "This observation holds true," says Dr. Turnbull, "in respect to creosote, which is one of the most powerful remedies in relieving pain at the stomach, and arresting sickness and vomiting ; and also in respect to pyroxilic spirit, another energetic antifermentative agent, which, we have seen,,stops sickness and vomiting, especially in phthisical cases. I have found that prussic acid, which is one of the remedies most commonly used to allay pain and irritability of the stomach, and vomiting, is a powerful agent in checking vinous fermentation. Nitrate of silver is another antifermentative agent which relieves dyspeptic pain and vomiting. It is well known that lime-water, and the alkalies which have considerable antifermentative power, allay irritability of the stomach and vomiting in many cases ; and the sulphite of soda, we have seen, to be the antifermentative agent which is most effective in stopping the acid vomiting of sarcina. Of the metallic antifermentative agents, the salts of mercury seem to be the most energetic ; and it is worthy of particular notice, that calomel is given to allay sickness, &c., in a variety of disordered states of the stomach and bowels. We give it in small doses, combined with opium, to stop the vomiting which so often accompanies the diarrhœa, or cholera of autumn ; and, on the other hand, where there is vomiting, with obstinate constipation, we give a large dose of calomel, with a pretty full dose of opium, and find, as in the case alluded to (at page 95), that there is no remedy or combination more generally effectual in settling the stomach, in frequently moving the bowels, and in enabling the stomach afterwards to retain other medicines.

"As so many of the most energetic antifermentative agents, organic as well as metallic, possess these powers, we are naturally led to conclude from these facts, that there is a connection between antifermentative power and the power of relieving pain at the stomach, and sickness, and vomiting ; and we may also regard it as not improbable, that any medicinal agent devoid of irritating properties, which is proved to have energetic antifermentative properties, will also be found to have more or less power in reference to the symptoms noticed."

The last chapter is devoted to the examination of diet in relation to the tendency of various articles of food and drink to promote or prevent fermentative actions, and to showing, that many condiments owe what value they possess to their antifermentative properties.

Such are the contents of a work which reflects great credit upon its author, and which must have the effect of leading the practitioner of medicine to view disorders of the stomach in a light in which they have been but little examined ; and also of proving, in some measure, that chemical facts admit of more extended practical application in the advancement of medical knowledge.

Recherches expérimentales sur la physiologie et la pathologie des Capsules Surrénales.
Par Dr. E. BROWN-SEQUARD. ("Archives Génerales de Med.," Oct. and Nov.,
1856.)
On Disease of the Supra-renal Capsules. By W. II. RANKING, M.D. ("ASSOC.
Med. Journal," Aug. 9th, 1856.)
Cases of Disease of the Supra renal Capsules. By Dr. ROOTES, Dr. ROBERTSON,
M. SECOND-FERREOL, M. TROUSSEAU, Dr. GIBBON, Dr. MONRO, and Dr. CHRISTIE.
("Medical Times and Gazette," June 7th, June 28th, Sept. 20th, and Oct. 4th,
1856. "Assoc. Med. Journal," Aug. 2d and Oct. 4th, 1856. "Gaz. Med. de
Paris," Aug. 30th and Sept. 6th, 1856.)

During the past half-year, several unequivocal cases of disease of the supra-renal
capsules (or "Addison's disease," as it has been called upon the Continent), have
been placed on record, and the bald clinical history of the disease has received much
light from the physiological investigations of M. Brown-Sequard. These investigations, indeed, are of extreme importance, for they show, very conclusively, that the
supra-renal capsules have a very important part to play in the animal economy—a
part which, if omitted, must lead to fatal results ; and thus they supply the evidence
which was wanting to complete the argument in Dr. Addison's monograph.

In this article, then, we propose to give the substance of M. Brown-Sequard's investigations, and to relate the cases which have occurred since our last report
("Abstract," XXIII), merely adding that the first case in our present list is the
case to which reference was made in this last report, as one in which the disease
under consideration would, in all probability, be found to exist after death.

The substance of M. Brown-Sequard's investigations may be stated in a few words.
Thus :

The supra-renal capsules are very sensitive.

As age advances, the supra-renal capsules are found to gain considerably, both
in weight and volume, and hence it appears that these organs are not exclusively
related, as is generally supposed, to embryonic life. This increase in weight and
volume, as age advances, was noticed in man and in all the mammifers examined.

The extirpation of both capsules destroys life with as much certainty, and with
greater rapidity, than the extirpation of the kidneys ; the mean duration of life in
more than sixty animals thus mutilated—rabbits, dogs, and cats, guinea-pigs, and
mice—being not more than eleven hours and a half.

The extirpation of a single organ even was invariably fatal, and in this case the
mean duration of life was not more than seventeen hours.

In all these experiments, it was fully proved, by experiments on other animals in
which hemorrhage or peritonitis was caused, or in which the kidney or liver was
injured, that the fatal results were not due to any of these causes.

After removing both capsules, the following phenomena were noticed :—feebleness, gradually passing into extreme prostration ; a respiration, first quickened,
then retarded, and lastly irregular and spasmodic ; a quick and weakened pulse ; a
gradual diminution of animal heat ; and lastly, vertigo, convulsions in various forms,
and occasionally coma.

When a single capsule was removed, all these phenomena became manifested,
after a short interval in which the animal seemed to rally from the operation. In
this case, the convulsions were generally more violent on the side operated upon,
and occasionally the animal performed the waltzing movement which is seen after
injury to the crus cerebri, the movement being towards the injured side.

The blood of rabbits about to die, in consequence of the removal of both supra-
renal capsules, proved almost immediately fatal when injected into the vessels of
another rabbit from which a single capsule had been removed a few hours previously ; whereas blood taken from a healthy rabbit would restore life for several hours
to a rabbit from which both capsules had been removed, even if the injection were
deferred until the animal was actually moribund.

It appears, also, from some former experiments of M. Brown-Sequard, that wounds
of certain parts of the spinal cord were followed by congestion with hypertrophy, or
else with rapidly fatal inflammation of the supra-renal capsules.

And, lastly, it is stated, that in Paris the rabbits have been decimated by an epi-
zootic malady in which the supra-renal capsules were found to be inflamed, and of

which the symptoms were in some measure similar to those produced by extirpation of these organs.

Instead of being organs of no importance in the economy, it would thus appear that the supra-renal capsules are essential to life, and that their removal or disorganization may lead, partly, to some injurious alteration in the blood, and, partly, to some injurious operation upon the nervous system—an operation which is illustrated in the fact, that the convulsive movements were chiefly confined to one side when a single capsule was operated upon. At any rate, it is evident from these investigations, that a serious disease may arise when the supra-renal capsules fail to discharge their appointed duty.

The cases we have to record are eight in number, and we relate them in the order in which they have occurred, without any comment, merely referring to our last volume for further information respecting the disease.

1. *Dr. Ranking's case.*—"The subject was a lady aged 58 years, of remarkably tall and robust frame, and of great obesity previously to the commencement of her fatal illness. Her habits of life were peculiar, especially in her partiality for fatty matters, and her abstinence from farinaceous diet. She was also a considerable consumer of porter and wine. When she first consulted me, in August, 1855, I was struck with the diminution of her bulk, and her great general prostration. Her chief complaint was of debility. Her appetite was bad, and she suffered from constant nausea and sinking at the pit of the stomach. She also incidentally called my attention to her color, being particularly dissatisfied with the appearance of her hands, which resembled those of a creole. I confess that, on this occasion, I paid no attention to this apparently unimportant symptom, being interested only in the endeavor to discover a cause for the emaciation and exhaustion. I examined the heart, the lungs, and, on a subsequent occasion, the urine, without finding any such disease as could explain the nature of the case. The heart's action was feeble, and its sounds sharp; and the only conclusion I could come to at the time was, that I had a case of general decadence of the digestive powers from over-stimulation, together with fatty degeneration of the heart. The latter suspicion was borne out by the results of the *post-mortem* examination.

"She paid me several visits, but made no satisfactory progress; and the discoloration of the skin gradually deepened, perplexing me as much as it annoyed the patient. At this time I noticed the first of a series of cases publishing in the 'Medical Times,' and I at once saw a clue to the enigma. I published the case at the time, and at once informed the friends of the peculiarity of the disease, and my conviction of its ultimate fatality. To be brief, the progress was, with some fluctuations, daily for the worse; and, in the month of March, there were the additional symptoms of pains in the joints, neck, and limbs, which continued to the time of her death. In the latter two months of her life, she emaciated rapidly; and in the final days, she had alternations of delirium and coma, the kidneys and bowels, however, acting naturally to the very last.

"The *post-mortem* examination exhibited the following appearances. The body was emaciated. The integuments, especially the face and hands, were of a deep bronzy color. The eyes were sunken; the conjunctiva pearly white. The subcutaneous fat, as well as that in the omentum and other internal parts, was firm, and of a deep chrome yellow. The head was not examined. The thoracic organs were healthy, with the exception of the heart, which was dilated, and in a state of fatty degeneration. The liver was softened, but otherwise healthy. The stomach was dilated, and its coats atrophied and destitute of rugæ. The spleen was of natural size and consistence. The intestines were healthy. The kidneys were congested and flabby. The supra-renal capsules were both enlarged, nodulated externally, and, when divided, were seen to be filled with tubercular deposit of various consistency, some portions being almost cartilaginous, others of the fluidity of scrofulous pus."

2. *M. Malherbe's case.*—A woman, named Ouvrard, æt. 48, was admitted into the Hôtel Dieu, at Nantes, on February 23d, 1856. She stated that she had been ill a year, and that she was very weak; but there were no symptoms of organic disease, excepting an enlargement of the cervical glands on the right side. She complained of wandering pains in the limbs and abdomen. There had been some loss of flesh, but the emaciation was not extreme. Her skin generally was noticed to be of a

remarkably earthy hue, but there was, nevertheless, an approach to the yellow pallor of some states of chlorosis, or of the last stage of organic disease. M. Malherbe was inclined to attribute the change in color to general anæmia, and accordingly prescribed a treatment by steel and nutritious diet. A few days after, the occurrence of a severe diarrhœa compelled the suspension of the medicine.

Shortly after her admission, the state of debility, which had previously been very well marked, increased greatly. The pulse, which was slow, became extremely feeble, and the stomach was so irritable, that all articles of food were rejected almost as soon as taken. M. Malherbe states, that it was at this juncture that he, for the first time, became acquainted, through the medium of M. Lasegue's translation in the "Archives Generales," with Dr. Addison's observations. On reading the description of the change in color of the skin which that physician had observed in association with a peculiar cachexia, he was at once forcibly reminded of his own patient.

On the 12th of March the woman died. By inquiring from her friends, it was now ascertained that her illness had commenced about eighteen months before, and had followed a severe mental emotion, since which she had grown languid and feeble, and her skin, previously very white, had acquired a gradually deepening shade of brown.

Autopsy.—The emaciation was not very marked. The smoked (*enfumée*) hue of the skin was rather less deep than it had been during life. It was deeper in the groins and axillæ than in other parts, but is perceptible everywhere. The lymphatic glands in all parts, were almost wholly transformed into masses of tubercle, but they did not form any noticeable swelling excepting in the right cervical and submaxillary region. Some of them were softening, others merely indurated. No tubercle existed in the lungs or any other of the viscera, excepting, as will be mentioned, in one kidney and the supra-renal capsules. The right kidney was somewhat increased in size and slightly congested. The left kidney was contracted and puckered, of scarcely half its natural size, and a grayish color. Its substance was crammed with encysted masses of tuberculous deposit of variable size. Some of them were of cheesy consistence, others hard, and a few had suppurated.

Supra-renal capsules.—The left preserved its natural shape, but was greatly increased in thickness. In its substance were two large masses of tubercle, not, as yet, commencing to soften. The right organ was completely altered in shape, having assumed that of a cylinder, somewhat tapered at its extremities, and placed transversely over the upper end of the kidney. It was throughout of lardaceous consistence, resembling crude tubercle, and presented also a great number of encysted deposits of tubercle, in a cheesy state, varying in size from that of a millet-seed to that of a pea.

3. *Dr. W. Symonds Rootes's case.*—"Mr. J. E——, æt. 54, by profession a solicitor, consulted me in February, 1852. He was a man of rather below middle height; of dark complexion; nearly black hair; stout, and inclined to corpulence; lame from early life from diseased hip-joint; of temperate habits, and of active life latterly, though in early life he had been kept close to the desk, and had worked hard as a clerk. Considered that he had always enjoyed good health; but said that for many years he had suffered from habitual looseness of the bowels, to the extent of three or four evacuations regularly every morning, and frequently as many during the rest of the day, and had occasionally had hemorrhoids slightly. He had also experienced some slight attacks of gout.

"Notwithstanding this habitual diarrhœa, he had got stout, and considered himself in very good health, till September 5th, 1851, when he was thrown out of his carriage, and sustained a severe scalp-wound, with concussion of the brain, with erysipelas following on the wound, and a paroxysm of gout succeeding to the latter.

"On coming under my observation he complained of feeling himself generally ill, but stated that he had no pain anywhere. He was still rather corpulent, but not nearly as much so as he had been. He had no headache; his mental powers were unimpaired; his memory (singularly retentive always) unaffected, his special senses perfect; he had no cough, no difficulty of breathing, no palpitation, no uneasiness of back. He had a very fair appetite, and enjoyed his food, but his diarrhœa still continued, and was very troublesome; and as soon as ever it became arrested by any means, so surely vomiting came on. He had also attacks of apparently causeless vomiting, of most uncertain occurrence, most frequently immediately after taking food, and even sometimes during a meal. There was one singular peculiarity in his aspect,—his skin was universally of a dirty chalky yellow hue, more marked on the exposed surfaces: in the face, of a deep yellowish-brown ; in the hands, of a tint resembling the stains of walnut juice, the conjunctivæ retaining their natural white color. The alteration of his outward appearance was, as I said, most marked and peculiar; it worried him, and he repeatedly asked me what it meant, and was constantly drawing my attention to it. He complained of general uneasiness, and of a sense of weariness and languor, and of muscular debility ; and complained more than would be expected from one still looking stout and robust. He laid great stress on the absence of pain ; appeared extremely solicitous to know what ailed him ; expressed much apprehension about himself, and manifested considerable dread of death, feebly attempting, at the same time, to make light of his condition. I submitted him to repeated and most careful physical examinations. I frequently inspected the evacuations from the bowels ; they were abundantly tinged with bile. I over and over again tested the urine (by heat and nitric acid)—it contained no albumen—there were no deposits, and with every care that I could bestow upon the case, could not find any evidence of disease in any organ. I was fairly puzzled to account for the symptoms. There was decidedly some serious derangement of the nutritive functions; but to the questions, Whence came it ? and Whither did it tend ? I could give no satisfactory answer. It was indeed well and pithily observed by his regular attendant, Mr. Thomson, of this town, ' throw a veil over his face, and pronounce him quite sound.'

" Meanwhile, week after week, and month after month rolled on, not only without any amendment, but with evident gradual aggravation of all his symptoms. The skin became still more changed in hue, till the casual passenger in the street would turn to gaze at him as he drove by ; he became thinner, but never emaciated, and his muscular power became more and more enfeebled. He took a variety of tonic and astringent medicines with no evident good result, although he thought himself better for a certain time, during which he took cod-liver oil, quinine, and opium simultaneously. At last, in August, he began to have slight transitory attacks of loss of consciousness, with convulsive disorder of the muscles of the face and left side of the body ; these were of irregular occurrence, but continued occasionally till the end of the month. In the night of the 30th he became violently delirious, and was very vociferous. This excitement passed rapidly into coma, and he died apoplectic on the morning of the 1st of September.

" I made an examination of the body after death, but permission was not given to examine the head. The discoloration of the skin was as evident in death as it had been during life ; there was even yet an abundant deposit of deep yellow-colored fat beneath the skin and in the omentum ; and the muscles were of a peculiar deep red color ; indeed the fat and flesh more resembled the flesh and fat of an Alderney cow, than that of a human being.

" I made a careful and strict search into the condition of all the organs of the thoracic and abdominal cavities, and I could find no trace of morbid change in any one of them, save the spleen and supra-renal capsules ; every other organ, so far as the scalpel can detect morbid conditions, was perfectly healthy ; and I say this the more positively, because I have, throughout the whole of my professional life, enjoyed great opportunities of studying morbid anatomy, and have made personally several hundred dissections. The spleen and supra-renal capsules were much changed ; the spleen was much enlarged, and so soft as to break down under very slight pressure ; and its interior resembled a mass of crushed mulberries. The supra-renal capsules were considerably enlarged, of firm consistence, and on division presented an appearance closely resembling a tuberculated gland."

4. *Dr. Tyndal Robertson's case.*—John Sumner, æt. 26, laborer, admitted into the Nottingham General Hospital, April 12th, 1856. A tall, good-looking, spare man, dark-haired ; temperate in his habits, and intelligent. Situation of abode healthy ; parentage healthy. Has never before had any serious illness.

Present illness commenced twenty-two months since, while he was at work, with pain in the legs, sickness, and vomiting. He was thus ill for a fortnight, and then returned to work. In a month the sickness returned, unaccompanied by the pain in the legs, and it continued at intervals until fifteen months since, when he began to suffer from pain in the right hypochondrium, of a pricking, darting character. This, with occasional remissions, has continued to the present time. About a year ago he began to change color, and, to use his own words, "has been jaundiced" since that time.

Present state.—The face, arms, hands, and chest are stained dark brown; the face and hands most notably, the arms and chest less distinctly so. The conjunctivæ are pearly, and very slightly tinged. The expression is pinched and anxious. Decubitus generally dorsal. Chest is equally resonant. Respiratory and heart's sounds perfectly normal. The heart's impulse is very feeble. The abdomen flat and retracted, not tender either on superficial or deep percussion. There is dulness on percussion on the right hypochondrium, extending two inches below the cartilages, and into the epigastrium. There is no notable flatulence. Tongue furred. Bowels confined. Stools whitish in color. Urine pale, copious, slightly acid, sp. gr. 1020; deposits no sediment, and contains nothing abnormal. Pulse 80, small, feeble. Appetite very bad. He was ordered 5 minims of nitro-muriatic acid, with inf. gent. co., three times a day; 2 grs. of blue pill, with 5 grs. of extract of dandelion, every night; and half a drachm of sulphate of magnesia in broth every morning.

April 20th.—He was not quite so well, from great sickness and inability to vomit. An ipecacuanha emetic was ordered, which relieved him very much; and this was repeated with the same effect.

May 2d.—Has had rather more pain in the side, and vomits generally every night and after taking food. To have a digestive pill before dinner, and an injection every other morning. To omit all other medicines, and take small quantities of nourishing food at frequent intervals.

9th.—Feels better, with the exception of great weakness. Has now no pain or vomiting. To have 2 grains of quinine, with inf. gentiana, three times a day, and half pint of beer daily.

12th.—Feels sick after the medicine. To take only half-doses.

15th.—Very feeble, and unable to take food. The bronzed character of the surface still continues. The epigastric swelling is softer, and the abdomen much retracted. There is distinct aortic pulsation visible to the left of the umbilicus. No murmur is heard on the light application of the stethoscope, but pressure elicits a strong blowing sound. There is dulness from the lower margin of the right ribs to a level with the umbilicus; percussion-note is resonant from the lower end of the sternum to the level of the ribs on the left side. Respiration very feeble. Heart's sounds indistinctly heard. Pulse 80. Tongue furred in centre, and dry. To have a mixture with ammonia and tincture of cardamoms; wine, ℥iv.

16th.—Was slightly delirious when he awoke this morning. He has had no pain, but frequent vomiting. Abdomen is extremely retracted; soft, except above the umbilicus. There is here an uneven hardness, elongated, and not movable. Bowels not open for two days. Tongue dry and tremulous. Pulse 84, extremely feeble; pupils contracted; great tremor of facial muscles. To continue the wine, and ammonia mixture, ℥ij. Gin with water, to relieve thirst.

17th.—At five A.M. he drank some gin-and-water, and said he felt better, but in about an hour he began to sink rapidly, and died about six o'clock.

Autopsy forty-eight hours after death.—Body emaciated. Abdominal walls greatly retracted. All the organs, carefully examined, gave little trace of disease. The lungs were healthy, with the exception of two or three small chalky deposits in the apex of the left one. The heart was rather small, and firmly contracted. Softish friable clots occupied both the left auricle and ventricle, the right ventricle, and extended into the pulmonary artery. The liver was marked with a few white spots on its convex surface. Gall-bladder distended partially. The stomach and small intestines nearly empty. The spleen apparently healthy. The transverse colon contained some lumpy fæcal matter; the rest of it, and the rectum, free. The brain was not examined, in consequence of the body being unexpectedly removed. The kidneys were apparently healthy. The supra-renal capsules were much enlarged. The left was cut across, and found to consist of a soft, cheesy mass, enveloped in a harder and rather more yellow-colored exterior. This could not be broken down with the finger, and, when sliced, was smooth, and somewhat glistening. The soft part was readily broken up, and a small stream of water at once detached it from the nidus in which it was placed. Under the microscope, it seemed to be composed of irregular cells, oil granules, and smaller portions of amorphous matter. Some of the cells contained one, some two or three nuclei. Acetic acid applied to a section of the firmer exterior part showed the same kind of cells, with the addition of some scattered fibrillæ. Not a particle of healthy structure was discernible in any part of the organs.

The right capsule, which seemed softer and further advanced in disintegration, was sent to the Pathological Society of London, through Dr. Quain, who has since furnished the following Report:

"The capsule, retaining much of its original form, was about the size of half a large hen-egg. On making a vertical section through the mass, it was seen to be composed of a thin capsule, containing a solid and semifluid mass of a yellow color. The solid substance, which was chiefly towards the surface, had the consistence of Gruyère cheese, and somewhat its appearance. The semifluid portion, which was evidently the result of a softening of the solid portion, had the consistence of thick cream.

"The solid and semifluid substances, under the microscope, presented very similar constituents—the difference being in the proportions of these constituents. The solid consisted of cells—small, abortive-like, and containing two or three small nuclei of broken-up cells, granular particles, and fatty matter. The more fluid portion contained more granules, more fat, and fewer cells. There were some traces of the original capsular structure in the wall of the anterior portion of the tumor.

"The deposit presented to my mind all the characters of scrofulous matter."

A little of the blood examined after death was rather thicker than usual. The colorless corpuscles were slightly in excess. The cretaceous deposit in the lung consisted of irregular corpuscles, phosphate of lime, and a few crystals of cholesterine.

5. *M. Cazenave's case.*—This case is reported by M. Second-Fereol. It is that of a man, æt. 35, of somewhat intemperate habits. The bronzed discoloration of the skin was noticed first of all in the countenance, and then, after passing off more or less completely on several occasions, it became considerably more marked, and at the same time it extended to the hands. For these symptoms, quinine and "l'eau d'Enghien" were given to him in the Hôpital Necker. In the commencement of 1856, he was admitted into the Hôpital St. Louis, under M. Cazenave, and at this time there were evident signs of pulmonary consumption. About the middle of February, he was discharged somewhat improved. Last of all he returned to die on the 17th of April, after having suffered for three weeks from diarrhœa, accompanied by frequent vomiting.

On examination after death, both supra-renal capsules were found to be evidently changed and voluminous, very hard, knobbed, or quasi-knobbed. Under the microscope, the only alteration was found to consist in the presence of some fat and pus globules.

The discolored portion of the skin, when examined microscopically, presented, as in the case of the negro, a very abundant layer of pigmentary granules under the epidermis; and, *apropos* of this remark, M. Second-Fereol says that the supra-renal capsules are usually more developed in the negro than in the white races. Is this so?

6. *M. Trousseau's case.*—A man, named Lavallee, æt. 30, the coachman of the Minister of the Interior, was admitted into the Salle Sainte-Agnès of the Hôtel Dieu, at Paris, under the care of M. Trousseau, on the 30th of July, 1856. As a child he had been rickety, and his legs exhibited the characteristic deformity of this disease; but he had enjoyed good and even robust health until about five months before his admission into the hospital, when he began to lose flesh. During these five months, according to his own statement, he has lost three-fourths of his former weight. Then his wife noticed a dark discoloration of his hands, which was at first referred to his work, but which was found to become darker the more he attempted to wash it off. Then his face and the rest of his body became affected, until his appearance differed very little from that of a quadroon. At the same time he experienced vague pains in the lumbar region, and every day his strength failed perceptibly.

On admission, the bronzed discoloration of the skin was very marked in several places, especially on the nipple, in the axilla, and on the penis and scrotum. The lips and gums were also discolored. The nails were blanched, as in extreme anæmia, and their whiteness contrasted in a very remarkable manner with the darkness of the hands. Although considerably emaciated, his muscles were not materially affected. The digestion was good, but there was a positive dislike for animal food. The chest was healthy; the pulse regular; the blood (examined by M. Robin) was that of a person slightly anæmic.

The treatment consisted principally of tonics, such as quinine and iròn, with a diet suited to his fancy, and under it he seemed to improve a short time, but only for a short time. On the 13th and 14th of August, there were some pains in the abdomen. On the 15th, there was a rigor of some hours' duration, and after this a copious diarrhœa. All food was refused. On the 16th, the diarrhœa continued, the skin became cool, the features changed, and the pulse small and frequent, the discoloration of the skin appearing more marked than ever. In the afternoon there was delirum. On the 17th, extreme prostration took the place of the agitation of the previous evening. The intelligence became obtuse, and the diarrhœa continued. On the 18th, the patient sank peacefully, and at 11 A.M., he died. M. Trousseau adds that there was nothing of the nature of cholera in the diarrhœa.

After death, the brain, the kidneys, the spleen, and the liver, were found to be in a perfectly healthy condition, and with the exception of a few tubercles in the lungs, the only disease that could be detected was in the supra-renal capsules. These organs were enlarged to the size of a hen's egg, and infiltrated with white kernels, which M. Brown-Sequard has shown to be composed of tubercular matter. Some of these kernels were softened.

7. *Dr. Gibbon's case.*—E. D—, æt. 52 years, a poor man, exposed very much to all weathers, was admitted in February into the London Hospital under the care of Dr. Parker. The man complained of general debility, loss of appetite, some slight cough, with some emaciation ; his skin was yellow but cool and moist ; some crepitus was detected at the posterior part of the chest. Pulse 94, soft, and weak ; bowels costive ; tongue furred. His urine was reported clear ; specific gravity 1·022, acid, and free from albumen. The treatment chiefly consisted of tonics ; he seemed to make very little way, but, on the contrary, to grow weaker and weaker. Dr. Gibbon took charge of the patient a week before his death, when he reported him in a low typhoid state, and, he believed, sinking from phthisis. Yet, after a careful examination, he could not detect the stethoscopic signs of phthisis. The symptoms were those rather of typhoid fever. From the yellowish-brown appearance of the skin, and the general cachectic state of the patient, Dr. Gibbon also diagnosticated disease of the supra-renal capsules. The poor man died apparently from exhaustion ; no treatment seemed of any use.

At the post-mortem examination, the yellowish color of the skin was most peculiar. There was great emaciation ; the lungs were healthy, as were also the heart, liver, spleen, and kidneys ; but on coming to the supra-renal capsules, they appeared both enlarged, and when laid open were seen to consist of simple membranous bags, with shreds of torn-up or disintegrated tissue. In one capsule some traces of healthy cortical structure were found ; but in the other the tissue of the capsule, whatever it is, whether glandular or otherwise, was completely gone.

8. *Dr. William Monro's case.*—Mrs. B—, æt. 40, wife of a clergyman, residing at Newport, Fifeshire, states that, about eight or nine years ago, she first observed a dark colored spot on her forehead, which gradually increased in size ; while other portions of her head, face, and neck, became similarly affected. At this time, her general health was pretty good, although, about fifteen years since, in consequence of having been obliged to leap from the top of a stage-coach, she suffered a good deal from some internal complaints. She understood that the uterus was displaced. She has been married sixteen years, but has had no children. When young, she was healthy, but never robust ; she has of late become very thin and weak. About eight months ago, while attending upon her husband, who was seriously ill, and being exposed to much mental anxiety and great bodily fatigue, the dark color of the skin became much deeper and more general, the whole surface of the body partaking more or less of the dark hue.

June 12th, 1856.—At present the patient is extremely emaciated. Her face in color nearly resembles that of a Lascar, or a native of the East Indies. When she

. sits up, she feels great weakness, sinking, and prostration, increased greatly by an attack, a few days ago, of diarrhœa. She has a dry short cough, with tough expectoration; she has been subject to a cough since childhood, when she had measles. Pulse 100, small, and compressible. Tongue whitish; very little appetite. Her sleep is much disturbed by the cough. The bowels are now regular. She has considerable thirst. The catamenia are regular. She complains of no pain. The chest sounds well on percussion, except for a space below the clavicle on each side, which is dull. The heart's action is normal. The abdomen is clung to the spine, which can be readily felt through the parietes of the abdomen, as can also the pulsation of the abdominal aorta. None of the abdominal viscera can, by a careful examination, be detected to be organically diseased. The urine is natural in quantity, and of a light straw color, specific gravity 1·012, free from albumen, and exhibiting under the microscope no unusual deposit. The uterus is in its normal position, and healthy. The blood examined under the microscope exhibited nothing unusual, no excess of white corpuscles. The color of the skin is particularly dark over both knees and elbow-joints, and also on the back of the neck. The palms of the hands and palmar surface of fingers are very little discolored, and contrast much with the posterior surface. She was recommended to try the use of tincture of muriate of iron, ten drops thrice a day; and, externally, the free use of olive oil to the skin; to pay attention to the bowels, and the state of the secretions; and to take a light nourishing diet.

June 17th.—She is no better. She has not been able to take the iron, but has used the oil. The cough is very troublesome. She was ordered to have a mixture with ipecacuanha and solution of muriate of morphia, and also to take the fluid extract of sarsaparilla. The appetite is bad; the bowels regular. She is evidently weaker.

She continued getting gradually worse until the evening of the 21st, when she died, remaining quite sensible to the last.

For the following interesting and minute post-mortem appearances, I am indebted to my friend Dr. William Aitken, late Assistant Pathological Commissioner to the Army in the East, to whom I beg to express my obligation for his kindness, and the interest he has taken in this case.

Post-mortem examination, June 23d, 1856.—In this case, the body was greatly emaciated. The chest and waist were greatly contracted, so much so that the waist could be embraced in the span of the two hands, the thumbs meeting in front, and the middle fingers behind, the girth being seventeen inches. The color of the skin was a dark bronze hue throughout, and in many places patches of a darker brown color were conspicuous. Such patches were more particularly obvious in the vicinity of the knees, and in the lateral and posterior regions of the neck. At the angles of the mouth, and round the lips, where the mucous membrane meets the skin, isolated deposits of pigment gave a dirty sordes-like appearance to the mouth. The body generally was anæmic. The heart was small and flabby; the lungs were adherent to their apices by old adhesions. A deposit of a tuberculous nature was also disseminated throughout the region of the apices on both sides, but not in any considerable quantity. The rest of the pulmonary substance appeared healthy. In the *abdomen*, the spleen, the liver, and the kidneys, were severally adherent to their surrounding connections; but the parenchyma of these organs appeared natural. The supra-renal capsules and the mucous membrane of the alimentary canal were alone the seat of marked morbid change. The supra-renal capsule on the right side presented a large mass, pressing up chiefly into the substance of the liver, a portion of whose tissue, altered by pressure, could not be separated from the morbid supra-renal body. The organ retained no part of its natural shape. It was enlarged to about four times its natural volume, and its enlargement assumed an irregular tuberculated form; while the shape of the mass was modified in some parts by surrounding structures on which it pressed. The side towards the vena cava had a deep groove in relation with that vein; and the texture of the vein, to the extent of half an inch, was so finely incorporated with the morbid supra-renal body, that the most careful dissection could not separate them. On careful removal from all its relations, the absolute weight of the right supra-renal body was 278 grains; its specific gravity, 1046. The supra-renal vein was very small, almost atrophic. The sympathetic nerves from the lesser splanchnic were greatly increased in size, and so were also some of the branches, as well as the ganglia of the solar plexus of nerves on that side, and in contact with the morbid organ. The texture of these nervous parts was of a rosy hue, as if under the influence of vascular excitement. No other change could be observed in them. The supra-renal capsule on the left side was an oblong rectangular body, and had retained so much of its original shape as to present its flattened form, and, on the whole, preserved its relations to surrounding parts. A nearly similar but less vascular condition of the nerves was apparent on this side also. The absolute weight of the body was 85 grains; its specific gravity, 1042.

Sectional and microscopic appearances.—A section in the longest axis of the organ showed two distinct appearances, namely, a part of a dense gristly hardness, and a part which evidently corresponded to the medullary part of the organ, which was chiefly occupied by a yellow deposit. In the medullary portion of the organs the morbid process appeared to have advanced the most, and to be in the greatest abundance. Deposition and subsequent softening of exuded matter of a marked and peculiar aspect, resembling very much what is usually called scrofulous, tubercular, or yellow cheesy-like matter, occupied the medullary portion of the capsule. The veins from the organ were generally diminished in size, and the cavity corresponding to the central venous sinus was entirely occupied by the yellow exudation, in various conditions as to softening. Small sacs of various sizes were scattered throughout the stroma (cortical) of the organ, and contained the same scrofulous-looking material, in various states of consistence. No true oval vesicles natural to the cortical substance of the viscus could be seen by the microscope; and the only structure of an elementary form, which could be observed and referred to the normal histological elements of the supra-renal body, consisted in the caudate and branched nucleated cells seen in the firmer parts of the yellow deposit, which involved the medullary portion of the organ. The gristly hard part was composed, microscopically, of fibrinous elements, in the form of elongated, fusiform, and spindle-shaped cells, with simple and compound nuclei, together with fine, filamentous fibres and granular matter. The yellow matter was made up of fine granular stroma, in which compound granular corpuscles, oil granules, and globules, together with crystals soluble in acetic acid, were most obvious and abundant. Clear and transparent cells, free of nuclei, together with club-shaped, caudate, and very irregularly-branched cells, with simple and compound nuclei, were also obvious constituents. The mucous membrane of the mouth was thin, pale, and bloodless, the labial and buccal glands shining prominently through. The stomach and substance of the intestinal tube were uniformly thin throughout. In the stomach, the solitary gastric glands were remarkably prominent, while the mucous membrane generally was wasted and atrophic. Microscopic sections from the jejunum and ileum showed the villi remarkably attenuated, and the mucous membrane very readily separated from the adjacent muscular part of the gut. The tubular glands of the mucous membrane were almost entirely gone, and their place was supplied by a granular amorphous material. The average specific gravity of the mucous membrane was 1040.

The greatly increased size and rosy hue of the nerves in contact with and passing into the morbid organs are worthy of notice; but whether these appearances were the result of an inflammatory condition of the capsules, or not, it would be unsafe to hazard an opinion.

Dr. Christie's case.—Betsy Tait, æt. 36, admitted into the Dundee Royal Infirmary, Aug. 2, 1856. This patient has always enjoyed good health up till about six months ago, when, after exposure to cold, she was seized with cough and expectoration. About two months after the commencement of illness, she had rigors, accompanied by pain of head and lumbar region, and, a few days after this attack, she observed her skin to become of a gradually increasing dusky color. She has been treated by a medical man for the last two months, but without any benefit.

State on admission.—She is emaciated, and her skin is of a bronze color; the right side of face is in a semi-paralyzed state, giving a great peculiarity of expression when she speaks. Complains of pain over the region of liver, and in the loins, aggravated on pressure, more especially in left lumbar region; in both of these situations there is evident fulness. She has also cough, accompanied by frothy, muco-purulent expectoration; but has no pain in chest, which, on examination, sounds dull over left lung, where harsh, cavernous respiration is heard. Puerile breathing audible over lower part of right lung, and harsh breathing at its apex. Her bowels are constipated; urine normal; tongue dry; pulse 108, feeble.

4th.—Some castor oil given yesterday operated well, bringing away a large quantity of very dark-colored fæces; but early this morning the patient sank into a comatose state, in which she continued till her death, at 10 A.M.

Sectio Cadaveris, 53 hours after death.—Body much emaciated; skin of a dark mahogany color all over body and legs. Extensive adhesions of old standing existed all round left lung, which also showed tubercle in all stages up to the large ulcerated cavity; the right lung was also tuberculous at its apex. Liver healthy; spleen healthy; heart small, and the muscular tissue rather flabby-looking; kidneys healthy. Supra-renal capsules rather larger than natural. On laying them open, each contained a series of cysts, filled with a thin, serous fluid, with small, floating flocculi, very little cortical substance remaining.

Inoculation des Eaux jambes du Cheval à l'Homme. Par M. PICHOT, de La Loupe, M. MANOURY, de Chartres, M. BOUSQUET, M. THOLAZAN. (Gaz. Médicale de Paris, May 31st, June 7th, June 14th, and June 21st, 1856.

On Inoculation of Man with the matter of "Grease." By MM. PICHOT, MANOURY, BOUSQUET, THOLAZAN.

On the 29th of April, in the present year, a communication was addressed to the Academie de Medecine, at Paris, by M. Manoury, surgeon to the Hôtel Dieu, at Chartres, and by M. Pichot, a physician at La Loupe, concerning a man who had been accidentally inoculated with matter proceeding from a horse affected with grease; and at the same time some of the matter obtained from the man was forwarded to M. Bousquet for experimental purposes. The account of the case is this. On Tuesday, the 5th of March, a farrier, named Brissot, aged 28, called upon Dr. Pichot, in consequence of a painful affection of his hands, and, on examination, these organs were found to be considerably swollen, and covered with *opaline and umbilicated pustules, which were confluent, and in every respect similar to vaccine pustules of the eighth or ninth day.* He had never been vaccinated, and he had not been near any cow, but he remembered to have shod a short time previously a horse affected with grease. This happened on the 11th of February. There are twenty-four days from the 11th of February to the 5th of March, but as at this latter date the pustules presented the appearance of vaccine pustules of the eighth or ninth day, it is necessary to conclude that the period of incubation had been fifteen days. The horse was seen by M. Bousergent, a pupil of the veterinary schools of Toulouse and Alfort, and found to be suffering from a true attack of grease.

Dr. Pichot obtained some matter from the back of the hands of the patient by puncturing the pustules with a lancet, and having placed it upon glass, some was sent to M. Manoury, at Chartres, and some to M. Bousquet. With the matter sent to him M. Manoury made a series of very exact experiments upon children, and in every case (the number is not given) the inoculation resulted in a well-defined pustule, of the size of a large lentil, umbilicated, surrounded with an areola, and not to be distinguished from a vaccine pustule. He also obtained similar pustules by inoculating other children with the matter obtained from these pustules. Some of this secondary matter was also sent by M. Manoury to M. Bousquet, and this gentleman inoculated a child at one and the same time with it and with the matter obtained directly from Brissot, and sent to him by Dr. Pichot. The right arm was inoculated with the one kind of matter, and the left arm with the other kind. The result was remarkable. The inoculation made with the matter obtained from the farrier failed altogether, producing neither congestion nor irritation; but in the inoculation made with the matter obtained secondarily from the child, the operation was perfectly successful, and every puncture was followed by a pustule which differed in no respect, either in its history or its appearance, from the common cow-pox.

These facts speak for themselves. There developed in the hands of this farrier a malady which has all the properties as well as all the appearances of cow-pox; and the only question is, as to how this malady originated. The man declares that he had not been near any cow, and he remembers to have shod a horse affected with grease fifteen days before the skin became affected—a horse which, when examined by a veterinarian, was found to be suffering in the foot and lower part of the leg from that cutaneous malady which is characterized by a discharge, at first serous and limpid, then yellowish, acrid, and fetid, with a reddish swelling of the skin and subcutaneous tissue, which the French call *défluxions, eaux-puanites, eaux aux jambes*, and which we call *grease*. Is there, then, that intimate relation between cow-pox and grease which appeared to be so probable to the illustrious discoverer of vaccination, and to some of his contemporaries, and which has since this time been almost or altogether overlooked? Jenner wrote, in 1798, that cow-pox was given to cows by farm servants from horses suffering from grease; and he succeeded in producing cow-pox in a cow and the vaccine pustule in a man, by inoculating them respectively with matter obtained from a horse thus affected. These experiments were repeated at the time, sometimes with success and sometimes without; and the cause of the uncertainty was not known until the subject was investigated by Mr. Loy, a surgeon living at Pickering, in Yorkshire. These investigations, which are models of scientific induction and deduction, were made in 1801. In the beginning of the year this gentleman was consulted by a farrier, whose hands were covered with an eruption, consisting of pustules, separated from each other, and surrounded by an inflammatory circle. These vesicles resembled those proceeding from a burn, only they were regularly rounded, and their centre exhibited a black spot which seemed to have been caused by some slight injury. This man had been engaged in dressing a horse suffering from grease. He had never suffered in the same way before; but he had had the small-pox. About the same period, a butcher living at Middleton, a place near Pickering, was attacked by painful ulcers on both hands, and especially about the roots of the nails. These ulcers became inflamed in the course of a few days, and a vesicle formed upon each of them. The lymphatics of the arms also became red and painful, and a tumor formed in one of the armpits. There was also a pustule on one of the eyebrows similar to the pustules upon the hands, which had to all appearance been communicated by touching or rubbing the part. In this case there was considerable fever. This patient, like the last, had been occupied in attending upon a horse suffering from grease, and was so occupied at the time he fell ill. He had not had small-pox.

In order to ascertain whether this malady was communicable by inoculation, Mr. Loy inserted some of the matter contained in the pustules into the arm of a brother of the man, who had never had small-pox. On the third day a vesicle had formed. Then there were some feverish symptoms. In the end the vesicle exhibited all the character of true cow-pox.

Cotemporaneously with this experiment some of the same matter was inserted, by means of a new lancet, into the teat of a cow. Nine days afterwards there was a vesicle, surrounded by a red areola. The teat also was hard to some distance from the puncture, and so painful that the animal would not allow it to be touched. A few days later a crust had formed upon the vesicle, and the inflammation had subsided.

An infant was inoculated with matter taken from the pustule which had formed upon the teat of this cow on the ninth day from its commencement, and the progress of the inoculation was watched with great attention, when it was found that the inflammation, the vesicles, and the formation of the crust, were not to be distinguished from the corresponding phenomena in ordinary vaccination. On the sixth day this infant was inoculated with the small-pox, and the puncture seemed to inflame until the third day; but this disturbance passed off without any further development, and the child escaped the disease.

Another infant was inoculated with matter taken from the butcher. On the third day there was a pimple on the part punctured; on the sixth day, this was surrounded with a pale inflammatory circle, and the borders were more elevated than the centre; on the eighth day there was a vesicle containing a limpid fluid; on the fourteenth, this vesicle had changed into a brown and hard crust. Shortly afterwards this child was inoculated with the small-pox without any result.

In addition to these experiments, Mr. Loy inoculated the nipple of a cow with a very limpid matter taken by a perfectly clean lancet, from the heel of a horse suffering from grease. On the fifth day the part punctured was elevated and surrounded with a pale redness. A few days afterwards a purple vesicle, containing a limpid fluid, had become formed, and the part was swollen and painful, but the general health of the animal did not appear to be affected.

Mr. Loy then inserted matter, which he had taken from the pustule of this cow, into the arm of an infant. On the sixth day afterwards there was considerable redness, and on the ninth a vesicle. Then this infant was inoculated in three different places with small-pox, and absolutely without result, either local or general.

Another infant was inoculated with matter taken from the heel of the horse which had been the occasion of the mischief. Three days afterwards there was a pustule surrounded with a small degree of inflammation; on the day following this pustule was more elevated; on the fifth day it had changed into a vesicle of a purple color; on the six and seventh days this vesicle had become larger and darker. These changes were accompanied by a considerable degree of fever, the onset of which was marked by shivering and vomiting. The variolous inoculation was tried in this case, also, but no impression was made by it.

Three other children were inoculated with matter obtained from this last-mentioned child on the sixth day after its inoculation; and on the tenth day they presented vesicles surrounded with some degree of erysipelatous redness. These vesicles at this time were beginning to dry, but they still contained a considerable quantity of limpid matter. The children were then inoculated with the matter of small-pox, and the only effect of this operation was to produce a slight degree of local inflammation, which disappeared on the fifth day.

It was only after several unsuccessful attempts that Mr. Loy was able to satisfy himself that the matter of grease would act upon the cow without having first passed through a metamorphosis in the human body. At last, however, he found that the inoculation was abortive unless the matter was taken from a horse in which the symptoms of grease were general as well as local, beginning with fever and ending with an eruption, not only in the heels, but upon other parts of the skin, the fever subsiding when the eruption made its appearance.

These observations of Mr. Loy are also confirmed in every respect by the observations of Signor Sacco, whose "Trattato de Vaccinazione con Osserv. sul Giavardo et Vajuolo Pecorine" were published in Milan in 1800.

M. Sacco says that his first attempts at inoculation with the matter of grease were very unsuccessful. Before reading Mr. Loy's treatise he had operated unsuccessfully upon twenty-seven cows and eighteen children, and before he succeeded he was still doomed to failure in several instances. At length his own horse was attacked with grease, and he repeated his experiment with the clear viscid and fetid serosity which escaped from a crack in the heel on the fourth day from the commencement of the symptoms. These experiments, which were made upon two children and one cow, failed as completely as the others. *But his groom, who had to dress the heels of this horse, was affected with five pustules,* three on the right hand and two on the left fore-arm; which pustules were precisely like those of the cow-pox. This man had not been inoculated. Unfortunately, however, these pustules were too much dried up to be serviceable for any experiment when they were first seen by M. Sacco. About the same time, the coachman of a gentleman called Clari, who had also had to dress a horse suffering from grease, and who had not had small-pox, had both his hands covered with a vesicular eruption, accompanied with fever and diarrhœa. These vesicles were perfectly similar to the vesicles of small-pox, and several children who were inoculated with matter obtained from them by a colleague of M. Sacco, M. Birago, went through the regular stages of the vaccine complaint. In addition to this, the same coachman was taken on the same day on which M. Birago made his experiments to the Foundling Hospital at Lembrate, and then M. Sacco inoculated nine children and one cow with matter obtained from him, the result being that the operation failed upon the cow and upon seven of the children, and succeeded upon the remaining two children. In these two children the complaint produced was absolutely undistinguishable from common cow-pox, and the matter obtained from these children has been subsequently used in a long series of vaccination.

Nor is this the only evidence connected with this subject. On the contrary, Jenner himself wrote, in January, 1801, of a farm servant on a neighboring estate near Berkeley, who was affected on one of his hands, after tending upon a horse affected with grease, with pustules which were not to be distinguished from those of cow-pox, and upon whom the inoculation with the matter of small-pox failed some three months afterwards. And in February of the following year Jenner writes of having seen, in the preceding summer, a pustule resembling cow-pox upon the hand of another farm servant, who had been employed in dressing a diseased horse. He says, moreover, that he made several attempts to vaccinate with matter procured from this pustule, but without producing any other effect than a slight and transitory redness. This failure, however, did not at all shake Jenner's confidence as to the relationship existing between grease and small-pox; and as explaining the failure by showing that the causes of success depend upon very subtle conditions, he remarks further that he had always failed to carry cow-pox by a lancet from one cow to the teat of another. He also says that oxen and bulls are never affected with cow-pox (this might be expected), and that vaccination succeeds readily upon calves of either sex.

Such, then, is the evidence upon which the analogy between grease and cow-pox must be made to rest, and hence the case of Brissot must be regarded as a very important contribution to the history of philosophical medicine.

II.

REPORT ON THE PROGRESS OF SURGERY.

On the effect of Chloroform upon the results of Surgical Operations. By JAMES ARNOTT, M.D. (Medical Times and Gazette, Oct. 25th, and Nov. 1st, 1856.)

THE announcement of "death from chloroform," does not now affect the professional reader in the manner it originally did. He regrets the individual occurrence, but he finds consolation in the reflection that such casualties are rare, and that they are much overbalanced by the favorable influence exerted by chloroform on the results of operations. Though a few may die, he says, from the immediate or direct effects of chloroform, many are saved by its ulterior agency.

He judges of the first circumstance—the number of sudden deaths—by the small number of reports which reach him; of the second, by the statistical investigations that have been instituted to determine the question.

On the first point, however, he is very apt to be deceived. Scarcely a hundred instances of sudden death from chloroform have as yet been reported, but there cannot be a doubt that by far the greater number have been concealed.

In some remarks on this subject, two years ago, it was stated, that although five cases of sudden death from chloroform had taken place in the London hospitals within the seven months preceding my publication, not one had been reported as occurring in the private practice of London during that period; and the same observation, it was stated, was applicable to a much longer time. Indeed, the author is not aware that more than two cases of sudden death from etherization have been published as happening in the private practice of London since its introduction. This evident concealment is neither extraordinary nor reprehensible. What family is there that would not endeavor to the utmost to avoid the horrors of a coroner's inquest, and the consequent newspaper report, where, as happens in the case of death from chloroform, there can be no suspicion of foul play? Nor can we blame the practitioner who would gladly escape from a criticism of his proceedings on such occasions. Useful as such modes of publicity may be on other accounts, they do not, in this instance, promote the advancement of medical knowledge. But many die from the direct effects of chloroform, and within a few hours of its administration, whose deaths are attributed to other causes. Dr. Mouat has recently drawn attention to such cases. He speaks of soldiers who were operated upon in the Crimea under chloroform, as gradually sinking under the peculiar state of nausea and depression which follows its use. "Reaction is never thoroughly established, the desire for food never returns, and the patient sinks as it were stealthily, and dies from exhaustion in from twelve to twenty-four hours." "These cases," he adds, "are far more numerous than is generally supposed, and many of them may fairly be termed 'deaths from chloroform,' but are never so returned."[*]

The second source of consolation on such occasions, we have said, is the opinion that the sudden deaths from chloroform are much overbalanced by saving properly as respects the results of operations. It has been asserted, in reference to certain amputations, that if five cases were to be killed by the direct agency of chloroform in every hundred operated upon, there would still be a saving of life by its ulterior agency. This is a most important point, about which there should be no doubt.

[*] "Medical Times and Gazette," September, 1856.

If the position that there is a saving of life upon the whole be incontestable, it ought, for the credit of the profession, to be brought more frequently forward, especially on such occasions as the recent inquest at St. Thomas's Hospital: if it be unfounded, the sooner it is contradicted the better. It is the purpose of this paper to renew the investigation of the subject.

The question whether chloroform saves life as well as prevents pain, can only be determined by statistics. To attempt to form a judgment from individual experience, would be scarcely less erroneous than to estimate the comparative proportion of the two sexes (now ascertained with such wonderful accuracy by the aid of statistics) by counting the males and females in the inquirer's own family. Nor would reasoning from the observation of the sensible effects on the system bring us nearer the truth. The absence of pain may be, and probably is, an advantage as respects the results of an operation, but it may be much overbalanced by the other effects of the anæsthetic; and the beneficial stimulus excited by chloroform may be followed by injurious prostration.* On the other hand, poisonous and depressing as the drug manifestly is in some cases, it may still possess some hidden virtues conducing to recovery. Whatever its ulterior agency may be, as this produces no peculiar symptoms, it is by results alone that its nature can be determined.

The writer whose inquiries on this subject have been most influential, is Dr. Simpson, of Edinburgh.

About two years after the introduction of etherization, and when surgeons were beginning to fear that the bad effects of chloroform might not be limited to the very time of its administration, but might seriously affect the results of operations, Dr. Simpson's statistical investigations respecting this point were published. They were prefaced by an ably written and lucid exposition of the value of statistics applied to this inquiry, which, with the manifest trouble he had had in collecting his materials, and the apparent care he had taken in arranging them, insured a ready and confiding reception to his investigations by the profession. From that time all anxiety about the ulterior effects of chloroform seemed to cease, and surgeons have continued to employ it without hesitation, under the conviction, that instead of there being a destruction of life as the price paid for the insensibility, a great saving of life is effected by it. The tables in which he condensed the results of his investigations, and which have just been reprinted in his collected works, have been as influential with surgeons as the Northampton Life Tables have been with Assurance Companies.

As these tables represent the mortality from amputations to have been 29 per cent. immediately before the introduction of etherization, and 23 per cent. after its introduction, and as the inference from them is that there has been a saving of life effected by the change to the amount of 6 per cent. (a number doubtless far exceeding that of the sudden deaths which have taken place during the administration of chloroform), it is no wonder that they should have been so often appealed to in discussions upon this subject, and that all theoretical objections to chloroform should have been refuted by them.

Nevertheless, these tables, when closely examined, are found to involve the greatest fallacies; they do not afford a particle of evidence that the introduction of chloroform has lessened the mortality after amputation.

The first, which professes to give the average mortality of thirty British hospitals, should have shown the number of operations, and their results, at each of these hospitals during precisely the same period of time; but, instead of this, while the period of observation, as respects the only large healthy hospital inserted in the list, is limited to two years, that of the large unhealthy hospitals of Edinburgh and Glasgow, the excessive mortality of which almost equals that of the Paris hospitals, extends to more than three times this duration. If an equal period of observation be taken to form this average (excluding two of the small hospitals, one healthy and the other unhealthy, on account of the period of observation respecting them being uncertain), the table, instead of showing a mortality of 29 per cent., would show

* The credit of a double advantage claimed for general anæsthesia, of preventing both pain and danger, is justly due to local anæsthesia from cold, and when used for other purposes as well as operations. Mr. Langston Parker, in his recent work on Cancer, speaks of our now being able to use caustic in its cure in consequence of the pain from it being removed by frigorific applications; but the prevention of erysipelas by intense cold is not of less importance, to say nothing of its own direct and efficacious curative agency in malignant disease.

one of only 24; and, if other large healthy hospitals, like that at Bristol, had been included—such as the Liverpool Royal Infirmary, where (as appears from a published return) the deaths from amputation during three consecutive years were only at the rate of 6 per cent.—the average mortality of the whole would probably have been considerably less than 20 per cent.

The second table involves no miscalculation so palpable as that in the first, but it leads to conclusions equally erroneous. It gives an account of the number of amputations in which ether was administered, with the results; but what the character of the cases was in which it was used—whether the patients were healthy or worn out with disease—we have no means of judging. In all probability the best cases were generally selected, for only a few were returned from each hospital; and it was natural and proper that at first the best cases should be chosen for trial; not only those free from serious organic disease of the vital parts (a class which were long excluded), but those in which the reparative powers were most conspicuous; and a clearer proof that this was the case cannot be adduced than the fact that the etherized cases from the eight London hospitals inserted in this list, show a mortality of more than 10 per cent. below that which (as we shall presently see) exists at the present day.

But as the prospect of recovery from amputation is good or bad, according to the general health of the patient, and other circumstances, if we could always select our cases, the usual mortality would probably be reduced to less than a half. As it is, all the advantage which the 302 etherized cases appear by the table to have over the non-etherized 618 of the other table (admitting the returns to be correct), does not amount to more than 1 per cent. To prove that there was not actually a loss of life, instead of a gain, from etherization, there should have been, assuming that the cases were generally selected, a much greater difference than this. A percentage of 23 deaths from amputation in the English provincial hospitals, even supposing that every case was etherized, would indicate a great increase of the usual rate of mortality before the introduction of etherization.

Another objection to the reception of this table as an argument in favor of the indiscriminate use of chloroform is, that it has reference principally to sulphuric ether as the means of producing anæsthesia, for very few operations had been performed under chloroform at the time of its publication. Now, chloroform, whatever other advantages it may possess over ether, has none as regards safety; and, what is of more importance in respect to this table, it has of late years been employed much more boldly than was formerly usual. Patients were then frequently only half intoxicated by the anæsthetic, and the intoxication was kept up but for a short time. A change in this practice had not yet been effected, by the singular argument, that, because a patient laboring under convulsions may be kept for a long time under the full influence of chloroform apparently without injury, the same proceeding can be adopted with impunity in the case of a patient exposed to the long-continued danger of a large amputation wound.

We shall now follow Dr. Arnott to the consideration of tables of a very different character to the above, as respects their construction, and which disclose facts of a very different import. Dr. Arnott writes:

"Although I had long felt convinced, from reflecting on the evidently poisonous character of chloroform, that the number of sudden deaths produced by it, whether reported or not reported, was by no means the measure of the whole mortality. I was unable to obtain satisfactory evidence of this. It was by statistics alone that this point could be determined, and I had no easy access to the repertories of the necessary facts preserved in hospitals. At last, my attention was directed to the Statistical Reports of Operations which have appeared for several years past in the 'Medical Times and Gazette,' by a reference to them in Sir Benjamin Brodie's recently published paper on Lithotrity. On examination, I found that these reports were all I could have desired. A monthly account is given of the whole of the operations during the last three years. Their accuracy is assured by the circumstantiality with which every case is mentioned, and by the fact that they were not drawn up with a view to the settlement of any particular question in practice. The reporters of these statistics have been under no conceivable bias; they have been actuated solely by a desire to promote surgical science. If their returns have a fault, it is certainly not the over-statement of the mortality; for, almost every month, a large number of cases are mentioned as being still under treatment; and although the fatal issue of a few of these is afterwards reported, it is probable that other deaths have happened in consequence of the operation, but at too long a period after it to be known to the reporter, or to be recorded by him. It might at first sight appear desirable to have reports for a longer period than three years, but were the period now extended, any such comparison as that we are now making between the results of operations, becomes imperfect or impossible, by the advancing improvements altering the circumstances.

"In the 'Medical Times and Gazette,' there are separate statistical reports both of the London and Provincial hospitals; but I shall restrict my attention to the first, for the following reasons. The principal is, that the hospitals in the provinces are too far apart, and differ from each other in too many circumstances, such as climate, site, and character of the patients frequenting them, to render it possible to form an estimate of their average mortality before etherization was introduced, from the very few published returns of the results of amputations in the provincial hospitals at that time. Another reason is, that I am not sure that the administration of chloroform has been so universal in operations in the country as it has been for many years past in the metropolis. In London, on the other hand, there are many large hospitals furnishing the requisite number of facts, and they are all under nearly the same kind of general management, surgical practice, &c. We have authentic returns, also, of the mortality after amputations in some of the large London hospitals before ether was introduced, from which, in consequence of the similarity of circumstances just alluded to, we can construct a sufficiently correct estimate of the general mortality for comparison with the present rate. The following table has been constructed from these returns.

TABLE I.

Showing the Average Mortality after Amputation of the Thigh, Leg, and Arm, in three London hospitals, before the introduction of Chloroform.

Hospitals.	Date of Observation.	Reporter.	Primary Amputations.		Secondary Amputations.		Total.	
			Cases.	Deaths.	Cases.	Deaths.	Cases.	Deaths.
University College,	1835–40	Mr. Potter.	8	3	50	7	58	10
St. Thomas's, . .	1842–47	Mr. South.	20	7	29	6	49	13
University College,	1841–46	Mr. Cadge.	7	4	38	10	45	14
St. Bartholomew's, .	1846	Mr. Haig.	8	1	14	3	22	4
							174	41

Percentage of deaths to cases (taking equal periods of observation), 21·9.

"The great diversity which appears in the above table between the two equal periods of observation at University College Hospital, is a striking illustration of what has been termed a run of good or bad luck in the practice of the same surgeon, for Mr. Liston was the principal operator at the hospital during both periods; and it shows, also, how unsafe it would be, unless for a very long period, to rely on any particular hospital as a standard. The return of deaths from amputations at St. Thomas's is heavy, and I might have been justified in rejecting it as being of too private a nature to have the requisite authority; but, in order to prevent any cavil, or appearance of selection, it is retained; and, for the same reason, I have omitted the only other return of amputations which I have been able to find, as respects the London hospitals: objection may be made to it, because the mortality is much below the usual average. This return is from Guy's Hospital, and is mentioned by Dr. Fenwick in his elaborate paper on the statistics of amputation, in the 'Edinburgh Journal of Medical Science' for 1847. The period of observation is from 1843 to 1845; the cases are 36, and the deaths 4, or at the rate of 11 per cent. Were this return added to the others in the table, it would reduce the average of the London mortality to less than 20 per cent., or 1 fatal result in 5 amputations.

"The present mortality of the London hospitals is shown by the following tables, into which the several returns in the 'Medical Times and Gazette' have been condensed.

TABLE II.

Showing the Mortality from Amputation of the Thigh, Leg, and Arm, performed under Chloroform in the London hospitals from June, 1855, to June, 1856, inclusive.

Hospitals.	Primary Amputations.		Secondary Amputations.		Total.	
	Cases.	Deaths.	Cases.	Deaths.	Cases.	Deaths.
St. Bartholomew's, ...	1	...	23	7	24	7
St. Thomas's, ...	4	3	12	3	16	6
Guy's, ...	15	10	34	3	49	13
London, ...	11	2	13	4	24	6
St. George's, ...	6	3	15	5	21	8
University College, ...	3	2	14	3	17	5
King's College, ...	1	1	8	3	9	4
Middlesex, ...	1	1	5	2	6	3
St. Mary's, ...	5	3	12	3	17	6
Westminster, ...	...	...	2	...	2	...
Charing Cross, ...	1	1	9	2	10	3
Metropolitan Free, ...	...	...	2	...	2	...
Hospital for Sick Children, . .	...	...	1	...	1	...
Seamen's, ...	...	...	5	...	5	...
Marylebone Infirmary, . . .	...	...	1	...	1	...
Total, ...	48	26	156	35	204	61

TABLE III.

Showing the Mortality from Amputation of the Thigh, Leg, and Arm, performed under Chloroform in the London hospitals during three years, from July, 1853, to June, 1856.

	Number of Cases.	Number of Deaths.
First year, ...	144	57
Second year, ...	150	50
Third year, ...	136	41
Total, ...	430	148

Average percentage of deaths, 34·4.*

"It appears, by comparing these with the foregoing table, that the mortality in the London hospitals has increased, since the introduction of etherization, from 21 to 34 per cent., or, to vary the expression, instead of amputation being fatal in a

* Several sudden deaths were reported as happening from chloroform in the London hospitals during this period, but none from its administration in amputations, though, in the accounts of cases in the journal, the fatal terminations are occasionally spoken of in such terms as these, "vomiting continued until death," "death from collapse followed," "sank from shock during the performance of a primary amputation," "sank almost immediately after artificial respiration and galvanism had been resorted to without success."

less proportion than 1 in 4 of those operated upon, it now proves fatal in 1 in 3. Is not so enormous a sacrifice of life too high a price to be paid for anæsthesia, even granting that this cannot be otherwise obtained with perfect safety? Is life to be held as nothing when compared to pain?

"If the above tables required confirmation, a reference might be made to other statistical statements, which, though the numbers constituting them are too small to have much weight by themselves, may be usefully considered in conjunction with others having a more extended basis. Of this kind are the tables respecting etherization, that were published four years ago in America ('American Journal of Medical Science' for 1852), and certain notices which we have received of the surgery of the Crimean campaign. It is generally understood that the results of amputations were unfavorable during this war; and, though several other causes were in operation, there can be now no doubt that this want of success may in some degree be attributed to the use of chloroform. Dr. Gordon, who had medical charge of the second division of the army (in which, however, chloroform was not so much used as in the other divisions), informs us (see the 'Report of the Proceedings of the Crimean Medical Society') that the result of amputations was very favorable in the preceding war in India, and before etherization was in use. Of twelve amputations performed in his regiment, during the Punjaub campaign, only one prove fatal.

"Allusion may also be made to a report of amputations performed under etherization, which was published in the 'Medical Gazette,' some years ago by Dr. Snow; and as its purpose was very different from recommending caution in the administration of chloroform, it may be here referred to; although under other circumstances the fact of its being a private unauthenticated report would, in such an inquiry as the present, render it inadmissible. Betrayed, apparently, by Dr. Simpson's erroneously high estimate of the mortality in British hospitals, before etherization was introduced, Dr. Snow did not hesitate to publish this report, in which the mortality from 55 amputations of the thigh, leg, and arm, amounts to 27 per cent., as a statement favorable to etherization. But when it is considered that none of the amputations in this list were primary, that at the commencement of the practice there was more selection of cases than has since obtained, and that several of them occurred in private practice—circumstances all highly favorable to recovery—the mortality from them must be deemed quite as high as that indicated by the reports in the 'Medical Times and Gazette.' Dr. Snow says he publishes this report in order to dispel the fears with which some surgeons may be troubled; as well might a recruiting sergeant encourage to enlistment by enumerating our losses at the Redan.

"Although I have not, for certain reasons assigned above, made so accurate an examination of the statistics of the results of amputation in the provinces as in London, I have ascertained that they show an equal, if not a greater, comparative increase of mortality. This operation, at some of the largest provincial hospitals, did not formerly prove fatal to 15 in 100; the average mortality for the last two years and nine months (the whole period embraced by the returns) is 30 in 100.

"I am perfectly aware that the inferences drawn from these tables and numerical statements will not be acceptable to many members of the profession, who have been using chloroform in every important operation; but I am unable to anticipate any valid objection that can be made to them. The point that was supposed established by Dr. Simpson's investigations, it must at once be acknowledged, is not so established; and, although there may be a difference of opinion regarding the exact correctness of the estimate, in my first table of the mortality in the London hospitals, before etherization was in use, this is a point of no importance. The great question is, not whether my table makes this estimate two or three per cent. higher or lower than it ought to be, but whether the mortality from amputation in the London hospitals, after all the improvement of late times, would have amounted steadily during the last three years to more than 30 per cent., or about a third of those operated upon, but for the continued agency of chloroform? If it be asserted that the mortality of the London hospitals has not increased, then it must follow that the returns we have had of the results of operations in former years have been most erroneous; that the long-boasted superior salubrity of the London over the Paris hospitals was not authorized by the truth; and that our surgeons, though well aware of the comparatively trifling mortality after amputation in the country or in well-ventilated hospitals, whither most of the patients might have been sent, recklessly persisted in this fearful sacrifice of life."

Dr. Arnott finds further illustration in the statistics of lithotomy. "The deaths from lithotomy, in adult patients, before the introduction of chloroform, were, according to our best authorities on the subject, in the proportion of 1 to 4½, or 22 per cent. of those operated upon. What they are now, will appear by the following tables.

TABLE IV.

Showing the Mortality from Lithotomy performed on the Adult and under Chloroform in the London hospitals during the last year, from July, 1855, to June, 1856.

Hospitals.	Cases.	Deaths.
St. Bartholomew's, ...	1	0
Guy's, ...	3	2
St. Thomas's, ...	2	1
London, ...	1	1
St. George's, ...	2	1
University College, ...	2	1
King's College, ...	3	2
St. Mary's, ...	2	1
Metropolitan, ...	1	0

Total cases, 17; deaths, 9; percentage of deaths, 52·9.

TABLE V.

Showing the Mortality from Lithotomy performed on Adults* in the London hospitals during the last three years.

	Cases.	Deaths.
First year, ...	10	7
Second year, ...	14	6
Third year, ...	17	9
Total, ...	41	22

Average percentage of deaths, 53·6.

"The fact that, instead of one in four operations proving fatal, the mortality should now be doubled, and amount to one half of those cut for stone, is so remarkable as to render any comment unnecessary."

Instead of being a means of saving life as well as of preventing pain, it would thus appear that chloroform has increased the hazard of amputation to so frightful an extent, as to make death probable in one out of every three cases, instead of in one out of four or five, as formerly, and to render recovery or death after lithotomy an equal chance. Nor is it necessary that the argument of an increase of the unfavorable results of operations under chloroform should be insisted upon, for if there be no sufficient proof of a decrease of these results as a compensation for the numerous deaths which proceed from the direct and immediate effect of chloroform, the recommendation of its use, especially in the large doses employed in late years, could hardly be justified.

* "I am not aware that more than one death from the direct effects of chloroform has been reported as occurring in the London hospitals, but the following notice in the statistical return in connection with one of these cases at Guy's Hospital nearly amounts to such a report: 'The man required an unusual quantity of chloroform. He never rallied well from the operation, and death took place next day.'"

The treatment of Cancerous Diseases by Caustics. A critical inquiry into the modern therapeutics of cancer; being the Address in Surgery delivered at Birmingham on the occasion of the twenty-fourth annual meeting of the Provincial Medical and Surgical Association. By LANGSTON PARKER, Surgeon to the Queen's Hospital, Birmingham, &c. (8vo. London, Churchill, 1856, pp. 40.)

In this address Mr. Parker opens a subject in some measure new to English surgical practice, viz., the treatment of cancerous diseases by caustic or enucleation. A subject of which the importance will be allowed when we consider the vast number of cases of cancerous and cancroid diseases which annually destroy life, and when we reflect upon the absolute failure of the present surgical means and appliances for giving even relief in a great number of these cases. Having indicated the nature of those local cancerous growths in which operative measures alone are to be employed, and having glanced at two out of three of those procedures which are recognized by modern surgeons in the treatment of cancer—excision or ablation and compression—Mr. Parker proceeds to speak of the principal caustics which have been used in the treatment of cancer, and of their effect.

"The *chloride of zinc* is perhaps the caustic best known in this country, and the one now most commonly, though too rarely, employed in the treatment of cancerous or cancroid diseases. This salt, as a caustic in the treatment of cancer, was first introduced by M. Canquoin of Paris, in 1834, who, in that year and the succeeding, addressed two communications to the Academy of Medicine, stating the success which he had obtained in removing cancerous growths without the aid of the knife. The preparation, at first known as Canquoin's plaster, was soon ascertained to consist of about equal parts of chloride of zinc and flour made into a paste of proper consistence with water. In 1838, M. Canquoin published a complete account of his remedy, by which 600 cases of cancerous disease had been treated with a confessedly great amount of success. M. Canquoin, in his work, gives four formulæ for the preparation of the chloride of zinc paste. 1. Equal parts by weight of zinc and flour. 2. Zinc one part, flour two parts. 3. Zinc one part, flour three parts. 4. Zinc one part, muriate of antimony one part, flour one part and a half. Water from twenty to thirty drops to the ounce for each of these preparations. The first preparation, applied four lines in thickness for forty-eight hours, destroys the parts to the depth of an inch and a half. The same preparation three lines thick, applied for the same period, acts to the depth of about an inch only.

"The pastes Nos. 2 and 3 are to be applied in carcinomatous ulcerations, which are not deep, but spread over a greater or less extent of surface. No. 3, on account of the greater dilution of the chloride of zinc, acts slowly and with a less amount of pain. No. 4 is combined with the chloride of antimony; this preparation when well made has the consistence of soft wax, and is particularly suited to growths which are uneven on the surface, to the inequalities of which it is easily moulded, and does not alter its form or run when applied. M. Velpeau* speaks very highly of the chloride of zinc as an application to cancerous ulcers and growths. It is a preparation easily manipulated; it possesses no action on the epidermis or on mucous membranes covered with epithelium; it may be moulded with the hand to any shape, form, or thickness; it does not fuse or run, its action being strictly limited to the surface to which it is applied. Its action again is expended on the parts which it touches; unlike the arsenical pastes, there is nothing to fear from absorption, its action being strictly limited to the local effects to which it gives rise.

"M. Maissoneuve, in his clinical lectures on cancerous diseases, gives very favorable testimony to the effects of the chloride of zinc, especially in reference to its application to large, fetid, bleeding cancerous or cancroid ulcers where the knife is utterly out of the question, and where the patient is sinking from local irritation and hemorrhage. M. Maisonneuve mentions a case in which an enormous cancer of this kind was entirely removed by the remedies I have mentioned. This case is quoted at page 63 of the first number of Maisonneuve's 'Clinical Lectures.'

* * * * * * * * *

"I have used the chloride of zinc paste in several cases, which I shall hereafter detail, with a gratifying amount of success. The two chief objections which may

* 'Traité des Maladies du Sein, et de la Region Mammaire, &c.' Par A. Velpeau. Paris, 1854.

be raised against the use of the chloride of zinc are the necessity of first destroying the epidermis before the remedy is applied ; and, secondly, the pain occasioned by the prolonged contact of the caustic with the disease, which varies from a period of from twelve to forty-eight hours, according to circumstances.

"The pain, however, may be vastly diminished, if not entirely removed, by the application of ice and salt on the plan recommended by Dr. J. Arnott. I removed, by means of the chloride of zinc paste, a growth of the size of a walnut from the back of a lady, who had been twice operated on before with the knife for the removal of a similar growth in the same situation, without the remedy causing anything like severe pain. The moment the burning power of the caustic was felt a large bladder of ice and salt was applied, which entirely removed it in a few seconds—this was continued for a short time, and then removed ; when the pain of the caustic began again, a fresh bladder similarly filled was applied, with similar effect, so that, although the caustic remained in contact with the skin for six hours, the pain experienced was of the most trivial character. I have tried this plan with other cases, with almost a uniform amount of success, and I believe some modification of this kind, properly carried out, will effectually remove the chief evil attendant on the application of caustic remedies to the destruction of cancerous growths, which is the amount of prolonged pain they occasion. The chloride of zinc may be applied with a degree of precision unattainable by any other remedy. It destroys the tissues in direct relation with the thickness of the layer of paste applied, and this with a little practice may be calculated to a great nicety ; it never runs or fuses ; it destroys only those parts which it covers, and these it divides from the surrounding structures as cleanly as though they had been cut with a knife. The crust of scab formed by this caustic is hard, dense, and white ; there is no sanguineous or other discharge produced by it. The eschar separates at the end of twelve or fourteen days, leaving a clean, healthy, granulating surface underneath.

"The *concentrated mineral acids* have been lately much employed as caustics in the treatment of cancerous diseases. I allude especially to the nitric and sulphuric acids. A set treatise on the use of one of these acids, the nitric, has been published by M. Rivallié, in which monohydrated nitric acid is made into a paste with scraped lint or charpie. This M. Rivallie describes as solidified nitric acid. Many successful cases are given by this surgeon of the total and rapid destruction of cancerous growths by his method. M. Velpeau and M. Maisonneuve speak favorably of this preparation ; the latter prefers it mixed with asbestos. It is neither so easily under command nor so destructive as the concentrated sulphuric acid.

"Concentrated sulphuric acid, made into a paste with saffron, has been described by Velpeau and others under the title of 'black caustic' (caustique noir).

"In speaking of this remedy, M. Velpeau says : 'No caustic has afforded me similar advantages; its action is prompt, energetic, and deep; it is easily manipulated, gives rise to no sanguineous oozing like the alkaline caustics, nor to inflammatory reaction or swelling. One is sometimes surprised,' says this surgeon, 'to see a vast fungoid surface secreting daily an immense quantity of blood and sanies, converted in a few hours into a black crust, from which issues no moisture whatever.' 'It is,' says M. Maisonneuve, 'our caustic (de predilection), of which I most frequently make use in the destruction of hard and large tumors.'

"'The day or day but one after its application, the surrounding integuments are neither red nor swelled, and hardly more sensible than the healthy skin. One would say, in fact, that the patient was already cured, and that the black crust reposed upon a cicatrix already formed.'—Velpeau, 666.

"The *alkaline caustics*, or those which have potass for their base, are powerful, effective, and manageable remedies in the treatment of many forms of cancer. The remedies chiefly applicable are the Vienna paste, or Heister's caustic, in the form of powder, composed of five parts of the hydrate of potass and six of quick-lime, rubbed together as a dry powder, and when applied mixed into a paste with a little spirit of wine ; or the same remedy, now much in vogue on the Continent, consisting of the same ingredients, though in different proportions, fused and run into leaden tubes, like nitrate of silver or potassa fusa. In this form the remedy is known on the Continent as the caustic of 'Filhos.'

"It is composed of two parts of potass and one of lime, and is a most convenient, active, and useful remedy. Its inventor chiefly employed it in destroying fungoid growths from the 'uterus,' what he terms 'fungoid ulcerations,' and which, according to the cases detailed by Dr. Filhos, appear to be varieties of epithelial cancers, some of them probably of the nature of what are termed 'cauliflower excrescence.'

"In a Clinical Lecture, reported in the 'Association Journal' for March 29, 1856, Dr. West reports a case of similar disease cured by the galvano-caustic, applied by Mr. Paget.

"This physician also remarks, in the same lecture, that the chief cancerous or cancroid growths, from the uterus, are of the epithelial kind, and it is to precisely this class of cases that the caustic of Dr. Filhos is suited. By the application of this remedy, which I have frequently used, the diseased mass may be gradually rubbed away into a kind of putrilage or soap, with a very trivial amount of pain.

"The amount of pain produced bears no relation to the activity and destructive agency of the caustic in such cases. All the alkaline caustics have the effect of producing a sanguineous oozing from the parts to which they are applied. They are unlike the chloride of zinc and the mineral acids in this respect, which have the effect of coagulating the blood in the smaller vessels in the immediate vicinity of cancerous growths, whilst the alkaline caustics give rise to a sanguineous discharge to a greater or less extent."

Mr. Parker then refers to the escharotic, which has been recently proposed by M. Llandolfi, and of which a notice will be found elsewhere in our present volume as well as in our last volume, and his judgment is more favorable than that of the commission of the French Academy. He says: "As a fluid caustic, used where pastes are inapplicable, I have had abundance of evidence of its utility."

The last-mentioned preparation is the arsenical caustic of M. Manec, of the Salpêtrière, at Paris,—a caustic, which consists of one part of arsenious acid to seven or eight of cinnabar, and four of burnt spunge, made into a paste with a few drops of water. This is a caustic of great importance, and all that may be done by remedies of this class may be done, in all probability, by it, and by the chloride of zinc, as modified by M. Canquoin. Even M. Lebert, not, in general, a great lover or advocate of caustics, speaks highly and confidently of the result of M. Manec's operation with caustics, and gives some instances of cases, supposed to be incurable, which were cured by him. Many cases are also on record in which arsenical pastes have succeeded after other caustics have failed, and this may probably be explained by the statement made by M. Manec, that the action of arsenic on cancerous tissue is not simply escharotic. According to this surgeon, indeed, arsenic has a peculiar destructive affinity for cancerous growths. "It is a remarkable fact," says he, "that this powerful remedy, which destroys thick morbid growths of compact structure, when applied in the same proportions to superficial corroding ulcers, only destroys the morbid growth; however then it may be, its action does not extend to the healthy textures." This is a very remarkable and interesting statement. "M. Manec directs, that the arsenical paste, when employed in the treatment of cancer, should not be applied to a surface of greater extent than the size of a two-franc piece (about the size of the English florin) at each application; the quantity of arsenic absorbed from such a surface never produces unpleasant symptoms. M. Lebert says, he never saw 'serious symptoms follow the prudent application of Manec's arsenical paste.' It produces, however, marked local effects, with which the generality of surgeons are little acquainted. A few hours after its first application, a moderately severe pain is felt, and the neighboring tissues swell and become inflamed; an erysipelatous blush surrounds the part; if the application is made on the face, the whole visage may assume a puffy appearance. These symptoms may remain for three or four days, and then gradually subside. The pain produced by the remedy may last longer, but this, I have shown, may be mitigated by the application, from time to time, of bladders containing ice and salt. The action of arsenic is not like that of other caustics, merely local; it pervades the whole system. Its presence, when applied in the form of paste to destroy a cancroid growth, may be detected in the urine in about twelve hours after its first application, and may continue to be detected during a period of eight or ten days; and it is not till it has totally disappeared from the urine prudent to reapply the paste, supposing a second application should become necessary. Thus any cumulative injurious effect of the remedy is entirely prevented. There are several formulæ extant for the preparation of arsenical pastes; I may especially mention those bearing the names of Frére Côme and Dupuytren. The latter, consisting of 2 parts of arsenious acid, and 200 parts of calomel, is generally too feeble as a destructive agent.* In fact, the form of Manec is the safest and the best, and the only one that ought to be employed, and may be used, with the precautions to which I have alluded, with advantage and safety. In speaking of the effects of arsenic, M. Velpeau makes use of these remarkable expressions: 'Two of the properties attributed to it,' says he, ' render its use preferable to that of all other remedies, supposing that such attributes are found correct. First, if it could be demonstrated as asserted by M. Manec, that its destructive action is concentrated on the abnormal or morbid tissues only, it must be the most precious of all caustics; and, second, if, when mixed with the blood, by absorption, as proved by its presence in the urine, it still preserved this elective action for the destruction of morbid cancerous tissues, would it not, by thus decomposing or destroying the ultimate molecules of the disease, thus place the patient out of the fear of future relapses?' Here, in fact, is the whole point on which the treatment of cancer hangs; it is not the extermination or destruction of the malady locally, which is so much the question, as the prevention of its reappearance. If this is ever to be done, it must and will be done by the action of chemical remedies on cancerous growths, and the subsequent mixture, by absorption, of these remedies with the blood; much has been proved in this respect, in reference to arsenic; for, M. Lebert tells us, that he carefully watched some of Manec's cases for several years, with this view, but no relapse took place. I must quote another passage from M. Velpeau, in support of this opinion. He says, ' It is not impossible, that the potential caustics may determine in the surrounding tissues an important modification, and it is equally not impossible that they may, consequently, better prevent the extension or return of the cancerous principle, than excision. Again, as they do not, so much as cutting operations, place the life of the patient in danger, I am far from rejecting their employment.' "—(Page 676.)

In pointing out in what class of diseases, in what situation of disease, in what stages of disease, caustics are particularly indicated, Mr. Parker says, "In most cases, where a cancerous tumor is circumscribed, movable, and uncomplicated, where the integuments covering such tumors are healthy, or only very slightly diseased, where the malady springs from the bone or periosteum, or where these are more or less implicated, in diseases which are of a cystic character, or those again which are placed in the vicinity of, or immediately connected with, large blood-vessels, the knife is preferable. These remarks apply also with greater force if the disease is primary.

"In open or ulcerated cancers, or cancroid growths generally, especially if situated on the skin, the lips, the tongue, or the uterus, where the patient appears sinking from the local symptoms of the disease, such as frequent hemorrhages, profuse and fetid discharges, where also a great extent of surface is destroyed, caustics are generally preferable; and numerous cases of success might be quoted from my own practice, and from the authorities I have referred to in the course of this address, where caustics have brought about the cicatrization of cancerous ulcers, when all interference with the knife was utterly out of the question." Contrary to an opinion expressed on a former occasion, Mr. Parker is now of opinion that caustics are perfectly applicable to the treatment of cancer or cancroid of the tongue. Again, caustics are eminently useful in secondary cancerous formations.

Mr. Parker does not advocate the use of caustics to the exclusion of the knife, but he evidently thinks that caustics are more likely to secure the destruction of cancerous growths, and so to prevent the return of the disease, than is the knife. In reference to this point, Mr. Parker quotes M. Velpeau, who says, " I have frequently employed caustics in the treatment of cancer, and I have frequently thought, I must confess, that they have more certainly prevented secondary cancerous affections in the neighboring lymphatic glands than extirpation with the knife."—(p. 659). "I have twice seen," continues M. Velpeau, "voluminous and indurated glands in the axilla diminish in a remarkable degree, during the period I was destroying a cancer of the breast by caustics, and I have observed the same effect in the sub-maxillary glands, whilst cancers or cancroid diseases of the lower lip were treated in a similar manner. The action of caustics is chemical and destructive, and doubtless their action extends to some distance into the surrounding

* Dupuytren varied these proportions. The late Mr. Samuel Cooper said 4 parts of arsenious acid and 90 of calomel. The latter employed it with complete success.—("Surgical Dictionary," Article —"Arsenic."

tissues beyond the exact line where their destructive agency is defined on the skin." Again, "M. Lebert, a great authority on cancer, speaks of what he terms a compound operation in the removal of cancerous and cancroid diseases, and this practice is evidently again a recognition of the principle I have just indicated, which shows that it is difficult and even impossible to remove the disease by excision; and therefore he says, speaking of cancer of the skin, in which he not only sanctions, but recommends the employment of caustics, 'The combination of excision and cauterization frequently brings about results which we obtain with difficulty by either method employed separately.' What this means is clearly, that after the bulk of the disease has been removed by excision, the surface thus exposed is to be treated by escharotics, with a view of destroying the cancerous nuclei or cells, which may be infiltrated through, or in process of formation in the neighboring or immediate surrounding tissues."

In concluding this very admirable and instructive address, Mr. Parker says, "I esteem very highly the class of remedies I have been considering, and I think many lives may be saved, and will be saved, by their judicious employ. I have used these remedies in many cases with a gratifying and encouraging amount of success. They can be used where the knife cannot, and in relapsed cancer they are especially serviceable."

On the use of Auscultation in Aural Surgery. By M. GENDRIN.
(Gazette Medicale de Paris, Sept. 6, 1856.)

The following letter describes a new and apparently happy application of auscultation for the detection of deep-seated mischief in the organ of hearing. It is addressed to the President of the Academie des Sciences by M. Gendrin.

Sir,—I beg to call the attention of the Academy to a mode of investigating deep-seated mischief in the ear which I have often put in practice during the last ten years—namely, direct or indirect auscultation over the ear itself. I apply the ear or else the stethoscope to the ear, and listen to the sounds produced in the interior of the organ by breathing, coughing, speaking, whistling, &c., and from the abnormal modifications of these sounds I form an opinion as to the nature of the mischief present, if mischief there be.

In the natural condition each expiration produces in the ear a low, soft, and distant "bruit de souffle," which dies out before the end of the expiratory movement. If the drum of the ear be perforated this sound becomes acute, dry, sometimes even sibilant, and always more prolonged. Is the Eustachian tube contracted? In that case the respiratory sound becomes as it were intermitted, and in the majority of cases the passage of the air, through mucus contained in the tube or in the cavity of the ear, causes the bruit to be accompanied by crepitation. Crepitation is also heard if there be caries of any of the parts belonging to or communicating with the internal ear.

These expiratory sounds are rendered more marked by the shock of coughing.

Inspiration does not produce any obvious sonorous vibrations in the healthy ear. But if the drum is perforated, the tube being permeable, one hears in the ear during inspiration, a very acute souffle sibilant accompanied with hurried crepitation, of which the patient himself is frequently conscious.

The voice, as it sounds in the ear, is deepened in tone and somewhat vibrating; and the words, and sometimes the syllables, sound as if detached from each other. But if the tube is contracted, or if the cavities of the ear are filled with mucus or pus, or otherwise obliterated, the voice degenerates into a confused and inarticulate murmur. If the tube is altogether obstructed, the voice fails altogether to reach the ear. On the other hand, it is whistling, and accompanied by crepitating rales if the drum be defective.

In the healthy ear the sound of whistling is heard as an acute souffle sibilant coming from far. If the Eustachian tube is narrowed, this souffle is enfeebled and interrupted by intervals of silence; if the tube is obliterated the souffle is entirely extinguished. But in cases where the tube is open, and the drum defective, the whistling becomes very acute and close—it seems to the auscultator as if the patient whistled in his ear.

In the majority of cases it is easy to ascertain the reality of these abnormal sounds by listening at the other ear, for it rarely happens that both ears are affected to the same extent. I have the honor to be, &c.

Deligation of the Abdominal Aorta. By Mr. SOUTH, Senior Surgeon to St. Thomas's Hospital. ("Lancet," July 12th and August 23d.)

Unquestionably, the operation of tying this great vessel is one of appalling magnitude, and so rarely is it adopted that we may hail it as an event in the annals of surgery whenever it is done. This was the celebrated operation of Sir Astley Cooper, which in his day created an interest of the most intense kind in the mind of every surgeon. It has not hitherto been selected in the cases that have been recorded, unless as a last resource, and justified by the most trying and urgent circumstances. Sir Astley Cooper was the first surgeon who applied a ligature to the aorta in the living subject—upon a porter, aged 38 years, at Guy's Hospital, in 1817. This case will ever stand as one of the most remarkable in the annals of surgical science. His patient survived forty hours. He made an incision, three inches long, in the linea alba, giving it a slight curve to the left, to avoid the umbilicus; one inch and a half was above, and the remainder below the navel. The peritoneum was then cut through, and, by scratching with his nail at the root of the mesentery, he was enabled to insulate the artery and carry a thread round it.

A precisely similar operation was performed by Mr. James, of Exeter, whose patient survived three hours and a half. In a third example of ligature of this great vessel, at the Cape of Good Hope, Dr. Murray tied it, without opening the peritoneum, making his incision from the jutting extremity of the tenth rib, continuing it downwards about six inches, and curving backwards to an inch from the upper front of the hip-bone. The aorta was easily reached, the peritoneum being separated with the flat of his hand from the internal iliac and psoas muscles. His patient survived twenty-three hours after the operation. In the "Abstract," vol. XVII, a fourth case is recorded, the operation being performed at Rio Janeiro, by Dr. C. B. Monteiro, the patient surviving till the tenth day, when he died from secondary hemorrhage from a small opening on the left side of the vessel immediately above the ligature. Mr. South's makes the fifth case, with a survival of forty-three hours. Monteiro's case, therefore, was the most successful. Three out of the five have been done in England—the first and the last at the Borough hospitals, where the preparations are to be seen in their respective museums.

The following were the forms of aneurism in the five cases for which this formidable operation was attempted: 1. Aneurism extending four inches above and as many below Poupart's ligament; affecting the left iliac artery. 2. Aneurism of the external iliac artery. 3. Very extensive iliac aneurism. 4. Spurious aneurism of the femoral artery, formed by the bursting of that vessel; a large swelling occupying a great portion of the right under part of the belly. 5. Aneurism of the external and common iliac arteries, occupying a very considerable portion of the right half of the abdomen.

The late Mr. Guthrie held that it is quite unnecessary to tie the aorta in any case, because, in an aneurism of the external or internal iliac arteries, the common iliac on the diseased side can always be got at—and if not there, yet on the healthy side —for the purpose of carrying a ligature around it. In these views the late Samuel Cooper coincided with Mr. Guthrie. If these cases are analyzed, it will be found that this operation was justifiable in this instance, as in Mr. South's patient only did the tumor extend absolutely pretty close up to the bifurcation of the trunk of the aorta; and to so great a magnitude had it arrived, that it would have been next to impossible to have tied the common iliac above the aneurism. This can be seen by a careful examination of the specimen in the museum of St. Thomas's Hospital. Several consultations were held by Mr. South, with his colleagues, on the urgency of the case, and the question was anxiously considered as to the propriety of the operation, and we believe most, if not all, inclined towards giving the poor man the benefit of the operation. In Sir Astley's case, the operation was a sort of forlorn hope, because the patient was reduced to the very point of death by hemorrhage from an iliac aneurism. In Mr. South's, this was not so; but the symptoms were becoming so urgent from other causes, that a suddenly fatal result might at any moment occur; immediate interference, therefore, became a matter of actual necessity. It is hardly possible to expect a permanently successful result from the operation, but circumstances may arise to justify its performance; thus prolonging life for a few hours or days, and giving the patient a little time to settle his worldly affairs.

CASE.—On the 21st of June, Mr. South ligatured the trunk of the abdominal aorta, a little above its bifurcation, for a large aneurism of the external and common iliac arteries of the right side, in a strong, healthy, and apparently robust young man, aged twenty-eight years. The aneurismal tumor filled the right iliac and lumbar regions, and occupied a considerable portion of the right half of the abdomen, rising above the umbilicus, nearly as high up as the cartilages of the ribs, and extending close to the median line. Pulsation in the tumor could be felt with great difficulty, but by the stethoscope a very distinct aneurismal bruit could be heard; sensation was almost completely lost in the whole of the right leg, in consequence of the pressure exercised by the tumor on the nerves emerging from the pelvis on that side. The aneurism had existed for some months, and the young man had been an inmate of St. Thomas's Hospital for the past few weeks. The early history of the case was somewhat obscure, but he had been subject to employment of a very laborious and fatiguing kind. During his stay in the hospital it had increased rapidly in size, and was extending in every direction; it became necessary, therefore, to have recourse to surgical measures without delay. The question of tying the common iliac was discussed by Mr. South, Mr. Green, and his colleagues, Mr. Solly, Mr. Simon, and Mr. Le Gros Clark. The uncertainty as to whether the common iliac was involved, and also the difficulty of getting at it, from the large size of the tumor, induced Mr. South to select the operation of deligating the aorta, which was done with the assistance of his colleagues, in presence of a large number of students from the various London hospitals, and many eminent members of the profession.

The left side of the abdomen was opened by an incision, commencing a little above the anterior superior spinous process of the ilium, and extending upwards to the cartilage of the tenth rib. The various intervening structures were severally cut through until the peritoneum was reached, which membrane was carefully raised by Mr. Green with his hands, and the wound kept open, whilst Mr. South passed a ligature around the aorta, from the right to the left side. There was very little time lost in the performance of this highly important operation, which was effected in a very beautiful and satisfactory manner, in consequence of the extremely quiet condition of the patient, who was completely under the influence of chloroform.

This was done at two o'clock on Saturday, the 21st of June. The young man went on remarkably well after it; but he died at nine o'clock on the morning of Monday, the 23d, having survived the operation forty-three hours. At the autopsy, the tumor was found to be a false and diffused aneurism, depending upon disease of the coats of the iliac artery, with, we believe, laceration.

Varicose Veins; their nature, consequences, and treatment, palliative and curative. By HENRY T. CHAPMAN, formerly Surgeon in the St. George's and St. James's Dispensary. (12mo. Churchill, pp. 99. 1856.)

This monograph, for the most part, consists of a reprint of several papers, which have already appeared in the "Medical Times and Gazette." It is divided into two parts. In the first part, the author concerns himself in succession with the definition of varix, the structure and function of the saphenæ, the origin and progress of the morbid changes of structure in, and the consequences of varix; and under each of these heads he presents us with an abstract of the most authentic details we possess on the subject. As one of the causes of varix, we may mention in passing, much stress is laid upon inflammation of the venous tissues, and very properly so. Passages are cited from Hasse and Rokitansky which clearly specify dilatation as an ordinary result of phlebitis; and others which speak no less positively of chronic phlebitis as a consequence of dilatation. In Hasse's work, however, the admissions are only to be found under the head of "Chronic Phlebitis," and there is no allusion to the malady as occurring in the chapter treating of the causes of varix. Rokitansky, it is true, includes inflammation of the vein in his catalogue of the cause of phlebectasis; but he mentions it quite incidentally, as a possible source of the disease. Indeed, Mr. Chapman is the first to *call* attention to the intimate connection which exists between dilatation and inflammation of the venous walls.

In the second part of the monograph, the subject of treatment is very carefully considered, and any practitioner may learn a good deal from what is there presented to his notice. In this part, the author sets himself to show, in the first place, that varix is not to be cured by obliterating the diseased vein; and after this he proceeds to speak of palliative and curative measures, the end of the argument being to show that the best means of curing varix is by wet strapping and bandaging. Plaste strapping is objected to as apt to heat, inflame, and excoriate the parts to which it is applied. Then (speaking of the curative treatment of simple uniform varix) the author says:

"I have for some years entirely abandoned plaster-strapping, in the treatment both of ulcers and of varicose veins, in favor of the following very simply constructed bandage, which possesses all the advantages of plaster-strapping without its inconveniences:

"Placing the patient on a low seat, and elevating the foot until the veins empty themselves by the gravitation of the blood towards the trunk, I apply wet straps of linen, or calico, precisely in the same manner as Mr. Scott applied adhesive plaster. The bands for this purpose should be from two to three inches in width, and from twelve to sixteen in length, stout enough to prevent them tearing easily, but not too thick. Adjusting the middle of one of the shorter and narrower of these bands, previously soaked in water, just above the heel, the two ends are brought forward over the ankles, drawn tightly, and crossed upon the instep. The middle of another is placed beneath the sole of the foot, its extremities brought up firmly over the instep, and laid down smoothly one upon the other. A third is applied, like the first, from behind forwards, but a little higher; and thus, ascending the leg, the process is repeated with the rest of the bands, each one in succession overlapping the upper half of that below it, until the limb is firmly and evenly cased to the knee. Over the straps a calico roller is carefully put on, the greatest attention being paid to its equable adjustment, so that the pressure may be uniformly distributed over the entire limb.

"Through its texture the course of the varicose veins should be moistened several times daily with cold water, diluted Goulard lotion, or solutions of alum, sulphate of zinc, or chloride of lime. Whenever the bandage is taken off for renewal, the dilated veins should be subjected to brisk friction, upwards, with the hand for some time, and a douche of cold water poured over them, the foot being kept in an elevated position until it is re-applied. In winter, and when patients are elderly, or delicate, the free application of cold water or lotions is not always safe, and this part of the treatment must of course be left to the discretion of the surgeon. It is better, under such circumstances, to confine the astringent influence of cold strictly to the vessels affected.*

"No one who has not tried this mode of bandaging can form an estimate of the power of adhesion possessed by the wet strapping, or the amount of steady, even support it is capable of affording. In these respects—as I have elsewhere stated, when advocating their employment in the treatment of ulcers and cutaneous eruptions on the leg—their action is in no degree inferior to that of plaster, at the same time that the softness of the material allows of its closer adaptation to the inequalities of the limb, and precludes all risk of cutting or excoriation, accidents so common when plaster-strapping is made use of, that its contact could never be borne long enough to produce any permanently good effect.

"The wet straps are especially serviceable in compressing the bulk of the soft parts before the application of the roller, and they give the latter a much better hold than it can take of the bare skin, or even of plaster, thus materially diminishing the chance of the roller slipping. Their greater permeability, again, admits of the more efficient use of lotions; and their cheapness, when compared with diachylon, or any other kind of plaster, is no slight recommendation. Unless displacement of its turns should occur earlier, or uneasiness be felt at any point, if the skin be sound the bandage need not be renewed before the fourth, fifth, or sixth day of its application: indeed I have frequently left it undisturbed for a fortnight or three weeks.

"In cold weather a flannel roller is preferable to one of calico in all respects. It is quite as elastic as Churton's cotton-web bandage, supports the veins more firmly and comfortably, and is not liable to rope. In summer, or with patients who find both flannel and calico heating, I employ rollers of coarse mull muslin, which are light and cool, and give as much support as calico.

"Although an elastic stocking, employed alone, may sometimes arrest the progress of varix in its earlier stages, it can never be regarded as a curative measure.

* A curious fact, mentioned by M. Parent Duchatelet, in his paper on the health of the "Débardeurs" of the Seine ("Annales d'Hygiène publique," t. iii), practically exemplifies the astringent influence of cold in maintaining the contractility of the venous tissues. Inquiring how far this class of workmen—whose legs are plunged in water for many hours daily—were subject to ulcer, he ascertained that, contrary to the general belief, they were not only unusually exempt from that troublesome complaint, but their lower extremities were also remarkably free from varicosities, œdema, and swelling.

In fact, the heating properties of the material rather augment the tendency to dilatation; and as the ordinary pressure exercised by it but partially empties the veins of blood, lateral expansion in a saccular or serpentine form will often go on beneath the stocking. When combined, however, with wet strapping, its efficiency is very considerably enhanced. But in order to derive the full advantage from this combination, the dimensions of the leg, for the stocking, must be taken after the wet strapping has been worn for some days, and the limb has been reduced a trifle below its natural size. Patients, accordingly, who are unable, or who will not take the trouble, to bandage a varicose leg in the manner set forth above, may adopt the alternative of an elastic stocking drawn on over a casing of wet strapping."

Afterwards, when speaking of the curative treatment of saccular, vesicular, and serpentine varix, the author adds:

" In cases of long standing and more aggravated character, where great tortuosity, saccular expansions of the main trunk and larger branches (numerous clusters often sprouting from these latter), and vesicular enlargements of the cutaneous veins exist, the support, distributed over the general surface of the limb by the wet straps and bandage alone, not entirely emptying the diseased veins, will do little more than palliate the complaint.

" To direct the pressure, therefore, effectually upon those points where it is most called for, I have recourse to compresses of lint, or spongiopiline, in combination with the bandage, large enough to cover the chief clusters and each of the sacculated portions of the vein separately, and thick enough to close their channels. These compresses, moistened in cold water or astringent lotions, are placed on the most salient dilatations, and the straps and bandage carried over them. Many of the varicosities rapidly disappear; others require the maintenance of the compression for a longer period; and in serpentine varix, especially, the process of reduction is occasionally very tedious.

" In saccular expansion and mulberry-like vesicular clusters in the skin, I seldom rely, for the completion of the cure, on the mere diversion of the circulation into other channels. Taking advantage of the known tendency of the lining membrane of the veins to adhesive inflammation, I endeavor to obliterate all lateral pouches, and vesicular protrusions through the skin, by submitting them to a high degree of pressure, so as to maintain their opposite surfaces forcibly in contact,—no 'very difficult matter when they happen to be situated over a bone; but when they lie upon the soft parts of the calf, as is most frequently the case, they recede beneath the pressure of the ordinary compresses, and require some more unyielding substance to close their cavities entirely. To meet this difficulty, I make use of the leather cones with which billiard cues are tipped, or smooth wooden or ivory buttons, choosing a size corresponding with that of the varicose pouch; and, for the blue cutaneous vesicles, glass or porcelain shirt-studs. The former are readily retained *in situ* by lint compresses and the bandage; the latter I insert into a small slit or button-hole in one of the wet straps, and carefully adjust it to the pit in the integument through which the vesicle has protruded; and, either by producing cohesion of their entire walls, or closure of the narrow neck connecting them with the vein, and coagulation of their contents, I generally succeed, ere long, in effacing both large and small cells.

" Whether the saphena in the thigh, as well as the branches below the knee, are diseased, the pressure from within upon the walls of the latter will be more than doubled by the superadded weight of the column of blood in the former. Until this dilating force from above be neutralized, no rational expectation of permanently reducing the enlarged veins to their natural size can be entertained. At the same time, therefore, that the several remedial measures described above are brought to bear upon the yielding branches, the dilated trunk ought also to be effectually supported. As, however, it is not possible, by any form of bandage, to exercise the same degree of equable compression upon the veins of the thigh as on those of the leg, I never attempt to carry the wet straps and roller above the knee; but, leaving them to counteract all undue accumulation below, I trust to Mr. Startin's elastic riband, wound spirally round the thigh from the knee to the groin, to divide the column of blood in the dilated trunk, and take off its downward pressure upon the branches; and I have more than once had occasion to observe that, by the time the veins of the leg are restored to a healthy condition, the dilatation of those of the thigh has, likewise, materially diminished."

These remarks are illustrated by some instructive cases.

III.

REPORT ON THE PROGRESS OF MIDWIFERY AND THE DISEASES OF WOMEN AND CHILDREN.

On the duration of Pregnancy, and the calculation of the date of Confinement. Is Dr. William Harvey or Dr. William Montgomery in the right? By J. MAT-THEWS DUNCAN, M.D. ("The Edinburgh Medical Journal," Nov., 1856.)

DR. DUNCAN's object in this article is to defend the opinions of Harvey, to re-affirm the conclusions at which he arrived in 1854 (*vide* "Abstract," XIX), on the ground of the data afforded by Dr. Montgomery, and to show that Dr. Montgomery's assumption of 280 days as the natural period of human gestation is, to say the least, unfounded.

The duration of pregnancy.—The period generally recognized under this name, and discussed by Dr. Montgomery, does not measure the real duration which extends from conception to parturition, but that other period extending from fruitful connection to parturition. It is this latter of which we now discourse.

Dr. Montgomery describes the natural period of human gestation as 280 days. Now, there is no such thing known to obstetricians to exist in nature, as a natural period of pregnancy, measuring a certain number of days. This interval between fruitful coitus and parturition, is known to us only as a variable period, of uncertain length, in different individuals, and in the same individual on different occasions. So far is Dr. Montgomery from having any authority for fixing 280 days as the natural period, that, in his own laborious collection of fifty-six cases, in which, he says, the day of fruitful intercourse was known, there are only four in which parturition certainly occurred on the 280th day. Obstetricians can only speak with propriety of an average duration. This is attainable by striking it from the largest collection of well-ascertained cases. This average is the nearest approximation that can be made to what may be called the natural period of gestation. The data afforded by Dr. Montgomery for arriving at this mean or average, or nearest accurate general statement of the interval between fruitful connection and parturition, the duration of pregnancy, are of different degrees of value.

The most trustworthy and valuable are undoubtedly those of a pregnancy which dates from a single coitus. They number twenty-five, and the duration of each is as follows :—263, 264, 265, 265, 267, 270, 271, 272, 273, 274, 274, 274, 274, 274, 275, 275, 276, 276, 275 or 277, 277, 278, 280, 280, 287, 291 to 293. Of these twenty-five cases the mean is 274 days. The best data accessible to Dr. Montgomery, then, give 274 days as the duration of pregnancy, not 280.

It appears that the next most valuable data for settling this point are to be found in the table of thirteen cases dating from the day of marriage. The interval between marriage and parturition in each of these cases was as follows :—261, 265, 268, 269, 270, 270, 271, 271, 271, 272, 273, 274, 279, 291. In regard to these, Dr. Montgomery himself says :—"The average interval between the day of marriage and that of labor was 272 days q. p., or thirty-nine weeks, minus one day; or, if we deduct the last case, which went to 291 days, the average interval would be 270½ days." Where, then, one naturally exclaims, are the grounds for saying that the natural duration of pregnancy is 280 days?

Dr. Montgomery's work presents us with another table of data. It consists of fifty-six cases, in which, he says, the day of fruitful intercourse was known. Now, to us, this table, at first sight, and before estimating the results of it, appeared to be of less value than either of the two former. Every case, almost, is invalidated, because we do not know the authority or grounds upon which it is said that the day of fruitful intercourse was known. We do not know even the observers' names. Dr. Montgomery has laboriously collected cases of protracted pregnancy, all of which, so far as available for this table, find place in it. The whole weight and importance of it is contributed by the distinguished obstetrician's name that publishes it. That authority is, undoubtedly, of the very highest, but can scarcely be communicable to cases derived from a promiscuous set of observers, whose reasons for decidedly fixing on a single day are not given. In an exact investigation like this, all cases should be rejected except those dating from a single coitus, or coitus on a single day. But let us examine and see what this table affords towards the solution of our question. Omitting six cases where a single day is not given, we have fifty where the interval between fruitful intercourse and parturition is said to be as follows :—242, 258, 258, 263, 265, 267, 267, 267, 267, 268, 269, 269, 272, 273, 273, 274, 274, 275, 275, 276, 277, 277, 278, 278, 279, 279, 279, 279, 279, 280, 280, 280, 280, 281, 283, 283, 284, 285, 286, 287, 287, 287, 288, 290, 291, 291, 292, 293, 293, 297. Of these fifty cases, all those satisfactorily known to Dr. Montgomery, the mean duration is 277 days. This table, framed under the conditions above described, yields a result opposed to the dogma of its author. Where, then, is the authority for stating 280 days as the natural period of gestation ? It is nowhere.

We agree with Dr. Montgomery in his opinion that there is no other satisfactory method of arriving at the solution of this question, but the one we have just followed, viz., the collection of well-ascertained facts, and their analysis. "Independently," says he, " of the very few cases in which we have satisfactory evidence of conception following casual intercourse, or perhaps a single coitus, we have no certain means of knowing exactly the commencement of gestation, and are obliged to form our calculation on one or other of three very fallacious grounds; which he then proceeds to consider."

The calculation of the day of confinement.—In the vast majority of cases this must be made from the termination of the last menstruation, for reasons which are well known. The average time to which a woman goes, after the last appearance of the menses, is 278 days (a period shorter than Dr. Montgomery's duration of pregnancy!) This average is obtained by the collection of single observations, and their subsequent analysis. If, then, we wish to ascertain the most probable day of a woman's confinement, we add 278 days to the last day of the last menstruation.

Dr. Montgomery gives no specific directions for making this important calculation. But it appears, from some passages occurring incidentally in his essay, that he adopts the following plan. Some day is selected after the last menstruation, as the most probable day of fruitful intercourse, and 280 days are added thereto. As the selection of this day must be, in almost every case, made on the most worthless and insufficient grounds, the resulting calculation must be similarly characterized. Besides, if there be any truth in the statistical data of Dr. Montgomery, and their analysis given above, which is partly his own, then this plan of his must lead to a putting off of the probable day of confinement to far too distant a time. For instance, we have in the table of observations dated from the day of marriage, thirteen cases on Dr. Montgomery's own authority. Now, in these, as already stated, the women went, on an average, only 272 days from the day of the nuptials. If a probable day of fruitful intercourse, after marriage, had been selected, and 280 days added thereto, in these cases, such a plan would have evidently led to a mass of errors in the way of putting off the predicted day of confinement far too long.

With the subject of this important calculation or prediction, Dr. Montgomery has confounded the question of the interval between insemination and conception. If such an interval existed, he says, "we should have no means of calculating the period of gestation with anything like an approximation to accuracy in any case." Now, if there be an interval in nature between insemination and conception, we must adopt it, whatever results it may lead to. If it truly exist, it can lead only to true and good results. It is not considered probable by Dr. Montgomery that any interval, or an interval of any importance, does exist. The highest authorities, however, on such a point, are unquestionably very strongly in favor of the belief in its

existence, and its being of considerable extent, say several days. But, in truth, this
question of a possible interval between insemination and conception has nought to do
with the calculation of the date of confinement. Its truth or untruth does not affect
such calculations, and no author but Dr. Montgomery, has, so far as Dr. Duncan
knows, discussed the two points as connected with one another in any way tending
to modify practical precepts.

Harvey's opinions.—Great men often seem to arrive at the truth, even in circumstances of complication and difficulty, by some process so simple that it appears like
an operation of instinct. The immortal Harvey's expressed opinions in regard to
the duration of pregnancy, and the calculation of the day of confinement, bear this
character, for we cannot discover the grounds on which he arrived at results so nearly
identical with those of modern science.

The interval between the festival of the Annunciation and the day of the Blessed
Nativity is that adopted by Harvey, as unquestionably the ordinary term of utero-
gestation. This is a period of 275 days, lady-day, or the festival of the Annunciation,
being on the 25th of March, or 80th day of the year, while the day of the Nativity
is the 25th of December, or 360th day of the year. It is remarkable, that the largest
recent collection of cases, made on certain or on the best grounds, gave also an
average result of 275 days. Harvey, it will be observed, does not speak of any
natural term, but only of the ordinary term, his correct appreciation of which is
clearly indicated.

Harvey guards, also, his rule for calculating the day of confinement from being
considered exact, by saying that those prudent matrons who follow it " are rarely
out of their reckoning." His statement is, that after ten lunar months have elapsed
from the commencement or appearance of last menstruation, they fall in labor the
very day the catamenia would have appeared had impregnation not taken place.
If the usual or average computation of the menstrual periods and intervals is
adopted, the period of Harvey is 280 days, including the number of days of the last
period. Ten times the usual interval and period of discharge, that is, ten times 28,
gives 280 days ; but as this includes the last period, of course the three, four, or
five days of that period have to be taken from the 280 days, if we wish to find the
interval he allowed between the end of last menses and parturition. Thus, Harvey
gives prudent matrons only an approximative calculation. The interval between
last menstruation and parturition, according to him, is something, a few days, less
than 280. The averge time found by modern calculations, as stated in an early
part of this paper, is 278 days, with which Harvey's rules are as nearly in accordance as can be expected in a subject altogether incapable of any exact statement.

Lectures on the Diseases of Women. By CHARLES WEST, M.D., F.R.C.S., Physician
   Accoucheur to St. Bartholomew's Hospital, Examiner in Midwifery to the Royal
   College of Surgeons of England, &c. Part I. Diseases of the Uterus. (8vo. Lon-
   don, Churchill, pp. 306. 1856.)

These lectures, Dr. West tells us, are a first instalment towards the discharge of
a debt which the opportunities of a hospital, and the responsibilities of a teacher
have imposed upon him, and as such they demand our careful consideration.

Passing over the first five lectures, then, which are devoted to diseases of menstruation, and which, though useful to medical students, contain nothing but what
all well-informed practitioners are acquainted with, we come to three lectures on
inflammation and ulceration of the womb ; six, on uterine displacements ; four, on
uterine fibrous tumors, and three (the last) on malignant uterine diseases. Now, as
the profession is pretty nearly united on the subject of cancerous complaints, we
shall not refer to that portion of Dr. West's work, nor to that on uterine tumors,
upon which opinions and practice are but little divided ; and we shall reserve our
space for two important subjects, upon which the profession is divided by conflicting
testimony,—uterine inflammation and uterine displacements.

One of our distinguished pathologists is gifted with so keen a power of vision,
that he can detect ganglia and nerves which are concealed from the view of other
anatomists, but whose sight seems to fail him when looking at the neck of the womb,
inasmuch as he affirms having never noticed any ulceration there, that was not
either syphilitic or scrofulous. But this is not the case with Dr. West, who finds

uterine lesions to be so frequent, that he considers them of comparatively little moment. The result of his experience on this point is set forth in the following table:

TABLE,

Showing the chief Results of the Examination of Sixty-five Uteri.

Uterus healthy in	36
" diseased in	29

Ulceration of os uteri in		17
" existed alone in	11	
" with diseased lining of uterus in . .	3	
" with induration of walls of uterus in .	3——17	
Induration of walls of uterus, without ulceration of os .		5
Disease of lining of uterus, without ulceration of os .		7

Total of diseased uteri, . . .	29

Dr. West's conclusions respecting the pathological import of uterine lesions are thus given:

"1st. Uterine pain, menstrual disorder, and leucorrhœal discharges—the symptoms ordinarily attributed to ulceration of the os uteri—are met with independently of that condition almost as often as in connection with it.

"2d. These symptoms are observed in both classes of cases with a vastly preponderating frequency at the time of the greatest vigor of the sexual functions, and no cause has so great a share in their production as the different incidents connected with the active exercise of the reproductive powers. But it does not appear that ulceration of the os uteri exerts any special influence either in causing sterility or in inducing abortion.

"3d. While the symptoms are identical in character in the two classes of cases, they seem to present a slightly increased degree of intensity in those cases in which ulceration of the os uteri exists.

"4th. In as far as could be ascertained by careful examination, four-fifths of the cases of either class presented appreciable changes in the condition of the uterus—such as misplacement, enlargement, and hardening of its tissue, while frequently several of these conditions coexisted. An indurated and hypertrophied state of the cervix uteri was, however, more frequent in connection with ulceration of the os uteri than independently of that condition.

"5th. The inference, however, to which the last-mentioned fact would seem to lead, as to the existence of some necessary relation—such as that of cause and effect—between ulceration of the os uteri and induration of its cervix, is in a great measure negatived by two circumstances.

"1. That in numerous instances an indurated cervix coexisted with a healthy os uteri.

"2. That while in many of the cases in which induration of the cervix existed, the ulceration of the os was very slight, induration was entirely absent in other instances where the ulceration was noticed as having been very extensive.

"Since, then, we find that a very great degree of resemblance exists between the two classes of cases; that women of the same age, in similar circumstances, present the same symptoms, leading to the same results, having the same duration, and attended with similar structural changes, whether ulceration of the os uteri is present or absent; it may fairly be inferred, that ulceration of the womb is neither a general cause of uterine disease, nor a trustworthy index of its progress; and it follows, I think, as a necessary corollary, that the endeavor by local remedies to remove this condition of the os is not the all-important object in the treatment of uterine disease, which the teaching and the practice of some physicians would lead us to imagine."

It seems to us that, as usual, when statistics are called in aid of medicine, great confusion lurks under an appearance of precision. There is no distinction made between the various degrees of ulceration of the neck of the womb, which is spoken of as one and the same pathological entity, and this absence of indispensable distinctions vitiates alike both Dr. West's statistics and his conclusions. That *slight* morbid lesions, such as erosions and superficial ulcerations of the neck of the womb, are generally of little moment, are of frequent occurrence, and are cured by nature alone, or aided by rest and constitutional measures, we agree with Dr. West; but should he pretend that *severe* lesions, deep or extensive ulcerations of the neck of the womb, do not produce most distressing, varied, and pertinacious symptoms,— symptoms ineffectually relieved by the best-directed constitutional measures, yielding, on the contrary, either to local treatment adopted alone, or to surgical treatment combined with constitutional measures, then we can only express our surprise, and leave the ultimate decision of this important question to the experience of future observers. Many pages are devoted to the consideration of the importance of uterine lesions, and the argument is conducted in a manner suggestive of comment. Struck by the fact that of late uterine polemics have degenerated into scurrilities, Dr. West has thought it advisable to differ in opinion with no individual authors, but he is strongly opposed to "some authors," to "some writers," &c. Does Dr. West allude to Dr. E. Kennedy, or Dr. F. Churchill, or to Mr. Whitehead, Dr. Murphy, Dr. Tilt, or Dr. Oldham? None of these gentlemen are called in question, but simply Dr. H. Bennet, whose book he has constantly in view, whose views he attacks, and whose statistics he even quotes, without once mentioning his name, except in a foot-note. Dr. West knows full well that, while all the distinguished practitioners, whose names we have cited, believe in the fatal effects of severe ulceration of the neck of the womb, none would be willing completely to adopt Dr. Bennet's opinion, nor his loosely expressed estimation of the frequency of uterine disease.

After perusing many pages, wherein the influence of uterine lesions in raking up constitutional diseases is sometimes admitted, as at page 114, and afterwards denied: after finding nitrate of silver objected to as being too weak an application, and potassa fusa c. calce, because it was too strong, we were agreeably surprised, on coming to the treatment, to find pages that might have been written by Dr. Bennet or Dr. Tilt, so judicious and numerous are the local modes of treatment recommended for the cure of uterine ulcerations. Thus does Dr. West's previous skirmishing not interfere with his practice; and, although, at page 126, the supposed perpetuation of uterine disease by local treatment is forcibly insisted on, he, nevertheless, recommends many plans of surgical treatment, with an inconsistency we willingly pardon. In like manner, at page 128, Dr. West is eloquent on the disadvantages of potassa fusa c. calce, but, when descending from the cloudy regions of discussion, he comes to treatment, he admits that strong caustics are sometimes required, and gives the preference to the acid nitrate of mercury.

It is so satisfactory to find authorities agreeing upon important practical points, that we willingly pass over this discrepancy between Dr. West's theory and his practice; but as he finds it sometimes necessary to cauterize ulcerations with the acid nitrate of mercury, it would have been well had he said something about the application of potassa fusa c. calce to deep and chronic ulcerations of the neck of the womb, for at page 129, he has merely spoken of it as a tissue-destroyer in chronic uterine induration. For the speedy cure of these lesions we know of no better application than its superficial cauterization with the potassa fusa c. calce. Has Dr. West tried it? and, if so, in how many cases, and with what results? A little statistical information on so important a point would not have been amiss. With regard to the treatment of uterine disease, Dr. West's observations, although judicious, present no novelty.

"The chapters on displacements of the womb are, perhaps, the best in the book. Dr. West shows himself well acquainted with what has been written on the subject by German and French, as well as by our own authors, and his materials are lucidly arranged. He is a decided opponent of Dr. Simpson's views on this point, and completely adopts the views long ago advocated by Dr. H. Bennet and Dr. Tilt, that deviations are, of themselves, harmless, though they forcibly attract attention on account of the uterine swelling, ulceration, or neuralgia by which they are accompanied; and with them and many French authorities, Dr. West believes that the principal indication of the treatment of deviations is to treat their complications. At page 122, Dr. West has briefly traced the rise and progress of the stem pessary, and at page 224, we find the following excellent reasons for neglecting its use.

"1st. The safe employment of the instrument requires that, as a general rule, its use should be continued for only a few hours at a time; a necessity which implies that every woman who is submitted to this mode of treatment shall undergo two vaginal examinations every day, the one for the introduction of the instrument, and the other for its withdrawal.

"2d. The quietude which its use imposes, and the restrictions to which the patient is compelled to submit in order to avoid severe suffering and the risk of serious danger, are at least as absolute in their kind, and as irksome to be borne, as those which any other mode of treatment involves, while it is necessary to continue them for as long a time.

"3d. In spite of all precautions, the treatment is generally painful, often dangerous, sometimes fatal; and the untoward accidents have not been by any means constantly attributable to want of prudence, either on the part of the practitioner or of his patient.

"4th. Cure, even by the long-continued employment of this means for several months, is uncertain, while relapses are very frequent after the mechanical support is discontinued; besides which the permanent cure of the misplacement is far from being always followed by the cessation of the symptoms."

These conclusions are certainly temperate, if Dr. Tilt be correct in his enumeration of the many fatal cases which are known to have occurred to women in the prime of life, from the use of the stem pessary at home and abroad, which will be found at page 259 of our last volume. This is a question of great importance, and it is deeply to be deplored that Dr. Simpson will not help to bring it to a satisfactory settlement. When the stem pessary was the subject of protracted discussion in the French Academy of Medicine, Dr. Depaul, the reporter of the commission, stated that he had written to Dr. Simpson asking him for cases, but that he had only received instruments; and when Dr. Simpson's papers were lately collected, under his supervision, by two of his own pupils and friends, he did not enable them to give the full results of his late as well as of his early experience of the dangers attending the use of the stem pessary. Dr. Simpson must be aware that the uterine stem pessary has fallen into disrepute in Germany, has been severely condemned in France, has never received the countenance of the profession in England, and that its value has even been strongly contested in Scotland; his silence, therefore, on the subject, ill becomes the midwifery professor of the Edinburgh University.

We regret that our space will not permit us to quote more largely from Dr. West's work, but we recommend it as one well calculated to give the student an insight into the literature of diseases of women, and we gladly enrol the author amongst the chosen band who are arduously endeavoring to advance our knowledge in such an important branch of medicine.

Records of Obstetric Consultation Practice; and a Translation of Busch and Moser on Uterine Hemorrhage (with notes and cases). By EDWARD COPEMAN, M.D., F.R.C.S., Physician to the Norfolk and Norwich Hospital, &c. (London, Churchill, 12mo., 1856, pp. 223.)

Dr. Copeman's object in publishing these "Records" is to convey a few practical exemplifications of certain subjects, rather than to enter into minute descriptions of them. Puerperal fever, the use of the vectis, the induction of premature labor, puerperal convulsions, and craniotomy, are the subjects occupying the first part; an essay on uterine hemorrhage, translated from Busch and Moser's "Handbuch der Geburtskunde," with additional notes and cases, forms the subject of the second part; while a case of placenta prævia and a case of fibrous tumor of the uterus, treated successfully, are added in an appendix. Such are the important subjects upon which Dr. Copeman has written in a manner which cannot fail to convey much sound information to all engaged in the arduous duties of obstetric practice.

For our own part, we are especially struck with what Dr. Copeman says upon the use of the vectis, and on the induction of premature labor; and it is to these points that we are wishful to direct the attention of our readers.

Of all the instruments employed in midwifery, Dr. Copeman believes the vectis to be the safest and most convenient, as well as the most efficient and the most general in its range of application, being applicable, not only to cases in which the short forceps are available, but also to such as require the long-forceps, and even to some in which no forceps could be used; and this belief is supported by the cases which are given.

"The instrument I have been in the habit of using," says Dr. Copeman, "and which I strongly recommend as being adapted to almost every variety of case requiring its employment, is 4½ inches long in the handle, and 8½ inches in the blade when straight; but the distance from the handle to the end of the blade when the proper curve has been made is 7½ inches. The fenestra begins at 4¾ inches from the handle, and there the blade is flattened, and 1¼ inch wide. The fenestra is ⅛ of an inch wide at its commencement, 1¼ inch across its middle, and a little wider than this nearer the end of the instrument, the widest part of the instrument being 2¼ inches, and that being about an inch from the end. The flattened iron border surrounding the fenestra is seven-sixteenths of an inch. The shaft of the instrument is round to the distance of 2¼ inches from the handle, and is then gradually bevelled off to the commencement of the fenestra, where the iron is about three-sixteenths of an inch thick at the inner border, and a little less at its outer margin, both being carefully rounded off. The round part of the shaft is rather more than an inch in circumference.

"The advantage of the peculiar curve of this instrument is, that it is sufficient to make a very effectual and powerful *hook*, and yet it is of a shape that will *fit* almost any part of the child's head; by which I mean that it can be kept in close contact with the child's head on whatever part it might be thought necessary to apply it; whereas, if it were a straighter instrument, it would either slip off the head, or must be used as a *lever* instead of a hook. which I think extremely objectionable; and if the curve were greater or more circular, it would be impossible to get so much of the instrument in close contact with the head; it would not have so much *bearing* upon the head, but would press upon it unequally, and require, therefore, more actual tractile force to obtain the same influence upon the head itself; because, of course, the greater the extent to which the blade is closely applied to the head, the greater mechanical power it will have to move it, and the less danger there will be of the force applied acting injuriously upon any one individual portion of the child's head.

"Its peculiar length also gives it advantages over many that I have seen, in not being too great to admit of the handle being a fixture; if the handle goes to screw on, it may be rather more convenient for the pocket, but more preparation is required to use it; and should it happen that the handle is by accident left at home (which I have known the case) the instrument might as well have been left too; and if, as in many I have seen, the handle has a hinge and button, it does not possess the necessary degree of firmness for satisfactory manipulation; for any movement or sound produced by the handle interferes with the delicacy of the sense of touch, and might confuse the operator. The instrument I have described is long enough and firm enough for every purpose for which it can be required, and yet not too long to be easy of application. Another advantage it possesses is the width of the blade, both as regards the whole instrument and also the flat margin around the fenestra; in both respects it is wider than usual, and therefore has a bearing over a larger extent of the child's head, making it less likely to press injuriously upon any particular point. I need scarcely observe that it should be well tempered, so as not to *give*, or alter its curve, during traction.

"In almost every notice of the vectis I have been able to find in books, it has met with no small share of abuse, not so much for any positive harm it has done as for being an inefficient and useless instrument; but the reason for this I have discovered to be, that those who have described it have not understood fully how to employ it, and have based their objections upon false views of its mechanical power and mode of operation. For instance, Baudelocque has written a long article upon the subject in depreciation of the instrument, and describes the manner of using it in a way that proves him to have been entirely ignorant of the principles which ought to guide its employment, of the nature of the mechanical power it ought to be made to exercise, and of the cases for which such an instrument as I describe is appropriate. It has been almost universally described as a lever of the first order, the child's head being the weight, the mother's pelvis, especially the arch of the pubes, the fulcrum, and the surgeon's hand the power; a mode of using it which I do not hesitate to say is far from safe, and which in but very few cases would, even if safe, be found successful. The mechanical power of the vectis I use, is that of a hook, so to speak,—that is to say, the blade should be passed so much over the head as to lie principally *behind* the part on which it is destined to act, and the principal moving power is that of *traction*: it is true, however, that simple traction might sometimes, perhaps often, cause some displacement of the instrument; and therefore something additional is required to keep it in its place, and this is a kind of pressure on the handle which keeps the blade in close proximity with the head, without making any part of the mother a fulcrum; a pressure, in fact, with the hand such as would be used were we attempting to bend the handle backwards upon the shaft or shank of the instrument, and a gradual elevation of the handle as the head descends in the pelvis. In fact, it ought to be used in much the same manner as the surgeon would employ his hand for the same purpose were there room to introduce it.

"By such a management of the vectis, the soft parts of the mother have to bear scarcely any more pressure than they must necessarily undergo during the passage of the child's head; the only difference being the thickness of the blade lying in close contact with the scalp; and this slight addition to the size of what has to pass through the pelvis is very amply compensated for by the much shorter time the parts have to suffer the pressure upon them. The child's head has, however, to bear the pressure of the instrument, and is not unfrequently a little marked by it; but this ought never to occur to any serious extent, and I have frequently seen the head more injured by the forceps than I have by the vectis. The occurrence of ruptured perinæum during the employment of the vectis is very rare indeed, and the reason is sufficiently obvious; for whatever dilating influence the vectis exercises upon the perineum is made *indirectly* through the medium of the globular head of the child, which is the *natural* mode of dilating it; whereas by using Assalini's forceps, the perineum is often put very much upon the stretch by the handles of the instrument, before it is touched by the head; and this pressure being exerted on two points only of its circumference, it is placed in circumstances the most favorable to rupture, and accordingly it is sometimes thus lacerated. The most essential pre-requisite in using the vectis (and the same may be said of every other instrument employed in midwifery) is a thorough knowledge of the position of the child's head, and of the direction to be given to it in order to facilitate in the greatest degree its expulsion or passage through the pelvis: there is no certain or invariable rule as to what part of the head it should be fixed upon; sometimes it should be the occiput, sometimes the brow, or the mastoid process, or the chin; and this is to be determined by the knowledge of the accoucheur as to the particular direction in which the head will most easily pass. It cannot be too strongly urged upon those who may be called upon to operate in midwifery, to make themselves thoroughly acquainted with the presentations of the head, and so to educate their sense of touch as to be able to determine, with as much certainty as possible, the points with which the finger during examination comes in contact, as well as the exact position in which the head in each case is placed. This, indeed, should be accurately made out in *every* case, whether natural or otherwise, for by constant practice it becomes easy; whereas if common cases are neglected because they are natural and will do well of themselves, and no preciseness of examination is attempted except where obstructions occur, it will be found exceedingly difficult to command, at once, a sufficient degree of tactile discrimination to ascertain with certainty what it will then be so desirable to know. I believe many of the failures attendant upon the use of the vectis arise from want of this precise knowledge of the position of the impacted head; and without it I feel sure no one can become an adept in the use of the instrument."

When speaking of the induction of premature labor, Dr. Copeman introduces the cases of two patients, in whom uterine contraction was induced by a method not usually adopted, but which appears to have several points to recommend it. This method arose out of the difficulty experienced, in the first case, in attempts to rupture the membranes. In this case the uterus was so high, that it was difficult to direct an instrument into it by the finger; and when the tube was passed in, it could not be made to rupture the membranes. The issue, however, proved that this was not necessary, and afterwards it was not attempted; for if the passing an œsophagus bougie or tube a distance into the uterus, between its inner wall and the chorion, will so disturb pregnancy as to induce labor, there is a very manifest advantage both to the child and the mother in resorting to this plan in preference to that of rupturing the membranes.

Case 1.—"March 5th, 1851.—Mrs. B—, æt. 36 years. The patient, it is estimated, is gone seven months and a week in her fifth pregnancy, and in consequence of her last three labors having proved destructive to the children from want of pelvic space, and the first, although a small child, requiring the use of the forceps, I met my friend Mr. — for the purpose of inducing premature labor. We found the external parts relaxed but very tender, and the pelvic arch too small to admit of the introduction of the hand. The os uteri was too high up to be reached satisfactorily by the finger; I could, however, just reach it with my middle finger, and introduce through it a flexible metallic bougie some way into the uterus, but without rupturing the membranes; so that it probably passed between them and the uterus, and it gave no pain in its introduction. We then agreed to wait awhile for the result of this proceeding, prescribing castor oil, rest, and warm fomentations to the external parts.

"6th.—Our proceedings yesterday were followed by no result, and to-day, with the aid of a speculum, I introduced a stomach pump tube easily several inches into the uterus, but could not rupture the membranes; it must, however, have separated them considerably from one side at least of the uterus, and we thought this might be sufficient to induce uterine contraction.

"March 10th.—She had had a little pain at times each day since the 6th; but early this morning labor pains set in in good earnest. At about 2 P.M. Mr. — saw her, and found the os uteri dilating; at six he was again summoned, and found the os quite dilated, the liq. amnii escaping at intervals as if the membranes were ruptured high up; the pains were very severe and frequent, and the head was pressing upon the brim of the pelvis. Finding no progress made in three hours with severe and forcing pains, he administered small quantities of chloroform, and sent for me at nine o'clock in the evening. The os uteri and other soft parts were in a favorable state for delivery; but the head was very high up, and covered by the membranes, which I ruptured, giving rise to a small escape of liq. amnii. With some difficulty I applied the vectis, by means of which I assisted the head into the pelvis, and, in about an hour, brought a living male child into the world, the labor having been very severe and difficult, owing to the small size of the pelvis. The child did not appear very active, and its forehead was marked by the vectis; but we congratulated ourselves in not having delayed inducing labor until a later period of pregnancy; for we felt that even another week's growth might have rendered it impossible to have saved the child.

"On the 6th of January, 1853, Mrs. B— being again pregnant, I accompanied Mr. — for the purpose of again bringing on premature delivery, and pursued the same plan as before; that is to say, we introduced the round end of a stomach pump tube seven or eight inches into the uterus, separating the membranes from the uterus to that extent without rupturing them. A few drops of bloody fluid escaped, but the introduction of the tube gave no pain. The vagina, as before, was extremely sensitive and painful under the use of the speculum, and the os uteri too much out of reach for convenient manipulation. Up to the 9th, no symptoms of labor had occurred, with the exception of there having passed on that day a little colored discharge; and at Mr. —'s request, I then introduced the tube again, and moved it about freely in the uterus, without occasioning pain.

"15th.—No pain having yet occurred, the tube was again introduced to-day.

"16th.—Still no symptoms of labor. A firmer tube, bent near its middle, was introduced to-day, and turned round in the uterus so as to describe a circle three inches in diameter.

"28th.—Labor not yet brought on, but she thinks she has some symptoms of its approach to-day. Tried to introduce the tube again to-day, but could not do so freely, owing, I believe, to its impinging upon some portion of the child; we therefore injected some warm water through it, hoping by this means to separate the membranes from the uterus to a greater extent.

"February 20th.—The patient had some uterine pain and slight indications of the approach of labor for a day or two after last report, but they went off again; and as the parts had become exceeding tender, and there was reason to fear we might excite inflammation of the uterus, we thought it right not to renew our efforts *to induce labor* at present.

" March 6th.—Summoned by Mr. — at two o'clock this morning. The patient had been in strong labor since nine the previous evening, and the head was still high up, having scarcely entered the pelvis. The membranes had not ruptured, but the uterus was fully dilated, and the soft parts were in a favorable state for delivery. The head presented with the anterior fontanelle towards the left ramus of the pubes. I passed the vectis over the occiput so as to get a purchase upon it by engaging it in the fenestra, and, by a little perseverance, turned the occiput towards the right ramus of the pubes, the head not being yet wedged into the pelvis. I then got the blade of the vectis over the child's right lower jaw near its angle, and, within an hour, succeeded in bringing into the world a small, living, uninjured boy. The labor was very painful, and the patient distressingly vociferous, notwithstanding the frequent administration of small quantities of chloroform. The placenta came away naturally, and we left her in a good state.

" Both mother and child lived.

" In this case, although we did not succeed in inducing labor at the time we desired, it appeared that our interference did in some way retard the growth of the child, which at the time of its birth was very much smaller than usual at the same period of pregnancy.

CASE 2.—" June 17th, 1854.—Mrs. —, æt. 29 years, having lost her three previous children, owing to want of pelvic space, was recommended to submit to the induction of premature labor in this her next pregnancy. She is now seven months gone, and at the request of my friend, Mr. —, I to-day introduced an œsophagus bougie into the uterus, and passed it up nearly its whole length without rupturing the membranes.

" 18th.—Tube introduced again to-day.

" 19th.—I again introduced the tube, and advised waiting a few days to see the effect of what had been done. The introduction of the tube hitherto had neither given pain nor ruptured the membranes ; but, to-day, I observed a nervous irritable condition of the patient, which led me to think uterine action would ere long ensue. Towards night she became uneasy ; the following day she had slight pains, and at nine o'clock in the evening of the 21st the waters broke, and at 11·30 a living female child was born, without other assistance than what the midwife could afford.

" She was doing well the next day, and had a very good recovery.

" July, 1855.—This patient being now again in the seventh month of pregnancy, Mr. — resorted to the same means of inducing labor. He introduced an œsophagus-tube on two successive days, and then once again after one day's interval. Labor commenced a few hours after this third introduction ; and, to the great delight of the mother, another living child was born after a natural though somewhat painful labor."

Cases of Rupture of the Womb, with remarks. By JAMES D. TRASK, A.M., M.D. of New York. (" American Journal of Medical Sciences," January, 1848 ; April, 1848 ; and July, 1856.)

In these papers Dr. Trask presents us with a careful and laborious analysis of no less than four hundred and seventeen cases of rupture of the womb, and with a lengthened summary, and of this analysis and summary we propose to give the principal results.

CAUSES OF RUPTURE.—A *diseased condition* of the womb is frequently met with in this accident. The condition of the womb is reported only in 67 cases out of the 417 cases. In 13 of these only is it reported healthy ; in 20, softened ; in 21, thinned ; in 1, both thinned and softened ; in 3, both thinned and thickened ; in 8, " diseased ;" in 1, thin and brittle.

As *conditions obstructing the progress of the child,* and in that way leading to rupture, we have in these 417 cases, *at least*—

74 cases of contracted pelvis.
12 " hydrocephalic fœtus.
6 " rigidity of the os.
6 " bands in the vagina.
1 case of enlarged ovary.

The proportion of each of these complications, compared with the whole number of cases, must be regarded as relatively very large, especially in the instance of contracted pelvis. We see that in at least one-fourth of the whole number of cases there is a disproportion between the head and the pelvis, or an obstruction from organized adhesions of the vagina. This estimate is exclusive of cases in which the head is noted as large and firmly ossified. We cannot, therefore, err in regarding this relation as one of cause and effect. That such obstructions existed in many cases in which it is not alluded to in the histories given, is rendered probable by considering the duration of labor previous to rupture.

Time from beginning of labor to rupture.—Taking the whole of our cases in which this is specified, we find that rupture occurred in—

6 hours and less from the beginning of labor in 38 cases.					
12 "	and over six	"	"	36	"
18 "	and over twelve	"	"	10	"
24 "	and over eighteen	"	"	20	"
36 "	and less	"	"	16	"
48 "	and less	"	"	14	"
Three days and less		"	"	11	"
Four days and less		"	"	2	"

Comparing these with the *duration* of labor in the 15,850 cases reported by Dr. Collins, we find that 13,412, or eighty per cent., terminated within six hours; 1672, or sixteen per cent., in from six to twelve hours; and that in corresponding periods of six hours beyond this, they were but from one to two per cent.

The table above embraces 34 cases of contracted pelvis, but, after deducting these, the relative periods remain but little changed. It will be seen that the duration of labor previous to rupture is very much greater on the average than the entire duration of ordinary labors, according to Dr. Collins. The obstacle to delivery presented by the disproportion between the head and the pelvis, &c., explains this fact ; and the probability that such hindrances to the progress of the child existed in many of our imperfectly reported cases, in which it is not noted, is strengthened by a consideration of the protracted character of the labors as a whole. But while the protracted character of the labor, under a continued succession of unavailing efforts to drive the head of the child through the pelvis, explains the frequent coexistence of such disproportion and rupture, there are not a few instances in which the duration of the labor was so short, or the character of the labor so little severe, that we cannot so readily trace any necessary connection between these and the relative size of the head and pelvis. In not a few instances, the first labor-pain was that causing the rupture.

Inordinate voluntary exertion deserves to be enumerated among the causes of rupture. It is prudent to persuade the patient to abstain from voluntary efforts, provided there be resistance to the progress of the child from any cause. We believe that no case of rupture has yet been published in which chloroform was used, which may be due to the fact, that voluntary effort is for the most part suspended under its influence.

Ergot had been given in five cases only.

SITUATION OF THE RUPTURE.—*During pregnancy* four involved the fundus ; these, added to thirteen in the fundus and body, before reported, make *seventeen* of the fundus and body, and *eight* involving, more or less, the cervix.

During labor.—Of the entire number of cases, *one hundred and ten* are distinctly spoken of as involving the cervix ; seventeen the fundus ; and *seventy-one* the body of the womb. Of these seventy-one, by far the larger part are reported as ruptures of the anterior or posterior part, or of the right or left side ; and in some of these it is highly probable that the rupture involved the cervix also.

It appears to be a fair inference from these facts, that labors in which ruptures occur are, as a class, protracted ; that the lesions of softening and thinning generally precede the rupture, and are, for the most part, a consequence of the delay ; but that, in a certain proportion of cases, as in those occurring during pregnancy and early in labor, these lesions must have existed before the expulsive action of the womb, was set up ; while in certain other cases, rupture appears to occur in the womb unaltered by morbid changes.

We copy the *table* of *ages*, with the additions, from the new cases :

Years.	Patients.	Years.	Patients.	Years.	Patients.
16	2	26	9	37	8
17	1	27	5	38	8
18	1	28	20	39	1
19	1	29	3	40	12
20	5	30	24	42 .	2
21	3	32	15	43	2
22	1	33	6	44	4
23	1	34	4	47	1
24	5	35	13	40—45	1
25	11	36	17		

The largest number were at the age of 30 years.

The largest number of cases delivered under Dr. Collins's supervision was also at the age of 30 years; viz., 2346 in a total of 16,414 cases.

The table showing the number of the pregnancy in which the rupture occurred :

No. of Pregnancy, .	1st.	2d.	3d.	4th.	5th.	6th.	7th.	8th.	9th.	10th	11th	12th	13th	Multi-parae.
No. of Patients, . .	31	25	30	27	21	25	14	7	7	12	8	5	2	25

SYMPTOMS OF RUPTURE.—The total, in which the character of the previous labor is stated, is 156. Of these—

> In 46, or 29·5 per cent., it was very severe.
> " 39, or 25·0 " " strong.
> " 46, or 29·5 " " moderate.
> " 11, or 7·0 " " feeble.
> " 14, or 9·0 " " "tedious,"

In *fifty-five* the pains ceased suddenly ; in *seventeen* they ceased gradually.

From this, it appears that liability to rupture is not confined to cases in which the labor is of great severity, and that it may sometimes happen when the pains from the outset are feeble. Its occurrence in the course of a labor of moderate severity appears to be quite as common as when the pains are very severe. We have also the contrast of extensive rupture and escape of the child with few and feeble pains, and a simple laceration of the muscular coat after labor of great severity.

The sudden cessation of the pains is one of the most characteristic symptoms of the accident ; but we learn that this is not of invariable occurrence, and that, in a small proportion of cases, the cessation of pains is gradual.

Again, the *recession of the presenting part* of the child takes place, as a general rule, upon the occurrence of the accident ; but the exceptions are of sufficiently frequent occurrence to deserve especial notice. In several cases the head did not recede ; and in a few the head remained within reach, and delivery was effected by the forceps or perforation. In a few the head receded when it was attempted to apply the forceps. In twenty-two the rupture was accompanied by a peculiar *sensation*. In four the rupture was audible to the bystanders. In two there was no sudden acute pain or tearing sensation, and in one the pains continued to recur after the uterus was empty and contracted. The early appearance of extreme depression after rupture was not seen in three cases. While the cessation of the pains, the sudden outcry of the patient, and the recession of the child, followed by symptoms of great prostration, in general render the diagnosis of the accident easy, the absence of any one of these is, as we have seen, not incompatible with the existence of rupture, and the knowledge that such exceptions occasionally exist may, in some cases, aid in the diagnosis.

INFLUENCE OF DELIVERY ON MORTALITY.—Total of all cases delivered, 207. Of these, 77 recovered, or 37 per cent.

Total of all cases undelivered, 115. Of these, 27 recovered, or 23·5 per cent.

But among the cases previously reported, were many in which the fœtus having escaped into the abdomen, was subsequently discharged after decomposition, and were reported as remarkable cases of recovery. Among the cases now related, of 26 undelivered, only 3 recovered, or about 11 per cent.

These results, however, are to be regarded only as approximating the relative proportion of cases saved and lost in actual practice; since we would naturally expect to find the larger proportion of cases published to have been cases of recovery.

But, if our statistics did not clearly exhibit a diminished mortality among those delivered, they show that life is prolonged by this measure, even in cases that do not recover.

We formerly showed that the average duration of life, after rupture, with those *delivered*, was *twenty-two* hours; and that of the *undelivered* but *nine* hours. By adding to those the new cases, we find that, of those *delivered fifty-four* per cent. survived beyond *twenty-four hours;* while of those dying *undelivered, twenty-seven* per cent. survived beyond the same period.

RELATIVE SUCCESS OF DIFFERENT MODES OF TREATMENT WHEN THE HEAD AND THE WHOLE OR PART OF THE BODY HAS ESCAPED INTO THE PERITONEAL CAVITY.

Summary of all the cases.

Gastrotomy,   saved 16, lost 4, or 20·0 per cent. lost.
Turning, &c.,   "   23, " 50, or 68·5   "   "
Abandoned,   "   15, " 44, or 75·0   "   "

RELATIVE SUCCESS OF DIFFERENT MODES OF TREATMENT WHEN THE PELVIS IS CONTRACTED.

Summary of all the cases.

Gastrotomy,   saved 6, lost 3, or 33·0 per cent. lost.
Perforation, &c.,   "   15, " 30, or 65·0   "   "
Abandoned,   "   0, " 11, or 100·0   "   "

Adding together these two classes, we get, as the comparative results of the different modes of treatment—

Gastrotomy, .   .   . saved 22, lost 7, or 24 per cent. lost.
Turning, perforation, &c.,   "   38, " 80, or 68   "   "
Abandoned, .   .   .   "   15, " 55, or 78   "   "

RESULT AS EFFECTED BY FACILITY OR DIFFICULTY IN DELIVERY.—Taking all the cases together in which this circumstance is alluded to, in *seventy* cases of *recovery, forty-eight* were delivered with ease, or 68·5 per cent. In *ninety-one* cases resulting in *death*, delivery was accomplished with ease in but *thirty-eight*, or 41·7 per cent.

We have included under *easy* deliveries those in which gastrotomy was performed; the term *easy* having reference to time occupied, as well as facility of execution. In all the cases of gastrotomy in which allusion is made to the point, delivery was accomplished very rapidly, and with comparatively little suffering.

If we deduct from each class just enumerated the cases of gastrotomy, we still find a preponderance of easy deliveries among recoveries, and of difficult deliveries among those who were lost. Thus, among *recoveries*, we get *twenty-six easy*, and *twenty-two difficult*, or 54 per cent. delivered with ease; and, among the deaths, *thirty-one easy*, and *fifty-three difficult*, or 37 per cent. delivered with ease. About gastrotomy, Dr. Trask says, "The relative success of gastrotomy is, as we have seen, greater than that of any other mode of delivery, and we believe that a more frequent resort to it would result in a diminished mortality to the accident. In short, *as a general rule, from whatever cause we might be led to anticipate a protracted and difficult delivery by the natural passages, gastrotomy will afford the best chance of recovery.* The only exception we would make is, when there is impaction of the head in the pelvic cavity or in the inferior strait."

There is a total of twenty-four cases of *hernia of the intestine* through the rent in the womb, and in one case death was attributed to strangulation of the bowel in the opening. In several cases there was injudicious interference or unjustifiable violence.

Vesico-vaginal Fistula cured in fourteen days by a new method of operating. By Mr. J. Baker Brown, Obstetric Surgeon to St. Mary's Hospital, &c. ("Lancet," November 15th, 1856.)

The method adopted by Mr. Brown in the following case was devised by Dr. Bozeneau, of Alabama, in America. It is very ingenious, and we quite agree with Mr. Brown in thinking that it will be found to answer in many cases which have hitherto proved intractable to treatment.

Case.—Deborah P—, æt. 22, was admittted into St. Mary's Hospital, under his care, September 22d, 1856. She stated that she was delivered of a still-born male child on the 15th of July, by instruments, after being forty-eight hours in labor. She was shortly afterwards seized with an attack of fever. Eight days after delivery she discovered that the urine dribbled away, after which it all seemed "to pass by the wrong passage." On examination per vaginam, he discovered a fistulous opening close up to the os uteri, about the size of an ordinary director, which instrument could readily be passed within the bladder, through the opening into the vagina. It appeared that all the urine passed through this opening, and none through the urethra; in fact that she was never able to retain any within the bladder, even within a short time. The health of the patient being carefully attended to, especially the removal of some long worms from the bowels, he (Mr. Brown) determined after consultation with some of his colleagues, to operate, after a method devised by Dr. Bozeneau, of Alabama, in America. Accordingly, on the 15th of October, the patient being placed under chloroform, and put in the position for lithotomy, a leg being held by each assistant; a firm retractor, being placed within the vagina, was held firmly backwards and downwards by a third assistant; and, each side of the vagina being held back by two other retractors, the bladder was seized, just at the juncture of its neck with the body, by a strong pair of Vulsellum forceps, and held firmly upwards and forwards by the right hand of the assistant holding the left leg. The fistulous opening was then with great difficulty brought into view, and the mucous membrane divided, by a sharp knife, completely around the opening, about the eighth of an inch in depth. Three silver-wire sutures, eighteen inches long, were then passed by a needle held by the porte-aiguille, and which are shown in fig. 5. The two ends of each wire were then brought together by an instrument, as represented in fig. 6, thus leaving the parts in apposition (fig. 7). A silver button, described in fig. 8, was then carefully passed over the end of each double suture, and a perforated shot passed over each wire, as shown in fig. 9, and pressed down upon the button, and then firmly pressed by a pair of long strong forceps. The wires were then cut off close to the shot, leaving the parts as represented in fig. 10. A piece of lint, dipped in sweet oil, was then introduced within the vagina, the patient placed in bed on a water cushion, on her side, and a bent catheter, with a bag attached to it, was inserted within the bladder, and allowed to remain there. Two grains of opium were given directly, and one grain every four hours afterwards for the first twenty-four hours, and afterwards one grain every six hours; and a generous diet, with wine, allowed daily. The lint was removed on the second day, and the vagina washed out night and morning with tepid water. All the urine passed freely through the catheter.

On the 24th he carefully removed the button and sutures, and found the most perfect union had taken place throughout the whole extent.

On the 26th the bowels were relieved, for the first time, by castor oil and enema, and the catheter was removed for three hours, at the end of which time she passed urine comfortably, with no escape per vaginam.

On the 27th the catheter was removed entirely, and she was allowed to sit up and walk about a little.

On the 28th she was up and about all day; she was able to retain the urine for four hours, and to pass it well.

On the 30th he made a most careful examination, and found the parts firmly united, and without the slightest escape of urine, even after a long and tedious investigation.

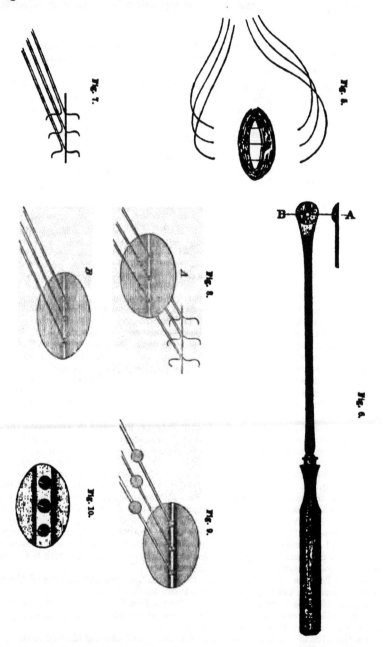

Mr. Brown observed that this method of operation had convinced him that cases hitherto intractable to treatment would be found to be curable by this operation.

IV.

REPORT ON PSYCHOLOGICAL MEDICINE.*

By C. LOCKHART ROBERTSON, M.B. Cantab., F.R.C.P., Edin. Honorary Secretary to the Association of Medical Officers of Asylums and Hospitals for the Insane.

§ I.—*Bibliography.*

I. *Elements of Psychological Medicine, being an introduction to the Practical Study of Insanity.* By DANIEL NOBLE, M.D. 2d Edition of Churchill, 1855.

II. *Medical Testimony and Evidence in cases of Lunacy (the Croonian Lectures, 1853); with an Essay on the Conditions of Mental Soundness.* By THOMAS MAYO, M.D., F.R.S. J. W. Parker and Son, 1854. Also a Supplement to these Lectures, by the Author, 1856.

III. *Lettsomian Lectures on Insanity.* By FORBES WINSLOW, M.D., D.C.D. Churchill, 1854. (Noticed fully in the Report on Practical Medicine, "Half-Yearly Abstract," January to July, 1856.)

IV. *Unsoundness of Mind in relation to Criminal Acts* (Sugden Prize Essay). By JOHN CHARLES BUCKNILL, M.D. Highley, 1854.

V. *The Progressive Changes in the Moral Management of the Insane.* By D. H. TUKE, M.D. (Prize Essay of the Society for Improving the Condition of the Insane.) Churchill, 1854.

VI. *On the Construction, Organization, and General Arrangements of Hospitals for the Insane.* By THOMAS KIRKBRIDE, M.D., Physician to the Pennsylvania Hospital for the Insane, Philadelphia, 1854.

VII. *Unsoundness of Mind in its Medical and Legal Considerations.* By J. W. HUME WILLIAMS, M.D. Churchill, 1856.

VIII. *Criminal Responsibility of the Insane, founded on the Trials of James Hill and William Dove.* By CALEB WILLIAMS, M.D. Churchill, 1856.

IX. *The Treatment of the Insane without Mechanical Restraints.* By JOHN CONOLLY, M.D., D.C.L. Smith, Elder & Co., 1856.

X. *Ninth and Tenth Annual Reports of the Commissioners in Lunacy to the Lord Chancellor.* (Ordered by the House of Commons to be printed.) 1855-6.

XI. *Seventh Report on the District Criminal and Private Lunatic Asylums in Ireland,* 1855. (Presented to both Houses of Parliament by Command of Her Majesty.)

XII. *Insanity, and Hospitals for the Insane; a Review.* Reprinted from the Dublin Quarterly Journal of Medical Science, Nov., 1855.

XIII. *Cases Illustrating the Pathology of Mania and Dementia.* By ALEXANDER JOHN SUTHERLAND, M.D. Reprinted from vol. xxxviii of the Medico-Chirurgical Transactions.

XIV. *William Tuke, the Founder of "The Retreat."* From the Journal of Psychological Medicine, Oct., 1855.

XV. *Criminal Lunatics, are they Responsible?* A Letter to the Lord Chancellor. By J. RUSSEL REYNOLDS, M.D. Churchill, 1856.

XVI. *An Address to the Trustees and Governors of the Warneford Lunatic Asylum.*

---

* The remainder of this Report, which is unfortunately deferred in consequence of the illness of the writer, will be given in the next volume.

By WILLIAM LEY, Esq., Medical Superintendent of the Oxford County Asylum. Oxford, 1856.

XVII. *Remarks on the Lunacy Laws of Scotland and France.* By JOHN WEBSTER, M.D. Reprinted from the Psychological Journal, 1856.

XVIII. *Du Suicide et de la Folie Suicidale.* Par A. Brière de Boismont, Paris, Balliere.

XIX. *The Journal of Psychological Medicine and Mental Pathology.* Edited by FORBES WINSLOW, M.D., D.C.L. Quarterly.

XX. *The Asylum Journal of Mental Science.* Published by authority of the Association of Medical Officers of Asylums and Hospitals for the Insane. Edited by JOHN CHARLES BUCKNILL, M.D. Quarterly.

XXI. *The American Journal of Insanity.* Edited by the Medical Officers of the New York State Asylum. Quarterly.

XXII. *Allgemeine Zeitschrift für Psychiatrie.* Unter der Redaction von Damerow, Flemming, und Roker. Quarterly.

XXIII. *Correspondenz-Blatt der Deutschen Gesellschaft für Psychiatrie.* Bi-monthly.

XXIV. *Annales Médico-Psychologiques.* Par MM. Baillanger, Brière de Boismont, and Cerise. Paris. Quarterly.

XXV. *Annual Reports of the following Lunatic Asylums: Devon, Oxford, Wilts, Bethlehem Hospital, Colney Hatch, and Hanwell; Dundee, Belfast, Perth, Essex, Clonmel, Kent, Suffolk, Hants, State Asylum Philadelphia, Salop and Montgomery, Surrey, R. Crichton's Institution, Aberdeen.*

§ II.—*The Present Condition of the Insane (Official Reports on).*

I. ENGLAND AND WALES.

The ninth and tenth Annual Reports of the Commissioners in Lunacy to the Lord Chancellor (31st March, 1855, and 31st March, 1856), contain much valuable information on the condition of the insane in England and Wales.

1. *New County Asylums.*—In the Report for 1855, the following interesting notice of no less than six new county asylums occurs.

"The six new county asylums, mentioned in our last report as having been recently opened, have, since their opening, been several times visited by the commissioners, and it may be well here to give a short statement of their progress, and present condition.

"The asylum for the county of Warwick was opened for the reception of patients in the month of June, 1852, and was first visited in the month of December, in the same year. At that time, the asylum contained only 125 patients, and seven entire wards were unoccupied and unfurnished. At the next visit, in October 1853, six wards were unoccupied, and at the last visit there still remained a large available space for the reception of patients, although some pauper patients belonging to the county of Gloucester had been received under a temporary contract.

"The reports as to the condition of this institution are of a favorable character. Instrumental restraint is never used, and seclusion appears to be rarely resorted to. A considerable number of patients of both sexes are employed, and a large proportion attend divine service on Sundays. The food is stated to be good, and the bedding and clothing comfortable. The ventilation, however, appears to be defective, and the visiting commissioners notice with regret the absence of open fireplaces in the galleries.

"Considerable progress has been made in bringing the land into cultivation, and in relaying many of the drains, the original construction of which appears to have been very bad.

"The Worcester County Asylum was opened in the month of August, 1852. It has been three times visited by the commissioners, and at the date of the last visit, in September, 1854, contained 215 patients, being eleven more than the asylum was originally calculated to accommodate.

"In this asylum the use of mechanical restraint, although not absolutely prohibited, is exceedingly rare, and only one instance is recorded since the opening. The patients have been generally healthy, and no disease of an epidemic character has prevailed.

"The asylum, although in most respects well conducted and in good order, is reported to be still deficient in appropriate furniture, and the stock of books, periodicals, and means of indoor amusement is insufficient. A better supply of clothing for the patients also appears to be required.

"The supply of water has been found to be quite insufficient for the wants of the asylum, but steps are about to be taken at once to remedy this defect.

"The building appears to be well adapted for its purpose. The wards are cheerful, spacious, and well ventilated. The various offices also are convenient. The justices propose shortly to erect a chapel, detached from the main building, and plans have already been approved by the secretary of state for the erection of new wards capable of accommodating eighty-two additional patients.

"The ground surrounding the asylum, although as yet in an unfinished state, is all that could be desired as regards situation and aspect; and although only a short distance from Worcester, the neighborhood is so retired, that the patients can at all times be taken out for exercise beyond the boundaries of the institution without inconvenience.

"The Lincoln County Asylum, which was opened in the month of August, 1852, contained, at the date of the commissioners' last visit in November, 1854, 246 patients, being within one of the number which the building was constructed to accommodate.

"It is probable that the building will, without crowding or inconvenience, contain more than 250 patients; but should this number be greatly exceeded, it is to be feared that the provision made for the pauper lunatics of the county will be found to be insufficient, and that some addition will become necessary.

"The total number of patients admitted up to the 1st of January, 1854, has been 383; within the same period 115 were discharged, of whom about half were recovered, and sixty-two patients have died. No disease of an epidemic character has prevailed.

"The condition of the patients, and the general management of the asylum, are reported by the visiting commissioners to be very satisfactory. The wards are clean and well ventilated, and the clothing and bedding of excellent quality. The dietary appears to be liberal.

"The whole of the land has been brought under cultivation, and as many as eighty of the male patients find regular occupation upon it.

"Nearly all the females are employed, and the average attendance at the chapel is 150.

"Instrumental restraint is never resorted to, and the instances of seclusion appear to be rare, and of short duration.

"The asylum occupies an elevated site at Bracebridge, in the neighborhood of Lincoln. Its principal galleries, day-rooms, and dormitories, have a southern aspect, and are cheerful and airy. The various offices are convenient and spacious.

"The amount of water afforded by the wells having been found to be insufficient, a contract was entered into with the Lincoln Waterworks Company, by whom an ample supply is now furnished.

"The Asylum for the County of Hants was opened in the month of December, 1852. It was built to accommodate 400, but has at no time contained quite 300 patients. The internal arrangements of the building are convenient. There are 105 acres of land belonging to the institution. The site is excellent, having a slope to the south. It is well wooded, and bounded on one side by a stream of water.

"The asylum has been visited four times by the commissioners; and at the last visit, they report, that considerable progress has been made towards the complete organization of the establishment. They state that the wards are, throughout, exceedingly clean and well ventilated; that the patients are well clothed and apparently comfortable, and that mechanical restraint is never employed.

"It is greatly to be regretted that so large an amount of excellent accommodation in this asylum, the whole of which is well furnished, and ready for the use of the patients, should remain unoccupied, whilst the numerous pauper lunatics belonging to the boroughs of Portsmouth and Southampton, which are not in union with the county, are sent to licensed houses near London, and are thus removed to a great distance from their friends, at a considerable expense, and sometimes, it is to be feared, to their serious injury.

"The Essex County Asylum is situate at Brentwood, and is surrounded by eighty-six acres of land. The building, the elevation of which is of a very pleasing character, and which is conveniently arranged, is constructed to accommodate 448 patients.

"At the last visit of the commissioners, in June, 1854, the asylum contained 137 male, and 174 female patients, thus leaving a very large amount of space unoccupied.

"The commissioners report that the patients were generally tranquil and orderly, that mechanical restraint had never been employed, and that seclusion, although occasionally resorted to, was very sparingly used; that the galleries and apartments were clean and well ventilated, and that the health of the patients was good. A considerable number of patients of both sexes are regularly employed, and about 220 of them attend Divine service in the chapel. The visiting commissioners conclude their report by stating, that, considering the short time during which the asylum has been opened, its condition is 'creditable and satisfactory.'

"The Asylum for the County of Bucks is situate at Stone, about four miles from Aylesbury. It was built for 200 patients, and would probably accommodate more than that number.

"The exterior is plain and unpretending. The wards are convenient and well arranged, and the situation agreeable. There are, however, only 20 acres of land belonging to the institution.

"The asylum has been three times visited by the commissioners, and their reports are favorable. The condition of the establishment is stated to be creditable to the superintendent and those engaged in its management.

"At the date of the last visit, on the 18th December, 1854, there were 169 patients in the asylum. The whole of the wards were found to be clean and well furnished, and presented a cheerful and comfortable appearance; but some of the galleries were cold, and the system of warming and ventilation, although very costly in construction, and extensively adopted, does not appear to answer its intended purpose, or compensate for the absence of open fire-places in many of the rooms.

"The whole of the land is under spade cultivation by the male patients, and a considerable number of the patients of both sexes are employed in various ways.

"Mechanical restraint has never been used, but seclusion in separate rooms is occasionally resorted to as a means for tranquillizing excited and violent patients.

"A large proportion of the patients walk out frequently beyond the boundaries of the institution.

"The supply of water has been very deficient; but, at the date of the last visit, pipes were being laid down to a neighboring well, from which it was hoped an abundant supply would be obtained.

"Owing to the small number of patients and the large staff of officers, the charge for pauper patients in this asylum is necessarily heavy."

2. *Army and Navy Lunatic Hospitals.*—The following notice of these institutions occurs in this report:

The excellent arrangements and liberal treatment for which Haslar Naval Hospital is distinguished, have been already sufficiently noticed in former reports.

"The Yarmouth Hospital ceased, in May, 1854, to be occupied as an hospital for military lunatics, possession of it having been resumed by the Board of Admiralty for the purposes of a general hospital for the sailors of the Baltic fleet. The improvements, therefore, which we anticipated in our last report as likely to arise from the appointment of Mr. Dartnell, as permanent medical superintendent of the institution, and which were in progress when the hospital ceased to receive lunatics, were only partially carried out. At that time the lunatic patients in Yarmouth Hospital consisted of nineteen officers, sixty-nine soldiers, and five women, for whom it became necessary to provide elsewhere, without delay. The Secretary at War having requested our opinion as to the best mode of providing for these inmates, we named Grove Hall, Bow, as a well-conducted asylum, and capable of affording proper accommodation for the soldiers and women, and we at the same time named Cotton Hill Lunatic Hospital (an institution under good management, near Stafford), for the officers. The patients were removed to these several establishments accordingly. But we trust that the arrangements thus made are merely of a temporary character, inasmuch as we should be unwilling to abandon the hope that a distinct asylum will be established for insane soldiers, for whom no public provision at present exists, except the very inadequate and unsuitable accommodation appropriated to them at Fort Pitt, Chatham."

"3. *Metropolitan Licensed Houses.*—With respect to the Metropolitan Licensed Houses, a manifest improvement has taken place in them, as compared with their condition at the time when they first came under the jurisdiction of the commissioners. 'No case of abuse or malversation, of such a nature as to call for public animadversion, has come under our cognizance in any of them in the course of the last year. A few of these houses which receive only patients of the wealthier classes continue to maintain a high standard of excellence.'

"In regard to licensed houses, however, both in the metropolitan and provincial districts, which receive pauper patients, and patients of the middle and humbler classes, we are of opinion that (with a few exceptions) they do not keep pace in the march of improvement, by which the county asylums of the first class are distinguished. Many of them are content to remain at a certain point of advancement; and require, indeed, the constant stimulus of official supervision to prevent their relapsing into the unsatisfactory condition from which, by great care and vigilance, they have been raised."

We take this opportunity of repeating, that the funds by which public asylums "are raised and supported," and the causes which influence those who have control over them, necessarily give them a great superiority over private establishments; and that we are fully convinced that the lunatic poor of England will never be altogether properly provided for until public asylums for all the pauper lunatics of the country shall have been erected.

4. *Increase of Insanity—its Causes and Extent.*—It appears from the summary contained in Appendix (A) annexed to this report, that the number of paupers under treatment as lunatics on the 1st of January, in the present year, amounted to 7,133 males, and 8,689 females, forming an aggregate of 15,822 patients, and that 13,324 of these were in lunatic asylums; 185 in registered hospitals; and 2,313 in licensed houses. From the same summary, it further appears, that 1,121 of these patients, being persons whose settlements could not be ascertained, were maintained at the expense of their respective counties or boroughs, under the provisions of the 98th section of the statute 16 and 17 Vict., cap. 97, so that the number of pauper lunatics then actually chargeable to unions or parishes as patients in asylums was 14,701.

On comparing these figures with those which are stated in the returns of previous years, under the corresponding heads, it will be found that there has been a large and progressive addition to the total number of paupers under treatment as insane—the increase, during the last eight years, commencing on the 1st of January, 1847, when they amounted to a total of 9,652, being no less than 6,170, or upwards of sixty-four per cent.; and that during the same period the relative proportions of those placed in asylums, registered hospitals, and licensed houses respectively have greatly altered; in particular, that since the 1st of January, 1847, when the total number of pauper patients in asylums was 5,247, the number of such patients has greatly more than doubled, while the number of paupers in registered hospitals has fallen from 384 to 185, and in licensed houses from 3,996 to 2,313.

The large addition which, as shown by these tables, has been of late years made to the total number of pauper lunatics, under treatment, may seem at first sight startling, and has led some observers to infer that insanity as a disease has been increasing in this kingdom in a greatly more rapid ratio than its population.

The facts, however, so far as we have been able to ascertain them, by no means necessarily warrant the inference; for a variety of causes, some of them of a temporary, others of a more permanent character, have been actively at work, the combined operation of which goes far towards explaining the result without our having recourse to so painful and disheartening a solution.

Independently of the facilities afforded for the due care of pauper lunatics by the greatly enlarged accommodation lately provided for them in public asylums in their own vicinity, and the encouragement held out by the legislature for placing all such lunatics under medical care in the earliest stage of their malady, it is impossible to doubt that the skill and kindness with which they are treated in such institutions have tended greatly to lengthen their lives, and have very materially diminished the average rate of mortality among them ; and, as a necessary consequence, have largely increased the number of chronic, and probably incurable cases with which all our asylums, even the most spacious, are rapidly becoming filled.

It is further to be observed, that the stringent provisions of the law, by which parochial and other local authorities are required to take immediate proceedings for placing all violent and recent cases under proper care, are being every day more rigidly and systematically enforced in proportion as the machinery for the purpose becomes better understood, and with the wholesome effect of transferring to lunatic asylums a great many insane paupers who have heretofore been harbored in workhouses, or allowed to live at large on a parish allowance with their relations, where, if they were not positively maltreated and abused, their mental disorder was utterly neglected.

It is obvious also, that the attention of medical practitioners (as well as of the public generally) has of late years been led to take a far more comprehensive, as well as scientific view of insanity in its various aspects, and to consider as properly falling under it many forms of the disease, which, from not exhibiting any strongly developed symptoms, were in former times wholly overlooked, although with a view to their cure, it might be of essential importance that the best remedial treatment should be applied to them with the utmost promptitude. It may be added, that the facilities of intercommunication supplied in these days by means of the post-office, the railway, and the press, bring to the cognizance of the humane many distressing cases of insanity among the poor which call for, and now receive, speedy relief, but which of old would probably have remained forever unnoticed and unknown.

A good deal may also be ascribed to, and more may hereafter be expected, from the exertions of the medical officers of the different unions, whose visits to chargeable lunatics, and the quarterly returns which they make of their visits, under the 66th section of 17 and 18 Vict., cap. 97, cannot fail to bring to light, and insure the early investigation, and if need be, the removal to a suitable asylum, of many of those numerous cases of lunacy and idiotcy, more or less intractable, which are to be found among paupers who are living at large with relatives or friends.

Moreover, as we have already had occasion to state in several of our former reports, our own efforts in the course of visitation have exercised a perceptible influence in the same direction; and seconded by the efforts of the Poor-Law Board, have tended strongly to inculcate on the guardians of unions and their subordinate functionaries the obligation, and to confirm them in the practice, of removing from the workhouses to a suitable asylum, with the least possible delay, and without exception, every case of insanity in which the attack is recent, or is attended with symptoms of violence, or in which, for any other reasons, it cannot be properly managed in the workhouse.

In some districts, too, a practice has sprung up, by which persons, who have never been themselves in receipt of parochial relief, and who are not unfrequently tradesmen, or thriving artisans, have been permitted to place lunatic relatives in the county asylums, as pauper patients, under an arrangement with the guardians for afterwards reimbursing to the parish the whole, or part of the charge for their maintenance.   This course of proceeding is stated to prevail to a considerable extent in the asylums of the metropolitan counties, and its effect in occupying with patients, not strictly or originally of the pauper class, the space and accommodations which were designed for others who more properly belong to it, has more than once been made the subject of complaint. It should, however, be borne in mind, that the language of the statute, the interpretation clause of which defines the term "pauper" to mean, "every person maintained, wholly or in part, by, or chargeable to any parish, union, or county," seems to countenance, if it does not actually justify, the practice; and that to insist upon a rigid observance of a different rule would, in most cases, either compel the party interposing, if legally liable for the maintenance of the lunatic, to throw himself, as well as the patient, on the parish for support; or, where he was not so liable, would induce him to decline undertaking any portion of the burden.

Another and somewhat analogous process is also steadily going on, by which many lunatics, who originally belonged to the class of private patients, are being continually withdrawn from it to swell the ranks of the pauper class. Nothing is more common in practice, than for the relatives or friends of a person who is suddenly stricken with insanity, while actively engaged in some laborious calling on which he depends for a livelihood, to undertake the cost of his maintenance and treatment as a private patient in a licensed house, for a few weeks or months, in the hope that a cure may be speedily wrought, and the necessity for resort to parochial aid may be avoided. But when that hope is disappointed, as too frequently it is, and their bounty becomes exhausted, the support of the patient is of course thrown on the parish, his name is placed upon the pauper list, and he is finally transferred, as soon as room can be found for him, to the public asylum of the district.

Indeed, it may be said with truth, that, except among what are termed the opulent classes, any protracted attack of insanity, from the heavy expenses which its treatment entails, and the fatal interruption which it causes to everything like active industry, seldom fails to reduce its immediate victims, and generally also their families with them, to poverty, and ultimately to pauperism. This is the main reason why, in our pauper lunatic asylums, many inmates are to be met with who have formerly held a respectable station in society, and who, in point of education and manners, are greatly superior to the inmates of a workhouse.

It is a significant fact, closely connected with the same subject, that the number of private patients, meaning by the term, patients who are maintained out of their own resources, or those of their near relatives, and nearly all of whom are now placed in registered hospitals or licensed houses, has increased at a much less rapid rate than the number of lunatic paupers,—the increase during the eight years between the 1st day of January, 1847, and the 1st of January, 1855, being from 4065 to 4671, or about 15 per cent. only.

If all these considerations are taken into account, it will excite little surprise that the strenuous efforts, which of late years have been made in England to provide for the insane poor in public asylums should have been unable to keep pace with the growing demand for such provision, and that a large, and every year an augmenting mass of chronic, and probably hopeless, cases, should become accumulated in these institutions, occupying much of the available accommodation there, to the exclusion, it is to be feared, of many other cases, to which, as being of recent date, the earliest remedial treatment would be most important.

5. *Removal of Patients on recommendation of Commissioners.*—The commissioners have adopted a plan of occasionally suggesting to the friends the removal of a patient to another asylum, when the treatment of the patients appeared to be unsuccessful or his condition unsatisfactory. They observe,—

" Independently of the benefit likely to arise from a different method of medical and moral treatment, it is found that the mere change of scene has invariably a tendency to interest the patient, dissociating him from those objects in connection with which his malady had continued, or perhaps increased, and placing him under the influence of new impressions, with all their attendant good consequences. Even in cases where the patient has not been removed pursuant to the recommendation, our interference has had the effect of attracting more attention to his case, and occasionally of inducing the adoption of remedies not previously resorted to, and has thus tended materially to his advantage.

" It is right to state, that our efforts in this respect have been generally seconded by the friends of the patient, who have, in almost every instance, acted upon our suggestion; and we have the gratification of adding that the visiting justices have in two instances, of their own accord, promoted the removal of patients who were resident in asylums subject to their supervision."

6. *Number of Insane Patients in England and Wales on the 1st of January,* 1856:

	Private.			Pauper.			Total Males.	Total Females.	Total Lunatics.
	M.	F.	Total.	M.	F.	Total.			
Asylums (County), ...	132	118	250	6066	7407	13,573	6298	7525	13,823
Hospitals, ...	773	743	1446	88	94	182	791	837	1628
Metropolitan Licensed Houses, .	687	603	1240	468	883	1351	1105	1436	2591
Provincial Licensed Houses, .	761	735	1506	615	480	1095	1386	1215	2601
	2343	2199	4442	7337	8864	16,201	9580	11,063	20,643
Royal Naval Hospital, ...	121	—	121	—	—	—	121	—	121
	2364	2199	4563	7337	8864	16,201	9701	11,063	20,764

7. *Licenses to non-professional Persons and Women.*—We subjoin, as so fully expressing our own opinion, the opening page of Dr. Bucknill's clever review of this Tenth Report of the Lunacy Commission in the "Asylum Journal" for October, 1856:

"The changes which have taken place in the licenses and proprietorships of licensed houses are no longer embodied in the report, but are set forth in an appendix. Our readers will be gratified to observe that all the *new* licenses have been granted to medical men. Ladies, it is true, still figure in four of the changes of proprietorship, but in three of these instances, they are the widows of the late proprietors. At Walton Lodge only the license has been transferred to Miss Eliza Squires. From these facts we gather that the evil of lady speculators in insanity is in process of cure. We say lady *speculators* advisedly, for ladies licensed to keep houses for the treatment of the insane can only be regarded as such. If insanity is a disease requiring medical treatment, ladies cannot legally or properly undertake that treatment. They are in a widely different position to medical men, who in the treatment of a special class of diseases are compelled by the law to take a license for the detention of their patients. Physicians or surgeons to whom licenses are granted are not necessarily more speculative in the maladies of their patients than any other class of medical men who invest money in their professional pursuits. The difference of position arises from the fact, that from the peculiar nature of the disease they are not medical attendants only, but also the custodians of their patients. Interference with the liberty of the subject demands the authority and surveillance of the State; and hence the need of a license. But with laymen and ladies the medical treatment of insanity is out of the question, and a license granted to them becomes merely a permission to speculate upon the profits of their maintenance. It is a remnant of the olden times when safe custody was everything, and medical treatment deemed absurd, or even an interference with the decrees of Providence; a remnant, however, of which we hope soon to see the last rag abolished. It may at first sight appear reasonable and just that upon the decease of a medical man who has invested much of his capital in purchasing or establishing a licensed house, his widow, or even his daughter should have the advantage thereof by transference of the license. But if, as a rule, lady licensees are objectionable, the fact of medical relationship cannot remove the objection. When a medical man in private practice pays the debt of nature, his widow is compelled to dispose of his interests on the best terms she can make. The license and proprietorship of a good private asylum is a very marketable commodity, and will always readily obtain a medical purchaser. If the public interests demands, as we hold they do, that all establishments for the treatment of the insane should be in the hands of medical men, private interests ought to give way. If private interests in such an important matter are to override public ones, the widow of a clergyman ought on the same principle to hold the rectory of her departed husband, and manage the parochial duties by means of curates."

II. SCOTLAND.

In the absence of any official report on the condition of the Scotch asylums, we are fortunate in having the trustworthy and carefully prepared notes of Dr. Webster's visit to the public lunatic asylums of Scotland ("Journal of Psychological Medicine," new series, 1, 2, and 3, January, 1856, *et seq.*) to refer to.

Dr. Webster's notes on the lunatic asylums of Scotland embrace six public institutions; respecting which some interesting statistical data, accompanied by various practical remarks, are laid before the profession. The several establishments examined were: Edinburgh, Glasgow, Perth, Dundee, Montrose, and Aberdeen.

8. *The Royal Edinburgh Asylum*—This institution, which is of modern construction, is situated at Morningside, about a mile and a half southwest of the Scottish metropolis. It contained 556 lunatic inmates, both private and pauper; of whom 273 were males, and 283 females. During the past year 212 new patients were admitted; 94 recovered, and 51 died; hence, the cures averaged 44·3 per cent., the deaths being 9·2 per cent., similarly calculated. Amongst the new admissions, acute mania was recognized in 50 cases, monomania affected 47 individuals, 33 were classed under dementia, 29 under melancholia, whilst 14 were examples of general paralysis; all being male patients. Intemperance figured as the most frequent cause, 33 persons, or one-seventh of the whole, having become insane in consequence of their excessive potations.

9. *Glasgow Royal Asylum.*—This establishment, only very recently constructed, is situated at Gant-Navel, about four miles northwest of the city. Its situation is very beautiful—so beautiful as to remind the spectator in some degree of Windsor Castle. Both private and pauper patients are received into this asylum; 296 out of 381 inmates being classed as indigents. During the past year, 240 new patients were received, comprising 123 male, and 117 female lunatics. Of those admitted, 107 were affected with mania, 83 exhibited monomania, including melancholia, and 50 labored under dementia. The numbers dismissed cured were 116, or about 48 per cent.; whilst the deaths amounted to 62, or 24 per cent.; the sexes showing nearly an equal mortality. Amongst the assigned causes, as in the case at Morningside, an intemperate use of alcoholic drinks stood forward as pre-eminent, 45 cases, or about one-fifth of the entire admissions, having been attributed to that baneful influence.

10. *Murray's Royal Asylum.*—This asylum occupies the northwestern declivity of Kinoull Hill, near Perth, enjoying a magnificent prospect of the Grampian and Strathearn hills, with the valley of the river Tay intervening. The Murray Asylum receives both private and pauper patients; the aggregate numbers being 141 when Dr. Webster visited the institution; 77 being males and 64 females. No inmate was under any bodily restraint, excepting two males, who wore strong leather gloves, temporarily, to prevent them destroying their clothes; and, as at Edinburgh and Glasgow, the strait-waistcoat appeared to have become a matter of history. During the past year, 36 new patients were admitted (23 male and 13 female), 17 (6 male and 11 female) were discharged cured; and 15 (7 male and 8 female) died, 7 of the deaths being from cholera. In addition to amusing and occupying the inmates, much attention is likewise paid (here as elsewhere) to intellectual culture; so that when the patients recover their mental equilibrium, the education thus imparted may be of use afterwards. Indeed, lectures, conversaziones, musical parties, and evening entertainments, are all carried out with as much spirit as in any other asylum in the kingdom.

11. *Dundee Royal Asylum.*—This institution, founded 43 years ago, has always enjoyed a high reputation throughout Scotland. It is situated close to the town. When first opened, in 1812, accommodation was only provided for 40 patients; at present, it could receive six times that number. This enlargement has enabled the authorities to dispense with various antiquated appliances, and so to substitute important improvements. When Dr. Webster visited the Dundee asylum, its total patients, private and pauper, amounted to 212 (93 males and 119 females). During the past year, 51 new patients were admitted (26 males and 25 females). The ratio of cures ranged 41 per cent.; that of deaths being 21·57 per cent., if calculated according to the total admissions. The form of disease manifested, appeared chiefly as mania and dementia. However much many arrangements at this insti-

tution seemed worthy of commendation, one feature, in Dr. Webster's opinion, appeared highly objectionable, namely, the regulation of requiring graduated fees to be paid by different classes of patients to the physician. In all public institutions the salaries of medical officers should be liberal, but fixed, and not varying according to the number of classes of inmates; whilst no premium ought ever to be held out for giving more professional attention to one patient than another. This system at the Dundee Asylum, in the Doctor's opinion, required amendment; and certainly the feature described seemed unprofessional.

12. *Montrose Royal Asylum.*—This establishment is the oldest public asylum for the insane in Scotland, having been founded 74 years ago; and chiefly through the exertions of Mrs. Carnegie, a benevolent lady residing in this neighborhood. When first opened, and during many years afterwards, it was the admiration of surrounding districts, and became almost a show-place, like Bethlem Hospital of olden times. Many changes and improvements have, however, taken place since its foundation, which would furnish an instructive history of every successive stage, characterizing the varied treatment of insanity in this country. Thus, the old, dark, and badly ventilated cells—considered so useful in 1780—the confined sleeping apartments of a later period; its alcoved dormitories, constructed in the early part of this century; the more airy rooms built about 21 years past; and lastly, the cross-windowed, thoroughly-ventilated, as also exceedingly cheerful dormitory completed only very recently, would each supply most instructive illustrations of the several different epochs, as of the varied modes of management pursued respectively. When inspected by Dr. Webster, the total inmates of the asylum amounted to 229; of whom 96 were males and 133 females. During last year, 39 male and 52 female patients were admitted. The cures amounted to 37 (the sexes being nearly equal); the deaths to 21. The very defective structure of this now venerable establishment being acknowledged—it having become almost surrounded, first, by a dock on one side, a ship-building yard opposite, a railway station on another side, and numerous buildings in its vicinity—this asylum has been condemned as no longer appropriate for receiving lunatic patients. A new building will therefore be speedily erected, in a salubrious, open, and elevated situation, not many miles from Montrose, called Sunnyside—an appropriate and truly descriptive appellation,—which, it is expected, must prove very different in many respects from its predecessor.

13. *Royal Asylum of Aberdeen.*—Although not so ancient as the institution at Montrose, this public asylum dates from 1800. Having gradually increased from an hospital, intended originally for only about 50 patients, to an average of 350; also, the existing structure displays correctly, in stone and lime, the progressive advances of the ideas entertained generally regarding receptacles for lunatics during the past half century; and hence this institution, in its various phases, presents much of interest to the psychological antiquary. When visited by Dr. Webster, the Aberdeen Asylum contained 133 male and 146 female lunatics. During the previous twelve months, 65 new patients had been admitted, 21 being male and 44 female lunatics; 11 males and 28 females were discharged cured, or 39 altogether; hence giving a ratio of 60 per cent. on the admissions. The deaths amounted to 19, consisting of 14 male and 5 female inmates, therefore, making the mortality 29·23 per cent., similarly calculated. Respecting the various special types of mental affections manifested by patients when first received, mania appeared the most frequent, almost half being of that description. Dementia and melancholia ranked next in frequency; both these varieties having each supplied nearly one-fifth respectively. Three cases were complicated with epilepsy, all females; and two males, laboring under dementia, also suffered from general paralysis. Regarding the influences exciting insanity, intemperance occupied a prominent position,—as it unfortunately does too often elsewhere;—childbirth and nursing proved a frequent cause; and hereditary predisposition embraced upwards of 38 per cent., which therefore seemed an unusually high proportion. Of the patients cured, mania constituted the largest number, 26 recoveries being of that category: of whom, half had not been affected beyond one month prior to their admission. Again, amongst the 19 deaths recorded, 12, or nearly three-fifths, were examples of dementia,—only 2 of these being females; whilst paralysis was also noted in half

the fatal cases last specified. No inmate was placed under any kind of personal restraint. Other interesting points were likewise specially commented upon by Dr. Webster; but one important feature seems to have attracted his special notice and approval, viz., the invariable rule which prevails throughout this institution, of leaving the doors of every day-room, communicating with its appropriate airing-court, or flower-garden, always *open* during daytime. Thus, no appearance of confinement prevailed; neither was any opening or shutting of door-locks required, nor marching out or in like soldiers at drill; but all seemed perfect freedom; hence the patients were treated almost as if sane. Of course, attendants were always present; whilst the judicious classification of inmates enabled the medical officers to carry out this excellent system more successfully. When concluding his notice of the Aberdeen Asylum, Dr. Webster alludes, in terms of deserved praise, to the permission afforded for students to attend the physician's practice, and to obtain clinical knowledge; which privilege, he wishes was accorded at all asylums; or, to quote his final phrase, *O ! si sic omnes.*

14. *Dr. Webster's Suggestions for the Amendment of several Details of Government in the Scotch Asylums.* (Psych. Journal, July, 1856.)

"Regarding the official staff in lunatic establishments, at several, some change in their position might be made most advantageously. For instance, the medical superintendent should have more administrative power than he often possesses, and be also better remunerated than sometimes happens. He ought to exercise *paramount* authority in everything appertaining to the management, and moral, medical, or physical treatment of patients. He should likewise attend all meetings of managing committees, although without the privilege of voting—from being a salaried officer—in order that he might give his opinion respecting the admission of new patients, or upon any professional questions which then arose; as also to prevent all future misunderstandings. The matron—who is sometimes too highly salaried, in relation to other officials, and her actual position—appears frequently not sufficiently subordinate. This objection has been felt elsewhere; and in France, for example, where they manage many things often so well in lunatic asylums, a lady matron is almost unknown. Throughout Scotland, as also in England, sufficient attention is not invariably paid to their qualifications in the character of housekeepers, head attendants, and as sick nurses, when the governors select for appointment this occasionally rather too self-important personage.

"Some institutions have consulting physicians; but other establishments are without such medical attendants. The system must be uniform; and there ought invariably to be both a consulting physician and surgeon whenever possible. These officers being called in consultation respectively, at the discretion and request of the medical superintendent; for which duty they ought to be remunerated liberally. There should further be always two resident medical officers in every asylum; one being the assistant, and subordinate to the resident physician. Besides which, but particularly at large establishments, I would appoint resident pupils, or 'internes,' as usually prevails in France. This constitutes one of the many good features characterizing various public insane asylumns of that country.

"Every building for the reception of lunatics should be disconnected with any other public establishment, whether infirmary, dispensary, or poor-house. Even in lay management, it is desirable that no kind of union obtains, much less any physical conjunction. Wherever this system exists, it may well be altered as unsuitable; from being apt to become, in various conceivable ways, disadvantageous to the lunatic institutions so situated.

"The two departments for private and pauper patients—very common in the public asylums of Scotland—as likewise the accommodation supplied in each of these divisions, must be properly distinguished, and always separate. Farther, the classification of inmates requires to be made, in the first place, more with reference to the phase of their mental malady, and less as to the pecuniary allowance received. This desirable object may not be always possible in limited or old-constructed dwellings; but henceforward, at every new asylum, which shall admit patients belonging to various social grades, special attention ought to be directed towards attaining separate buildings, like those now at Morningside, having gardens attached; instead of making—which occasionally happens—a common class composed of the poorest private patients and pauper inmates. In truth, the educated and refined should never be indiscriminately mixed among the debased and unpolished, when afflicted with such calamity as poverty, conjoined to mental alienation. I would further remark, that the impression produced on my mind, whilst visiting particular asylums was, the distinctions adopted amongst patients sometimes appeared too much based on a system of money classification—each inmate deriving advantages according to their respective payments. Hence, individuals paying similar rates, although in a different mental condition, were often associated together, irrespective of their nosological peculiarities.

"At an asylum I lately inspected abroad, a totally opposite method was adopted: but which, however, carried the treatment too far the reverse. Patients in that establishment were usually classified according to their diseased mental condition, so that inmates paying a high board became associated with those of a lower scale; the chief advantages obtained by the higher-paying classes being a better kind of fare, in the same dining-hall with the others, and from having superior furniture in their private apartments. This mode of classification, though better in some respects than the Scottish system, has, nevertheless, a tendency to depreciate the condition of the upper class, by making them live, while in a similar mentally weak condition, with persons often of inferior education, of different habits, and varied acquirements. Both plans seem disadvantageous: but a combination of the two would be followed by fewer objections, in comparison, with the one usually adopted in North Britain."

15. *Dr. Webster's testimony to the general Character of the Scotch Public Asylums.*—"Notwithstanding the brief notice in former pages, apparently censuring some regulations now in force at particular institutions, readers must, however, always remember that it was in Scotland, where one of the earliest public asylums for the reception of lunatics, and improved treatment of mental diseases, was first founded throughout the entire United Kingdom. Besides this creditable distinction, when contrasted with other countries, it should likewise be recollected that of late considerable progress has been made in their management, highly honorable to many official functionaries. Indeed, I can justly say, in addition to occupying, amusing, and physically treating insane residents, in a manner very superior to the system pursued during former times, the intellectual culture of such patients—often previously much neglected—has been materially advanced; not only greatly to the lunatics' present comforts, but also their future advantage when discharged from the asylum. Hence, these proceedings reflect considerable credit on the gentlemen by whom such praiseworthy tasks—often most beneficial—are undertaken."

III. IRELAND.

The Seventh Report of the Inspectors of Asylums in Ireland is a very able document. Our limits oblige us to confine our attention to the central criminal asylum at Dundrum. The criminal asylum for England is still *in futuro*.

16. *General Abstract of the Mental State of the Patients in the Central Lunatic Asylum, on the 31st March*, 1855.

Offences.	Males.	Females.	Total.	Mental Condition.	Males.	Females.	Total.
Homicide, ...	33	5	38	Recovered, ...	15	13	28
Infanticide, ...	—	11	11	Improved, ...	10	8	18
Violent Assaults. . . .	26	6	32	Insane, ...	54	17	71
Burglary, Arson, &c. &c.,	25	20	45	Idiots, ...	5	4	9
Total, ...	84	42	126	Total, ...	84	42	126

From the preceding analysis it appears that twenty-eight, or nearly a fourth of the whole number of patients, are recovered or convalescent, fifteen of whom have become so within the last two years. Had these twenty-eight been ordinary inmates of an asylum, they would have been set free, each after a probation of about six weeks; but in the Dundrum Asylum their sojourn is much more lengthened and indefinite, as even under the most favorable circumstances we would not submit the proposition of. a discharge without an unbroken restoration of mind, coupled with exemplary good conduct, for a twelvemonth, as the very shortest period.

"One patient alone, a respectabble married female, who destroyed her infant whilst laboring under puerperal mania, has been liberated since the date of our last report. We shall have occasion, however, in the course of the present year, to lay before his Excellency the Lord Lieutenant, for his consideration, seven or eight cases as fit subjects for freedom. Of these cases three were acquitted of homicide; but being now for over four years under our immediate supervision, and certified by the attendant physicians to be free of every symptom of mental derangement, at the same time that they have been uniformly quiet, industrious, and well conducted, we feel justified in the course we propose—the more so as they undertake to emigrate ; two having already received money for the passage out to join their families.

"Independent of the exercise of clemency itself—in a moral point of view—the very fact of opening the gates of an asylum, such as the Dundrum, and affording egress to objects deemed worthy of it, produces a beneficial and tranquillizing influence over those who remain behind, and who, if finding no prospective hope of freedom or recovery, but obliged to regard their future doom as the companions of madmen, might, from their very numbers, become most dangerous and difficult to control. There are two individuals, both respectably connected, acquitted of very aggravated assaults, who being now, and, indeed, since their transference to the asylum, quite well, might be liberated; but as the parties on whom the assaults were committed (one the father, the other a solicitor) object to their enlargement, in deference, to strong personal apprehensions, and aware of the responsibility we might incur, if anything untoward subsequently took place, we are unwilling to interfere. In the course of time, however, should those justifiable fears subside, or if some arrangement can be effected by us, between the various parties, we trust they may then participate in the same consideration extended by government to others."

§ III. *Moral Management of the Insane without Mechanical Restraints.*

I. DR. CONOLLY ON THE PRINCIPLES OF THE MORAL MANAGEMENT OF THE INSANE.

Dr. Conolly's new work "On the Treatment of the Insane without Mechanical Restraint" bears on its pages all the marks of that great, good man, as for years we have now known him, in his simple truthfulness and warm sympathy with the wretched. The finished diction and eloquence, rising often to the pathetic, are the same as in a former report ("Half-Yearly Abstract," vol. vii) we found in his valuable monograph on the construction and government of lunatic asylums. This present publication is his legacy to the profession. The record of his life's work in the cause of humanity and of science, and the story it tells will indeed be a grand monument for his children, and children's children to point to.

In the opening chapter he well observes, "When the close of active professional exertion is felt to be approaching, and the pressure of that period, *aut jam urgentis aut certe adventantis senectutis*, becomes perceptible, a natural wish arises in the mind of any man who has been specially engaged in what he regards as a good and useful work, to leave the work, if not finished, yet secure ; or, if not yet secure, at least advanced by his labors, and as little incomplete as the shortness of his life and the limitation of his opportunities permit. The accordance of such a privilege must have imposed obligations which his imperfect powers never can have fulfilled satisfactorily ; and consolation under consciousness of deficient performance, can only arise from a trust in that Higher Power which allows men to be the instruments in any kind of good. Influenced by some feelings of this kind, I am anxious, in these pages, to explain, as distinctly as I am able, the nature, as well as the rise and progress, of that method of treating the insane which is called the Non-restraint System ; so as to contribute to its preservation and further improvement, and perhaps to its wider adoption ; or, at least, to prevent its being abandoned or imperfectly acted upon, or misrepresented, when those by whom it has been steadily maintained in its early days of trial and difficulty can no longer describe or defend it."

Dr. Conolly divides his work into six parts, viz.:

Part I. The Last Days of the Old Method of Treatment.
    II. The First Days of the New or Non-Restraint System.
    III. The New System in Private Asylums.
    IV. Abolition of Mechanical Restraints in Hanwell in 1839.
    V. Gradual adoption of the Non-Restraint System in the Large Asylums of
        England after 1839.
    VI. Progress of the New System on the Continent.

We consider this work of Dr. Conolly's as of such infinite practical importance and permanent value, that we have no hesitation in devoting a portion of our limited space to a consideration of each of the several parts.

17. *The last days of the Old Method of Treatment.*—Dr. Conolly concludes his historical sketch of the past treatment of the insane with the following well-advised remarks: "What the old system of treatment by restraint really was, ought, therefore, not to be forgotten, nor should palliations of it be unreflectingly admitted. Its evils were not imaginary, but real and dreadful. In the clean, quiet, orderly galleries of well-managed asylums, the visitor now sees nothing indicative of the condition to which the apologists of restraints look back as scarcely objectionable. In the gloomy mansions in which hands and feet were daily bound with straps or chains, and wherein chains of restraint and baths of surprise, and even whirling chains were blended, all was constantly bad. The patients were a defenceless flock, at the mercy of men and women who were habitually severe, often cruel, sometimes brutal. The evidence of this stands on record, and can neither be denied nor explained away. Cold apartments, beds of straw, meagre diet, scanty clothing, scanty bedding, darkness, pestilent air, sickness and suffering, and medical neglect—all these were common; and they must remain common, however disguised, wherever the system of restraint remains the subject of eulogy. Before the appointment of commissioners, armed with power to inspect these receptacles of madness, there was so much security and concealment, that the aggravation of loathsome dirt, of swarming vermin, and of the keeper's lash, were safely added. No mercy, no pity, no decent regard for affliction, for age, or for sex, existed. Old and young, men and women, the frantic and the melancholy, were treated worse, and more neglected, than the beasts of the field. The cells of an asylum resembled the dens of a squalid menagerie. The straw was raked out, and the food was thrown in through the bars; and exhibitions of madness were witnessed which are no longer to be found, because they were not the simple product of malady, but of malady aggravated by mismanagement."

18. *The first days of the new or Non-restraint System.*—Dr. Conolly here gives a graphic description of the first influences of a well-conducted asylum on a newly admitted patient, and points out, with great clearness, the remedial value of seclusion, and of the padded room; and then enters into many interesting details of the non-restraint system as fully carried out. Thus, he observes, "In the greater number of recent cases of mental malady the patient is unable to sleep; the days are tolerably tranquil, but in the night restless distraction comes. Whoever has known the affliction of a restless night must know that his affliction would have received no abatement from his being tied down to his bed; and that fresh air, cold water, sitting up awhile, and diversion of mind, are the things to which he would resort for relief. The poor lunatic, equally restless, equally sleepless, and with a brain more excited, should not be deprived of these alleviations, all of which form a part of the true non-restraint system; but none of which are regarded where restraints are employed, which are indeed utterly incompatible with them. The attendant, who has fastened down his troublesome and sleepless patients in bed, retires with a satisfied mind to his supper and his rest. The patients may suffer from heat and thirst, and may shout and yell in their dispair—he heeds them not; or, if he does, it is only to visit them in an angry mood, and to punish them as he chooses. The attendant, where restraints are not used, cannot leave his patients so neglected, or punish them at will. If a patient cannot lie down without distress, he is not compelled to lie down, but allowed to walk about; being supplied with soft warm shoes, and other clothing, to prevent his suffering from being out of bed. If he knocks at the door of his room, the reason of his doing so is inquired into; if he is thirsty,

he has water given to him; if he has been restless, and his bed is discomposed, the bed is made comfortable again; the patient's face and hands are cooled with water; perhaps a cup of tea or coffee, or beef-tea, or arrowroot—kept in readiness by the night attendants—is given to him, or sometimes a little tobacco; and thus the patient is refreshed in body and soothed in mind, blesses his visitors, bids them good night, and falls asleep; and thus the cries and howls which disturbed the wards so often are heard no more.

"The old system placed all violent or troublesome patients in the position of dangerous animals. The new system regards them as afflicted persons, whose brain and nerves are diseased, and who are to be restored to health, and comfort, and reason. This simple difference of view it is, which influences every particular in the arrangement of every part of an asylum for the insane."

Dr. Conolly traces throughout the several influences exerted on the insane by a comprehensive system of non-restraint; and so (he adds), "by these various appliances, some of them simply of small significance, and perhaps almost wearisome in detail, but conjointly, forming a complete system directed to one object,—the whole constitution of an asylum, and the transactions and incidents of every-day life are made remedial. Everything done by every officer, and every word spoken by the sane to the insane, is in conformity to one plan; directed by a chief physician, carried out in all its details by efficient and faithful officers, and having for its sole object the happiness of the patients, the relief or cure of all the griefs and troubles of the heart, and the restoration of composure and power to the mind. *These, in their union, constitute the system of managing the insane without mechanical restraints.*"

19. *The New System in Private Asylums.*—Dr. Conolly gives the following graphic account of the private asylums as they were under the old régime,—as we ourselves have seen them,—as, indeed, the extracts we made in a former section from the Commissioners' last Report, show that they still are. "Such houses were generally distinguishable from all the houses in the neighborhood by their dismal appearance; their exterior was as gloomy as their interior was dirty. Heavy gates, a neglected shrubbery, windows heavily barred, doors clumsily locked, prepared the visitor for rooms which, though rooms of reception, had an air of cold discomfort and shabby finery; and, whilst the friends of the patient were shown into them, the patient himself, ushered by men of repulsive aspect, disappeared into long passages, closed to the curiosity of those who brought him there in the hope that change of scene and specific skill and kindness would promote his speedy recovery.

"From that time, and commonly for a long period, the visits of all his friends were jealously interdicted; although the patient often grieved no less than they did at each absolute and prolonged denial of what might have been a consolation to both. If the patient had previously been violent, or had on any occasion acted in a manner to excite a suspicion of a suicidal tendency, it was not unusual to resort to restraint at once, and he passed his first dreadful night in the asylum fast bound in a strait-waistcoat. In the morning he awoke to find himself in a strange apartment, watched, rather than waited upon, by rude, ungentle keepers; all the details of his dressing disregarded, and his morning meal brought to him with little care. An ill-furnished, ill-cleaned room; a half darkened window, looking into a wretched yard; and a scanty fire, rendered less efficient for warmth by a heavy fire-guard advancing far into the room; were the characteristics of the apartment in which he was to pass the day, either in solitude, or with some other patients more or less afflicted than himself. If he went out for exercise, it was into a dolorous space of ground; the grass-plots and borders of walks half trodden into clay, unadorned by flowers, and disfigured, rather than ornamented, by torn and withering shrubs and trees. The hour of dinner brought no comfortable meal; and no social or rational conversation, and no amusements of any kind, diversified the evening. Beyond the boundaries of the lofty walls, no exercise was allowed; and within them there was no variety and no companionship, nor anything calculated to cheer the mind or soothe the feelings; so that by degrees even the hope of change and liberation became faint, and almost died away. Such I know—from observation made when the access of visitors to such establishments was difficult, and my own visits were only permitted because an official appointment qualified me to demand it.—was the general condition of insane persons in the old asylums; in which the doctrine of non-restraint was years afterwards received with derision and defiance, and made the groundwork of every kind of misrepresentation; and into which the full principle of non-restraint can scarcely yet be said to have found a willing admission."

As a contrast, we subjoin the following description of a private asylum, conducted on the non-restraint principle, gladly bearing testimony to our acquaintance with many such, both near London and in the provinces:

"The outward appearance of such houses is indicative of comfort; highly cultivated grounds and gardens surround them, and nothing is suggestive of a place of confinement. The patient is received as a visitor, proper refreshment is placed before him, friendly words are addressed to him, and he retires at night to a bed-room where cleanliness and all arrangements fitting his station in life reconcile him to being its occupant. If his case requires that an attendant should be near him in the night, or even in the same room with him, it is represented to him that this is done for his own safety, or for his comfort, in a strange house. In the morning, he is persuaded to get up, without threats and rough words; and his dressing is attended to as carefully as if he were in his own house. On coming down stairs, he finds a cheerful breakfast prepared for him, either with a few other patients, or with one of the proprietors or officers of the establishment. He can read the morning paper, or walk out in the grounds, or look over the new books from the library, or adjourn to the billiard-room, or join one of the walking parties or carriage parties. On returning, he is allowed, within limits of prudence and of rules necessary for the preservation of health, to choose what luncheon he will take—a small privilege, but productive of a feeling of liberty not to be undervalued. The remainder of the morning is passed much according to his own inclination. The visits of friends to himself or the other patients, or to the proprietors, and from conversation with whom he is not debarred, diversifies much of the time, and serves to introduce new ideas without any formality of device; and at dinner-time he sits down with the proprietor or the resident physician, and perhaps a lady acting as matron, and with several of the patients, who are gentlemen of his own station, and whose neatness of dress reminds him of the propriety of his making some alteration in his own before that meal. A table well appointed, an excellent and varied dinner, wine in moderation, a dessert, and agreeable conversation, make him almost unmindful of being the inmate of an asylum; and in the evening, a party in the drawing-room, and music, and chess, and backgammon, and cards, make the hours pass agreeably until it is time to retire.

"Such, then, is the non-restraint system: by which it is found to be no less practicable, and safe, and advantageous, to control and govern, and in many cases to contribute to the cure, and in all to the improvement of the insane, in private than in public asylums: a system which meets all the difficulties arising out of the condition of the most highly endowed creature in the universe when deprived of guiding reason, and when, in proportion to his higher faculties and gifts, he has fallen from being either in reason noble, or in faculty infinite, to a condition in which he is merely the most mischievous, and dangerous, and miserable of animals. In the illustrative cases already given, the applicability of this system, which excludes all forms of mechanical coercion, has, I think, been shown in relation to every form of mental imbecility, derangement, depression, and decay. The general results are open to all observation in all our larger asylums; the increased individual comfort, the diminution of individual suffering, and the banishment of all the most repulsive features of institutions set apart for the reception of human beings disqualified for ordinary life; but now placed amidst circumstances promotive in the utmost degree of their comfort, and, in proportion to the possibilities in each case, of mental amendment and recovery."

Part IV.—*Abolition of Mechanical Restraint at Hanwell in* 1839.

Dr. Conolly gives in this part a very interesting historical record of the great movement at Hanwell, illustrated by copious extracts from his several Annual Reports for the years 1839–49.

He thus introduces the subject:

"These pages are prepared for publication at a time when no inducement exists, on my part, to introduce matter of a merely personal nature, or which does not appear to me likely to be of some use to the reader. If, therefore, I now more particularly allude to the subject of the abolition of mechanical restraints with reference to the Hanwell Asylum, it is certainly with no design of claiming for that institution, or for myself, more than, or even so much as has been already accorded by public opinion and the kindness of the medical profession. But the change of treatment adopted there seventeen years ago, and gradually effected, including the entire disuse of restraints, having been accomplished in the face of many difficulties, all of which must be incidental to such an attempt, wherever made; and the annual reports, in which all the principles of the new system were successively laid down, and the progress of the experiment was carefully recorded, being now not to be procured; I think it most desirable to give some extracts from those made by me in the first seven years of that period, which may be regarded as having been peculiarly years of trials."

Part V treats of the gradual adoption of the non-restraint system in the large asylums of England after 1839.

20. *Gradual Advance of the New System:*
"The gradual advance of the new system has perhaps been marked by no circumstances more striking than by that of the opening of at least ten English county asylums, of considerable size, within the last few years, without any preparation being considered necessary or desirable, in any one of them, for any application of mechanical restraints. These asylums have been erected to receive, altogether, about 4000 patients; patients of all descriptions—the violent, the melancholic, and those rendered nearly intractable by long misery. It is among the glories of medical philosophy, which no false splendor enhances, and which therefore attracts little popular regard, that the physicians selected to govern these new institutions undertook to do so by moral and intellectual means alone. So much more confident were they, indeed, of the efficacy of these means than of the effects of the old measures of force, that they did not even require the windows of their asylums to be guarded; and scarcely demanded strong dresses, and the other substitutes for restraints, which had become in every successive year less required at Hanwell, and were found to be scarcely required at all in the more modern asylums in which restraints had never been known.
"The statements and sentiments contained, indeed, in every report now issued from the English county asylums, become, in every year, more uniformly gratifying."

21. *Introduction of the New System into the Private Asylums.*—Dr. Conolly, on this point, has spoken out with a boldness that does him credit:
"In the preceding record (he says) of the progressive practice of non-restraint in the English asylums, reference has chiefly been made to the large public institutions; but the example set in them has forced some degree of reform into every institution for insane persons, however private. Even in workhouses, although still deficient in the proper means of treating the many recent cases almost unavoidably sent to them, the principles of treatment are better understood than formerly, so that the number of furious cases brought into the county asylums is probably less than it used to be. The old method of at once, and indiscriminately, fastening down every troublesome patient, made many frantic who are now preserved from that dreadful aggravation of their malady, and preserved by the kindness and judgment of the medical officers of parish unions. The very great improvement in private asylums has been mainly promoted by the indefatigable industry of the Commissioners in Lunacy during the last ten years; but some of the improvement, it is but just to say, has been spontaneous on the part of the proprietors of the most respectable of such establishments, men of high character and education, and not without a considerable sacrifice of money.
"It is yet to be regretted that licenses cannot in all cases be restricted to persons so qualified and disposed; and that the most specious appearances, including prompt and wonderful unfastenings and dressings of the astonished patients, are too successfully employed to make the inspection of the Commissioners futile. As too many of the private asylums are still deficient in the means of non-restraint, and either superintended or visited by medical men who have taken no pains to acquaint themselves with the practice of large asylums, I have never ventured to say that.

mechanical restraints can be wholly abolished in them. It occasions, therefore, no great surprise, to find that the managers of only thirty-seven private asylums, out of eighty-four from which returns were made to the Commissioners, had contrived to conduct their houses without mechanical restraints when the Eighth Report was published. There is too much to fear, that, in the forty-four other private asylums from which no returns were made, the discreet silence proves the preservation of most of the old abuses. The excuses offered, in the answers from some of the private establishments, for their adherence to the use of restraints, are such as would be considered unsatisfactory, and even frivolous, in any public asylum in which the system of non-restraint is understood. They consist, for the most part, of the old arguments as to the calming influence of restraints, and the economy of using them. By precisely the same arguments the employment of chains was anciently defended. It is deserving of observation, that restraints appear chiefly to be resorted to in the smaller private asylums; and that the patients are in many such establishments extremely neglected I have had most convincing proofs, some of which have been furnished in houses of considerable pretension. The most sensible of the patients in these ill-conducted places are, indeed, well treated, and are sometimes taught to praise the proprietor, or, to use the language of one of them to me, 'to show how happy they are.' They are seen by their friends in the best apartments, and addressed in terms of endearment; whilst the rest, those who are occasionally excited and abusive, those who are imbecile, or apathetic and silent, are kept in wretched abandonment. Some of these unfortunate beings, when removed to a better asylum, are found to have been in a sort of half-starved state for a length of time, and the cleanliness of the person quite neglected, the very hair being matted together for want of washing and combing. In such abandonment they cannot improve; and yet in many of these cases recovery is found to be possible under proper treatment. I have invariably found that the use of restraints in private establishments was associated with these neglects; and, as far as my own observation has extended, I have never known all the patients properly attended to so long as even a few of them were habitually subjected to mechanical coercion. Restraints and neglect may be considered as synonymous, for restraints are merely a general substitute for the thousand attentions required by troublesome patients. The obstinate adherence to a system so objectionable creates, doubtless, the strongest argument against private asylums, and in favor of their suppression. But it is too certain that, if there were no private asylums, the richer patients would be generally secluded, shut up in upper stories, or in small habitations, and under the care of mere attendants. Happily, also, there are private asylums in which the richer patients enjoy all those advantages which are found so favorable to recovery in county asylums for the poor, combined with all the more extensive means applicable to the insane of the most cultivated classes of society. The exceptions, it is to be hoped, will gradually cease to exist."

22. *General Summary of Progress:*
Upon the whole, however, in this country, there is nothing left of the old system calculated to discourage the expectation, not only that the manner of treating insane persons without ever having recourse to restraints will soon be so far understood and appreciated as to be almost universally adopted, but that the old deceptions and abuses in private asylums and private houses must soon exist no more.
" The accomplishments and general character of the candidates for appointments in our county asylums; the admirable reports issuing every year from those institutions, recording every variety of improvement and progress; the clinical instruction already given in some of them; the generous desire evinced by the majority of the county magistrates to make proper provision for the insane poor: together with the continual and even minute attention given by the Commissioners in Lunacy to all that passes in both public and private asylums, are among the circumstances justifying very sanguine hopes of the conservation and extension of all good principles of asylum management. Frequent and liberal discussion of the various subjects connected with lunacy, and with asylums, has also lately been productive of benefits which will go on increasing.
" The varied contents of the 'Psychological Journal' established by Dr. Forbes Winslow, and conducted with great talent and energy, have attracted the attention

of many general, as well as professional readers, to considerations more or less connected with the welfare of the insane. Still more recently, the formation of an association of the medical officers of asylums, has been an indication of their sincere
wish to profit by the experience of each other, and to unite in advancing an elevated
branch of pathology and therapeutics ; for which the establishment of ' The Asylum
Journal,' now so ably edited by Dr. Bucknill, affords every facility, by the diffusion
of information, interesting and instructive to all readers whose duties, whether medical, or magisterial, or general, have any relation to insane persons. The general
character of our public asylums, conducted chiefly by members of that association,
is already honorable to us as a nation ; furnishes an example which is 'a globe of
precepts ;' justifying the expectation that no false economy, and no delusive theories,
will ever lead to the abandonment of the non-restraint system, which comprehends
and binds together all the details of sound principle and humane practice. The system, as now established, will form no unimportant chapter in the history of medicine in relation to disorders of the mind. It has been carried into practical effect
in an intellectual and practical age, unostentatiously, gradually, and carefully ; and
is, I trust, destined to endure as long as science continues to be pursued with a love
of truth and a regard for the welfare of man. No longer residing in the Hanwell
Asylum, and no longer superintending it, or even visiting it, I continue to live within
view of the building, and its familiar trees and grounds. The sound of the bell that
announces the hour of the patients' dinner still gives me pleasure, because I know
that it summons the poorest creature there to a comfortable, well-prepared, and sufficient meal ; and the tones of the chapel bell, coming across the narrow valley of the
Brent, still remind me, morning and evening, of the well-remembered and mingled
congregation of the afflicted, and who are then assembling, humble yet hopeful, and
not forgotten, and not spiritually deserted.

" The contemplation of the vast exterior of the wings of the asylum still deepens
the happy impression, that through all that extent of ward and gallery, kindness
and watchfulness ever reign. And when my thoughts are transferred from this, my
home asylum, with its thousand patients, to nearly forty large public institutions for
the insane in this great country, in which are more than 13,000 patients, to whom
similar comforts are afforded, and throughout which the same system prevails, I
find a reward for any share I have had in promoting these things, beyond my deserving ; a consolation in years of comparative inactivity, and a happiness far over-
balancing the pains and troubles incidental to my life, as to that of all mortal men."

§ IV. *Pathology of Mental Disease.*

a. MORBID ANATOMY.

33. *Dr. Bucknill's Researches into the Morbid Anatomy of the Brain.*—One of
the most important additions which has of late years been made to the pathology
of insanity, is an original communication in the 25th No. of the "British and
Foreign Medico-Chirurgical Review," by Dr. John Charles Bucknill, the physician
of the Devon Asylum. Dr. Bucknill's views on the nature of insanity are strictly
somatic. He shows that mental disease frequently does depend upon purely physical conditions ; and that it is illogical and unnecessary to refer to metaphysical
and speculative theories for the production of phenomena for which a sufficient
cause is thus ascertained. Dr. Bucknill states that for ten years he has been in the
habit of examining, yearly, the bodies of about 30 persons dying insane; that during the first six years of this period, the only impression made upon his mind was
a belief in the justice of Esquirol's opinion, that no cerebral changes were observable in the insane, which were not also to be found in others in whom no insanity
had existed. He gradually, however, became aware of the leading fact, that the
brains of all persons dying insane, some epileptics excepted, presented well-marked
appearances of degraded and deficient nutrition. For the purpose of testing this,
he carefully ascertained the specific gravity of brains; and he published the first
series of "Pathological Observations," in which the specific gravity of brain was
noted in each case, in the year 1851. This mode of observation has been subsequently followed by many observers, but without adding to the single result—obtained by Dr. Bucknill—that in many cases the brain substance acquires a lower

specific gravity in consequence of fatty degeneration. For the purpose of accurately
ascertaining the amount of cerebral atrophy, Dr. Bucknill compared the quantity of
water which was required to fill the cavity of the cranium, with the quantity of water
which the brain-substance, when removed from the body, was capable of displacing.
The difference of the two quantities gives the amount of atrophy, which varies, in
the 64 cases that are tabulated in the article, from nothing up to 15 oz., the latter
representing nearly one-third of the entire bulk of the brain. The average amount
of shrinking in the whole number of cases was 5¼ oz.; that of the epileptic cases
was only 3¹₇ oz. In epilepsy, unaccompanied by dementia, there was no atrophy.
The author remarks that, in the examination of 33 brains of epileptics, he has only once
found a spiculum of bone projecting from the cranium; this is usually, but erroneously, taught to be a frequent cause of epilepsy. Cerebral atrophy increases with
age; in 13 patients whose age exceeded 65 years, the average amount of atrophy
was 8⅛ oz., or more than 50 per cent. above that of the whole number. An interesting case is detailed of a patient who suffered from cerebral hemorrhage after the
brain had fallen into a state of atrophic shrinking; the patient survived the attack of
apoplexy nine months. On examination, after death, a sanguineous effusion, which
had become fibrinous and tough, was found *completely enveloping the cerebrum*, and
extending about two inches down the spine. It was in the cavity of the arachnoid,
and over the vortex of the sides of the brain it was half an inch thick. This enormous amount of cerebral hemorrhage could not have found space except around a
brain previously atrophied : and a much smaller effusion of blood, pressing upon an
otherwise healthy brain, usually causes death in a few hours. But in this case the
blood only displaced so much serum, which was probably accommodated within the
spinal sac, and thus the brain escaped a fatal pressure.

Opinions on the ultimate nature of the nutritive defect, which results in cerebral
atrophy and insanity, must, necessarily, be speculative, since the ultimate nature of
nutrition itself is unknown to us. Its apparent and exciting causes may be classified as follows :

1 In predisposed persons it may depend upon poverty of blood, since it is producible by deficient food and by diseases interfering with the alimentative processes;
and since an analogous train of symptoms occurs during starvation.

2. It is probable that in other cases it may depend upon some derangement of
" the intimate connection between the nervous and vascular systems, through which
their most important functions are performed." Because it is sometimes found to
be accompanied by extensive disease of the minute cerebral capillaries, the coats of
which can be shown to be subject to fatty or earthy decay.

3. A third class of cases would appear to be producible by the molecular change
effected by blows or violent concussions, and followed by atrophy, owing to some
process as yet unknown to us. Atrophy of a testicle from a blow, without inflammation, presents an analogous instance.

4. Another class of cases are those following inflammation, and perhaps, also,
following frequent or long-continued congestion. The basis of inflammatory action
is an abnormal state in the mutual relationship between the blood and the tissues.
That this state effects changes in the tissues which, if not speedily repaired, must
be followed by conditions of degraded nutrition, is proved by the pathology of every
organ in the body. The brain certainly offers no exception. The capillaries become blocked up, or their coats become spoiled for the purposes of nutritive regeneration of the tissue. It also appears probable that, during inflammatory or
congestive conditions, albuminous matter or serous fluid may be effused by the
capillary network into the intimate structure of the brain ; thus separating its vesicles and tubules from the capillaries, and preventing the due nutrition of the
elements of nerve-structure. For this form of atrophy, Dr. Bucknill suggests the
prefix of *relative*, as it may exist where there is no shrinking of the brain ; atrophy
with shrinking being termed *positive*. The two, however, may, and frequently do,
coexist.

5. The most numerous class, however, is that which depends upon want of rest,
and the special period of nutrition of the brain—namely, sleep. Want of refreshing
sleep he believes to be the origin of numerous cases of insanity, dependent upon
moral causes. Dr. Bucknill thinks it very probable that morbid degeneration of
the brain-substance, like that of muscular tissue, takes place by the running to-

gether of its organic elements into forms of hydro-carbon. It may be that the microscope will remain incompetent to detect undoubted indications of such a change in the whole of the encephalon, since death may be inevitable before changes can occur in the intimate structure of the whole organ, grave enough to be appreciable by the assisted sight. But when portions only of the brain have undergone degenerative change, he has repeatedly and easily seen an abnormal quantity of oil globules; and in several such instances he has observed abundance of the peculiar crystals of cholesterine. The brain appears to afford no exception to the law, that one stage of regressive metamorphosis of animal tissues is that of fatty or oily compounds. The recent researches of Meckel and Henle, on the formation of specviolet (a combination of cholesterine and other fats) during cerebral decay, afford strong confirmation of this opinion. We are unable to find space for the author's observations on the microscopic examinations of the brain, or those on the relation between sleep and nutritive repair. The table containing the weights and measurements of the encephalic organs of 63 cases of insanity examined with special reference to cerebral atrophy, is drawn up with great care and skill. One column records the breadth of the gray matter of the convolutions in each case. This was ascertained by measuring, with a pair of hair-dividers inspected through a lens, the average breadth of the least oblique, that is, the narrowest sections, made by a perpendicular slice through the hemispherical ganglion. In five cases the breadth was $\frac{3}{30}$ths of an inch. Of these, two were cases of epilepsy, one of general paralysis, one of dementia, one of melancholia. In one of these cases the cerebral shrinking was as much as 8½ oz., in another as little as 2 oz. In four of these cases the brains were above the average weight. In 38 instances the breadth of the gray matter was $\frac{3}{30}$ths of an inch; in the remainder it was $\frac{8}{30}$ths.

24. *Dr. Boyd's Researches on the same subject.*—In the thirty-ninth volume of the "Medico-Chirurgical Transactions," published Dec., 1856, there is a communication from Dr. Boyd, of the Somerset Asylum, on Atrophy of the Brain, with cases in which there were remarkable inequalities of the cerebral hemispheres, attended with hemiplegia and contraction of the limbs on the side opposite the atrophied hemisphere.

25. *Dr. Sutherland's Researches into the Pathology of the Urine in cases of Mania and Dementia.*—In the thirty-eighth volume of the "Medico-Chirurgical Transactions," we find an able statement, by Dr. Sutherland, of cases illustrating the pathology of mania and dementia, in a paper read before the Society on the 26th of June, 1855. Dr. Sutherland considered that it might not be uninteresting to the Fellows of the Society, if he laid before them the analysis of the mixed phosphates of the urine in cases of mania and dementia (which was undertaken at his request by Dr. Beale, of King's College), and if he were to compare it with the evidence of the pathology of these diseases which we derive from other sources.

" It is necessary," he continues, " to premise that in these analyses the following method was pursued. After the reaction which each specimen exhibited had been noticed, and the specific gravity taken, 500 grains of the urine were evaporated to dryness over a water-bath, and the dry residue was exposed over sulphuric acid *in vacuo* for several hours, when it was carefully weighed : the weight being multiplied by 2 gave the quantity of solid matter in 1000 parts. A weighed portion of the dry extract was incinerated, and perfectly decarbonized, the saline residue was weighed, and the proportion of salts existing in the total quantity of solid matter calculated from the results of experiment.

"Another portion of urine, consisting of 1000 grains, was poured into a glass, and a quantity of solutions of chloride of calcium and ammonia were added, sufficient to precipitate the whole of the phosphoric acid as phosphate of lime. After standing for six hours, the glass being covered to exclude the air, the precipitate was thrown on a filter, well washed with water, dried, and ignited, and when the ash had become nearly white it was weighed. The proportion which the amount of salts and phosphate bore to 100 grains of solid matter was then calculated, in order that the results of each analysis might be compared with the rest. A comparison may be made between the results obtained in each case, quite independent of the variations in density of the several specimens examined.

"It is quite true that no accurate comparison can be made, unless the whole quantity of the urine passed in the twenty-four hours be obtained, and a specimen of this submitted to analysis; but in by far the greater number of cases, more especially in those of insanity, this is quite impossible, and it is also equally difficult to obtain specimens from the various patients at any particular time of the day; the only method, therefore, by which accurate conclusions can be deduced from the results of experiment is by comparing the quantities of phosphate corresponding to 100 grains of the solid matter present in each specimen of urine. I have, however, given both results in the following tables; but in order that I might compare them with those of Dr. Bence Jones, I have referred to the first table in the remarks which I have made as to the amount of phosphates found in the different cases. I might have strengthened my case had I referred to the other table; for if the proportion of phosphate to 100 grains of solid matter be compared with the symptoms existing at the time of the analysis in the different cases, we shall find that a larger proportional amount of mixed phosphates was shown by Table II to have existed in cases of acute mania. I might also have referred to Table II in the cases of J. H. and J. W., patients suffering under general paralysis, but I have found that where the specific gravity is very low, as in the case of J. H., where it was only 1008, the first table is rather to be relied on.

"The great source of fallacy in the quantitative analysis of the phosphates in the urine originates in variations of diet, particularly in the quantity of bread taken at meal time, which contains a large proportion of alkaline phosphates; but in an hospital where all the patients have the same diet this fallacy is avoided.

"The ordinary diet of the patients in St. Luke's Hospital, at the time the analysis was made, was as follows: For male patients, 2 pints of milk-and-water gruel, and 2 oz. of bread for breakfast; 12 oz. of cooked meat, 12 oz. of potatoes, and 6 oz. of bread, and 1 pint of beer for dinner; 8 oz. of bread, 2 oz. of cheese or butter, and 1 pint of beer for supper. For females, 1½ pint of milk and gruel, and 2 oz. of bread for breakfast; 8 oz. of cooked meat, 8 oz. of potatoes, and 6 oz. of bread, and ¾ of a pint of beer for dinner; 8 oz. of bread, 2 oz. of cheese or butter, and ¾ of a pint of beer for supper. It will be seen that the allowance of bread was the same for males and females.

"The urine was selected from patients laboring under different forms of the disease in the following proportions, viz.: 5 cases of acute mania with paroxysms, 4 of common mania, 2 of intermittent mania, 1 of remittent mania, 2 of hysterical mania, 3 of puerperal mania, 5 of acute dementia, 1 of acute dementia with catalepsy, 5 of paralysis of the insane, 3 of chronic mania, and 3 of chronic dementia; making in all 34 cases."

Remarks.—We observe that in the five cases of acute mania the proportion of phosphates to 1000 grs. was, in four, above the mean quantity found in health, and in one the proportion was nearly of the healthy standard. In Case 47 the phosphates were as high as 9·73, the specific gravity of the urine being 1033; but while we see that this amount of the phosphates is nearly equal to what Dr. Bence Jones has found in certain cases of delirium, and inflammatory action from fracture at the base of the skull, and in violent delirium at the end of phthisis, we must not too hastily conclude that acute inflammation is present in acute mania, because this theory is refuted by the analysis of the blood, by our post-mortem examinations, and by the effect of treatment.

"In Case 47 the analysis of the urine was made three days after the admission of the patient, the disease having existed only six days; in Cases 21 and 24 the analysis was made four days after the admission of the patients, the disease in both cases having existed three months; and in Case 51 the analysis was made on the day after the symptoms had changed from tranquillity to excitement, the paroxysm having broken out in the hospital. The analysis in 49 and 59 were made in one case seventeen days, in the other eighteen days, after the admission of the patient; whilst that of Case 4 was made after the paroxysm had lasted nine weeks, and when the patient was much exhausted from its effects. It would appear, therefore, that if the urine be analyzed at the commencement of a paroxysm of acute mania, a plus quantity of the phosphates will be found to exist—in some instances equal in extent to the quantity found in encephalitis; that this large secretion of the salt lasts but for a short period; and that it is modified, as in Case 49, by refusal of food, and the

Form of Dise			Chronic Mania.			Chronic Dementia.		
Initials of patient,	C. C.	J. W.	E. K.	J.C.C.	J. S.	A. M.	H.	S. H.
Number,	87	15	16	27	53	3	28	57
Date,	June 9	May 20	May 20	June 2	July 8	May 3	May 27	July 15
Reaction,	Acid	Acid	Very acid	Acid	Acid	Feebly acid	Feebly acid	Feebly acid
Specific Grav	10·17	10·21	10·27	10·22	10·25	10·24	10·11	...
Water,	959·00	958·00	944·40	949·80	929·20	...	978·4	973·00
Solid matter,	41·00	42·00	55·60	50·20	70·80	...	21·60	27·00
Fixed salts,.	13·13	16·82	17·95	19·48	9·15	...	8·88	10·16
Phosphate Lime preci tated by Cl. and N.	2·95	4·83	7·56	2·76	4·02	4·10	2·68	1·26
Solid matter the urine,	100·00	100·00	100·00	100·00	100·00	100·00	100·00	100·00
Fixed salts,	32·02	35·28	32·28	38·80	12·92	...	41·11	37·62
Phosphate o lime precip tated by C Cl. and N.	7·19	10·30	13·59	5·50	5·67	...	12·40	4·66

Form of Dise	Mania.		Remittent.	Puerperal Mania.			Hysterical Mania.	
Initials of the	E. H.	S. H.	M. D.	C. P.	S. P.	A. C.	A. G.	E. W.
Number,	58	32	36	14	30	50	55	28
Date,	July 15	June 2	June 9	May 20	June 2	July 5	July 15	June 2
Reaction,	Acid	Acid	Acid	Very acid	Acid	Acid	Acid	Acid
Specific gravi	...	10·25	10·18	10·26	10·20	10·18	...	10·27
Water,	965·40	938·00	946·4	941·60	957·20	965·2	931·00	924·4
Solid matter,	34·60	62·00	53·6	58·40	42·80	34·8	69·00	75·6
Fixed salts,	13·37	12·91	7·91	10·32	15·62	18·71	12·48	17·00
Phosphate of	1·80	3·57	8·23	7·72	2·60	1·23	4·96	5·66
Solid matter	100·00	100·00	100·00	100·00	100·00	100·00	100·00	100 00
Fixed salts,	12·83	20·82	14·75	17·67	36·49	53·76	18·08	22·48
Phosphate of	5·24	5·75	6·02	13·21	6·07	8·53	7·18	7·48

prolongation of the paroxysm; and that the exhaustion, which is the effect of the paroxysm, is accompanied, as in Case 4, by a minus quantity of the phosphates, as small, indeed, as that found by Dr. Bence Jones in certain cases of delirium tremens.

"The question, then, which is forced upon the mind from these results, is this: Is the amount of phosphates found in the urine a measure of inflammatory action? Is it not rather a measure of the consumption of nerve-force? To this question we shall return in the sequel. In the four cases of common mania, and in the case of remittent mania, no symptoms of paroxysmal excitement were present when the analysis of the urine was made, and the amount of phosphates in the urine was in all below the average of health. In Case 34 the health was much broken, in consequence of previous habits of intoxication; and E. H—, Case 58, was admitted in a very weak and emaciated condition, the insanity being accompanied with scrofulous disease of the ankle-joint; besides which, the digestion was much impaired, and he took very little food; these circumstances may in some measure account for the quantity of the phosphates being as low as 1·80. In Case 32 there were well-marked symptoms of the stage of exhaustion, indeed the case was nearly allied to one of acute dementia; upon admission, the reaction of the urine was alkaline, with deposit of the triple phosphate crystals, and as the symptoms improved the urine regained its acid reaction; this may be considered by some to favor the opinion, to which I shall afterwards have to refer, that in cases of mania the urine is generally found to be alkaline; but it is an exception to the general rule which I shall have to lay down, viz.; that in the majority of cases of mania, the reaction of the urine is acid.

"In the cases of puerperal mania the analysis was made in Case 14, before the stage of excitement had passed off, about a month after the commencement of the attack, and eleven days after the patient was admitted into the hospital: and the quantitative analysis gave the amount of phosphates as 7·72. In Case 30, the analysis was made during the stage of exhaustion, nine weeks after the admission of the patient, and nineteen weeks after the commencement of the disease, and the amount of phosphates was 2·60. While in Case 50, where the disease occurred after prolonged lactation, although the patient, at the time the analysis was made, was taking abundance of food with two ounces of brandy and two pints of porter daily, to prevent her sinking into a state of collapse, the amount of phosphates was 1·23. These cases appear to confirm the results met with in the above cases of acute mania, and would lead us to infer that, in the acute stage of mania, there is a plus quantity—in the stage of exhaustion a minus quantity, of the phosphates present in the urine.

"In the two cases of hysterical mania it was interesting to compare the manner in which the disease manifested itself in constitutions so dissimilar, the cause of the illness being the same in both. In Case 28, that is, in the anæmic weaver, we find that the phosphates amounted to 5·66; and, in the hyperæmic case, to 4·96; in the second table we find that the amount of phosphates was very nearly of the healthy standard, being in A. G—, 7·18; in E. W—, 7·48.

"In the cases of acute dementia we find the amount of phosphates to be remarkably deficient in quantity in the first table, and below the average of health in five of the analyses. When the first analysis of the urine was made, in Case 6, the patient was unconscious of the calls of nature, and inattentive to all that was passing around him; when the second analysis was made, in the same case (No. 17), there was some improvement in the symptoms; and we find the quantity of the phosphates to be 3·95, i. e., 2·43 higher than in the first analysis. In Case 18, when the powers of the mind were in abeyance, the proportion of phosphates was 2·49; when they began to be again exercised, the proportion was 5·10: as a contrast to this we have the case of C. B—, 35, in which we find the proportion of phosphates, June 2d, to be 5·23; and, as the disease advanced, and when she was unable to comprehend what was said to her, the proportion was 2·37.

"The analysis of the urine of those suffering from paralysis of the insane corresponds with that made by Dr. Bence Jones, who was the first to point out the great deficiency of phosphates in this disease; and as the cases from which he derived the specimens of urine, in 1845, were under my care in the hospital, I am able to compare the two analyses with the particular symptoms in all the cases.

" The first case in our analysis, F. B—, 1, had a fair average amount of phosphates when the urine was examined in May and June: this patient recovered. The second case, J. C. T—, 2 and 42, is interesting as showing that, when the disease was in the first stage, the proportion of phosphates was 3·42, and the reaction of the urine was acid ; and a month afterwards, when the disease was in the transition stage, the amount was 1·57, and the reaction of the urine was alkaline. In the third case, J. H—, 9 and 33, although the urine was examined at the commencement of a paroxysm, the proportion of phosphates amounted only to 2·90 ; and after the excitement had passed off, and the urine was again examined, it was 2·86 ; this patient was discharged uncured. In the fourth case, C. C—, 12 and 37, the amount of phosphates was at first 4·46, and, afterwards, when he became worse, it was 2·95. I should say, however, that soon after the second examination of the urine was made, a large boil appeared on his side, after which the symptoms began to improve, and he ultimately recovered. In the fifth case, the examination was made during the stage of excitement, and the proportion of phosphates was 4·33 : this patient likewise recovered.

" In the first case referred to in Dr. Bence Jones's analysis, the proportion of phosphates was 6·90, and the patient was well enough to be discharged on trial about a month afterwards ; he, however, relapsed, and was readmitted into the hospital, August 8th ; and when Dr. Jones again examined the urine, the phosphates amounted to 4·14 ; this patient was discharged uncured. In the second case, the patient was admitted March 7th, the paralysis became rapidly worse, and when the urine was analyzed, on June 16th, the proportion of phosphates was only 2·02. Case 3 and 4, in Dr. Jones's analysis, refer to the same patient ; and although the urine was examined the second time during a paroxysm, the amount of phosphates was only 1·30. Case 5, in Dr. Bence Jones's analysis, was one where the patient had labored under paralysis of the insane for many years, and the disease had passed into dementia ; here the amount of phosphates was as low as 1·35. In these cases we observe a diminution in the amount of phosphates corresponding with the progress of the disease ; and in the two analyses we have evidence that in two cases where the analysis was made during the existence of a paroxysm, it was, in Case 9, 2·90 ; and in Dr. Jones's second case, 2·02 : if, therefore, the amount of the mixed phosphates be any measure of the expenditure of nerve-force, as the above analyses appear to me to prove, we have here evidence of the small amount of phosphoric acid possessed by the atrophied brain in white softening, or œdema of that organ ; and we might ask, whether there be not something analogous to this in those cases of delirium tremens where an equally small amount of the phosphates is found in the urine ; and whether it be not the atrophy and œdema of the brain which is the cause of such diminution, and not the peculiar action of alcohol upon nervous matter, which action is, in all probability, neutralized by the vital power of the brain itself.

" The cases of chronic mania, and chronic dementia, are so far interesting, as they exhibit an amount of the phosphate below the average in every case but one, viz., that of E. K—, 16, whose powers of mind were very little impaired by the existence of her disease, and who was discharged 'on trial' from the hospital on the 22d instant.

" If we compare the reaction of the urine in the above cases of acute mania, and chronic dementia, we shall find that in recent cases of mania it was acid seventeen times, feebly acid twice, neutral once ; whereas, in chronic cases, and those complicated with general paralysis, it was acid nine times, feebly acid four times, neutral once, and feebly alkaline once. Erlenmayer has stated that the urine is generally alkaline in recent cases of mania (' De Urina Maniacorum,' 1844) : this does not correspond with my experience ; I find that in 125 cases of recent mania admitted during two years under my care into St. Luke's Hospital, the urine was acid in 111 cases, neutral in 1, alkaline in 13 ; being in the proportion of 88⅔ per cent. acid, 10⅓ alkaline, and, omitting fractions, 1 neutral ; whereas in 100 cases of chronic mania and dementia, under my care at the same time, the urine was acid in 61, neutral in 6, alkaline in 33 ; and in 25 cases of paralysis of the insane, the reaction of the urine was acid in 12, neutral in 1, alkaline in 12.

" But we must not infer that it is always a bad symptom when we find the urine alkaline, or an alternation of the acid and alkaline reaction, as in the cases of fracture of the spine, mentioned by Sir B. Brodie; as it is not an evidence of the existence of organic disease of the brain in cases of mania, but rather of exhaustion of the nervous centres; and in this respect it is analogous to the urine of fever; for, as Simon has observed, 'in proportion as fever assumes a torrid character, and the vital powers become depressed, the urine becomes clearer, loses its acidity, becomes neutral, and in a very short time alkaline.'

"If we compare the analysis of the urine in the above cases of mania and dementia, with that of the brain and the blood, it will appear that they correspond in a very interesting manner: we find in the brain of infancy and old age, according to L'Heritie, a minus quantity of albumen, cerebral fat, and phosphorus, as compared with that of adults, and a minus quantity of the same substances in the brains of idiots; whereas there is a plus quantity of phosphorus, according to M. Couerbe, in the brains of those suffering from acute mania. In the quantitative analysis of the blood of acute mania, published by Hittorf, we find a deficiency of blood corpuscles, and a slight increase of fibrin and albumen; and Michea states that, in cases of paralysis of the insane, he found the albumen to be remarkably deficient in the blood in nearly one-third of the cases, and that there was an augmentation of the blood globules, and an absolute diminution of the fibrin. The tissue from which the phosphates are eliminated is the albuminous, and in the urine we find a plus quantity of the mixed phosphates at the commencement of the paroxysm, and a minus quantity in acute dementia, and in the third stage of paralysis of the insane.

"This result corresponds also with the symptoms which we observe during life; for in dementia, when the brain is in a passive state, there is less interference with the functions of the nerves of organic life, and digestion goes on much as in health; but in acute mania there is great disturbance in the functions of primary and secondary assimilation, as is evident from the symptoms of constipation, the unhealthy evacuations, and the deposits of uric acid and urate of ammonia in the urine; the emaciation also which takes place during the acute stage of mania is sometimes very great; and the patients at St. Luke's Hospital sometimes weigh many pounds heavier at the time of their discharge, as compared with their weight upon admission. The fat appears to be absorbed from all parts of the body to supply the brain; for, in acute mania, the production of nerve-force is very rapid, the increased flow of blood, which is the result, at first stimulates the intellect beyond its ordinary power, when ideas pass through the mind with unaccustomed rapidity; as the disease advances, incoherence is the result, in consequence of the multiplicity of thoughts which pass through the patient's mind making it impossible for him to give utterance to all; the cell-nuclei are thrown into a state of unhealthy activity, there is little repose night or day, and want of sleep, as is well known, is one of the most common symptoms; there is a constant demand upon the blood for the albuminous and oleaginous principles; the whole nervous system partakes of this activity, and feels its influence, and is thrown into a state analogous to that of electric tension; not only are the hemispheric ganglia involved, but the fibrous structure conveys the impulse to the peripheral extremities of the nerves, producing hyperæsthesia and pseudæsthesia: the nerves of organic life likewise sympathize; the false perceptions of the nerves of special sense, and those of sensation, and the errors of nutrition and secretion, are sufficient evidence of this; and when the disease arrives at its highest point, and a paroxysm occurs, we have then to deal with another force, which becomes equally unmanageable—I mean the force developed by muscular contractions—which, as Matteucci has shown, is quite independent of the nervous system; these two forces acting and reacting upon each other, produce such a state of nervous erethism, that I have seen patients with symptoms resembling those of an animal poisoned by strychnine; the fury of the passions and the movements of the limbs are quite beyond their control; and the muscular force is developed to such an extent, that they sometimes perform feats of strength which they would have been quite unequal to when well.

"The symptoms of acute dementia form a striking contrast to the paroxysm of mania. The patient never speaks, he is apparently unconscious of all that passes around him, and his movements are automatic: the pulse is weak, sometimes scarcely perceptible; the extremities are cold and livid; the respiration is chiefly abdominal, and slower than in health. In a case at present under my care, the index of Dr. Quain's stethometer showed that the thorax was raised during each inspiration only five degrees instead of fifty, while the abdominal respiration ranged from thirty to forty-five degrees; the number of respirations being sixteen in the minute. In these cases there is little consumption of nervous force, whereas in the dementia of general paralysis there is little supply; for the atrophy and œdema of the brain must prevent the cell-nuclei from being formed in sufficient quantity, and the blood, as has been shown, is not able to furnish the requisite amount of albumen. But this happens in the last stage of the disease; for if the nervous system and the blood were affected in the same way in every case, we should not be able, as in some of the cases given above, to quote instances of recovery; and medical treatment would be of no avail. The fact has been overlooked, that there is more than one species of paralysis of the insane; the scrofulous species differs from that which is the result of delirium tremens; that which is accompanied with anæmia and local congestion differs from that with hyperæmia and hypertrophy of the left ventricle of the heart; and that species which is the result of atheromatous and bony deposits of the bloodvessels of the brain, no less than the hardening, differs from the softening of the brain found in these cases, in our post-mortem examinations. Probably the reason why Dr. Conolly has spoken so strongly as to the incurable nature of paralysis of the insane is, that patients laboring under this disease are seldom admitted into Hanwell during its first stage.

"If, then, we compare the plus quantity of the mixed phosphates secreted in the commencement of the paroxysm of acute mania, and the minus quantity found in acute dementia, and in the third stage of paralysis of the insane, with the symptoms during life, it gives us, to a certain extent, a measure of the expenditure of nervous force. We know that this force is intimately associated with all the operations of the mind; we believe it to be the connecting link in its relation with matter, being probably the highest form in which matter is found; over-exertion of intellect exhausts its energies, no less than over-exertion of body tends to impair its supplies. It is now generally admitted, that the cell-nuclei found in the nervous centres, and at the extremities of the afferent nerves, are the sources of nervous force, and that this force is correlated with electricity; therefore, the subject of electricity becomes of greater importance to us in our investigations, whether physiological or pathological. It has long been observed that sudden variations in the temperature and weight of the atmosphere exert a powerful influence upon all nervous disorders; and that the partial distribution of light and heat have favored the production of insanity on the northern side of mountainous districts. The effects, also, of the Siroc of the Mediterranean, and of the viento norte of Buenos Ayres, are well known; and we are able to trace a connection between disorders of the nervous system and epidemic diseases. But whether the magnetic variations have any influence upon nervous disorders, is still a problem to be solved by future investigations. Schwabe has proved that the epochs of maxima and minima in the variations of the solar spots, are identical with those which have been assigned to the magnetic variations; but Colonel Sabine has shown that he has not been able to derive, from the indications of the thermometer and barometer, any sensible connection between climatic conditions and the number of spots."

The conclusions which may be drawn from the above analysis of the mixed phosphates in the urine of cases of mania and dementia, and the comparison of this analysis with that of the brain and of the blood, and of the symptoms in similar cases, are as follows:

"1. A plus quantity of phosphates exists in the urine in the paroxysms of acute mania.

"2. A minus quantity exists in the stage of exhaustion in mania, in acute dementia, and in the third stage of paralysis of the insane.

"3. The plus and minus quantities of phosphates in the urine correspond with the quantitative analysis of the brain and of the blood; for a plus quantity of phosphorus is found in the brain, and a slight excess of albumen in the blood, of maniacal patients: and a minus quantity of phosphorus and albumen are found in the brains of idiots, and a minus quantity of albumen in the blood of paralysis of the insane.

"4. The plus quantity of phosphates in the urine of cases of acute mania, denotes the expenditure of nervous force, and is not a proof of the existence of acute inflammation in this disease."

(To be continued.)

INDEX TO NO. XXIV.

Lightning Source UK Ltd.
Milton Keynes UK
UKHW010804110119
335238UK00008B/738/P